RN Adult Medical Surgical Nursing
REVIEW MODULE EDITION 10.0

P9-DJU-444

Contributors

Norma Jean E. Henry, MSN/Ed, RN

Mendy McMichael, DNP, MSN

Janean Johnson, MSN, RN, CNE

Agnes DiStasi, DNP, RN, CNE

Brenda S. Ball, MEd, BSN, RN

Honey C. Holman, MSN, RN

Carrie B. Elkins, DHSc, MSN

Mary Jane Janowski, RN, MA

Robin A. Hertel, EdS, MSN, RN, CMSRN

Marsha S. Barlow, MSN, RN

Peggy Leehy, MSN, RN

Terri Lemon, DNP, MSN, RN

Consultants

Susan Adcock, RN, MS

Tracey Bousquet, BSN, RN

Katrina Coggins, MSN, RN, CNE

Anne L. Coonrad, JD, MS, RN

Sara Hoffmann, MSN, RN

Deb Johnson-Schuh, RN, MSN, CNE

Donna Russo, RN, MSN, CCRN, CNE

Ranee Seastrom, MSN, MHA, RN–BC

Pam DeMoss, MSN, RN

Betty Daniel, MSN Nursing Education, RN

Lakeisha Wheless, MSN, RN

Director of content review: Kristen Lawler

Director of development: Derek Prater

Project management: Janet Hines, Nicole Burke

Coordination of content review: Norma Jean E. Henry, Mendy McMichael

Copy editing: Kelly Von Lunen, Derek Prater

Layout: Spring Lenox, Randi Hardy

Illustrations: Randi Hardy

Online media: Morgan Smith, Ron Hanson, Nicole Lobdell, Brant Stacy

Cover design: Jason Buck

Interior book design: Spring Lenox

IMPORTANT NOTICE TO THE READER

User's Guide

Welcome to the Assessment Technologies Institute® RN Adult Medical Surgical Nursing Review Module Edition 10.0. The mission of ATI's Content Mastery Series® Review Modules is to provide user-friendly compendiums of nursing knowledge that will:
- Help you locate important information quickly.
- Assist in your learning efforts.
- Provide exercises for applying your nursing knowledge.
- Facilitate your entry into the nursing profession as a newly licensed nurse.

This newest edition of the Review Modules has been redesigned to optimize your learning experience. We've fit more content into less space and have done so in a way that will make it even easier for you to find and understand the information you need.

ORGANIZATION

This Review Module is organized into units covering the foundations of nursing care (Unit 1), body systems and physiological processes (Units 2 to 13), and perioperative nursing care (Unit 14). Chapters within these units conform to one of three organizing principles for presenting the content.
- Nursing concepts
- Procedures
- System disorders

Nursing concepts chapters begin with an overview describing the central concept and its relevance to nursing. Subordinate themes are covered in outline form to demonstrate relationships and present the information in a clear, succinct manner.

Procedures chapters include an overview describing the procedure(s) covered in the chapter. These chapters provide nursing knowledge relevant to each procedure, including indications, nursing considerations, interpretation of findings, and complications.

System disorders chapters include an overview describing the disorder(s) and/or disease process. These chapters address assessments, including risk factors, expected findings, laboratory tests, and diagnostic procedures. Next, you will focus on patient-centered care, including nursing care, medications, therapeutic procedures, interprofessional care, and client education. Finally, you will find complications related to the disorder, along with nursing actions in response to those complications.

ACTIVE LEARNING SCENARIOS AND APPLICATION EXERCISES

Each chapter includes opportunities for you to test your knowledge and to practice applying that knowledge. Active Learning Scenario exercises pose a nursing scenario and then direct you to use an ATI Active Learning Template (included at the back of this book) to record the important knowledge a nurse should apply to the scenario. An example is then provided to which you can compare your completed Active Learning Template. The Application Exercises include NCLEX-style questions, such as multiple-choice and multiple-select items, providing you with opportunities to practice answering the kinds of questions you might expect to see on ATI assessments or the NCLEX. After the Application Exercises, an answer key is provided, along with rationales.

NCLEX® CONNECTIONS

To prepare for the NCLEX-RN, it is important to understand how the content in this Review Module is connected to the NCLEX-RN test plan. You can find information on the detailed test plan at the National Council of State Boards of Nursing's website, www.ncsbn.org. When reviewing content in this Review Module, regularly ask yourself, "How does this content fit into the test plan, and what types of questions related to this content should I expect?"

To help you in this process, we've included NCLEX Connections at the beginning of each unit and with each question in the Application Exercises Answer Keys. The NCLEX Connections at the beginning of each unit point out areas of the detailed test plan that relate to the content within that unit. The NCLEX Connections attached to the Application Exercises Answer Keys demonstrate how each exercise fits within the detailed content outline.
These NCLEX Connections will help you understand how the detailed content outline is organized, starting with major client needs categories and subcategories and followed by related content areas and tasks. The major client needs categories are:
- Safe and Effective Care Environment
  - Management of Care
  - Safety and Infection Control
- Health Promotion and Maintenance
- Psychosocial Integrity
- Physiological Integrity
  - Basic Care and Comfort
  - Pharmacological and Parenteral Therapies
  - Reduction of Risk Potential
  - Physiological Adaptation

An NCLEX Connection might, for example, alert you that content within a unit is related to:
- Reduction of Risk Potential
  - Diagnostic Tests
    - Monitor the results of diagnostic testing and intervene as needed.

QSEN COMPETENCIES

As you use the Review Modules, you will note the integration of the Quality and Safety Education for Nurses (QSEN) competencies throughout the chapters. These competencies are integral components of the curriculum of many nursing programs in the United States and prepare you to provide safe, high-quality care as a newly licensed nurse. Icons appear to draw your attention to the six QSEN competencies.

Safety: The minimization of risk factors that could cause injury or harm while promoting quality care and maintaining a secure environment for clients, self, and others.

Patient-Centered Care: The provision of caring and compassionate, culturally sensitive care that addresses clients' physiological, psychological, sociological, spiritual, and cultural needs, preferences, and values.

Evidence-Based Practice: The use of current knowledge from research and other credible sources, on which to base clinical judgment and client care.

Informatics: The use of information technology as a communication and information-gathering tool that supports clinical decision-making and scientifically based nursing practice.

Quality Improvement: Care related and organizational processes that involve the development and implementation of a plan to improve health care services and better meet clients' needs.

Teamwork and Collaboration: The delivery of client care in partnership with multidisciplinary members of the health care team to achieve continuity of care and positive client outcomes.

ICONS

Icons are used throughout the Review Module to draw your attention to particular areas. Keep an eye out for these icons.

(N) This icon is used for NCLEX Connections.

(G) This icon indicates gerontological considerations, or knowledge specific to the care of older adult clients.

Qs This icon is used for content related to safety and is a QSEN competency. When you see this icon, take note of safety concerns or steps that nurses can take to ensure client safety and a safe environment.

Qpcc This icon is a QSEN competency that indicates the importance of a holistic approach to providing care.

Qebp This icon, a QSEN competency, points out the integration of research into clinical practice.

Qi This icon is a QSEN competency and highlights the use of information technology to support nursing practice.

Qqi This icon is used to focus on the QSEN competency of integrating planning processes to meet clients' needs.

Qtc This icon highlights the QSEN competency of care delivery using an interprofessional approach.

M◇ This icon appears at the top-right of pages and indicates availability of an online media supplement, such as a graphic, animation, or video. If you have an electronic copy of the Review Module, this icon will appear alongside clickable links to media supplements. If you have a hard copy version of the Review Module, visit www.atitesting.com for details on how to access these features.

FEEDBACK

ATI welcomes feedback regarding this Review Module. Please provide comments to comments@atitesting.com.

Table of Contents

UNIT 3

Nursing Care of Clients Who Have Respiratory Disorders

UNIT 8   *Nursing Care of Clients Who Have Renal Disorders*

ⓃNCLEX® Connections

When reviewing the following chapters, keep in mind the relevant topics and tasks of the NCLEX outline, in particular:

Client Needs: Health Promotion and Maintenance

HEALTH PROMOTION/DISEASE PREVENTION
Identify risk factors for disease/illness.

Educate the client on actions to promote/ maintain health and prevent disease.

Client Needs: Physiological Adaptation

HEMODYNAMICS: Intervene to improve the client's cardiovascular status.

ILLNESS MANAGEMENT: Educate the client about managing illness.

MEDICAL EMERGENCIES: Apply knowledge of pathophysiology when caring for a client experiencing a medical emergency.

UNIT 1 FOUNDATIONS OF NURSING
CARE FOR ADULT CLIENTS

CHAPTER 1 *Health, Wellness, and Illness*

Health and wellness combine to form a state of optimal physical functioning and a feeling of emotional and social contentment. Wellness involves the ability to adapt emotionally and physically to a changing state of health and environment.

Illness is an altered level of functioning in response to a disease process. Disease is a condition that results in the physiological alteration in the composition of the body.

Nurses must understand the variables affecting health, wellness, and illness, and how they relate to clients' individual perceptions of health needs.

Health and wellness

The level of health and wellness is unique to each individual and relative to the individual's usual state of functioning. For example, a person who has rheumatoid arthritis, a strong support system, and positive outlook might consider himself healthy while functioning at an optimal level with minimal pain.

VARIABLES Qpcc
- **Modifiable:** Can be changed, such as smoking, nutrition, access to health education, sexual practices, and exercise
- **Nonmodifiable:** Cannot be changed, such as sex, age, developmental level, and genetic traits

ASPECTS OF HEALTH AND WELLNESS

- **Physical:** Able to perform activities of daily living
- **Emotional:** Adapts to stress; expresses and identifies emotions
- **Social:** Interacts successfully with others
- **Intellectual:** Effectively learns and disseminates information
- **Spiritual:** Adopts a belief that provides meaning to life
- **Occupational:** Balances occupational activities with leisure time
- **Environmental:** Creates measures to improve standards of living and quality of life

ENVIRONMENT

- A client's state of health and wellness is constantly changing and adapting to a continually fluctuating external and internal environment.
- THE EXTERNAL ENVIRONMENT
  - **Social:** Crime vs. safety, poverty vs. prosperity, peace vs. social unrest, and presence vs. absence of support from social networks
  - **Physical:** Access to health care, sanitation, availability of clean water, and geographic location
- THE INTERNAL ENVIRONMENT includes cumulative life experiences, cultural and spiritual beliefs, age, developmental stage, gender, emotional factors, and perception of physical functioning.

DESIRED OUTCOMES

- Desired outcomes are to obtain and maintain optimal state of wellness and function through access to and use of health promotion, wellness, and illness prevention strategies.
- Health and wellness can be achieved through health education and positive action (stress management, smoking cessation, weight loss, immunizations, seeking health care).

ILLNESS-WELLNESS CONTINUUM

The Illness–Wellness Continuum is an assessment tool used to measure the level of wellness to premature death.
- It can be useful as an assessment guide or tool to set goals and find ways to improve a client's state of health or to have the client return to a previous state of health, which can include an illness within optimal wellness. The health care professional can assist the client to see where he is at on the continuum and seek ways to move toward optimal wellness.
- At the center of the continuum is the client's normal state of health.
- The range of wellness to illness runs from optimal wellness to severe illness.
- The degree of wellness is relative to the usual state of wellness for a client and is achieved through awareness, education, and personal growth.

Illness

- Illness is the impairment of a client's physical, social, emotional, spiritual, developmental, or intellectual functioning.
- Illness encompasses the effects of a disease on a client. However, illness and disease are not synonymous.

Response to illness can be influenced by
- Degree of physical changes as a result of a disease process.
- Perceptions by self and others of the illness, which can be influenced by various reliable and unreliable sources of information, such as friends, magazines, TV, and the Internet.
- Cultural values and beliefs.
- Denial or fear of illness.
- Social demands, time constraints, economic resources, and health care access.

HEALTH PROMOTION AND DISEASE PREVENTION

Use health education and awareness to reduce risk factors and promote health care.

HEALTH/WELLNESS ASSESSMENT

- Physical assessment
- Evaluating health perceptions
- Identifying risks to health/wellness
- Identifying access to health care

Identifying obstacles to compliance and adherence
- Perceptions of illness: awareness of the severity of the illness
- Confidence in the provider
- Belief in the prescribed therapy
  - A client who has had a negative experience with the health care system might not trust the provider and might not follow the advice or comply with the treatment prescribed.
  - Cultural or religious beliefs might not align with prescribed treatment.
- Availability of support systems
- Family role and function: One family member might be the family caregiver but neglect caring for herself.
- Financial restrictions that can lead to prioritized health care
  - Prescription medication costs
  - A parent might seek medical care for children, but not for herself

NURSING CARE

Evaluate the health needs of a client and create strategies to meet those needs. Qpcc

INTERVENTIONS

- Provide resources to strengthen coping abilities. Qpcc
- Identify and encourage use of support systems during times of illness and stress.
- Identify obstacles to health and wellness and create strategies to reduce these obstacles.
- Identify ways to reduce health risks and improve compliance.
- Develop health education methods to improve health awareness and reduce health risks.

Application Exercises

1. A nurse is caring for an older adult client who has a new diagnosis of type 2 diabetes mellitus and reports difficulty following the diet and remembering to take the prescribed medication. Which of the following actions should the nurse take to promote client compliance? (Select all that apply.)

   A. Ask the dietitian to assist with meal planning.

   B. Contact the client's support system.

   C. Assess for age-related cognitive awareness.

   D. Encourage the use of a daily medication dispenser.

   E. Provide educational materials for home use.

2. A nurse in a health care clinic is evaluating the level of wellness for clients using the illness-wellness continuum tool. The nurse should identify which of the following clients as being at the center of the continuum?

   A. A college student who has influenza

   B. An older adult who has a new diagnosis of type 2 diabetes mellitus

   C. A new mother who has a urinary tract infection

   D. A young male client who has a long history of well-controlled rheumatoid arthritis

3. A nurse is evaluating clients at a health fair for modifiable variables affecting health and wellness. The nurse should identify which of the following variables as modifiable? (Select all that apply.)

   A. Smoking on social occasions

   B. BMI of 28

   C. Alopecia

   D. Trisomy 21

   E. History of reflux

4. A nurse is caring for a client who was just told she has breast cancer. The nurse evaluates the client's response. Which of the following statements by the client reflects a lack of understanding of an illness perspective?

   A. "I have no family history of breast cancer."

   B. "I need a second opinion. There is no lump."

   C. "I am glad we live in the city near several large hospitals."

   D. "I will schedule surgery next week, over the holidays."

PRACTICE Active Learning Scenario

A nurse in a clinic is caring for a client who continues to smoke despite numerous attempts to quit and has a family history of cardiovascular disease. What nursing interventions should the nurse use to meet the health needs of this client? Use the ATI Active Learning Template: Basic Concept to complete this item.

RELATED CONTENT: Include one statement identifying the goal.

UNDERLYING PRINCIPLES: Include one statement regarding health promotion and disease prevention.

NURSING INTERVENTIONS: Include a minimum of four.

Application Exercises Key

1. A. **CORRECT:** The nurse provides resources to strengthen coping abilities by asking the dietitian to assist the client with meal planning. This will improve client compliance.

   B. **CORRECT:** With the client's consent, the nurse can contact members of the client's support system and encourage the client to use this support during times of illness and stress to improve compliance.

   C. Assessing the client for age-related cognitive awareness is important but it is not an appropriate intervention that enhances the client's compliance.

   D. **CORRECT:** The nurse encourages the use of a daily medication dispenser to reduce health risks and improve medication compliance by the client.

   E. **CORRECT:** The nurse provides educational materials to the client to improve health awareness and reduce health risks after discharge.

   Ⓝ *NCLEX® Connection: Physiological Adaptation, Alterations in Body Systems*

2. A. The client who has influenza is measured on the continuum by the level of health to illness in comparison to the norm for the client.

   B. The client who is newly diagnosed with type 2 diabetes mellitus is measured by the level of health to illness in comparison to the norm for the client.

   C. The client who has a urinary tract infection is measured on the continuum by the level of health to illness in comparison to the norm for the client.

   D. **CORRECT:** The client who has well-controlled rheumatoid arthritis is measured at the center of the continuum, which is the client's normal state of health.

   Ⓝ *NCLEX® Connection: Health Promotion and Maintenance, Developmental Stages and Transitions*

3. A. **CORRECT:** The nurse identifies smoking as a modifiable variable that a client can change. The nurse should provide the client with educational materials and information on smoking cessation.

   B. **CORRECT:** The nurse identifies a BMI of 28 as a modifiable variable that a client can change. The nurse should provide the client with educational materials and information on weight reduction and exercising.

   C. The nurse identifies alopecia as a nonmodifiable variable because alopecia is a genetic disorder.

   D. The nurse identifies Trisomy 21 as a nonmodifiable variable because Trisomy 21 is genetic in origin.

   E. **CORRECT:** The nurse identifies reflux as a modifiable variable that a client can change. The nurse should provide the client with step-by-step educational information about treatment.

   Ⓝ *NCLEX® Connection: Health Promotion and Maintenance, Health Promotion/Disease Prevention*

4. A. The client's lack of a family history of cancer can influence the client's response to the new diagnosis, but it does not reflect a lack of understanding of an illness perspective.

   B. **CORRECT:** The client's statement of denial reflects a lack of understanding of the illness perspective and can influence the client's acceptance of the diagnosis.

   C. Access to health care resources can influence the client's response to the new diagnosis, but it does not reflect a lack of understanding of an illness perspective.

   D. Time constraints can influence a client's response to the diagnosis, but it does not reflect a lack of understanding of an illness perspective.

   Ⓝ *NCLEX® Connection: Health Promotion and Maintenance, Health Screening*

PRACTICE Answer

Using the ATI Active Learning Template: Basic Concept

RELATED CONTENT:
Identifying obstacles for compliance and adherence

UNDERLYING PRINCIPLES:
Health promotion and disease prevention are influenced by many factors that a nurse should address for a client success.

NURSING INTERVENTIONS
- Provide the client with resources to strengthen coping abilities.
- Encourage use of support systems (e.g. family, support group).
- Identify ways to improve compliance.
- Develop health education methods to reduce health risks.
- Identify the client's obstacles to health and wellness.
- Create strategies to reduce the client's obstacles.

Ⓝ *NCLEX® Connection: Health Promotion and Maintenance, High Risk Behaviors*

CHAPTER 2

CHAPTER 2 *Emergency Nursing Principles and Management*

Emergency nursing principles are the guidelines that nurses follow to assess and manage emergency situations for a client or multiple clients.

Nurses must have the ability to identify emergent situations and rapidly assess and intervene when life-threatening conditions exist. Emergent conditions are common to all nursing environments.

Emergency nursing principles: triage, primary survey, the ABCDE principle, poisoning, rapid response team, cardiac emergency, postresuscitation. Q_EBP

Emergency departments often implement the five-level system of triage: resuscitation (level one), emergent (level two), urgent (level three), less urgent (level four), and nonurgent (level five). Time and experience are required for the nurse to become an effective member of the triage team. The nurse, provider, and other members of the health care team work together in the triage area to determine the needs of the client.

Resuscitation triage requires immediate treatment to prevent death.

Nonurgent is a non-life-threatening condition requiring simple evaluation and care management.

PRIMARY SURVEY

- A primary survey is a rapid assessment of life-threatening conditions.
- The primary survey should be completed systematically so life-threatening conditions are not missed.
- Standard precautions—gloves, gowns, eye protection, face masks, and shoe covers—must be worn to prevent contamination with bodily fluids.
- The ABCDE principle guides the primary survey.

ABCDE PRINCIPLE

AIRWAY/CERVICAL SPINE

- This is the most important step in performing the primary survey. If a patent airway is not established, subsequent steps of the primary survey are futile. As a result of hypoxia, brain injury or death will occur within 3 to 5 min if the airway is not patent. Q_s
- If a client is awake and responsive, the airway is open.
- If a client's ability to maintain an airway is lost, it is important to inspect for blood, broken teeth, vomitus, or other foreign materials in the airway that can cause an obstruction.
- If the client is unresponsive without suspicion of trauma, the airway should be opened with a head-tilt/chin-lift maneuver. Q_s
  - Do NOT perform this technique on clients who have a potential cervical spine injury.
  - To perform the head-tilt/chin-lift maneuver, the nurse should assume a position at the head of the client, place one hand on his forehead, and place the other hand underneath the client's chin. His head should be tilted while his chin is lifted upward and forward. This maneuver lifts the tongue away from the laryngopharynx and provides for a patent airway. Q_s
- If the client is unresponsive with suspicion of trauma, the airway should be opened with a modified jaw thrust maneuver.
  - The nurse should assume a position at the head of the client, and place both hands on either side of the client's head. Locate the connection between the maxilla and the mandible. Lift the jaw superiorly while maintaining alignment of the cervical spine.
- Once the airway is opened, it should be inspected for blood, broken teeth, vomitus, and secretions. If present, obstructions should be cleared with suction or a finger-sweep method if the object is clearly visible.
- The open airway can be maintained with airway adjuncts, such as an oropharyngeal or nasopharyngeal airway.
- A bag valve mask with a 100% oxygen source is indicated for clients who need additional support during resuscitation until an advanced airway is established.
- A nonrebreather mask with 100% oxygen source is indicated for clients who are spontaneously breathing.

BREATHING

Once a patent airway is achieved, the nurse should assess for the presence and effectiveness of breathing.

BREATHING ASSESSMENT

- Auscultation of breath sounds
- Observation of chest expansion and respiratory effort
- Notation of rate and depth of respirations
- Identification of chest trauma
- Assessment of tracheal position
- Assessment for jugular vein distention

If a client is not breathing or is breathing inadequately, manual ventilation should be performed by a bag valve mask with supplemental oxygen or mouth-to-mask ventilation until a bag valve mask can be obtained.

CIRCULATION

- Once adequate ventilation is accomplished, circulation is assessed.
- Nurses should assess heart rate, blood pressure, peripheral pulses, and capillary refill for adequate perfusion.
- Nurses should consider cardiac arrest, myocardial dysfunction, and hemorrhage as precursors to shock and leading to ineffective circulation.

INTERVENTIONS

- **Interventions geared toward restoring effective circulation:**
  - CPR Qᴾᶜᶜ
  - Assess for external bleeding.
  - Hemorrhage control — Apply direct pressure to visible, significant external bleeding.
  - Obtain IV access using large-bore IV catheters inserted into the antecubital fossa of both arms, unless there is obvious injury to the extremity.
  - Infuse isotonic IV fluids such as lactated Ringer's and 0.9% sodium chloride, and/or blood products.
- Shock can develop if circulation is compromised. Shock is the body's response to inadequate tissue perfusion and oxygenation. It manifests with an increased heart rate and hypotension and can result in tissue ischemia and necrosis.

- **Interventions to alleviate shock** Qᴾᶜᶜ
  - Administer oxygen.
  - Apply pressure to obvious bleeding.
  - Elevate lower extremities to shunt blood to vital organs.
  - Administer IV fluids and blood products.
  - Monitor vital signs.
  - Remain with the client, and provide reassurance and support for anxiety.

DISABILITY

Disability is a quick assessment to determine the client's level of consciousness.
- The AVPU mnemonic is useful. **(2.1)** Qᴱᴮᴾ
- The Glasgow Coma Scale is another widely used method. **(2.2)** Qᴱᴮᴾ
- Neurologic assessment must be repeated at frequent intervals to ensure immediate response to any change.

EXPOSURE

- The nurse removes the client's clothing for a complete physical assessment. The nurse might need to cut off the client's clothing to accomplish this task.
- Clothing is always removed during a resuscitation situation to assess for additional injuries or those related to chemical and thermal burns involving the clothing.
- The nurse should preserve items of evidence, such as clothing, bullets, drugs, or weapons.
- Hypothermia is a primary concern. Hypothermia occurs when the client's core temperature is 35 °C (95 °F) or less.
- Victims of trauma are at risk for hypothermia due to exposure, unwarmed oxygen, and cold IV fluids.
- Hypothermia can lead to eventual coma, hypoxemia, and acidosis.

To prevent hypothermia:
- Remove wet clothing from the client.
- Cover the client with warm blankets.
- Increase the temperature of the room.
- Use a heat lamp to provide additional warmth.
- Infuse warmed IV fluids.

2.1 AVPU mnemonic

A Alert
V Responsive to voice
P Responsive to pain
U Unresponsive

2.2 Glasgow Coma Scale

EYE-OPENING RESPONSE		➕ VERBAL RESPONSE		➕ MOTOR RESPONSE	
Spontaneous	4	Oriented	5	Obeys commends	6
To voice	3	Confused	4	Localizes pain	5
To pain	2	Inappropriate words	3	Withdraws	4
None	1	Incomprehensible sounds	2	Flexion	3
		None	1	Extension	2
				None	1

A low score of 3 indicates a client who is totally unresponsive, and a high score of 15 indicates a client who is within normal limits neurologically.

POISONING

Poisoning is exposure to a toxic agent.
- Medications, illicit drugs, ingestion of a toxic agent
- Environmental (e.g., pollutants, snake and spider bites)

Poisoning is considered a medical emergency and requires rapid management therapy.
- Obtain a client history to identify the toxic agent.
- Implement supportive care.
- Determine type of poison.
- Prevent further absorption of the toxin.
- Extract or remove the poison.
- Administer antidotes when necessary.
- A snakebite from a venomous snake is a medical emergency.
  - Children ages 1 to 9 are at highest risk for snakebites.
  - The nurse should be familiar with indigenous snakes in the community.
  - Generally, ice, tourniquets, heparin, and corticosteroids are contraindicated in the first 6 to 8 hr after the bite.
  - Antivenom based on the type and severity of a snake bite is most effective if administered within 4 to 12 hr.

Interventions to manage the clinical status of the client exposed to or who ingested a toxic agent
- Provide measures for respiratory support (oxygen, airway management, mechanical ventilation).
- Monitor compromised circulation (resulting from excess perspiration, vomiting, diarrhea).
- Restore fluids with IV fluid therapy.
- Monitor blood pressure, cardiac monitoring, ECG.
- Assess for tissue edema every 15 to 30 min if bitten by a snake or spider.
- Administer opioid medications for pain due to snake or spider bite.
- Monitor ABGs, blood glucose levels, coagulation profile.
- For ingested poison, three procedures are available: activated charcoal, gastric lavage (if done within 1 hr of ingestion), and aspiration. Syrup of ipecac is no longer recommended.
- Administer diazepam if seizures occur.
- Reverse heroin and other opiate toxicity with naloxone.
- Implement dialysis and an exchange blood transfusion as a nonpharmacologic technique to remove toxic agents.

RAPID RESPONSE TEAM

- The team is a group of critical care experts (ICU nurse, respiratory therapist, a critical care provider, hospitalist). Q EBP
- Responds to an emergency call from nurses or family members when a client exhibits indications of a rapid decline.
- Provides early recognition and response before a respiratory or cardiac arrest or stroke occurs.
- Policies and procedures are established in a health care setting.
- Training for personnel is provided about criteria for calling for assistance when a client's condition changes toward a crisis situation.
- SBAR (Situation, Background, Assessment, Recommendation) communication techniques are used for contacting the team and documentation of event.
- Implement follow-up, education, and sharing of information (debriefing) for participants after the call.
- Discuss information to identify system failures (not recognizing a crisis, lack of adequate communication, failure in the plan of care).
- Retrieve more information at www.ihi.org.

CARDIAC EMERGENCY

Cardiac arrest: the sudden cessation of cardiac function caused most commonly by ventricular fibrillation or ventricular asystole.

Ventricular fibrillation (VF): a fluttering of the ventricles causing loss of consciousness, pulselessness, and no breathing. This requires collaborative care to defibrillate immediately using ACLS protocol.

Pulseless ventricular tachycardia (VT): an irritable firing of ectopic ventricular beats at a rate of 140 to 180/min. The client over time will become unconscious and deteriorate into VF.

Ventricular asystole: a complete absence of electrical activity and ventricular movement of the heart. The client is in complete cardiac arrest and requires implementation of BLS and ACLS protocol.

Pulseless electrical activity (PEA): a rhythm that appears to have electrical activity but is not sufficient to stimulate effective cardiac contractions and requires implementation of BLS and ACLS protocol.

2.3 Common causes of pulseless electrical activity

5 H's	5 T's
Hypovolemia	Toxins (accidental or deliberate drug overdose)
Hypoxia	
Hydrogen ion accumulation, resulting in acidosis	Tamponade (cardiac)
	Tension pneumothorax
Hyperkalemia or hypokalemia	Thrombosis (coronary)
Hypothermia	Thrombosis (pulmonary)

2.4 Receptor sites and responses

Alpha$_1$
Activation of receptors in arterioles of skin, viscera and mucous membranes, and veins lead to vasoconstriction

Beta$_1$
Heart stimulation leads to increased heart rate, increased myocardial contractility, and increased rate of conduction through the atrioventricular (AV) node.

Activation of receptors in the kidney leads to the release of renin.

Beta$_2$
Bronchial stimulation leads to bronchodilation.

Activation of receptors in uterine smooth muscle causes relaxation.

Activation of receptors in the liver causes a breakdown of glycogen into glucose.

Skeletal muscle receptor activation leads to muscle contraction, which can lead to tremors.

Dopamine
Activation of receptors in the kidney cause the renal blood vessels to dilate.

EMERGENCY NURSE CERTIFICATIONS

- Basic Life Support (BLS), Advanced Cardiac Life Support (ACLS), and Pediatric Advanced Life Support (PALS) are certifications required for nurses practicing in United States emergency departments.
- BLS involves a hands-on approach for assessment and management to restore airway, breathing, and circulation.
- ACLS builds on the BLS assessment and management skills to include advanced concepts.
  - Cardiac monitoring for specific resuscitation rhythms
  - Invasive airway management
  - Electrical therapies (defibrillation or cardioversion)
  - Obtaining IV access
  - Administration of IV antidysrhythmic medications
  - Management of the client postresuscitation
- PALS is built on the BLS protocol for neonatal and pediatric assessment and management skills to include advanced concepts for resuscitation of children.
- Certification courses are based on evidence-based practice management theory, and the basic concepts and techniques for cardiopulmonary resuscitation (CPR). Q EBP
- Current BLS and ACLS guidelines are available from the American Heart Association (AHA) at www.americanheart.org.

2.5 Food interactions

MAOIs promote the release of norepinephrine from sympathetic nerves and thereby prolong and intensify the effects of epinephrine and can cause hypertensive crisis.

NURSING INTERVENTIONS: Avoid the use of MAOIs in clients who are receiving epinephrine.

Tricyclic antidepressants block the uptake of epinephrine, which will prolong and intensify the effects of epinephrine.

NURSING INTERVENTIONS: Clients taking these medications concurrently can need a lower dose of epinephrine.

General anesthetics can cause the heart to become hypersensitive to the effects of epinephrine, which leads to dysrhythmias.

NURSING INTERVENTIONS

Perform continuous ECG monitoring.

Notify the provider if the client experiences chest pain, dysrhythmias, or an elevated heart rate.

Beta-adrenergic blocking agents, such as propranolol, block the action at beta receptors.

NURSING INTERVENTIONS: Propranolol may be used to treat chest pain, hypertension, myocardial infarction, and dysrhythmias.

Diuretics promote the beneficial effect of dopamine.

NURSING INTERVENTIONS: Monitor for therapeutic effects.

AHA ACLS PROTOCOLS

VF or pulseless VT

- Initiate the CPR components of BLS. Q EBP
- Defibrillate according to BLS guidelines.
- Establish IV access.
- Administer IV antidysrhythmic medications, such as epinephrine or vasopressin, according to ACLS guidelines.
- Consider the following medications.
  - Amiodarone hydrochloride
  - Lidocaine hydrochloride
  - Magnesium sulfate

Pulseless electrical activity (PEA)

- Initiate the CPR components of BLS.
- If shockable rhythm, defibrillate according to BLS guidelines.
- Establish IV access.
- Consider the most common causes. **(2.3)** Q EBP
- Administer epinephrine 1 mg IV push every 3 to 5 min.
- Asystole
  - Initiate the CPR components of BLS.
  - Establish IV access.
  - Give epinephrine 1 mg IV push every 3 to 5 min.
  - Consider reversible causes.
  - Asystole is often the final rhythm as the electrical and mechanical activity of the heart has stopped. The provider should consider ceasing resuscitation if asystole persists.

POSTRESUSCITATION

PHARMACOLOGICAL MANAGEMENT

- Medication therapy following a successful cardiac arrest includes IV medications that cause a catecholamine adrenergic agonist's effect.
- Catecholamine adrenergic agonists cannot be taken by the oral route, do not cross the blood-brain barrier, and have a short duration of action.
- Medications include epinephrine, dopamine, and dobutamine.
- These medications respond to an identifiable receptor and produce specific effects.

CONTRAINDICATIONS/PRECAUTIONS

- Pregnancy Risk Category C: epinephrine, dopamine, dobutamine
- These medications are contraindicated in clients who have tachydysrhythmias and ventricular fibrillation.
- Use cautiously in clients who have hyperthyroidism, angina, history of myocardial infarction, hypertension, and diabetes mellitus.

NURSING INTERVENTIONS AND CLIENT EDUCATION

- Medications must be administered by continuous IV infusion.
- Use IV pump to control infusion.
- Titrate dosage based on blood pressure response and/or heart rate response (these medications affect heart rate and blood pressure).
- Stop the infusion at the first sign of infiltration. Extravasation can be treated with a local injection of an alpha-adrenergic blocking agent, such as phentolamine.
- Assess/monitor the client for chest pain. Notify the provider if the client experiences chest pain.
- Provide continuous ECG monitoring. Notify the provider if the client experiences tachycardia or dysrhythmias.

2.6 Emergency medications

RECEPTORS	PHARMACOLOGICAL ACTION	THERAPEUTIC USE	ADVERSE EFFECTS	NURSING ACTIONS
Epinephrine				
Alpha$_1$	Vasoconstriction	Slows absorption of local anesthetics Manages superficial bleeding Reduces congestion of nasal mucosa Increases blood pressure	Vasoconstriction from activation of alpha$_1$ receptors in the heart can lead to hypertensive crisis.	Provide continuous cardiac monitoring. Report changes in vital signs to the provider.
Beta$_1$	Increases heart rate Strengthens myocardial contractility Increases rate of conduction through the AV node	Treatment of AV block and cardiac arrest	Beta$_1$ receptor activation in the heart can cause dysrhythmias. Beta$_1$ receptor activation also increases the workload of the heart and oxygen demand, leading to the development of angina.	Provide continuous cardiac monitoring. Monitor closely for dysrhythmias, change in heart rate, and chest pain. Monitor for hyperglycemia in clients who have diabetes mellitus. Notify the provider if the client experiences dysrhythmias, an elevated heart rate, or chest pain, and treat per protocol.
Beta$_2$	Bronchodilation	Asthma	The activation of beta$_2$ receptors in the liver and skeletal muscles can cause hyperglycemia from the breakdown of glycogen.	
Dopamine				
Dopamine	Low dose – dopamine (2 to 5 mcg/kg/min) Renal blood vessel dilation	Shock Heart failure Acute kidney injury		
Beta$_1$	Moderate dose – dopamine (5 to 10 mcg/kg/min) Renal blood vessel dilation Increases: • Heart rate • Myocardial contractility • Rate of conduction through the AV node • Blood pressure		Beta$_1$ receptor activation in the heart can cause dysrhythmias. Beta$_1$ receptor activation also increases the workload of the heart and oxygen demand, leading to the development of angina.	Provide continuous cardiac monitoring. Monitor closely for dysrhythmias, change in heart rate, and chest pain. Notify the provider of signs of dysrhythmias, elevated heart rate, and chest pain, and treat per protocol. Monitor for urinary output less than 30 mL/hr. Do not confuse dopamine with dobutamine.
Beta$_1$ Alpha$_1$	High dose – dopamine (greater than 10 mcg/kg/min) Renal blood vessel vasoconstriction Increases: • Heart rate • Myocardial contractility • Rate of conduction through the AV node • Blood pressure • Vasoconstriction		Necrosis can occur from extravasation due to high doses of dopamine.	Infuse dopamine into the central line. Monitor the IV site carefully. Discontinue the infusion at first sign of irritation.
Dobutamine				
Beta$_1$	Increases: • Heart rate • Myocardial contractility • Rate of conduction through the AV node	Heart failure	Increased heart rate	Provide continuous cardiac monitoring. Report changes in vital signs to the provider. Monitor for urinary output less than 30 mL/hr. Do not confuse dobutamine with dopamine.

Application Exercises

1. A nurse on a medical-surgical unit is caring for a group of clients. The nurse should notify the rapid response team for which of the following clients?

   A. Client who has an ulceration of the right heel whose blood glucose is 300 mg/dL

   B. Client who reports right calf pain and shortness of breath

   C. Client who has blood on a pressure dressing in the femoral area following a cardiac catheterization

   D. Client who has dark red coloration of left toes and absent pedal pulse

2. A nurse is caring for a client who has ingested a toxic agent. Which of the following actions should the nurse plan to take? (Select all that apply.)

   A. Induce vomiting.

   B. Instill activated charcoal.

   C. Perform a gastric lavage with aspiration.

   D. Administer syrup of ipecac.

   E. Infuse IV fluids.

3. A nurse in the emergency department is caring for a client who fell through the ice on a pond and is unresponsive and breathing slowly. Which of the following actions should the nurse take? (Select all that apply.)

   A. Remove wet clothing.

   B. Maintain normal room temperature.

   C. Apply warm blankets.

   D. Apply a heat lamp.

   E. Infuse warmed IV fluids.

4. A nurse in the emergency department is assessing a client who is unresponsive. The client's partner states, "He was pulling weeds in the yard and slumped to the ground." Which of the following techniques should the nurse use to open the client's airway?

   A. Head-tilt, chin-lift

   B. Modified jaw thrust

   C. Hyperextension of the head

   D. Flexion of the head

5. A nurse is reviewing the common emergency management protocol for clients who have asystole. Which of the following actions should the nurse plan to take during this cardiac emergency?

   A. Perform defibrillation.

   B. Prepare for transcutaneous pacing.

   C. Administer IV epinephrine.

   D. Elevate the client's lower extremities.

PRACTICE Active Learning Scenario

A nurse in the emergency department (ED) is implementing triage using the five-level system. Use the ATI Active Learning Template: Basic Concept to complete this item.

RELATED CONTENT: Identify the five levels of the ED triage system.

UNDERLYING PRINCIPLES: Define each of the five triage levels.

NURSING INTERVENTIONS: Describe a client who meets the criteria for each of the five triage levels.

Application Exercises Key

1. A. The nurse should notify the provider. The situation does not indicate the beginning of a rapid decline in the client's condition.

   B. **CORRECT:** The nurse should identify that the client is at risk for respiratory arrest due to a possible embolism. The nurse should call the rapid response team because the manifestations can indicate the beginning of a rapid decline in the client's condition.

   C. This assessment does not indicate the beginning of a rapid decline in the client's condition at this time. The nurse should reassess the client and notify the provider if the bleeding increases.

   D. The nurse should notify the provider. The situation does not indicate the beginning of a rapid decline in the client's condition.

   Ⓝ NCLEX® Connection: Physiological Adaptation, Medical Emergencies

2. A. Vomiting places the client at risk for aspiration.

   B. **CORRECT:** This is an appropriate action by the nurse because activated charcoal adsorbs toxic substances, and the charcoal does not pass into the bloodstream.

   C. **CORRECT:** This is an appropriate action by the nurse because gastric lavage with aspiration removes the toxic substance when the instilled fluid is suctioned from the gastrointestinal tract.

   D. Administering syrup of ipecac is not recommended because it induces vomiting, which increases the client's risk for aspiration.

   E. **CORRECT:** This is an appropriate action by the nurse because intravenous fluids help dilute the toxic substances in the bloodstream and promote elimination from the body through the kidneys.

   Ⓝ NCLEX® Connection: Physiological Adaptation, Medical Emergencies

3. A. **CORRECT:** This is an appropriate action by the nurse because the body temperature can rise more quickly when heat is applied to dry skin.

   B. The nurse should increase the temperature of the room to help return the client to a normal body temperature.

   C. **CORRECT:** This is an appropriate action by the nurse because the client's body temperature can rise more quickly when warm blankets are applied.

   D. **CORRECT:** This is an appropriate action by the nurse because the client's body temperature can rise more quickly when a heat lamp is safely applied.

   E. **CORRECT:** This is an appropriate action by the nurse because the client's body temperature can rise more quickly when warmed IV fluids are infused.

   Ⓝ NCLEX® Connection: Physiological Adaptation, Medical Emergencies

4. A. **CORRECT:** The nurse should open the client's airway by the head-tilt, chin-lift because the client is unresponsive without suspicion of trauma.

   B. The nurse should not open the client's airway with the modified jaw thrust because this method is used for a client who is unresponsive with suspected traumatic neck injury.

   C. The nurse should not open the client's airway with hyperextension of the head because hyperextension of the head can close off the airway and cause injury.

   D. The nurse should not open the client's airway with flexion of the head because flexion of the head does not open the airway.

   Ⓝ NCLEX® Connection: Physiological Adaptation, Medical Emergencies

5. A. Defibrillation is not indicated for asystole, because this is not considered a shockable cardiac rhythm.

   B. Transcutaneous pacing is not indicated for the treatment of asystole.

   C. **CORRECT:** Administering epinephrine during asystole is an appropriate action by the nurse because it increases heart rate, improves cardiac output, and promotes bronchodilation.

   D. Elevating the client's lower extremities is indicated for the treatment of a client who is in shock, rather than asystole.

   Ⓝ NCLEX® Connection: Physiological Adaptation, Medical Emergencies

---

PRACTICE Answer

Using the ATI Active Learning Template: Basic Concept

RELATED CONTENT
- Resuscitation
- Emergent
- Urgent
- Less Urgent
- Nonurgent

UNDERLYING PRINCIPLES
- Resuscitation: The client needs immediate treatment to prevent death.
- Emergent: The client requires time sensitive treatment for a problem that has the potential to become a life or limb-threatening situation.
- Urgent: The client requires treatment but the situation is not life-threatening.
- Less Urgent: The client is able to wait for a period of time without immediate treatment.
- Nonurgent: The client requires simple evaluation and minor management of care.

NURSING INTERVENTIONS
- Resuscitation: A client who is experiencing cardiac arrest, stroke, pulmonary emboli, or drug overdose.
- Emergent: A client who has sustained a traumatic amputation, head or neck injury, snake or spider bite.
- Urgent: A client who has a kidney stone, gallbladder colic, or fracture.
- Less Urgent: A client who has a bladder infection, laceration, or infected toe.
- Nonurgent: A client who has a rash, minor cut, or backache.

Ⓝ NCLEX® Connection: Physiological Adaptation, Medical Emergencies

NCLEX® Connections

When reviewing the following chapters, keep in mind the relevant topics and tasks of the NCLEX outline, in particular:

Client Needs: Basic Care and Comfort

NON-PHARMACOLOGICAL COMFORT INTERVENTIONS: Provide non-pharmacological comfort measures.

MOBILITY/IMMOBILITY: Assess the client for mobility, gait, strength, and motor skills.

NUTRITION AND ORAL HYDRATION
Evaluate client intake and output and intervene as needed.

Evaluate the impact of disease/illness on nutritional status of a client.

Client Needs: Pharmacological and Parenteral Therapies

ADVERSE EFFECTS/CONTRAINDICATIONS/SIDE EFFECTS/INTERACTIONS: Assess the client for actual or potential side effects and adverse effects of medications.

EXPECTED ACTIONS/OUTCOMES: Evaluate client response to medication.

PHARMACOLOGICAL PAIN MANAGEMENT
Assess client need for administration of a PRN pain medication.

Administer pharmacological measures for pain management.

Client Needs: Reduction of Risk Potential

DIAGNOSTIC TESTS: Compare client diagnostic findings with pretest results.

POTENTIAL FOR COMPLICATIONS OF DIAGNOSTIC TESTS/TREATMENTS/PROCEDURES: Use precautions to prevent injury and/or complications associated with a procedure or diagnosis.

THERAPEUTIC PROCEDURES: Apply knowledge of related nursing procedures and psychomotor skills when caring for clients undergoing therapeutic procedures.

UNIT 2 **NURSING CARE OF CLIENTS WHO HAVE NEUROSENSORY DISORDERS**
SECTION: DIAGNOSTIC AND THERAPEUTIC PROCEDURES

CHAPTER 3 *Neurologic Diagnostic Procedures*

Neurologic assessment and diagnostic procedures are used to evaluate neurologic function by testing indicators such as mental status, motor functioning, electrical activity, and intracranial pressure.

Neurologic assessment and diagnostic procedures that nurses should be knowledgeable about include cerebral angiography, cerebral computed tomography (CT) scan, electroencephalography (EEG), Glasgow Coma Scale, intracranial pressure monitoring, lumbar puncture (spinal tap), magnetic resonance imaging (MRI), positron emission tomography, single-photon emission computed tomography, and radiography (x-ray).

Cerebral angiography

Cerebral angiography provides visualization of the cerebral blood vessels.
- Digital subtraction angiography hides the bones and tissues from the images, providing x-rays with only the vessels apparent.
- The procedure detects defects, narrowing, or obstruction of arteries or blood vessels in brain.
- The procedure is performed within the radiology department because iodine-based contrast dye is injected into an artery during the procedure.

INDICATIONS

Cerebral angiography is used to assess the blood flow to and within the brain, identify aneurysms, and define the vascularity of tumors (useful for surgical planning). It is also used therapeutically to inject medications that treat blood clots or to administer chemotherapy.

CONSIDERATIONS

PREPROCEDURE

If the client is pregnant, a determination of the risks to the fetus versus the benefits of the information obtained by this procedure should be made.

NURSING ACTIONS
- Instruct the client to refrain from consuming food or fluids for 4 to 6 hr prior to the procedure.
- Assess for allergy to shellfish or iodine, which would require the use of a different contrast media.
- Any history of bleeding or taking anticoagulant medication requires additional considerations and additional monitoring to ensure clotting after the procedure. Qs
- Assess BUN and serum creatinine to determine kidney's ability to excrete the dye.
- Ensure that the client is not wearing any jewelry.
- A mild sedative for relaxation is occasionally administered prior to and during the procedure, and vital signs are continuously monitored during the procedure.

CLIENT EDUCATION
- Instruct the client about the importance of not moving during the procedure and about the need to keep the head immobilized.
- Instruct the client to void immediately before the test.
- Warn the client about a metallic taste in the mouth, and a warm sensation over the face, jaw, tongue, lips, and behind the eyes from the dye injected during procedure.

INTRAPROCEDURE
- The client is placed on a radiography table, where the client's head is secured.
- A catheter is placed into an artery (usually in the groin or the neck), dye is injected, and x-ray pictures are taken.
- Once all pictures are taken, the catheter is removed and an arterial closure device is used or pressure is held over the artery to control bleeding by thrombus formation sealing the artery.

POSTPROCEDURE

NURSING ACTIONS
- Closely monitor the area to ensure that clotting occurs.
- Movements are restricted depending on the type of procedure used to seal the artery to prevent rebleeding at the catheter site.

COMPLICATIONS

There is a risk for bleeding or hematoma formation at the entry site.

NURSING ACTIONS
- Check the insertion site frequently.
- Check the affected extremity distal to the puncture site for adequate circulation (e.g., color, temperature, pulses, and capillary refill).
- If bleeding occurs, apply pressure over the artery and notify the provider. QEBP

Cerebral computed tomography scan

A CT scan provides cross-sectional images of the cranial cavity. A contrast media can be used to enhance the images.

INDICATIONS

CT scanning can be used to identify tumors and infarctions, detect abnormalities, monitor response to treatment, and guide needles used for biopsies.

CONSIDERATIONS

PREPROCEDURE

If the client is pregnant, a determination of the risks to the fetus versus the benefits of the information obtained by this procedure should be made.

NURSING ACTIONS
- If contrast media and/or sedation is expected:
  - Instruct the client to refrain from consuming food or fluids for at least 4 hr prior to the procedure.
  - Assess for allergy to shellfish or iodine, which would require the use of a different contrast media.
  - Assess renal function (BUN and creatinine), because contrast media is excreted by the kidneys. Qs
- Because this procedure is performed with the client in a supine position, placing pillows in the small of the client's back can assist in preventing back pain. The head must be secured to prevent unnecessary movement during the procedure.
- Ensure that the client's jewelry is removed prior to this procedure. In general, clients wear a hospital gown to prevent any metals from interfering with the x-rays.

INTRAPROCEDURE

- The client must lie supine with the head stabilized during the procedure.
- Although CT scanning is painless, sedation can be provided.

POSTPROCEDURE

NURSING ACTIONS
- There is no follow-up care associated with a CT scan.
- If contrast media is injected, monitor for allergic reaction and changes in kidney function.
- If sedation is administered, monitor the client until stable.

Electroencephalography

This noninvasive procedure assesses the electrical activity of the brain and is used to determine if there are abnormalities in brain wave patterns. An EEG provides information about the ability of the brain to function and highlights areas of abnormality.

INDICATIONS

EEGs are most commonly performed to identify and determine seizure activity, but they are also useful for detecting sleep disorders and behavioral changes.

CONSIDERATIONS

PREPROCEDURE

NURSING ACTIONS: Review medications with the provider to determine if they should be continued prior to this procedure.

CLIENT EDUCATION
- Instruct the client to wash his hair prior to the procedure and eliminate all oils, gels, and sprays.
- If indicated, instruct the client to be sleep-deprived because this provides cranial stress, increasing the possibility of abnormal electrical activity, such as seizure potentials, occurring during the procedure.
- Increased electrical activity can be stimulated with exposure to bright flashing lights, or by requesting the client to hyperventilate for 3 to 4 min.
- Instruct the client to avoid taking any stimulant or sedative medication 12 to 24 hr prior to the procedure.

INTRAPROCEDURE

- The procedure generally takes 1 hr.
- There are no risks associated with this procedure.
- With the client resting in a chair or lying in bed, small electrodes are placed on the scalp and connected to a brain wave machine or computer.
- Electrical signals produced by the brain are recorded by the machine or computer in the form of wavy lines. This documents brain activity.
- Notations are made when stimuli are presented or when sleep occurs. (Flashes of light or pictures can be used during the procedure to assess the client's response to stimuli.)

POSTPROCEDURE

CLIENT EDUCATION: Instruct the client that normal activities may be resumed.

Glasgow Coma Scale

This assessment concentrates on neurologic function and is useful to determine the level of consciousness and monitor response to treatment. The Glasgow Coma Scale (GCS) is reported as a number that allows providers to immediately determine if neurologic changes have occurred.

INDICATIONS

GCS scores are helpful in determining changes in the level of consciousness for clients who have head injuries, space-occupying lesions or cerebral infarctions, and encephalitis. This is important because complications related to neurologic injuries can occur rapidly and require immediate treatment.

CONSIDERATIONS

GCS scores are calculated by using appropriate stimuli (a painful stimulus can be necessary) and then assessing the client's response in three areas. Q EBP

- **Eye opening (E):** The best eye response, with responses ranging from 4 to 1
  - 4 = Eye opening occurs spontaneously.
  - 3 = Eye opening occurs secondary to sound.
  - 2 = Eye opening occurs secondary to pain.
  - 1 = Eye opening does not occur.
- **Verbal (V):** The best verbal response, with responses ranging from 5 to 1
  - 5 = Conversation is coherent and oriented.
  - 4 = Conversation is incoherent and disoriented.
  - 3 = Words are spoken, but inappropriately.
  - 2 = Sounds are made, but no words.
  - 1 = Vocalization does not occur.
- **Motor (M):** The best motor response, with responses ranging from 6 to 1
  - 6 = Commands are followed.
  - 5 = Local reaction to pain occurs.
  - 4 = There is a general withdrawal to pain.
  - 3 = Decorticate posture (adduction of arms, flexion of elbows and wrists) is present.
  - 2 = Decerebrate posture (abduction of arms, extension of elbows and wrists) is present.
  - 1 = Motor response does not occur.

Responses within each subscale are added, with the total score quantitatively describing the client's level of consciousness. **E + V + M = Total GCS**

- In critical situations, where head injury is present and close monitoring is required, subscale results may also be documented. Thus, a GCS may be reported as either a single number, indicating the sum of the subscales (3 to 15), or as 3 numbers, one from each subscale result, and the total (E3 V3 M4 = GCS 13). This allows providers to determine specific neurologic function.
- Intubation limits the ability to use GCS summed scores. If intubation is present, the GCS may be reported as two scores, with modification noted. This is generally reported as "GCS 5t" (with the t representing the intubation tube).

INTERPRETATION OF FINDINGS

- The best possible GCS score is 15. In general, total scores of the GCS correlate with the degree or level of coma.
- A score less than 8 is associated with severe head injury and coma.
- A score of 9 to 12 indicates a moderate head injury.
- A score greater than 13 is associated with minor head trauma.

Intracranial pressure monitoring

An intracranial pressure (ICP) monitor is a device inserted into the cranial cavity that records pressure and is connected to a monitor that shows a picture of the pressure waveforms. Qs

- Monitoring ICP facilitates continual assessment and is more precise than vague manifestations.
- The insertion procedure is performed by a neurosurgeon in the operating room, emergency department, or critical care unit. This procedure is rarely used unless the client is comatose, so there is minimal need for pain medication and preprocedural client teaching.

Three basic types of ICP monitoring systems

- **Intraventricular catheter** (also called a ventriculostomy): A fluid-filled catheter is inserted into the anterior horn of the lateral ventricles (most often on the right side) through a burr hole. The catheter is connected to a sterile drainage system with a three-way stopcock that allows simultaneous monitoring of pressures by a transducer connected to a bedside monitor and drainage of cerebrospinal fluid (CSF).
- **Subarachnoid screw or bolt:** A hollow, threaded screw or bolt is placed into the subarachnoid space through a twist-drill burr hole in the front of the skull, behind the hairline. The bolt is connected by fluid-filled tubing to a transducer leveled at the approximate location of the lateral ventricles.
- **Epidural or subdural sensor:** A fiber-optic sensor is inserted into the epidural space through a burr hole. The fiber-optic device measures changes in the amount of light reflected from a pressure-sensitive diaphragm in the catheter tip. The cable is connected to a precalibrated monitor that displays the numerical value of ICP. This method of monitoring is noninvasive because the device does not penetrate the dura.

INDICATIONS

- ICP monitoring is useful for early identification and treatment of increased intracranial pressure. Clients who are comatose or have GCS scores of 8 are candidates for ICP monitoring.
- Manifestations of increased ICP include severe headache, deteriorating level of consciousness, restlessness, irritability, dilated or pinpoint pupils, slowness to react, alteration in breathing pattern (Cheyne-Stokes respirations, central neurologic hyperventilation, apnea), deterioration in motor function, and abnormal posturing (decerebrate, decorticate, flaccidity).

CONSIDERATIONS

PREPROCEDURE

The head is shaved around the insertion location. The site is then cleansed with an antibacterial solution.

INTRAPROCEDURE

- Local anesthetic can be used to numb the area if the client's GCS indicates some level of consciousness (GCS 8 to 11).
- Insertion and care of any ICP monitoring device requires surgical aseptic technique to reduce the risk for CNS infection.

POSTPROCEDURE

NURSING ACTIONS
- Maintain system integrity at all times. There is a risk of serious, life-threatening infection.
- Inspect the insertion site at least every 24 hr for redness, swelling, and drainage. Change the sterile dressing covering the access site per facility protocol. Qs
- ICP monitoring equipment must be balanced and recalibrated per facility protocols.
- After the insertion procedure, observe ICP waveforms, noting the pattern of waveforms and monitoring for increased ICP (a sustained elevation of pressure greater than 15 mm Hg).
- Assess the client's clinical status and monitor routine and neurologic vital signs every hour as needed.

INTERPRETATION OF FINDINGS

Normal ICP is 10 to 15 mm Hg. Persistent elevation of ICP extinguishes cerebral circulation, which will result in brain death if not treated urgently.

COMPLICATIONS

The insertion and maintenance of an ICP monitoring system can cause infection and bleeding.

NURSING ACTIONS QEBP
- Follow strict surgical aseptic technique.
- Perform sterile dressing changes per facility protocol.
- Keep drainage systems closed.
- Limit monitoring to 3 to 5 days.
- Irrigate the system only as needed to maintain patency.

Lumbar puncture (spinal tap)

A lumbar puncture is a procedure during which a small amount of CSF is withdrawn from the spinal canal and then analyzed to determine its constituents.

INDICATIONS

This procedure is used to detect the presence of some diseases (multiple sclerosis, syphilis, meningitis), infection, and malignancies. A lumbar puncture may also be used to reduce CSF pressure, instill a contrast medium or air for diagnostic tests, or administer medication or chemotherapy directly to spinal fluid.

CONSIDERATIONS

PREPROCEDURE

The risks versus benefits of a lumbar puncture should be discussed with the client prior to this procedure.
- A lumbar puncture can be associated with rare but serious complications, such as brain herniation, especially when performed in the presence of increased ICP.
- Lumbar punctures for clients who have bleeding disorders or who are taking anticoagulants can result in bleeding that compresses the spinal cord.

NURSING ACTIONS
- Ensure that all of the client's jewelry is removed and that the client is wearing only a hospital gown.
- Instruct the client to void prior to the procedure.
- Clients should be positioned to stretch the spinal canal. This can be done by having the client assume a "cannonball" position while on one side. (3.1)

INTRAPROCEDURE

- The area of the needle insertion is cleansed, and a local anesthesia is injected.
- The needle is inserted and the CSF is withdrawn, after which the needle is removed.
- A manometer can be used to determine the opening pressure of the spinal cord, which is useful if increased pressure is a consideration.

POSTPROCEDURE

CSF is sent to the pathology department for analysis.

- NURSING ACTIONS: Monitor the puncture site. The client should remain lying for several hours to ensure that the site clots and to decrease the risk of a post-lumbar puncture headache, caused by CSF leakage. Q EBP
- CLIENT EDUCATION: Once stable, advise the client that normal activities may be resumed.

COMPLICATIONS

If clotting does not occur to seal the dura puncture site, CSF can leak, resulting in a headache and increasing the potential for infection.

NURSING ACTIONS

- Encourage the client to lie flat in bed. Provide fluids for hydration, and administer pain medication.
- Prepare the client for an epidural blood patch to seal the hole in the dura if the headache persists.

Magnetic resonance imaging scan

An MRI scan provides cross-sectional images of the cranial cavity. A contrast media may be used to enhance the images.

- Unlike CT scans, MRI images are obtained using magnets, thus the consequences associated with radiation are avoided. This makes this procedure safer for women who are pregnant.
- The use of magnets precludes the ability to scan a client who has an artificial device (pacemakers, surgical clips, intravenous access port). Qs
- Use MRI-approved equipment to monitor vital signs and provide ventilator/oxygen assistance to clients undergoing MRI scans.

INDICATIONS

- MRI scans are used to detect abnormalities, monitor response to treatment, and guide needles used for biopsies.
- MRIs are capable of discriminating soft tissue from tumor or bone. This makes the MRI scan effective in determining tumor size and blood vessel location.

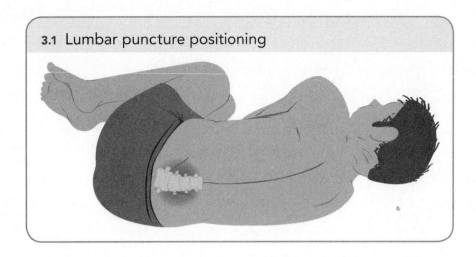

3.1 Lumbar puncture positioning

CONSIDERATIONS

PREPROCEDURE

NURSING ACTIONS

- Remove any transdermal patches with a foil backing, as these can cause burn injuries. Qs
- Ensure that the client's jewelry is removed prior to this procedure. The client should wear a hospital gown to prevent any metals from interfering with the magnet.
- If sedation is expected, the client should refrain from food or fluids for 4 to 8 hr prior to the procedure.
- Determine if the client has a history of claustrophobia, and explain the tight space and noise.
- Ask the client about any implants containing metal (e.g., pacemaker, orthopedic joints, artificial heart valves, intrauterine devices, aneurysm clips).
- All people in the scanning area while the magnet is on must remove all jewelry, electronics, and phones to prevent damage to themselves or the magnet.
- Because this procedure is performed with the client in a supine position, placing pillows in the small of the client's back can assist in preventing back pain. The head must be secured to prevent unnecessary movement during the procedure.

INTRAPROCEDURE

- The client must lie supine with the head stabilized.
- MRI scanning is noisy, and earplugs or sedation may be provided.

POSTPROCEDURE

NURSING ACTIONS

- If contrast media is injected, monitor the site to ensure that clotting has occurred and monitor for any indications of an allergic reaction.
- If sedation is administered, monitor the client until stable.

PET and SPECT scans

Positron emission tomography (PET) and single-photon emission computed tomography (SPECT) scans are nuclear medicine procedures that produce three-dimensional images of the head. These images can be static (depicting vessels) or functional (depicting brain activity).

- A glucose-based tracer is injected into the blood stream prior to the PET scan. This initiates regional metabolic activity, which is then documented by the PET scanner. A radioisotope is used for SPECT scanning.
- A CT scan may be performed after a PET/SPECT scan, as this provides information regarding brain activity and pathological location (e.g., brain injury, death, neoplasm).

INDICATIONS

A PET/SPECT scan capture of regional metabolic processes is most useful in determining tumor activity and/or response to treatment. PET/SPECT scans are also able to determine the presence of dementia, indicated by the inability of the brain to respond to the tracer.

CONSIDERATIONS

PREPROCEDURE

PET/SPECT scans use radiation, thus the risks and benefits to a client who might be pregnant must be discussed.

NURSING ACTIONS: Assess for a history of diabetes mellitus. While this condition does not preclude a PET/SPECT scan, alterations in the client's medications can be necessary to avoid hyperglycemia or hypoglycemia before and after this procedure. Qs

INTRAPROCEDURE

- While the pictures are being obtained, the client must lie flat with the head restrained.
- This procedure is not painful and sedation is rarely necessary.

POSTPROCEDURE

NURSING ACTIONS
- If radioisotopes are used, assess for allergic reaction.
- There is no follow-up care after a PET/SPECT scans.
- Because the tracer is glucose-based and short-acting (less than 2 hr), it is broken down within the body as a sugar, not excreted.

Radiography (x-ray)

An x-ray uses electromagnetic radiation to capture images of the internal structures of an individual.

- A structure's image is light or dark relative to the amount of radiation the tissue absorbs. The image is recorded on a radiograph, which is a black-and-white image that is held up to light for visualization. Some are recorded digitally and available immediately.
- X-rays are interpreted by a radiologist, who documents the findings.

INDICATIONS

X-ray examinations of the skull and spine can reveal fractures, curvatures, bone erosion and dislocation, and possible soft tissue calcification, all of which can damage the nervous system.

CONSIDERATIONS

PREPROCEDURE

NURSING ACTIONS
- There is no specific preprocedure protocol for x-rays that do not use contrast. X-rays are often the first diagnostic tool used after an injury (e.g., rule out cervical fracture in head trauma), and they can be done without any preparation.
- Determine if female clients are pregnant.
- Ensure that the client's jewelry is removed and that no clothes cover the area.

CLIENT EDUCATION: Explain that the amount of radiation used in contemporary x-ray machines is very small.

INTRAPROCEDURE

CLIENT EDUCATION: Instruct the client to remain still during the procedure.

POSTPROCEDURE

NURSING ACTIONS: No postprocedure care is required.
CLIENT EDUCATION: Inform the client when results will be available.

Application Exercises

1. A nurse is caring for a client who is postprocedure following lumbar puncture and reports a throbbing headache when sitting upright. Which of the following actions should the nurse take? (Select all that apply.)

    A. Use the Glasgow Coma Scale when assessing the client.

    B. Assist the client to a supine position.

    C. Administer an opioid medication.

    D. Encourage the client to increase fluid intake.

    E. Instruct the client to perform deep breathing and coughing exercises.

2. A nurse is caring for a client who experienced a traumatic head injury and has an intraventricular catheter (ventriculostomy) for ICP monitoring. The nurse should monitor the client for which of the following complications related to the ventriculostomy?

    A. Headache

    B. Infection

    C. Aphasia

    D. Hypertension

3. A nurse is assessing a client for changes in the level of consciousness using the Glasgow Coma Scale (GCS). The client opens his eyes when spoken to, speaks incoherently, and moves his extremities when pain is applied. Which of the following GCS scores should the nurse document?

    A. E2 + V3 + M5 = 10

    B. E3 + V4 + M4 = 11

    C. E4 + V5 + M6 = 15

    D. E2 + V2 + M4 = 8

4. A nurse is developing a plan of care for a client who is scheduled for cerebral angiography with contrast dye. Which of the following statements by the client should the nurse report to the provider? (Select all that apply.)

    A. "I think I might be pregnant."

    B. "I take warfarin."

    C. "I take antihypertensive medication."

    D. "I am allergic to shrimp."

    E. "I ate a light breakfast this morning."

5. A nurse is providing education to a client who is to undergo an electroencephalogram (EEG) the next day. Which of the following information should the nurse include in the teaching?

    A. "Do not wash your hair the morning of the procedure."

    B. "Try to stay awake most of the night prior to the procedure."

    C. "The procedure will take approximately 15 minutes."

    D. "You will need to lie flat for 4 hours after the procedure."

PRACTICE Active Learning Scenario

A nurse is developing a plan of care for a client who is scheduled for a magnetic resonance imaging (MRI) scan with contrast dye. What should the nurse include in the plan of care? Use the ATI Active Learning Template: Diagnostic Procedure to complete this item.

PROCEDURE NAME: Define this diagnostic test.

NURSING INTERVENTIONS (PRE, INTRA, POST): Identify three preprocedure actions, one intraprocedure action, and one postprocedure action.

Application Exercises Key

1. A. The Glasgow Coma Scale is used to assess a client's level of consciousness and is not necessary following a lumbar puncture.

   B. **CORRECT:** The nurse should assist the client to a supine position, which can relieve a headache following a lumbar puncture.

   C. **CORRECT:** The nurse should administer an opioid medication for a client's report of headache pain.

   D. **CORRECT:** The nurse should encourage an increased fluid intake to maintain a positive fluid balance, which can relieve a headache following a lumbar puncture.

   E. Coughing can increase ICP, which can result in an increase in the client's headache.

   Ⓝ *NCLEX® Connection: Reduction of Risk Potential, Potential for Complications of Diagnostic Tests/Treatments/Procedures*

2. A. The nurse should monitor a client who has increased ICP for a headache, but a headache does not indicate a complication directly related to the ventriculostomy.

   B. **CORRECT:** The nurse should monitor a client who has a ventriculostomy for infection, which is a complication. The nurse should use strict asepsis to avoid this life-threatening condition, which can result in meningitis.

   C. The nurse should monitor a client who has increased ICP for aphasia related to the head injury, but this not a complication directly related to the ventriculostomy.

   D. The nurse should monitor a client who has increased ICP for hypertension, but this is not a complication directly related to the ventriculostomy.

   Ⓝ *NCLEX® Connection: Reduction of Risk Potential, Potential for Complications of Diagnostic Tests/Treatments/Procedures*

3. A. The calculation is incorrect. E2 represents eyes opening secondary to pain, V3 represents verbal response with words spoken inappropriately, and M5 represents motor response to pain with a local reaction.

   B. **CORRECT:** The client's score is calculated correctly, indicating moderate head injury. E3 represents opening eyes secondary to voice stimulation, V4 represents verbal conversation that is incoherent and disoriented, and M4 represents motor response as a general withdrawal to pain.

   C. The client's score is calculated incorrectly. E4 represents eyes opening spontaneously, V5 represents verbal conversation as coherent and oriented, and M6 indicates a client is able to follow commands.

   D. The client's score is calculated incorrectly. E2 represents eyes opening secondary to pain, V2 represents verbal response by the client making sounds but speaking no words, and M4 is a motor response with a general withdrawal to pain.

   Ⓝ *NCLEX® Connection: Reduction of Risk Potential, Diagnostic Tests*

4. A. **CORRECT:** The nurse should report the client's statement of possible pregnancy to the provider because the contrast dye can place the fetus at risk.

   B. **CORRECT:** The nurse should report that the client is taking warfarin to the provider due to the potential for bleeding following angiography.

   C. There is no contraindication related to contrast dye for a client who is taking antihypertensive medication.

   D. **CORRECT:** The nurse should report a client's report of allergy to shrimp, which is a shellfish, to the provider due to a potential allergic reaction to the contrast dye.

   E. **CORRECT:** The nurse should report a client's intake of food to the provider since the client should remain NPO for 4 to 6 hr prior to the procedure.

   Ⓝ *NCLEX® Connection: Reduction of Risk Potential, Diagnostic Tests*

5. A. The nurse should teach the client to wash her hair on the morning of the procedure to remove oils, gels, and sprays, which can affect the EEG readings.

   B. **CORRECT:** The nurse should teach the client to remain awake most of the night to provide cranial stress and increase the possibility of abnormal electrical activity.

   C. The nurse should teach the client that the procedure will take approximately 1 hr.

   D. The nurse should teach the client that normal activity can resume immediately following the procedure.

   Ⓝ *NCLEX® Connection: Reduction of Risk Potential, Therapeutic Procedures*

PRACTICE Answer

Using the ATI Active Learning Template: Diagnostic Procedure

PROCEDURE NAME: Magnetic resonance imaging (MRI) scan relies on magnetic field to take multiple images of the body.

NURSING INTERVENTIONS (PRE, INTRA, POST)
- Preprocedure
  - Remove all client jewelry.
  - Determine if the client has claustrophobia.
  - Question the client concerning implants containing metal.
  - Question the client regarding allergies.
- Intraprocedure: Stabilize the client's head
- Postprocedure: Monitor for allergic reaction to the contrast dye used during the MRI.

Ⓝ *NCLEX® Connection: Reduction of Risk Potential, Diagnostic Tests*

CHAPTER 4

CHAPTER 4 *Pain Management*

Effective pain management includes the use of pharmacological and nonpharmacological pain management therapies.

Clients have a right to adequate assessment and management of pain. Nurses are accountable for the assessment of pain. Professional organizations and The Joint Commission have mandates requiring pain assessment and management. The nurse's role is that of an advocate, member of the health care team, and educator for effective pain management.

Nurses have a priority responsibility for the continual assessment of the client's pain level and to provide individualized interventions. They should assess the effectiveness of the interventions 30 to 60 min after implementation. Qᴘᴄᴄ

Assessment challenges can occur with clients who are cognitively impaired, critically ill, or on a ventilator.

PHYSIOLOGY

- Transduction is the conversion of painful stimuli to an electrical impulse through peripheral nerve fibers (nociceptors).
- Transmission occurs as the electrical impulse travels along the nerve fibers, where neurotransmitters regulate it.
- Perception or awareness of pain occurs in various areas of the brain, with influences from thought and emotional processes
- Modulation occurs in the spinal cord, causing muscles to contract reflexively, moving the body away from painful stimuli.
- The pain threshold is the point at which a person feels pain.
- Pain tolerance is the amount of pain a person is willing to bear.

Substances that increase pain transmission and cause an inflammatory response include substance P, prostaglandins, bradykinin, and histamine.

Substances that decrease pain transmission and produce analgesia include serotonin and endorphins.

ASSESSMENT

Pain is whatever the person experiencing it says it is, and it exists whenever the person says it does. The client's report of pain is the most reliable diagnostic measure of pain. Self-report using standardized pain scales is useful for clients over the age of 7 years. Specialized pain scales are available for use with younger children. Qᴘᴄᴄ

- Assess and document pain (the fifth vital sign) according to the client's condition and agency guidelines. Pain is categorized by duration (acute or chronic) or by origin (nociceptive or neuropathic). **(4.1)**
- Use a focused assessment to obtain subjective data. **(4.2)**

4.1 Pain categories

Acute pain

Acute pain is protective, temporary, usually self-limiting, and resolves with tissue healing.

Physiological responses (sympathetic nervous system) are fight-or-flight responses (tachycardia, hypertension, anxiety, diaphoresis, muscle tension).

Behavioral responses include grimacing, moaning, flinching, and guarding.

The nurse should be aware that a client not exhibiting physiological or behavioral responses does not mean that pain is absent.

Interventions include treatment of the underlying problem.

Chronic pain

Chronic pain is not protective. It is ongoing or recurs frequently, lasting longer than 3 months and persisting beyond tissue healing.

Physiological responses do not usually increase vital signs. The client's vital signs can actually be lower than normal in response to chronic pain. Clients can have depression, fatigue, decreased level of functioning, or disability.

Chronic pain might not have a known cause, and it might not respond to interventions.

Management aims at pain relief.

Chronic pain can be classified as chronic cancer pain or chronic noncancer pain.

Nociceptive pain

Nociceptive pain arises from damage to or inflammation of tissue other than that of the peripheral and central nervous systems.

Nociceptive pain is the activation of normal processing of painful stimuli.

It is usually throbbing, aching, and localized.

This pain typically responds to opioids and nonopioid medications.

TYPES OF NOCICEPTIVE PAIN

Somatic: in bones, joints, muscles, skin, or connective tissues.

Visceral: in internal organs such as the stomach or intestines. It can cause referred pain in other body locations separate from the stimulus.

Neuropathic pain

Neuropathic pain arises from abnormal or damaged pain nerves.

It differs from nociceptive pain as it is the abnormal processing of painful stimuli.

It includes phantom limb pain, pain below the level of a spinal cord injury, and diabetic neuropathy.

Neuropathic pain is usually intense, shooting, burning, or described as "pins and needles."

This pain typically responds to adjuvant medications (antidepressants, antispasmodic agents, skeletal muscle relaxants).

4.2 Focused pain assessment

Location

USE ANATOMICAL TERMINOLOGY AND LANDMARKS TO DESCRIBE LOCATION.

Ask: *"Where is your pain?"*

Ask: *"Does it radiate anywhere else?"*

Ask clients to point to the location.

Quality

QUALITY REFERS TO HOW THE PAIN FEELS: sharp, dull, aching, burning, stabbing, pounding, throbbing, shooting, gnawing, tender, heavy, tight, tiring, exhausting, sickening, terrifying, torturing, nagging, annoying, intense, or unbearable.

Ask: *"What does the pain feel like?"* Give more than two choices (*"Is the pain throbbing, burning, or stabbing?"*).

Measures

INTENSITY, STRENGTH, AND SEVERITY ARE "MEASURES" OF THE PAIN. Use visual analog scales (description scale, number rating scale) to measure pain, monitor pain, and evaluate the effectiveness of interventions.

Ask: *"How much pain do you have now?"*

Ask: *"What is the worst/best the pain has been?"*

Ask: *"Rate your pain on a scale of 0 to 10."*

Timing

ONSET, DURATION, FREQUENCY.

Ask: *"When did it start?"*

Ask: *"How long does it last?"*

Ask: *"How often does it occur?"*

Ask: *"Is it constant or intermittent?"*

Setting

HOW THE PAIN AFFECTS DAILY LIFE OR HOW ACTIVITIES OF DAILY LIVING (ADLS) AFFECT THE PAIN.

Ask: *"Where are you when the symptoms occur?"*

Ask: *"What are you doing when the symptoms occur?"*

Ask: *"How does the pain affect your sleep?"*

Ask: *"How does the pain affect your ability to work and do your job?"*

Associated manifestations

DOCUMENT ASSOCIATED MANIFESTATIONS: fatigue, depression, nausea, anxiety.

Ask: *"What other symptoms do you have when you are feeling pain?"*

Aggravating/relieving factors

Ask: *"What makes the pain better?"*

Ask: *"What makes the pain worse?"*

Ask: *"Are you currently taking any prescription, herbal, or over-the-counter medications?"*

RISK FACTORS

Risk factors for undertreatment of pain
- Cultural and societal attitudes
- Lack of knowledge
- Fear of addiction
- Exaggerated fear of respiratory depression

Populations at risk for undertreatment of pain
- Infants
- Children
- Older adults
- Clients who have substance use disorder

Causes of acute and chronic pain
- Trauma
- Surgery
- Cancer (tumor invasion, nerve compression, bone metastases, associated infections, immobility)
- Arthritis
- Fibromyalgia
- Neuropathy
- Diagnostic or treatment procedures (injection, intubation, radiation)

Factors that affect the pain experience
- Age
  - Infants cannot verbalize or understand their pain.
  - Older adult clients can have multiple pathologies that cause pain and limit function. Ⓒ
- Fatigue can increase sensitivity to pain.
- Genetic sensitivity can increase or decrease pain tolerance.
- Cognitive function: Clients who are cognitively impaired might not be able to report pain or report it accurately.
- Prior experiences can increase or decrease sensitivity depending on whether clients obtained adequate relief.
- Anxiety and fear can increase sensitivity to pain.
- Support systems can decrease sensitivity to pain.
- Culture can influence how clients express pain or the meaning they give to pain.

EXPECTED FINDINGS

- Behaviors complement self-report and assist in pain assessment of nonverbal clients.
  - Facial expressions (grimacing, wrinkled forehead), body movements (restlessness, pacing, guarding)
  - Moaning, crying
  - Decreased attention span
- Blood pressure, pulse, and respiratory rate can temporarily increase with acute pain. Eventually, increases in vital signs will stabilize despite the persistence of pain. Therefore, physiologic indicators might not be an accurate measure of pain over time.

PATIENT-CENTERED CARE

NONPHARMACOLOGICAL PAIN MANAGEMENT

- Cutaneous (skin) stimulation: transcutaneous electrical nerve stimulation (TENS), heat, cold, therapeutic massage Qᴾᶜᶜ
  - Interruption of pain pathways
  - Cold for inflammation
  - Heat to increase blood flow and to reduce stiffness
- Distraction: includes ambulation, deep breathing, visitors, television, and music
- Relaxation: includes meditation, yoga, and progressive muscle relaxation
- Imagery
  - Focusing on a pleasant thought to divert focus
  - Requires an ability to concentrate
- Acupuncture: vibration or electrical stimulation via tiny needles inserted into the skin and subcutaneous tissues at specific points
- Reduction of pain stimuli in the environment
- Elevation of edematous extremities to promote venous return and decrease swelling

PHARMACOLOGICAL INTERVENTIONS

Analgesics are the mainstay for relieving pain. The three classes of analgesics are nonopioids, opioids, and adjuvants.

Nonopioid analgesics

Nonopioid analgesics (acetaminophen, nonsteroidal anti-inflammatory drugs [NSAIDs], including salicylates) are appropriate for treating mild to moderate pain. Nonopioid analgesics also have antipyretic and anti-inflammatory properties.

- Be aware of the hepatotoxic effects of acetaminophen. Clients who have a healthy liver should take no more than 4 g/day. Make sure clients are aware of opioids that contain acetaminophen, such as hydrocodone bitartrate 5 mg/acetaminophen 500 mg. Qˢ
- Monitor for salicylism (tinnitus, vertigo, decreased hearing acuity).
- Prevent gastric upset by administering NSAIDs with food or antacids.
- Monitor for bleeding with long-term NSAID use. NSAIDs can increase the effects of warfarin.

Opioid analgesics

Opioid analgesics, such as morphine, fentanyl, and oxycodone, are appropriate for treating moderate to severe pain. The term "narcotic" is not synonymous with opioid analgesics. Narcotics can also refer to illegal substances such as cocaine.

- Managing acute severe pain with short-term (24 to 48 hr) around-the-clock administration of opioids is preferable to following a PRN schedule.
- The parenteral route is best for immediate, short-term relief of acute pain. The oral route is better for chronic, nonfluctuating pain. Opioids are available in transdermal, transmucosal, and buccal routes.
- Consistent timing and dosing of opioid administration provide consistent pain control.
- It is essential to monitor and intervene for adverse effects of opioid use.
  - Constipation: Use a preventative approach (monitoring of bowel movements, fluids, fiber intake, exercise, stool softeners, stimulant laxatives, enemas).
  - Orthostatic hypotension: Advise clients to sit or lie down if lightheadedness or dizziness occur. Instruct clients to avoid sudden changes in position by slowly moving from a lying to a sitting or standing position. Provide assistance with ambulation.
  - Urinary retention: Monitor I&O, assess for distention, administer bethanechol, and catheterize.
  - Nausea/vomiting: Administer antiemetics, advise clients to lie still and move slowly, and eliminate odors.
  - Sedation: Monitor level of consciousness, and take safety precautions. Sedation usually precedes respiratory depression. Qˢ
  - Respiratory depression: Monitor respiratory rate prior to and following administration of opioids. Initial treatment of respiratory depression and sedation is generally a reduction in opioid dose. If necessary, administer naloxone to reverse opioid effects.

Adjuvant analgesics

Adjuvant analgesics enhance the effects of nonopioids, help alleviate other manifestations that aggravate pain (depression, seizures, inflammation), and are useful for treating neuropathic pain.

- Adjuvant medications include the following.
  - Anticonvulsants: carbamazepine
  - Antianxiety agents: diazepam
  - Tricyclic antidepressants: amitriptyline
  - Antihistamine: hydroxyzine
  - Glucocorticoids: dexamethasone
  - Antiemetics: ondansetron

Patient-controlled analgesia (PCA)

PCA is a medication delivery system that allows clients to self-administer safe doses of opioids.

- Small, frequent dosing ensures consistent plasma levels.
- Clients have less lag time between identified need and delivery of medication, which increases their sense of control and can decrease the amount of medication they need.
- Morphine and hydromorphone are typical opioids for PCA delivery.
- Clients should let the nurse know if using the pump does not control the pain.
- To prevent inadvertent overdosing, the client is the only person who should push the PCA button.

Other strategies

- Other strategies for effective pain management include the following.
    - Taking a proactive approach by giving analgesics before pain becomes too severe. It takes less medication to prevent pain than to treat pain.
    - Instructing clients to report developing or recurrent pain and not wait until pain is severe (for PRN pain medication).
    - Explaining misconceptions about pain. Qpcc
    - Helping clients reduce fear and anxiety.
    - Creating a treatment plan that includes both nonpharmacological and pharmacological pain-relief measures.
- Strategies specific for relieving chronic pain include the above interventions, plus:
    - Administering long-acting or controlled-release opioid analgesics (including the transdermal route).
    - Administering analgesics around the clock rather than PRN.

COMPLICATIONS

- Undertreatment of pain is a serious complication and can lead to increased anxiety with acute pain and depression with chronic pain. Assess clients for pain frequently, and intervene as appropriate.
- Sedation, respiratory depression, and coma can occur as a result of overdosing. Sedation always precedes respiratory depression. Qs
    - Identify high-risk clients (older adult clients). Ⓖ
    - Carefully titrate doses while closely monitoring respiratory status.
    - Stop the opioid and give the antagonist naloxone if respiratory rate is below 8/min and shallow, or the client is difficult to arouse.
    - The nurse should closely monitor the client following administration of naloxone. The duration of the certain opioids can last longer than the effectiveness of the naloxone creating a need for additional doses.
    - Identify the cause of sedation.
    - Use a sedation scale in addition to a pain rating scale to assess pain, especially when administering opioids.

Application Exercises

1. A nurse is assessing the pain level of a client who came to the emergency department reporting severe abdominal pain. The nurse asks the client whether he has nausea and has been vomiting. The nurse is assessing which of the following components of a pain assessment?

    A. Presence of associated manifestations

    B. Location of the pain

    C. Pain quality

    D. Aggravating and relieving factors

2. A nurse is assessing a client who is reporting pain despite analgesia. Which of the following actions should the nurse take to assess the intensity of the client's pain?

    A. Ask the client what precipitates his pain.

    B. Question the client about the location of his pain.

    C. Offer the client a pain scale to measure his pain.

    D. Use open-ended questions to identify the sensation of his pain.

3. A nurse is caring for a client who is receiving morphine via a patient-controlled analgesia (PCA) infusion device after abdominal surgery. Which of the following client statements indicates that the client understands how to use the device?

    A. "I'll wait to use the device until it's absolutely necessary."

    B. "I'll be careful about pushing the button so I don't get an overdose."

    C. "I should tell the nurse if the pain doesn't stop after I use this device."

    D. "I will ask my son to push the dose button when I am sleeping."

4. A nurse is discussing pain assessment with a newly licensed nurse. Which of the following information should the nurse include?

    A. Most clients exaggerate their level of pain.

    B. Pain must have an identifiable source to justify the use of opioids.

    C. Objective data are essential in assessing pain.

    D. Pain is whatever the client says it is.

5. A nurse is monitoring a client who is receiving opioid analgesia. Which of the following findings should the nurse identify as adverse effects of opioid analgesics? (Select all that apply.)

    A. Urinary incontinence

    B. Diarrhea

    C. Bradypnea

    D. Orthostatic hypotension

    E. Nausea

PRACTICE Active Learning Scenario

A nurse on a medical-surgical unit is reviewing with a group of newly licensed nurses the various types of pain the clients on the unit have. Use the ATI Active Learning Template: Basic Concept to complete this item.

UNDERLYING PRINCIPLES: List the four different types of pain, their definitions, and characteristics.

Application Exercises Key

1. A. **CORRECT:** Nausea and vomiting are common manifestations clients have when they are in pain.

   B. The location of the pain is where the client feels the pain.

   C. Pain quality is what the pain feels like, such as throbbing and dull.

   D. Aggravating and relieving factors are what might make the pain better or worse.

   Ⓝ *NCLEX® Connection: Pharmacological and Parenteral Therapies, Pharmacological Pain Management*

2. A. Assessment of pain triggers will provide valuable information to help select pain-control interventions, but it does not provide information about the intensity of pain.

   B. Identification of the location of the client's pain provides valuable information to help select pain-control interventions, but it does not provide information about the intensity of pain.

   C. **CORRECT:** The nurse should use a pain scale to help the client measure the amount of pain he has and its intensity.

   D. Asking open-ended questions is important in pain assessment, but it does not provide for quantification of pain intensity.

   Ⓝ *NCLEX® Connection: Pharmacological and Parenteral Therapies, Pharmacological Pain Management*

3. A. The client may use the device when he begins to feel pain. It will help prevent unnecessary worsening of the pain and more doses of analgesia to provide relief.

   B. A feature of PCA devices is the timing control or lockout mechanism, which enforces a preset minimum interval between medication doses. This safety feature is one means of preventing an overdose because the client cannot self-administer another dose of medication until that time interval has passed.

   C. **CORRECT:** The nurse should identify that PCA is a method of delivering pain medication through an electronic infusion device that allows the client to self-administer pain medication on an as-needed basis. If the client is not achieving adequate pain control, he should let the nurse know so that she can initiate a reevaluation of the client's pain management plan.

   D. The client is the only one who should operate the PCA pump. In situations where the client is not able to do so, the provider may authorize a nurse or a family member to operate the pump.

   Ⓝ *NCLEX® Connection: Pharmacological and Parenteral Therapies, Pharmacological Pain Management*

4. A. A misconception about pain is that clients exaggerate their pain level.

   B. Clients can have pain without being able to identify the source.

   C. Objective data are not always present when clients have pain.

   D. **CORRECT:** The nurse should identify that pain is a subjective experience, and the client is the best source of information about it.

   Ⓝ *NCLEX® Connection: Pharmacological and Parenteral Therapies, Pharmacological Pain Management*

5. A. Urinary retention, not urinary incontinence, is a common adverse effect of opioid analgesia.

   B. Constipation, not diarrhea, is a common adverse effect of opioid analgesia.

   C. **CORRECT:** Respiratory depression, which causes respiratory rates to drop to dangerously low levels, is a common adverse effect of opioid analgesia.

   D. **CORRECT:** Dizziness or lightheadedness when changing positions is a common adverse effect of opioid analgesia.

   E. **CORRECT:** Nausea and vomiting are common adverse effects of opioid analgesia.

   Ⓝ *NCLEX® Connection: Pharmacological and Parenteral Therapies, Expected Actions/Outcomes*

PRACTICE Answer

Using the ATI Active Learning Template: Basic Concept

UNDERLYING PRINCIPLES

Acute pain
- Definition: Protective, temporary, usually self-limiting, resolves with tissue healing
- Physiological responses: Tachycardia, hypertension, anxiety, diaphoresis, muscle tension
- Behavioral responses: Grimacing, moaning, flinching, guarding

Chronic Pain
- Definition: Not protective; ongoing or recurs frequently, lasts longer than 3 months, persists beyond tissue healing, can be chronic cancer pain or chronic noncancer pain.
- Physiological responses: No change in vital signs, depression, fatigue, decreased level of functioning, disability

Nociceptive pain
- Definition: Arises from damage to or inflammation of tissue other than that of the peripheral and central nervous systems, is usually throbbing, aching, localized; pain typically responds to opioids and nonopioid medications
- Types of nociceptive pain
  - Somatic: In bones, joints, muscles, skin, or connective tissues
  - Visceral: In internal organs such as the stomach or intestines, can cause referred pain

Neuropathic pain
- Definition: Arises from abnormal or damaged pain nerves (phantom limb pain, pain below the level of a spinal cord injury, diabetic neuropathy), usually intense, shooting, burning, or "pins and needles"
- Physiological responses to adjuvant medications (antidepressants, antispasmodic agents, skeletal muscle relaxants)

Ⓝ *NCLEX® Connection: Pharmacological and Parenteral Therapies, Pharmacological Pain Management*

UNIT 2 **NURSING CARE OF CLIENTS WHO HAVE NEUROSENSORY DISORDERS**
SECTION: CENTRAL NERVOUS SYSTEM DISORDERS

CHAPTER 5 *Meningitis*

Meningitis is an inflammation of the meninges, which are the membranes that protect the brain and spinal cord.

Viral, or aseptic, meningitis is the most common form of meningitis and commonly resolves without treatment. Fungal meningitis is common in clients who have AIDS. Bacterial (or septic) meningitis is a contagious infection with a high mortality rate. The prognosis depends on how quickly care is initiated.

There are three vaccines for different pathogens that cause bacterial meningitis. One is available for high-risk populations, such as residential college students.

HEALTH PROMOTION AND DISEASE PREVENTION

Haemophilus influenzae type b (Hib) vaccine
Ensure infants receive vaccine for bacterial meningitis on schedule. A series of four doses is recommended beginning at 2 months of age, with the final dose at 12 to 15 months.

Pneumococcal polysaccharide vaccine (PPSV)
Though primarily intended to prevent respiratory infection, this immunization also decreases the risk for CNS infections. Vaccinate adults who are immunocompromised, have a chronic disease, smoke cigarettes, or live in a long-term care facility. Follow CDC guidelines for reimmunization. Give one dose to adults older than 65 who have not previously been immunized nor have history of disease.

Meningococcal vaccine (MCV4) (Neisseria meningitidis)
Ensure that adolescents receive the vaccine on schedule and prior to living in a residential setting in college. Individuals in other communal living conditions (e.g., military) also should be immunized. An initial dose is recommended for healthy children between the ages of 11 to 12, with a booster administered at age 16.

ASSESSMENT

RISK FACTORS

Viral meningitis
- Viral illnesses such as the mumps, measles, herpes, and arboviruses (West Nile).
- There is no vaccine against viral meningitis.

Fungal meningitis: Fulminant fungal-based infection of the sinuses are from the organism *Cryptococcus neoformans*.

Bacterial meningitis: Bacterial-based infections, such as otitis media, pneumonia, or sinusitis, in which the infectious micro-organism is *Neisseria meningitidis*, *Streptococcus pneumoniae*, or *Haemophilus influenzae*

Immunosuppression

Direct contamination of spinal fluid

Invasive procedures, skull fracture, or penetrating wound.

Environment: Overcrowded living conditions.

EXPECTED FINDINGS

SUBJECTIVE DATA
- Excruciating, constant headache
- Nuchal rigidity (stiff neck)
- Photophobia (sensitivity to light)

OBJECTIVE DATA: Physical Assessment Findings
- Fever and chills
- Nausea and vomiting
- Altered level of consciousness (confusion, disorientation, lethargy, difficulty arousing, coma)
- Positive Kernig's sign (resistance and pain with extension of the client's leg from a flexed position)
- Positive Brudzinski's sign (flexion of the knees and hips occurring with deliberate flexion of the client's neck)
- Hyperactive deep tendon reflexes
- Tachycardia
- Seizures
- Red macular rash (meningococcal meningitis)
- Restlessness, irritability

LABORATORY TESTS

- **Urine, throat, nose, and blood culture and sensitivity**: Perform culture and sensitivity of various body fluids to identify possible infectious bacteria and an appropriate broad-spectrum antibiotic. Not definitive for meningitis but can guide initial selection of antimicrobial.
- **CBC**: Elevated WBC count

DIAGNOSTIC PROCEDURES

Cerebrospinal fluid (CSF) analysis

- CSF analysis is the most definitive diagnostic procedure. CSF is collected during a lumbar puncture performed by the provider.
- Results indicative of meningitis
  - Appearance of CSF: cloudy (bacterial) or clear (viral)
  - Elevated WBC
  - Elevated protein
  - Decreased glucose (bacterial)
  - Elevated CSF pressure
- Counterimmunoelectrophoresis (CIE) can be done on CSF to determine whether the infectious agent is viral or protozoa. This diagnostic study is also indicated if the client received antibiotics before CSF was collected.

CT scan and MRI: A CT scan or an MRI can be performed to identify increased intracranial pressure (ICP) and/or an abscess.

PATIENT-CENTERED CARE

NURSING CARE

- Isolate the client as soon as meningitis is suspected.
- Maintain isolation precautions per hospital policy.
  - The nurse should initiate droplet precautions, which require a private room. Continue droplet precautions until antibiotics have been administered for 24 hr and oral and nasal secretions are no longer infectious. Clients who have bacterial meningitis might need to remain on droplet precautions continuously. Qs
  - Standard precautions are implemented for all clients who have meningitis.
- Implement fever-reduction measures, such as a cooling blanket, if necessary.
- Report meningococcal infections to the public health department.
- Decrease environmental stimuli.
- Provide a quiet environment.
- Minimize exposure to bright light (natural and electric).
- Maintain bed rest with the head of the bed elevated to 30°.
- Monitor for increased ICP.
- Tell the client to avoid coughing and sneezing, which increase ICP.
- Maintain client safety, such as seizure precautions. Qs
- Replace fluid and electrolytes as indicated by laboratory values.
- Older adult clients are at an increased risk for secondary complications, such as pneumonia. ©

MEDICATIONS

- **Ceftriaxone or cefotaxime in combination with vancomycin**: Antibiotics given until culture and sensitivity results are available. Effective for bacterial infections.
- **Phenytoin**: Anticonvulsants given if ICP increases or client experiences a seizure.
- **Acetaminophen, ibuprofen**: Analgesics for headache and/or fever. Nonopioid to avoid masking changes in the level of consciousness.
- **Ciprofloxacin, rifampin, or ceftriaxone**: Prophylactic antibiotics given to individuals in close contact with the client.

COMPLICATIONS

Increased ICP

Meningitis can cause ICP to increase, possibly to the point of brain herniation.

NURSING ACTIONS

- Monitor for indications of increasing ICP (decreased level of consciousness, pupillary changes, impaired extraocular movements).
- Provide interventions to reduce ICP (positioning with head of the bed elevation at 30° and avoidance of coughing and straining). Qs
- Mannitol can be administered via IV.

SIADH

SIADH can be a complication of meningitis due to abnormal stimulation to the hypothalamic area of the brain, causing excess secretion of antidiuretic hormone (vasopressin).

NURSING ACTIONS

- Monitor for manifestations (dilute blood, concentrated urine).
- Provide interventions, such as the administration of demeclocycline and restriction of fluid.
- Monitor the client's weight daily.

Septic emboli

- Septic emboli can form during meningitis and travel to other parts of the body, particularly the hands, but can occur in the feet as well.
- Development of gangrene can necessitate an amputation.
- Septic emboli can lead to disseminated intravascular coagulation or stroke.

NURSING ACTIONS

- Monitor circulatory status of extremities and coagulation studies.
- Report any alterations immediately to the provider.

Application Exercises

1. A nurse is assessing a client who reports severe headache and a stiff neck. The nurse's assessment reveals positive Kernig's and Brudzinski's signs. Which of the following actions should the nurse perform first?

   A. Administer antibiotics.

   B. Implement droplet precautions.

   C. Initiate IV access.

   D. Decrease bright lights.

2. A nurse is assessing for the presence of Brudzinski's sign in a client who has suspected meningitis. Which of the following actions should the nurse take when performing this technique? (Select all that apply.)

   A. Place client in supine position.

   B. Flex client's hip and knee.

   C. Place hands behind the client's neck.

   D. Bend client's head toward chest.

   E. Straighten the client's flexed leg at the knee.

3. A nurse is planning care for a client who has meningitis and is at risk for increased intracranial pressure (ICP). Which of the following actions should the nurse plan to take? (Select all that apply.)

   A. Implement seizure precautions.

   B. Perform neurological checks four times a day.

   C. Administer morphine for the report of neck and generalized pain.

   D. Turn off room lights and television.

   E. Monitor for impaired extraocular movements.

   F. Encourage the client to cough frequently.

4. A nurse is reviewing the use of the meningococcal vaccine (MCV4) for the prevention of meningitis with a newly licensed nurse. Which of the following information should the nurse include?

   A. The vaccine is indicated to reduce the risk of respiratory infection.

   B. The vaccine is administered in a series of four doses.

   C. The vaccine is recommended for adolescents before starting college.

   D. The vaccine is initially given at 2 months of age.

5. A nurse is planning care for a client who has bacterial meningitis. Which of the following actions should the nurse include in the plan of care? (Select all that apply.)

   A. Monitor for bradycardia.

   B. Provide an emesis basin at the bedside.

   C. Administer antipyretic medication.

   D. Perform a skin assessment.

   E. Keep the head of the bed flat.

PRACTICE Active Learning Scenario

A nurse is reviewing the plan of care for a client who has bacterial meningitis. Use the ATI Active Learning Template: System Disorder to complete this item.

ALTERATION IN HEALTH (DIAGNOSIS): Define bacterial meningitis.

MEDICATIONS: Identify three medications, their actions, and the reason for administration.

COMPLICATIONS: Describe two complications of meningitis.

Application Exercises Key

1. A. The nurse should administer antibiotics to stop the micro-organisms from multiplying, but this is not the priority action.

    B. **CORRECT:** When using the urgent vs. nonurgent approach to care, the nurse determines the priority action is to initiate droplet precautions when meningitis is suspected to prevent spread of the disease to others.

    C. The nurse should initiate IV access to allow IV medication and fluid administration, but this is not the priority action.

    D. The nurse should decrease bright lights because of the client's sensitivity to light, but this is not the priority action.

    (N) *NCLEX® Connection: Safety and Infection Control, Standard Precautions/Transmission-Based Precautions/Surgical Asepsis*

2. A. **CORRECT:** The nurse should place the client in supine position when assessing for Brudzinski's sign.

    B. The nurse should flex the client's hip and knee when assessing for Kernig's sign.

    C. **CORRECT:** The nurse should place her hands behind the client's neck when assessing for Brudzinski's sign, in order to flex the client's neck.

    D. **CORRECT:** The nurse should bend the client's head toward the chest when assessing for Brudzinski's sign.

    E. The nurse should straighten the client's flexed leg at the knee when assessing for Kernig's sign.

    (N) *NCLEX® Connection: Reduction of Risk Potential, Diagnostic Tests*

3. A. **CORRECT:** The client is at risk for seizures due to possible increased ICP. Therefore, the nurse should implement seizure precautions to reduce the client's risk for injury.

    B. The nurse should perform neurological checks at least every 2 hr for a client who is at risk for increased ICP.

    C. The nurse should avoid administering opioids to a client who is at risk for increased ICP. Opioids can mask changes in the client's level of consciousness.

    D. **CORRECT:** The nurse should turn off room lights and the television because they can increase neuron stimulation and cause a seizure when a client is at risk for increased ICP.

    E. **CORRECT:** The nurse should monitor for impaired extraocular movements because this finding can indicate increased ICP.

    F. The nurse should instruct the client to avoid coughing because this action can cause increased ICP.

    (N) *NCLEX® Connection: Physiological Adaptation, Alterations in Body Systems*

4. A. The pneumococcal vaccine is primarily indicated to reduce the risk of respiratory infection. However, it also reduces the risk of CNS infection.

    B. The HIB vaccine is administered to infants in a series of four doses.

    C. **CORRECT:** The nurse should identify that the meningococcal vaccine is recommended for adolescents prior to starting college due to the increased risk for infection in communal living facilities.

    D. The initial dose of the HIB vaccine is recommended for infants at 2 months of age.

    (N) *NCLEX® Connection: Safety and Infection Control, Standard Precautions/Transmission-Based Precautions/Surgical Asepsis*

5. A. The nurse should plan to monitor for tachycardia when a client has meningitis.

    B. **CORRECT:** The nurse should provide an emesis basin at the bedside because the client who has meningitis can have nausea and vomiting.

    C. **CORRECT:** The nurse should plan to administer antipyretic medication for fever to a client who has meningitis.

    D. **CORRECT:** The nurse should perform a skin assessment to determine whether the client has a red macular rash associated with meningococcal meningitis.

    E. The nurse should elevate the head of the client's bed 30° to promote venous drainage from the head and prevent increased ICP.

    (N) *NCLEX® Connection: Physiological Adaptation, Illness Management*

PRACTICE Answer

Using the ATI Active Learning Template: System Disorder

ALTERATION IN HEALTH (DIAGNOSIS): Bacterial meningitis is a bacterial infection that causes an inflammation of the meninges, the membranes that protect the brain and spinal cord.

MEDICATIONS
- Ceftriaxone with vancocin: antibiotics administered to treat the infection.
- Acetaminophen: an antipyretic used to treat a fever.
- Phenytoin: an anticonvulsant given to prevent the client from experiencing a seizure when at risk of ICP.

COMPLICATIONS
- Increased ICP, which can lead to seizures, coma, and death.
- Syndrome of inappropriate antidiuretic hormone (SIADH), which is due to pressure from inflammation abnormally stimulating the hypothalamus, causing increased secretion of antidiuretic hormone (vasopressin).
- Septic emboli can occur as a result of meningitis. This complication can lead to disseminated intravascular coagulation, stroke, or gangrene.

(N) *NCLEX® Connection: Physiological Adaptation, Illness Management*

CHAPTER 6   # Seizures and Epilepsy

Seizures are abrupt, abnormal, excessive, and uncontrolled electrical discharge of neurons within the brain that can cause alterations in the level of consciousness and/or changes in motor and sensory ability and/or behavior.

Epilepsy is the term used to define chronic recurring abnormal brain electrical activity resulting in two or more seizures. Seizures resulting from identifiable causes, such as substance withdrawal or fever, are not considered epilepsy.

The International Classification of Epileptic Seizures uses three broad categories to describe seizures: generalized, partial, and unclassified.

ASSESSMENT

RISK FACTORS

- **Genetic predisposition:** Absence seizures are more common in children and tend to occur in families.
- **Acute febrile state:** Particularly among infants and children younger than 2 years old.
- **Head trauma:** Can be early or late onset (up to 9 months), and incidence is increased when the head trauma includes a skull fracture.
- **Cerebral edema:** Especially when it occurs acutely and seizure activity tends to disappear when the edema is successfully treated.
- **Abrupt cessation of antiepileptic drugs (AEDs)**: As a rebound activity.
- **Infection:** If intracranial, a result of increased intracranial pressure; if systemic, a result of the persistent febrile state.
- **Metabolic disorder:** A result of insufficient or excessive chemicals within the brain, such as occurring with hypoglycemia or hyponatremia.
- **Exposure to toxins:** Especially those associated with pesticides, carbon monoxide, and lead poisoning.

- **Stroke:** Most likely to occur within the first 24 hr following a stroke as a result of increased intracranial pressure.
- **Heart disease:** Common cause of new-onset seizures in older adults.
- **Brain tumor:** If benign, seizures caused by the increased bulk associated with the tumor; if malignant, associated with the ability of the brain tissue to function.
- **Hypoxia:** Results in a decreased oxygen level of the brain; necessary for neuronal activity.
- **Acute substance withdrawal:** Dehydration accompanies withdrawal, creating a toxic level of the substance in the body.
- **Fluid and electrolyte imbalances:** Results in abnormal levels of nutrients required for neuronal function.
- With older adult clients, increased seizure incidence is associated with cerebrovascular diseases. ©

TRIGGERING FACTORS
- Increased physical activity
- Excessive stress
- Hyperventilation
- Overwhelming fatigue
- Acute alcohol ingestion
- Excessive caffeine intake
- Exposure to flashing lights
- Substances such as cocaine, aerosols, and inhaled glue products

EXPECTED FINDINGS

Generalized seizures
Generalized seizure involves both cerebral hemispheres. Generalized seizures can begin with an aura (alteration in vision, smell, hearing, or emotional feeling).
Clients can experience five types of generalized seizures.
- **Tonic-clonic seizure**
  - A tonic-clonic seizure begins for only a few seconds with a tonic episode (stiffening of muscles) and loss of consciousness.
  - A 1- to 2-min clonic episode (rhythmic jerking of the extremities) follows the tonic episode.
  - Breathing can stop during the tonic phase and become irregular during the clonic phase.
  - Cyanosis can accompany breathing irregularities.
  - Biting of the cheek or tongue can occur during clonic phase.
  - Incontinence can also accompany a tonic-clonic seizure.
  - During the postictal phase, a period of confusion and sleepiness follows the seizure.
- **Tonic seizure**
  - Only the tonic phase is experienced.
  - Clients suddenly lose consciousness and experience sudden increased muscle tone, loss of consciousness, and autonomic manifestations (e.g., arrhythmia, apnea, vomiting, incontinence, salivation).
  - The seizure usually lasts 30 seconds to several minutes.

- **Clonic seizure**
  - Only the clonic phase is experienced.
  - The seizure lasts several minutes.
  - During this type of seizure, the muscles contract and relax.
- **Myoclonic seizure**
  - Myoclonic seizures consist of brief jerking or stiffening of the extremities, which can be symmetrical or asymmetrical.
  - This type of seizure lasts for seconds.
- **Atonic or akinetic seizure**
  - Atonic or akinetic seizures are characterized by a few seconds in which muscle tone is lost.
  - The seizure is followed by a period of confusion.
  - The loss of muscle tone frequently results in falling.

Partial or focal/local seizure

Partial or focal/local seizure involves only one cerebral hemisphere.

Clients can experience two types of partial seizures.

- **Complex partial seizure**
  - Complex partial seizures have associated automatisms (behaviors that the client is unaware of, such as lip smacking or picking at clothes).
  - The seizure can cause a loss of consciousness or blackout for several minutes.
  - Amnesia can occur immediately prior to and after the seizure.
- **Simple partial seizure**
  - Consciousness is maintained throughout simple partial seizures.
  - Seizure activity can consist of unusual sensations, a sense of déjà vu, autonomic abnormalities such as changes in heart rate and abnormal flushing, unilateral abnormal extremity movements, pain, or offensive smell.

Unclassified or idiopathic seizures

Unclassified or idiopathic seizures do not fit into other categories. These types of seizures account for half of all seizure activity and occur for no known reason.

LABORATORY TESTS

Tests should include alcohol and illicit substance levels, HIV testing, and, if suspected, screen for the presence of excessive toxins.

DIAGNOSTIC PROCEDURES

- Electroencephalogram (EEG) records electrical activity and can identify the origin of seizure activity.
- Magnetic resonance imaging (MRI), computed tomography (CT) imaging/computed axial tomography (CAT) scan, positron emission tomography (PET) scan, cerebrospinal fluid (CSF) analysis, and skull x-ray can be used to identify or rule out potential causes of seizures.

PATIENT-CENTERED CARE

NURSING CARE

During a seizure
- Protect the client's privacy and the client from injury (move furniture away, hold head in lap if on the floor). Qs
- Position the client to provide a patent airway.
- Be prepared to suction oral secretions.
- Turn the client to the side to decrease the risk of aspiration.
- Loosen restrictive clothing.
- Do not attempt to restrain the client.
- Do not attempt to open the jaw or insert airway during seizure activity (can damage teeth, lips, and tongue).
- Do not use padded tongue blades.
- Document onset and duration of seizure and findings (level of consciousness, apnea, cyanosis, motor activity, incontinence) prior to, during, and following the seizure.

After a seizure
- This is the postictal phase of the seizure episode.
- Maintain the client in a side-lying position to prevent aspiration and to facilitate drainage of oral secretions.
- Check vital signs.
- Assess for injuries.
- Perform neurological checks.
- Allow the client to rest if necessary.
- Reorient and calm the client, who might be agitated or confused.
- Determine if client experienced an aura, which can indicate the origin of seizure in the brain.
- Try to determine possible trigger (e.g., fatigue).

MEDICATIONS

Administer prescribed antiepileptic drugs (AEDs), such as phenytoin.

NURSING CONSIDERATIONS
- Initial goal is to control seizure activity using one medication. If the chosen medication is not effective, either the dose is increased, or another medication is added or substituted.
- Therapeutic levels are determined by blood tests. These are performed on a routine schedule to ensure compliance and effectiveness of the medication. Qebp
- The client should take medications at the same time every day to enhance effectiveness.
- Allergic reactions to these medications are rare, yet can occur immediately or late in therapy. If the client is allergic, another medication may be substituted.
- Be aware of adverse effects and interactions with food or other medications. These are specific to the medication.
- Some antiepileptic medications cause oral gum overgrowth. Routine oral hygiene and dental visits can minimize this adverse effect.
- When using phenytoin, specific instructions should include avoidance of oral contraceptives, as this medication decreases their effectiveness. Warfarin should also not be given with this medication, as phenytoin can decrease absorption and increase metabolism of oral anticoagulants.

INTERPROFESSIONAL CARE

- Initiate a social services referral to aid in obtaining medications if cost will affect the client's ability to adhere to the medication routine.
- If employment is affected by seizure activity, refer to social agencies for financial support and vocational evaluation.
- If seizure activity affects a school-age child's performance in the classroom, this condition should be reported to the disability office, which can develop specialized interventions or facilitate an Individualized Education Program (IEP).
- Discrimination on the basis of epilepsy is illegal in all states.

THERAPEUTIC PROCEDURES

Vagal nerve stimulation and conventional surgical procedures can be helpful for clients whose seizures are not controlled with medication therapy.

Vagal nerve stimulator

- Vagal nerve stimulation is indicated for treatment of partial seizures.
- The vagal nerve stimulator is a device implanted into the left chest wall and connected to an electrode placed on the left vagus nerve.
- This procedure is performed under general anesthesia.
- The device is then programmed to administer intermittent stimulation of the brain via stimulation of the vagal nerve, at a rate specific to the client's needs.

CLIENT EDUCATION

- In addition to routine stimulation, the client may initiate vagal nerve stimulation by holding a magnet over the implantable device, at the onset of seizure activity. This either aborts the seizure, or lessens its severity.
- Avoid diagnostic procedures, such as MRI, ultrasound diathermy, and the use of microwave ovens and shortwave radios.

Conventional surgical procedures

- Conventional surgical procedures are available for clients who experience partial or generalized seizures.
- Prior to surgery, AEDs are discontinued and the specific area of the seizure activity is identified through the use of EEG monitoring. Surgically implanted electrodes can also be used.
- The affected area of the brain can be excised if it is determined that vital brain function will not be affected.
  - An intracarotid amobarbital (Wada) test can help determine if language or memory would be affected.
  - Neuropsychological testing can help determine if visuospatial function, memory, language, or cognitive function would be affected.
- Partial corpus callosotomy can be used for clients who are not candidates for conventional surgical procedures. The procedure resects the corpus callosum, preventing neuronal discharges across hemispheres and reduces the severity and frequency of seizures.
- These procedures have associated morbidities, including infection, loss of cerebral function, and a lack of success in preventing seizures. Qs

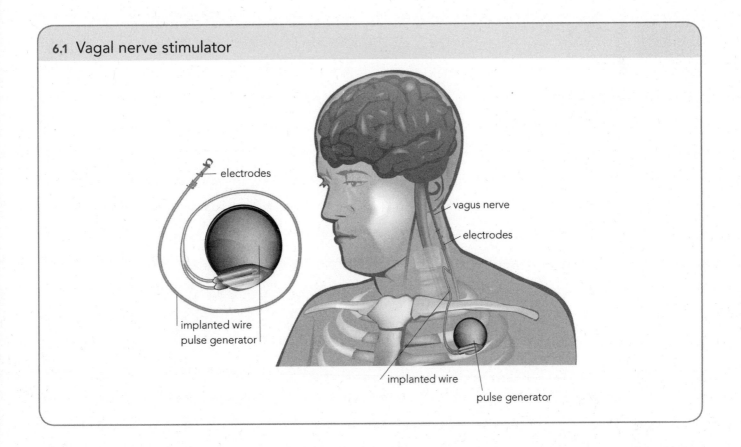

6.1 Vagal nerve stimulator

electrodes

implanted wire
pulse generator

vagus nerve

electrodes

implanted wire

pulse generator

NURSING ACTIONS

- Provide client education regarding seizure management.
  - Importance of monitoring AED levels and maintaining therapeutic medication levels
  - Possible medication interactions (decreased effectiveness of oral contraceptives)
- Encourage the client to wear a medical identification tag at all times.
- Instruct clients who have a history of seizures to research state driving laws. Some states restrict or limit driving for individuals who have a recent history of seizures. Qs

COMPLICATIONS

Status epilepticus

This is repeated seizure activity within a 30 min timeframe or a single prolonged seizure lasting more than 5 min. The complications associated with this condition are related to decreased oxygen levels, inability of the brain to return to normal functioning, and continued assault on neuronal tissue. This acute condition requires immediate treatment to prevent permanent loss of brain function.

The usual causes are substance withdrawal, sudden withdrawal from AEDs, head injury, cerebral edema, infection, and metabolic disturbances. Qᴛᴄ

NURSING ACTIONS

- Maintain an airway, provide oxygen, establish IV access, perform ECG monitoring, and monitor pulse oximetry and ABG results.
- Administer diazepam or lorazepam IV push followed by IV phenytoin or fosphenytoin.

Application Exercises

1. A nurse is assessing a client who has a seizure disorder. The client reports he thinks he is about to have a seizure. Which of the following actions should the nurse implement? (Select all that apply.)

   A. Provide privacy.

   B. Ease the client to the floor if standing.

   C. Move furniture away from the client.

   D. Loosen the client's clothing.

   E. Protect the client's head with padding.

   F. Restrain the client.

2. A nurse is caring for a client who just experienced a generalized seizure. Which of the following actions should the nurse perform first?

   A. Keep the client in a side-lying position.

   B. Document the duration of the seizure.

   C. Reorient the client to the environment.

   D. Provide client hygiene.

3. A nurse is providing discharge instructions to a female client who has a prescription for phenytoin. Which of the following information should the nurse include?

   A. Consider taking oral contraceptives when on this medication.

   B. Watch for receding gums when taking the medication.

   C. Take the medication at the same time every day.

   D. Provide a urine sample to determine therapeutic levels of the medication.

4. A nurse is reviewing trigger factors that can cause seizures with a client who has a new diagnosis of generalized seizures. Which of the following information should the nurse include in this review? (Select all that apply.)

   A. Avoid overwhelming fatigue.

   B. Remove caffeinated products from the diet.

   C. Limit looking at flashing lights.

   D. Perform aerobic exercise.

   E. Limit episodes of hypoventilation.

   F. Use of aerosol hairspray is recommended.

5. A nurse is completing discharge teaching to a client who has seizures and received a vagal nerve stimulator to decrease seizure activity. Which of the following statements should the nurse include in the teaching?

   A. "It is safe to use microwaves that are 1,200 watts or less.".

   B. "You should avoid the use of CT scans with contrast.".

   C. "You should place a magnet over the implantable device when you feel an aura occurring."

   D. "It is recommended that you use ultrasound diathermy for pain management."

PRACTICE Active Learning Scenario

A nurse is planning care for a client who is experiencing status epilepticus. What concepts should the nurse include in the plan of care? Use the ATI Active Learning Template: Basic Concept to complete this item.

RELATED CONTENT: Define the condition.

UNDERLYING PRINCIPLES: Describe four possible causes.

NURSING INTERVENTIONS: Describe five actions the nurse should plan to take.

Application Exercises Key

1. A. **CORRECT:** The nurse should implement privacy to minimize the client's embarrassment.

   B. **CORRECT:** The nurse should ease the client to the floor to prevent falling and injury.

   C. **CORRECT:** The nurse should move the furniture away from the client to prevent injury.

   D. **CORRECT:** The nurse should loosen the client's clothing to minimize restriction of movement.

   E. **CORRECT:** The nurse should protect the client's head from injury by placing the client's head in her lap or using a pillow or blanket under the head during a seizure.

   F. The nurse should not restrain the client. Restraint can increase the client's risk for injury or more seizure activity.

   ℕ *NCLEX® Connection: Physiological Adaptation, Alterations in Body Systems*

2. A. **CORRECT:** The greatest risk to the client is aspiration during the postictal phase. Therefore, the priority intervention is to keep the client in a side-lying position so secretions can drain from the mouth keeping the airway patent.

   B. The nurse should document the duration of the seizure in the client's medical record, but there is another action that the nurse should take first.

   C. The nurse should reorient the client to the environment because the client can feel confused, but there is another action that the nurse should take first.

   D. The nurse should provide client hygiene if the client experienced incontinence during the seizure, but there is another action that the nurse should take first.

   ℕ *NCLEX® Connection: Physiological Adaptation, Alterations in Body Systems*

3. A. The nurse should not instruct the client to take oral contraceptives, because contraceptive effectiveness is decreased when taking phenytoin.

   B. The nurse should instruct the client that phenytoin causes overgrowth of the gums.

   C. **CORRECT:** The nurse should instruct the client to take phenytoin at the same time every day to enhance effectiveness.

   D. The nurse should instruct the client to have periodic blood tests to determine the therapeutic level of phenytoin.

   ℕ *NCLEX® Connection: Pharmacological and Parenteral Therapies, Medication Administration*

4. A. **CORRECT:** The nurse should instruct the client to avoid overwhelming fatigue, which can trigger a seizure by stimulating abnormal electrical neuron activity.

   B. **CORRECT:** The nurse should instruct the client to remove caffeinated products from the diet, which can trigger a seizure by stimulating abnormal electrical neuron activity.

   C. **CORRECT:** The nurse should instruct the client to refrain from looking at flashing lights, which can trigger a seizure by stimulating abnormal electrical neuron activity.

   D. The nurse should instruct the client to avoid vigorous physical activity, which can help to avoid triggering a seizure.

   E. The nurse should instruct the client to limit excess hyperventilation, which can trigger a seizure by stimulating abnormal electrical neuron activity.

   F. The nurse should instruct the client to avoid using aerosol hairspray, which can trigger a seizure by stimulating abnormal electrical neuron activity.

   ℕ *NCLEX® Connection: Physiological Adaptation, Alterations in Body Systems*

5. A. The nurse should instruct the client to avoid using a microwave, regardless of wattage, which can affect the function of the stimulator.

   B. The nurse should instruct the client to avoid MRIs, which can affect the function of the stimulator.

   C. **CORRECT:** The nurse should instruct the client to hold a magnet over the implantable device when an aura occurs so as to decrease seizure activity.

   D. The nurse should instruct the client to avoid the use of ultrasound diathermy for pain management because of its effect on the function of the stimulator.

   ℕ *NCLEX® Connection: Reduction of Risk Potential, Therapeutic Procedures*

PRACTICE Answer

Using the ATI Active Learning Template: Basic Concept

RELATED CONTENT: Status epilepticus is repeated seizure activity within a 30-min time frame or a single prolonged seizure lasting more than 5 min.

UNDERLYING PRINCIPLES
- Substance withdrawal
- Withdrawal from antiepileptic medication
- Infection
- Head injury
- Cerebral edema
- Metabolic disturbances

NURSING INTERVENTIONS
- Maintain a patent airway.
- Perform ECG monitoring.
- Review ABG results.
- Establish IV access.
- Provide oxygen.
- Monitor pulse oximetry.
- Administer lorazepam or diazepam.
- Administer phenytoin or fosphenytoin.

ℕ *NCLEX® Connection: Physiological Adaptation, Alterations in Body Systems*

CHAPTER 7 *Parkinson's Disease*

Parkinson's disease (PD) is a progressively debilitating disease that grossly affects motor function. It is characterized by four primary symptoms: tremor, muscle rigidity, bradykinesia (slow movement), and postural instability. These symptoms occur due to overstimulation of the basal ganglia by acetylcholine.

The secretion of dopamine and acetylcholine in the body produce inhibitory and excitatory effects on the muscles respectively.

Overstimulation of the basal ganglia by acetylcholine occurs because degeneration of the substantia nigra results in decreased dopamine production. This allows acetylcholine to dominate, making smooth, controlled movements difficult.

Treatment of PD focuses on increasing the amount of dopamine or decreasing the amount of acetylcholine in a client's brain.

ASSESSMENT

RISK FACTORS

- Onset of symptoms between age 40 to 70
- More common in men
- Genetic predisposition
- Exposure to environmental toxins and chemical solvents
- Chronic use of antipsychotic medication

EXPECTED FINDINGS

- Report of fatigue
- Report of decreased manual dexterity over time

PHYSICAL ASSESSMENT FINDINGS

- Stooped posture
- Slow, shuffling, and propulsive gait
- Slow, monotonous speech
- Tremors/pill-rolling tremor of the fingers
- Muscle rigidity (e.g., rhythmic interruption, mildly restrictive, or total resistance to movement)

M◇ Online Video: Assessment Findings with Parkinson's Disease

- Bradykinesia/akinesia
- Masklike expression
- Autonomic symptoms (orthostatic hypotension, flushing, diaphoresis)
- Difficulty chewing and swallowing
  - Drooling
  - Dysarthria
  - Progressive difficulty with ADLs
  - Mood swings
  - Cognitive impairment (dementia)

LABORATORY TESTS

- There are no definitive diagnostic procedures.
- Diagnosis is made based on manifestations, their progression, and by ruling out other diseases. (7.1)

PATIENT-CENTERED CARE

NURSING CARE

- Administer medications at prescribed times. Monitor medication effectiveness, and make recommendations for changes in dosage and time of administration to provide best coverage.
- Monitor swallowing, and maintain adequate nutrition and weight. Consult speech and language therapist to assess swallowing if the client demonstrates a risk for choking. Qs
  - Consult the client's dietitian for appropriate diet, which often includes semisolid foods and thickened liquids.
  - Document the client's weight at least weekly.
  - Keep a diet intake log.
  - Encourage fluids and document intake.
  - Provide smaller, more frequent meals.
  - Sit the client upright to eat or drink.
  - Consult with occupational therapist for adaptive eating devices. Qtc
  - Evaluate need for high-calorie, high-protein supplements to maintain the client's weight.
- Maintain client mobility for as long as possible.
  - Encourage exercise, such as yoga (can also improve mental status).
  - Encourage use of assistive devices as disease progresses.
  - Encourage range-of-motion (ROM) exercises.
  - Teach the client to stop occasionally when walking to slow down speed and reduce risk for injury.
  - Pace activities by providing rest periods.
  - Assist with ADLs as needed (hygiene, dressing).

7.1 The five stages of Parkinson's disease involvement

As Parkinson's disease is a progressive disease, there are five stages of involvement.

STAGE I:	STAGE II:	STAGE III:	STAGE IV:	STAGE V:
Unilateral shaking or tremor of one limb.	Bilateral limb involvement occurs, making walking and balance difficult.	Physical movements slow down significantly, affecting walking more.	Tremors can decrease but akinesia and rigidity make day-to-day tasks difficult.	Client unable to stand or walk, is dependent for all care, and might exhibit dementia.

- Promote client communication for as long as possible.
  - Teach the client facial muscle strengthening exercises.
  - Encourage the client to speak slowly and to pause frequently.
  - Use alternate forms of communication as appropriate.
  - Refer client to a speech-language pathologist.
- Monitor mental and cognitive status
  - Observe for signs of depression and dementia.
  - Provide a safe environment (no throw rugs, encourage the use of an electric razor). Qs
  - Assess personal and family coping with the client's chronic, degenerative disease.
  - Provide a list of community resources (support groups) to the client and family.
  - Refer the client to a social worker or case manager as condition advances (financial issues, long-term home care, and respite care). Qᴛᴄ

MEDICATIONS

- Can take several weeks of use before improvement of symptoms is seen.
- While the client is taking a combination of medications, maintenance of therapeutic medication levels is necessary for adequate control.

Dopaminergics

- When given orally, medications such as levodopa are converted to dopamine in the brain, increasing dopamine levels in the basal ganglia.
- Dopaminergics may be combined with carbidopa to decrease peripheral metabolism of levodopa, requiring a smaller dose to make the same amount available to the brain. Side effects are subsequently less.
- Due to medication tolerance and metabolism, the dosage, form of medication, and administration times must be adjusted to avoid periods of poor mobility.
- NURSING CONSIDERATIONS: Monitor for the "wearing-off" phenomenon and dyskinesias (problems with movement), which can indicate the need to adjust the dosage or time of administration or the need for a medication holiday.

Dopamine agonists

Dopamine agonists, such as bromocriptine, ropinirole, and pramipexole, activate release of dopamine. May be used in conjunction with a dopaminergic for better results.

NURSING CONSIDERATIONS: Monitor for orthostatic hypotension, dyskinesias, and hallucinations. Qs

Anticholinergics

Anticholinergics, such as benztropine and trihexyphenidyl, help control tremors and rigidity.

NURSING CONSIDERATIONS: Monitor for anticholinergic effects (dry mouth, constipation, urinary retention, acute confusion).

Catechol O-methyltransferase (COMT) inhibitors

COMT inhibitors, such as entacapone, decrease the breakdown of levodopa, making more available to the brain as dopamine. Can be used in conjunction with a dopaminergic and dopamine agonist for better results.

NURSING CONSIDERATIONS
- Monitor for dyskinesia/hyperkinesia when used with levodopa.
- Assess for diarrhea.
- Dark urine is a normal finding.

Monoamine oxidase type B (MAO-B) inhibitors

MAO-B inhibitors, such as selegiline and rasagiline, inhibit monoamine oxidase type B activity and increase dopamine levels. They reduce the wearing-off phenomenon when administered concurrently with levodopa.

NURSING CONSIDERATIONS
- Teach the client to avoid foods high in tyramine, which can cause hypertensive crisis. Qs
- Severe reactions can occur when these medications are administered with sympathomimetics, meperidine, and fluoxetine.

Antivirals

Antivirals, such as amantadine, stimulate release of dopamine and prevent its reuptake.

NURSING CONSIDERATIONS
- Monitor for discoloration of the skin that subsides when amantadine is discontinued.
- Client might experience anxiety, confusion, and anticholinergic effects.

THERAPEUTIC PROCEDURES

Stereotactic pallidotomy or thalamotomy

- Strict eligibility criteria generally includes those who have not responded to other therapies.
- Stereotactic pallidotomy and thalamotomy causes the destruction of a small portion of the brain within the globus pallidus or thalamus through the use of brain imaging and electrical stimulation.
- Target area is identified with a CT scan or an MRI.
- Mild electrical stimulation is provided through a burr hole to a target area.
- Client is assessed for a decrease in tremors and muscle rigidity.
- When a decrease is elicited, a temporary lesion is formed and the client is reassessed.
- If symptomatic relief is demonstrated (e.g., alleviation of tremors and rigidity), a permanent lesion is made.

NURSING ACTIONS: Assess for a neurological impairment and brain hemorrhage postoperatively.

Deep brain stimulation

- An electrode is implanted in the thalamus.
- A current is delivered through a small pulse generator implanted under the skin of the upper chest. Electrical stimulation from DBS impulses decreases tremors and involuntary movements, and can decrease medications required to control PD.

NURSING ACTIONS: Monitor for infection, brain hemorrhage, or stroke-like symptoms.

INTERPROFESSIONAL CARE

- Because PD is a degenerative neurological disorder, long-term treatment and care must be accommodated.
- During the later stages of the disorder, the client needs referrals to and support from disciplines such as speech therapists, occupational therapists, physical therapists, and social service/case management.

COMPLICATIONS

Aspiration pneumonia

As PD advances in severity, alterations in chewing and swallowing worsen, increasing the risk for aspiration.

NURSING ACTIONS
- Use swallowing precautions to decrease the risk for aspiration. Qs
- Develop individual dietary plan based on the speech therapist's recommendations.
- Have a nurse in attendance when the client is eating.
- Encourage the client to eat slowly and chew thoroughly before swallowing. Qs
- Feed the client in an upright position and have suction equipment on standby.
- Evaluate need for enteral feedings to maintain weight and prevent aspiration as PD progresses.

Altered cognition (dementia, memory deficits)

Clients in advanced stages of PD can exhibit altered cognition in the form of dementia and memory loss.

NURSING ACTIONS
- Acknowledge the client's feelings.
- Provide for a safe environment.
- Develop a comprehensive plan of care with the family, client, and interprofessional team. Qtc

Application Exercises

1. A nurse is caring for a client who displays signs of stage III Parkinson's disease. Which of the following actions should the nurse include in the plan of care?

   A. Recommend a community support group.
   B. Integrate a daily exercise routine.
   C. Provide a walker for ambulation.
   D. Perform ADLs for the client.

2. A nurse is developing a plan of care for the nutritional needs of a client who has stage IV Parkinson's disease. Which actions should the nurse include in the plan of care? (Select all that apply.)

   A. Provide three large balanced meals daily.
   B. Record diet and fluid intake daily.
   C. Document weight every other week.
   D. Place the client in Fowler's position to eat.
   E. Offer nutritional supplements between meals.

3. A nurse is reinforcing teaching with a client who has Parkinson's disease and has a new prescription for bromocriptine. Which of the following instructions should the nurse include in the teaching?

   A. Rise slowly when standing.
   B. Expect urine to become dark-colored.
   C. Avoid foods containing tyramine.
   D. Report any skin discoloration.

4. A nurse is assessing a client for manifestations of Parkinson's disease. Which of the following are expected findings? (Select all that apply.)

   A. Decreased vision
   B. Pill-rolling tremor of the fingers
   C. Shuffling gait
   D. Drooling
   E. Bilateral ankle edema
   F. Lack of facial expression

5. A nurse is caring for a client who has Parkinson's disease and is starting to display bradykinesia. Which of the following is an appropriate action by the nurse?

   A. Teach the client to walk more quickly when ambulating.
   B. Complete passive range-of-motion exercises daily.
   C. Place the client on a low-protein, low-calorie diet.
   D. Give the client extra time to perform activities.

Application Exercises Key

1. A. The client/family should be involved in a community support group at the onset of the disease process to enhance coping mechanisms.

    B. The client should perform daily exercises with the onset of the disease process to promote mobility and independence for as long as possible.

    C. **CORRECT:** The client should use a walker for ambulation in stage III of Parkinson's disease because movement slows down significantly and gait disturbances occur.

    D. The client loses ability to perform ADLs during stage V of Parkinson's disease and is dependent on others for care at that time. During earlier stages, the client should be encouraged to remain as independent as possible.

    (N) *NCLEX® Connection: Safety and Infection Control, Accident/Error/Injury Prevention*

2. A. The nurse should plan to provide small frequent meals during the day to maintain adequate nutrition.

    B. **CORRECT:** The nurse should record the client's diet and fluid intake daily to assess for dietary needs and to maintain adequate nutrition and hydration.

    C. The nurse should document the client's weight weekly to identify weight loss and intervene to maintain the client's weight.

    D. The nurse should ensure that the client is sitting upright for meals rather than in a supported Fowler's position, where the client's head is elevated to 45 to 60°.

    E. **CORRECT:** The nurse should offer nutritional supplements between meals to maintain the client's weight.

    (N) *NCLEX® Connection: Basic Care and Comfort, Nutrition and Oral Hydration*

3. A. **CORRECT:** Orthostatic hypotension is a common adverse effect of bromocriptine, a dopamine receptor agonist. Therefore, rising slowly when standing up will decrease the risk of dizziness and lightheadedness.

    B. The client should expect urine to turn dark when taking entacapone, a COMT inhibitor. Dark urine is not an expected finding when taking bromocriptine.

    C. The client should avoid tyramine in the diet when taking selegiline, a monoamine type B inhibitor. However, bromocriptine does not interact with foods that contain tyramine.

    D. Skin discoloration is an adverse effect of amantadine, an anti-viral medication. However it is not an adverse effect of bromocriptine.

    (N) *NCLEX® Connection: Pharmacological and Parenteral Therapies, Adverse Effects/Contraindications/Side Effects/Interactions*

4. A. Decreased vision is not an expected finding in a client who has PD.

    B. **CORRECT:** The client who has PD can manifest pill-rolling tremors of the fingers due to overstimulation of the basal ganglia by acetylcholine, making controlled movement difficult.

    C. **CORRECT:** The client who has PD can manifest shuffling gait because of overstimulation of the basal ganglia by acetylcholine, making controlled movement difficult.

    D. **CORRECT:** The client who has PD can manifest drooling because of overstimulation of the basal ganglia by acetylcholine, making the controlled movement of swallowing secretions difficult.

    E. Bilateral ankle edema is not an expected finding in a client who has PD, but can be an adverse effect of certain medications used for treatment.

    F. **CORRECT:** The client who has PD can manifest a lack of facial expressions due to overstimulation of the basal ganglia by acetylcholine, making controlled movement difficult.

    (N) *NCLEX® Connection: Physiological Adaptation, Pathophysiology*

5. A. The client who has PD develops a propulsive gait and tends to walk increasingly rapidly. The client should be reminded to stop occasionally when walking to prevent a propulsive gait and decrease the risk for falls.

    B. The nurse should encourage active, not passive, range-of-motion exercises to promote mobility in the client who has PD and is displaying bradykinesia.

    C. The client who has PD often requires high-calorie, high-protein supplements between meals in order to maintain adequate weight.

    D. **CORRECT:** Bradykinesia is abnormally slowed movement and is seen in clients who have PD. The client should be given extra time to perform activities and should be encouraged to remain active.

    (N) *NCLEX® Connection: Reduction of Risk Potential, System Specific Assessments*

PRACTICE Active Learning Scenario

A nurse is preparing a plan of care for a client who has a new diagnosis of Parkinson's disease. What should the nurse include in the plan of care? Use the ATI Active Learning Template: System Disorder to complete this item.

ALTERATION IN HEALTH (DIAGNOSIS): Define Parkinson's disease.

COMPLICATIONS: Identify four.

NURSING CARE: Describe six nursing actions.

PRACTICE Answer

Using the ATI Active Learning Template: System Disorder

ALTERATION IN HEALTH (DIAGNOSIS): Parkinson's disease is a debilitating condition that progresses to complete dependent care. The disease involves a decrease in dopamine production and an increase in secretion of acetylcholine, causing resting tremor, slowed movement, and muscular rigidity.

COMPLICATIONS
- Aspiration due to pharyngeal muscle involvement making swallowing difficult
- Orthostatic hypotension, slow movement, and muscle rigidity
- Change in speech pattern: slow, monotonous speech
- Altered emotional changes that can include depression and fear

NURSING CARE
- Add thickener to liquids to prevent aspiration.
- Consult with a dietitian about appropriate diet.
- Encourage periods of rest between activities.
- Allow adequate time to rise slowly from a sitting to standing position.
- Encourage slower speech when expressing thoughts.
- Observe for signs of depression and dementia.

(N) *NCLEX® Connection: Physiological Adaptation, Illness Management*

CHAPTER 8 *Alzheimer's Disease*

Alzheimer's disease (AD) is a nonreversible type of dementia that progressively develops over many years. A framework made up of seven stages has been designed to categorize the disease and its manifestations. The framework is based on three general stages: early stage, mid stage, and late stage.

Dementia is defined as multiple cognitive deficits that impair memory and can affect language, motor skills, and/or abstract thinking. The percentage of dementia attributable to AD ranges from 60% to 90%.

The mean duration of survival after diagnosis is approximately 10 years, but some people can live with the disease for up to 20 years.

AD is most likely to occur in clients in their 60s and 70s. However, it can be diagnosed as early as 40. Age is the No. 1 known risk factor for AD, which usually occurs after the age of 65. ©

AD is characterized by memory loss, problems with judgment, and changes in personality. As the disease progresses, severe physical decline occurs along with deteriorating cognitive functions.

ASSESSMENT

Mini Mental State Examination (MMSE) is used.

RISK FACTORS

- Advanced age
- Chemical imbalances
- Family history of AD or Down syndrome
- Genetic predisposition, apolipoprotein E
- Environmental agents (herpes virus, metal, or toxic waste)
- Previous head injury
- Sex (female)
- Ethnicity (African Americans greater risk; Hispanics develop AD earlier)

EXPECTED FINDINGS

AD progression and manifestations are categorized into seven stages. (8.1)

LABORATORY TESTS

- No specific lab test can definitively diagnose AD.
- Several lab can rule out other causes of dementia.
- Genetic test for the presence of apolipoprotein can determine if there is an increased risk of AD, but it does not specifically diagnose AD. The presence of the protein increases the likelihood that dementia is due to AD.

DIAGNOSTIC PROCEDURES

- There is no definitive diagnostic procedure, except brain tissue examination upon death.
- Magnetic resonance imaging (MRI), computed tomography (CT) imaging/computed axial tomography (CAT) scan, positron emission tomography (PET) scan, and electroencephalogram (EEG) may be performed to rule out other possible causes of findings.
- A lumbar puncture may be performed for laboratory testing of cerebral spinal fluid for soluble beta protein precursor (sBPP). Beta amyloid protein normally assists in growth and protection of nerve cells. The presence of low levels of sBPP supports the diagnosis of AD.

PATIENT-CENTERED CARE

NURSING CARE

- Assess cognitive status, memory, judgment, and personality changes.
- Initiate bowel and bladder program based on a set schedule.
- Encourage the client and family to participate in an AD support group.
- Provide a safe environment. Qs
  - Frequent monitoring/visual checks.
  - Keep client from stairs, elevators, exits.
  - Remove or secure dangerous items in the client's environment.
- Provide frequent walks to reduce wandering.
- Maintain a sleeping schedule, and monitor for irregular sleeping patterns.
- Provide verbal and nonverbal ways to communicate with the client.
- Offer snacks or finger foods if the client is unable to sit for long periods of time.
- Check skin weekly for breakdown.
- Provide cognitive stimulation.
  - Offer varied environmental stimulations, such as walks, music, or craft activities.
  - Keep a structured environment and introduce change gradually (client's daily routine or a room change).
  - Use a calendar to assist with orientation.
  - Use short directions when explaining an activity or care the client needs, such as a bath.
  - Be consistent and repetitive.
  - Use therapeutic touch.

- Provide memory training.
  - Reminisce with the client about the past.
  - Use memory techniques, such as making lists and rehearsing.
  - Stimulate memory by repeating the client's last statement.
- Avoid overstimulation. (Keep noise and clutter to a minimum, and avoid crowds.)
- Promote consistency by placing commonly used objects in the same location and using a routine schedule.
  - Reality orientation (early stages)
  - Easily viewed clock and single-day calendar
  - Pictures of family and pets
  - Frequent reorientation to time, place, and person
- Validation therapy (later stages)
  - Acknowledge the client's feelings.
  - Don't argue with the client; this will lead to the client becoming upset.
  - Reinforce and use repetitive actions or ideas cautiously.
- Promote self-care as long as possible. Assist with activities of daily living as appropriate.
- Speak directly to the client in short, concise sentences.
- Reduce agitation. (Use calm, redirecting statements. Provide a diversion.)
- Provide a routine toileting schedule.

MEDICATIONS

- Most medications for clients who have dementia attempt to target behavioral and emotional problems, such as anxiety, agitation, combativeness, and depression.
- These medications include antipsychotics, antidepressants, and anxiolytics. Closely monitor clients receiving these medications for adverse effects.
- AD medications temporarily slow the course of the disease and do not work for all clients.
  - Pharmacotherapeutics is based on the theory that AD is a result of depleted levels of the enzyme acetyltransferase, which is necessary to produce the neurotransmitter acetylcholine.
  - Benefits for clients who do respond to medication include improvements in cognition, behavior, and function.
- If a client fails to improve with one medication, a trial of one of the other medications is warranted.
  - **Donepezil** prevents the breakdown of acetylcholine (ACh), which increases the amount of ACh available. This results in increased nerve impulses at the nerve sites.
  - **Cholinesterase** inhibitors help slow this process.

NURSING CONSIDERATIONS

- Observe for frequent stools or upset stomach.
- Monitor for dizziness or headache. The client can feel lightheaded or have an unsteady gait.
- Use caution when administering this medication to clients who have asthma or COPD, as lung problems can worsen.

THERAPEUTIC PROCEDURES

ALTERNATIVE THERAPY

- Estrogen therapy for women can prevent Alzheimer's disease, but it is not useful in decreasing the effects of existing dementia.
- Ginkgo biloba, an herbal product taken to increase memory and blood circulation, can cause a variety of side effects and medication interactions. If a client is using ginkgo biloba or other nutritional supplements, that information should be shared with providers.

INTERPROFESSIONAL CARE

- Encourage the client and family to seek legal counsel regarding advanced directives, guardianship, or durable medical power of attorney.
- Refer the client and family to social services and case managers for possible adult day care facilities or long-term care facilities.
- Refer the client and family to the Alzheimer's Association and community outreach programs. This can include family support groups, in-home care, or respite care.
- Review the resources available to the family as the client's health declines. Include long-term care options. A variety of home care and community resources, such as respite care, can be available to the family in many areas of the country. Some respite care allows the client to remain at home rather than in a facility.

CLIENT EDUCATION

- Refer to social services and case managers for long-term/home management, Alzheimer's Association, community outreach programs, and support groups
- Educate family/caregivers about illness, methods of care, medications, and adaptation of the home environment.
- Home safety measures to be implemented can include: **Qs**
  - Removing scatter rugs.
  - Installing door locks that cannot be easily opened, and placing alarms on doors.
  - Keeping a lock on the water heater and thermostat, and keeping the water temperature at a safe level.
  - Providing good lighting, especially on stairs.
  - Installing handrails on stairs and marking step edges with colored tape.
  - Placing the mattress on the floor.
  - Removing clutter and clearing hallways for walking.
  - Securing electrical cords to baseboards.
  - Keeping cleaning supplies in locked cupboards.
  - Installing handrails in the bathroom, at bedside, and in the tub; placing a shower chair in the tub.
  - Having the client wear a medical identification bracelet if living at home with a caregiver.
    - Enroll in Safe Return Home Program (www.alz.org).
  - An exercise program to maintain mobility.
  - Care for seizures that can happen late in the disease.
  - Strategies to reduce caregiver stress.

8.1 Alzheimer's disease stages and manifestations

Mild Alzheimer's (early stage)

NO IMPAIRMENT
- Normal function
- Manifestation: No memory problems.

VERY MILD COGNITIVE DECLINE
- (Can be normal age-related changes or very early signs of AD)
- Manifestations
  - Forgetfulness, especially of everyday objects (eyeglasses or wallet).
  - No memory problems evident to provider, friends, or coworkers.

MILD COGNITIVE DECLINE
- (Problems with memory or concentration can be measurable in clinical testing or during a detailed medical interview)
- Mild cognitive deficits, including losing or misplacing important objects.
- Manifestations
  - Decreased ability to plan.
  - Short-term memory loss noticeable to close relatives.
  - Decreased attention span.
  - Difficulty remembering words or names.
  - Difficulty in social or work situations.

Moderate Alzheimer's (middle stage)

MODERATE COGNITIVE DECLINE
- Medical interview will detect clear-cut deficiencies.
- Manifestations
  - Personality changes: appearing withdrawn or subdued, especially in social or mentally challenging situations.
  - Obvious memory loss.
  - Limited knowledge and memory of recent occasions, current events, or personal history.
  - Difficulty performing tasks that require planning and organizing (paying bills or managing money).
  - Difficulty with complex mental arithmetic.

MODERATELY SEVERE COGNITIVE DECLINE
- Manifestations
  - Increasing cognitive deficits emerge.
  - Inability to recall important details such as address, telephone number, or schools attended, but memory of information about self and family remains intact.
  - Assistance with ADLs becomes necessary.
  - Disorientation and confusion as to time and place.

Severe Alzheimer's (late stage)

SEVERE COGNITIVE DECLINE
- Manifestations
  - Memory difficulties continue to worsen.
  - Loss of awareness of recent events and surroundings.
  - Can recall own name, but unable to recall personal history.
  - Significant personality changes are evident (delusions, hallucinations, and compulsive behaviors).
  - Wandering behavior.
  - Requires assistance with ADLs such as dressing, toileting, and grooming.
  - Normal sleep/wake cycle is disrupted.
  - Increased episodes of urinary and fecal incontinence.

VERY SEVERE COGNITIVE DECLINE
- Manifestations
  - Ability to respond to environment, speak, and control movement is lost.
  - Unrecognizable speech.
  - General urinary incontinence.
  - Inability to eat without assistance and impaired swallowing.
  - Gradual loss of all ability to move extremities (ataxia).

Application Exercises

1. A nurse is providing teaching to the partner of an older adult client who has Alzheimer's disease and has a new prescription for donepezil. Which of the following statements by the partner indicates the teaching is effective?

   A. "This medication should increase my husband's appetite."

   B. "This medication should help my husband sleep better."

   C. "This medication should help my husband's daily function."

   D. "This medication should increase my husband's energy level."

2. A nurse working in a long-term care facility is planning care for a client in stage V of Alzheimer's disease. Which of the following interventions should be included in the plan of care?

   A. Use a gait belt for ambulation.

   B. Thicken all liquids.

   C. Provide protective undergarments.

   D. Assist with ADLs.

3. A nurse is making a home visit to a client who has AD. The client's partner states that the client is often disoriented to time and place, is unsteady on his feet, and has a history of wandering. Which of the following safety measures should the nurse review with the partner? (Select all that apply.)

   A. Remove floor rugs.

   B. Have door locks that can be easily opened.

   C. Provide increased lighting in stairwells.

   D. Install handrails in the bathroom.

   E. Place the mattress on the floor.

4. A nurse is caring for a client who has AD and falls frequently. Which of the following actions should the nurse take first to keep the client safe?

   A. Keep the call light near the client.

   B. Place the client in a room close to the nurses' station.

   C. Encourage the client to ask for assistance.

   D. Remind the client to walk with someone for support.

5. A nurse is caring for a client who has Alzheimer's disease. A family member of the client asks the nurse about risk factors for the disease. Which of the following should be included in the nurse's response? (Select all that apply.)

   A. Exposure to metal waste products

   B. Long-term estrogen therapy

   C. Sustained use of vitamin E

   D. Previous head injury

   E. History of herpes infection

Application Exercises Key

1. A. Donepezil does not affect appetite.

   B. Donepezil does not affect sleep or sleep patterns.

   C. **CORRECT:** Donepezil helps slow the progression of AD and can help improve behavior and daily functions.

   D. Donepezil does not affect energy levels.

   Ⓝ *NCLEX® Connection: Pharmacological and Parenteral Therapies, Medication Administration*

2. A. Ambulation is affected as the client advances into stage VII of Alzheimer's disease.

   B. Impaired swallowing is a finding as the client advances into stage VII of Alzheimer's disease.

   C. The client in stages VI and VII of Alzheimer's disease experiences episodes of urinary and fecal incontinence.

   D. **CORRECT:** A client in Alzheimer's disease stage V requires assistance with ADLs as increasing cognitive deficits emerge.

   Ⓝ *NCLEX® Connection: Safety and Infection Control, Home Safety*

3. A. **CORRECT:** Removing floor rugs can decrease the risk of falling.

   B. Easy-to-open door locks increase the risk for a client who wanders to get out of his home and get lost.

   C. **CORRECT:** Good lighting can decrease the risk for falling in dark areas, such as stairways.

   D. **CORRECT:** Installing handrails in the bathroom can be useful for the client to hold on to when his gait is unsteady.

   E. **CORRECT:** By placing the client's mattress on the floor, the risk of falling or tripping is decreased.

   Ⓝ *NCLEX® Connection: Health Promotion and Maintenance, Developmental Stages and Transitions*

4. A. Keeping the call light within the client's reach is an appropriate action, but not the first action because the client might not remember to use it.

   B. **CORRECT:** Using the safety and risk reduction priority-setting framework, placing the client in close proximity to the nurses' station for close observation is the first action the nurse should take.

   C. Encouraging the client to ask for assistance is an appropriate action, but not the first action because the client might not remember to ask for assistance.

   D. Reminding the client to walk with someone is an appropriate action, but not the first action because the client might not remember to call for assistance.

   Ⓝ *NCLEX® Connection: Safety and Infection Control, Home Safety*

5. A. **CORRECT:** Exposure to metal and toxic waste is a risk factor for Alzheimer's disease.

   B. Long-term estrogen therapy can prevent Alzheimer's disease.

   C. Long-term use of vitamin E is not a risk factor for Alzheimer's disease.

   D. **CORRECT:** A previous head injury is a risk factor for Alzheimer's disease.

   E. **CORRECT:** A history of herpes infection is a risk factor for Alzheimer's disease.

   Ⓝ *NCLEX® Connection: Health Promotion and Maintenance, Health Promotion/Disease Prevention*

PRACTICE Active Learning Scenario

A nurse educator in a long-term care facility is preparing a program for assistive personnel about caring for a client who has Alzheimer's disease. What should be included in this program? Use the ATI Active Learning Template: System Disorder to complete this item.

NURSING CARE: Describe three nursing interventions for each of the following areas.
- Providing cognitive stimulation
- Providing memory training

PRACTICE Answer

Using the ATI Active Learning Template: System Disorder

NURSING CARE
- Providing cognitive stimulation
  - Offer varied environmental stimulations, such as walks, music, and craft activities.
  - Keep a structured environment. Introduce change slowly.
  - Use a calendar to assist with orientation.
  - Use short directions when explaining care to be provided, such as a bath.
  - Be consistent and repetitive.
  - Use therapeutic touch.
- Providing memory training
  - Reminisce about the past.
  - Help the client make lists and rehearse.
  - Repeat the client's last statement to stimulate memory.

Ⓝ *NCLEX® Connection: Health Promotion and Maintenance, Developmental Stages and Transitions*

CHAPTER 9 *Brain Tumors*

Brain tumors occur in any part of the brain and are classified according to the cell or tissue of origin. Cerebral tumors are the most common.

Types of brain tumors include benign and malignant. Examples include malignant gliomas (neuroglial cells), benign meningiomas (meninges), pituitary adenomas, and acoustic neuromas (acoustic cranial nerve).

A secondary classification, supratentorial tumors occur in the cerebral hemispheres above the tentorium cerebelli. Those below the tentorium cerebelli, such as tumors of the brainstem and cerebellum, are classified as infratentorial tumors.

Brain tumors apply pressure to surrounding brain tissue, resulting in decreased outflow of cerebrospinal fluid, increased intracranial pressure, cerebral edema, and neurological deficits. Tumors that involve the pituitary gland can cause endocrine dysfunction.

Malignant brain tumors are associated with a high overall mortality rate. Primary malignant brain tumors originate from neuroglial tissue and rarely metastasize outside of the brain. Secondary malignant brain tumors are lesions that are metastases from a primary cancer located elsewhere in the body. Cranial metastatic lesions are most common from breast, kidney, lung, and gastrointestinal tract cancers.

Benign brain tumors develop from the meninges or cranial nerves and do not metastasize. These tumors have distinct boundaries and cause damage either by the pressure they exert within the cranial cavity and/or by impairing the function of the cranial nerve.

MⓄOnline Media: *Nystagmus, Testing for Romberg Sign, Babinski Reflex*

HEALTH PROMOTION/ DISEASE PREVENTION

There are no routine screening procedures to detect brain tumors.

ASSESSMENT

RISK FACTORS

The cause is unknown, but several risk factors have been identified.
- Genetics
- Environmental agents
- Exposure to ionizing radiation
- Exposure to electromagnetic fields
- Previous head injury

EXPECTED FINDINGS

PHYSICAL ASSESSMENT FINDINGS
- Dysarthria
- Dysphagia
- Positive Romberg sign
- Positive Babinski sign
- Vertigo
- Hemiparesis
- Cranial nerve dysfunction (inability to discriminate sounds, loss of gag reflex, loss of blink response)
- Papilledema

MANIFESTATIONS SPECIFIC TO SUPRATENTORIAL BRAIN TUMORS
- Severe headache (worse upon awakening but improving over time)
- Visual changes (blurring, visual field deficit)
- Seizures
- Loss of voluntary movement or the inability to control movement
- Change in cognitive function (memory loss, language impairment)
- Change in personality, inability to control emotions
- Nausea with or without vomiting
- Paralysis

MANIFESTATIONS SPECIFIC TO INFRATENTORIAL BRAIN TUMORS
- Hearing loss or ringing in the ear
- Visual changes
- Facial drooping
- Difficulty swallowing
- Nystagmus, crossed eyes, or decreased vision
- Autonomic nervous system (ANS) dysfunction
- Ataxia or clumsy movements
- Hemiparesis
- Cranial nerve dysfunction (inability to discriminate sounds, loss of gag reflex, loss of blink response)

LABORATORY TESTS

- CBC and differential to rule out anemia or malnutrition
- Blood alcohol and toxicology screen to rule out these as possible causes of altered physical assessment findings
- TB and HIV screening if social conditions warrant

DIAGNOSTIC PROCEDURES

- X-ray, computed tomography (CT) imaging scan, magnetic resonance imaging (MRI), brain scan, position emission tomography (PET) scan, and cerebral angiography are used to determine the size, location, and extent of the tumor.
- Lumbar puncture (LP) and electroencephalography (EEG) can provide additional information about the tumor.
- LP should not be done if the client has or shows signs of increasing intracranial pressure (ICP) to prevent brain herniation.
- Lab tests can be done to evaluate endocrine function, renal status, and electrolyte balance.
- Cerebral biopsy identifies cellular pathology.
  - This procedure may be performed in the surgical suite or in a radiology specialty suite.
  - Diagnostic procedure may be used to guide the biopsy, such as a CT or MRI scan. Image guiding systems, which use CT or MRI scan information, may be used in the surgical suite.
  - A piece of cerebral tissue that appears abnormal on the CT/MRI scan is obtained. This tissue is then sent to pathology, where diagnostic tests are performed.
  - Benefit: Biopsy is minimally disruptive to the rest of the brain, provides a decreased recovery time, and is not associated with the risks of an open craniotomy.
  - Negative: Biopsy does not remove or debulk the tumor, the diagnostic determination by pathology can be inconclusive (related to insufficient tissue), and a misdiagnosis can occur if the tumor contains many types of tissue or the specimen is taken from one site.

CLIENT EDUCATION: Include specific instruction regarding medications.

- If the client is on antiepileptic medications, these must be continued to prevent seizure activity. **Qs**
- If the client is on aspirin products, these should be discontinued at least 72 hr prior to the procedure to minimize the risk of intracerebral bleeding.
- Other medications may be withheld prior to the procedure.
- Normally, preprocedure activities may be resumed after the client recovers from the general anesthetic. Care of the incision should include keeping the area clean and dry. If sutures are in place, they need to be removed 1 to 7 days later. Driving or other dangerous activities should be avoided until follow-up appointment occurs and diagnosis is known.

PATIENT-CENTERED CARE

NURSING CARE

- Maintain airway (monitor oxygen levels, administer oxygen as needed, monitor lung sounds).
- Monitor neurological status — in particular, assessing for changes in level of consciousness, neurological deficits, and occurrence of seizures.
- Maintain client safety. (Assist with transfers and ambulation, provide assistive devices as needed.) **Qs**
- Implement seizure precautions.
- Administer medications as prescribed.

MEDICATIONS

- **Nonopioid analgesics** are used to treat headaches.
  - Opioid medications are avoided because they tend to decrease level of consciousness.
- **Corticosteroids** are used to reduce cerebral edema.
  - Corticosteroid medications quickly reduce cerebral edema and may be rapidly administered to maximize their effectiveness.
  - Chronic administration is used to control cerebral edema associated with the presence or treatment of benign or malignant brain tumors.
- **Anticonvulsant medications** are used to control or prevent seizure activity.
  - Anticonvulsant medications suppress the neuronal activity within the brain, which prevents seizure activity.
  - There are several classifications of antiepileptic medications, each specifically designed to treat specific seizure behavior.
- **H_2-antagonists** are used to decrease the acid content of the stomach, reducing the risk of stress ulcers.
  - H_2-antagonists are administered during acute or stressful periods, such as after surgery, at the initiation of chemotherapy, or during the first several radiation therapy treatments.
  - The effect of these treatments, together with the necessity of corticosteroids, places the client at risk for stress ulcers. This is primarily preventative treatment.
- **Antiemetics** are used if nausea (with or without vomiting) is present.
  - Nausea and vomiting can be present as a result of the increased ICP, the site of the tumor, or the treatment required.
  - These medications are administered as prescribed, and may be provided as a preventative intervention, especially when the treatment is associated with nausea and/or vomiting.

INTERPROFESSIONAL CARE

- Initiate appropriate referrals (social services, support groups, medical equipment, and physical, speech, and occupational therapy).
- Treatments include steroids, surgery, chemotherapy, conventional radiation therapy, stereotactic radiosurgery, and clinical trials. Chemotherapy and/or conventional radiation therapy may be administered prior to surgery to reduce the bulk of the tumor, or after surgery to prevent tumor recurrence.
- In most cases when the tumor is benign, surgery is a curative treatment. However, these tumors can regrow. Radiation and/or chemotherapy may be provided to prevent recurrence.
- Some tumors can be malignant by location, meaning that while the pathology is benign, the location makes the mortality rate associated with them high.
- In cases where the tumor is a metastatic lesion from a primary lesion elsewhere in the body, treatments are palliative. These treatments may consist of surgery, radiation, and chemotherapy, in any combination, and are aimed at controlling intracerebral lesions.

THERAPEUTIC PROCEDURES

Craniotomy: complete or partial resection of brain tumor through surgical opening in the skull

PREOPERATIVE NURSING ACTIONS

- Explain the procedure to the client, answering all appropriate questions and providing emotional support.
- Questions regarding the surgery and its outcomes should be written, in an effort to ensure all questions are answered.
- The client's partner should be present to hear the responses and avoid miscommunication.
- If the client takes aspirin, this medication needs to be stopped at least 72 hr prior to the procedure.
- No alcohol, tobacco, anticoagulants, or NSAIDs for 5 days prior to surgery.
- If the client uses alternative/complementary medications or treatments, make these known to the provider.
- A living will and durable power for health care decisions should be completed.
- Administer medications as prescribed. An antianxiety or muscle relaxant medication can be administered, if requested, and provided by the provider.

POSTOPERATIVE NURSING ACTIONS

- Closely monitor vital signs and neurological status, including using the Glasgow Scale.
- Treat pain adequately.
- Elevate the head of the client 30° for clients who had supratentorial surgery and in a neutral position to prevent increased ICP. Turn the client to the side or supine to decrease risk of pressure ulcers and pneumonia. Qs
- Infratentorial craniotomy clients lie flat and side-lying. Turn side to side every 2 hr for 24 to 48 hr.
- Straining activities (moving up in bed and attempting to have a bowel movement) should be avoided to prevent increased ICP. Postoperative bleeding and seizure activity are the greatest risks.
- Periorbital edema and ecchymosis is not unusual. Treat with cold compresses
- Assess head dressing every 1 to 2 hr for drainage.

COMPLICATIONS

Syndrome of inappropriate antidiuretic hormone

Syndrome of inappropriate antidiuretic hormone (SIADH) is a condition where fluid is retained as a result of an overproduction of vasopressin or antidiuretic hormone (ADH) from the posterior pituitary gland.

- SIADH occurs when the hypothalamus has been damaged and can no longer regulate the release of ADH.
- Treatment consists of fluid restriction, administration of oral conivaptan, and treatment of hyponatremia.
- If SIADH is present, the client can have disorientation, headache, vomiting, muscle weakness, decreased LOC, irritability, loss of thirst, and weight gain.
- If severe or untreated, this condition can cause seizures and/or a coma.

Diabetes insipidus

Diabetes insipidus (DI) is seen most often after supratentorial surgery, especially when involving the pituitary gland or hypothalamus.

- This is a condition where large amounts of urine are excreted as a result of a deficiency of ADH from the posterior pituitary gland.
- The condition occurs when the hypothalamus has been damaged and can no longer regulate the release of ADH.
- Treatment of DI consists of massive fluid replacement, careful attention to laboratory values, and replacement of essential nutrients as indicated.

Application Exercises

1. A nurse is caring for a client who is having surgery for the removal of an encapsulated acoustic tumor. Which of the following potential complications should the nurse monitor for postoperatively? (Select all that apply.)

   A. Increased intracranial pressure

   B. Hemorrhagic shock

   C. Hydrocephalus

   D. Hypoglycemia

   E. Seizures

2. A nurse is caring for a client who has just undergone a craniotomy for a supratentorial tumor. Which of the following postoperative prescriptions should the nurse clarify with the provider?

   A. Dexamethasone 30 mg IV bolus BID

   B. Morphine sulfate 2 mg IV bolus PRN every 2 hr for pain

   C. Ondansetron 4 mg IV bolus PRN every 4 to 6 hr for nausea

   D. Phenytoin 100 mg IV bolus TID

3. A nurse is completing an assessment of a client who has increased intracranial pressure (ICP). Which of the following are expected findings? (Select all that apply.)

   A. Disoriented to time and place

   B. Restlessness and irritability

   C. Unequal pupils

   D. ICP 15 mm Hg

   E. Headache

4. A nurse is reviewing a prescription for dexamethasone with a client who has an expanding brain tumor. Which of the following are appropriate statements by the nurse? (Select all that apply.)

   A. "It is given to reduce swelling of the brain."

   B. "You will need to monitor for low blood sugar."

   C. "You may notice weight gain."

   D. "Tumor growth will be delayed."

   E. "It can cause you to retain fluids."

5. A nurse is caring for a client who has a benign brain tumor. The client asks the nurse if he can expect this same type of tumor to occur in other areas of his body. Which of the following is an appropriate response by the nurse?

   A. "It can spread to breasts and kidneys."

   B. "It can develop in your gastrointestinal tract."

   C. "It is limited to brain tissue."

   D. "It probably started in another area of your body and spread to your brain."

6. A nurse is reviewing the health record of a client who has a malignant brain tumor and notes the client has a positive Romberg sign. Which of the following actions should the nurse take to assess for this sign?

   A. Stroke the lateral aspect of the sole of the foot.

   B. Ask the client to blink his eyes.

   C. Observe for facial drooping.

   D. Have the client stand erect with eyes closed.

PRACTICE Active Learning Scenario

A nurse is completing preoperative teaching for a client who has a brain tumor and will undergo a craniotomy. What should be included in the teaching? Use the ATI Active Learning Template: Therapeutic Procedure to complete this item.

DESCRIPTION OF PROCEDURE

NURSING INTERVENTIONS: Describe three preoperative and three postoperative interventions.

Application Exercises Key

1. A. **CORRECT:** A client who has had a craniotomy should be monitored postoperatively for increased ICP.

   B. Although hypovolemic shock can occur secondary to SIADH, hemorrhagic shock is not a concern.

   C. **CORRECT:** Following a craniotomy, the client should be monitored for the development of hydrocephalus.

   D. An alteration in glucose metabolism is not usually a postoperative concern after this surgery.

   E. **CORRECT:** Seizures is a postoperative complication that should be monitored following a craniotomy.

   Ⓝ *NCLEX® Connection: Physiological Adaptation, Unexpected Response to Therapies*

2. A. Dexamethasone is given to prevent cerebral edema and has no CNS depressant effects.

   B. **CORRECT:** Narcotic analgesics should be avoided postoperatively due to their CNS depressant effects.

   C. Ondansetron is prescribed to manage nausea and has no CNS depressant effects.

   D. Phenytoin is prescribed to prevent seizures and has no CNS depressant effects.

   Ⓝ *NCLEX® Connection: Pharmacological and Parenteral Therapies, Adverse Effects/Contraindications/Side Effects/Interactions*

3. A. **CORRECT:** Changes in level of consciousness are an early indicator of increased ICP.

   B. **CORRECT:** Increased ICP can cause behavior changes, such as restlessness and irritability.

   C. **CORRECT:** Unequal pupils indicates pressure on the oculomotor nerve secondary to increased ICP.

   D. An ICP of 15 mm Hg is within the expected reference range.

   E. **CORRECT:** A headache is a manifestation of increased ICP.

   Ⓝ *NCLEX® Connection: Physiological Adaptation, Unexpected Response to Therapies*

4. A. **CORRECT:** Dexamethasone is a common steroid prescribed to reduce cerebral edema.

   B. The client can experience hyperglycemia as an adverse effect of dexamethasone.

   C. **CORRECT:** Weight gain is an adverse effect of dexamethasone.

   D. Dexamethasone does not affect tumor growth. It is given to prevent cerebral edema.

   E. **CORRECT:** Fluid retention is an adverse effect of dexamethasone.

   Ⓝ *NCLEX® Connection: Pharmacological and Parenteral Therapies, Medication Administration*

5. A. Metastases of a benign brain tumor do not occur.

   B. Metastases of a benign brain tumor do not occur.

   C. **CORRECT:** Benign brain tumors develop from the meninges or cranial nerves and do not metastasize.

   D. Benign brain tumors develop from the meninges or cranial nerves and are not secondary to other types of tumors.

   Ⓝ *NCLEX® Connection: Physiological Adaptation, Alterations in Body Systems*

6. A. A Babinski sign is elicited by stroking the lateral aspect of the sole of the foot.

   B. Asking the client to blink his eyes assesses cranial nerve function and is not part of the Romberg test.

   C. Observing for facial drooping assesses cranial nerve function and is not part of the Romberg test.

   D. **CORRECT:** A positive Romberg sign is indicated when a client loses his balance while attempting to stand erect with his eyes closed.

   Ⓝ *NCLEX® Connection: Reduction of Risk Potential, Diagnostic Tests*

PRACTICE Answer

Using the ATI Active Learning Template: Therapeutic Procedure

DESCRIPTION OF PROCEDURE: A craniotomy is a surgical opening in the skull to expose brain tissue. It involves a complete or partial resection of the brain tumor.

NURSING INTERVENTIONS

Preoperative
- Explain the procedure, answer appropriate questions, and provide emotional support.
- Provide written explanations.
- Include the client's partner in teaching.
- Remind client to stop taking aspirin at least 72 hr prior to the procedure, if appropriate.
- Review use of alternative/complementary therapies, and report their use to the provider.
- Review the need for a living will and durable power for health care decisions.
- Administer medications (anxiolytics, muscle relaxants) as prescribed.

Postoperative
- Monitor vital signs and neurological status to include use of Glasgow Scale.
- Maintain client's head elevated to 30° and in a neutral position to prevent increased ICP.
- Monitor for postoperative bleeding and seizures.
- Prevent client performing any straining activities (moving up in bed, attempting to have a bowel movement).

Ⓝ *NCLEX® Connection: Reduction of Risk Potential, Therapeutic Procedures*

CHAPTER 10 *Multiple Sclerosis*

Multiple sclerosis (MS) is a neurological disease that typically results in impaired and worsening function of voluntary muscles.

MS is an autoimmune disorder that affects nerve cells in the brain and spinal cord. It is characterized by development of plaque in the white matter of the central nervous system (CNS). This plaque damages the myelin sheath and interferes with impulse transmission between the CNS and the body.

MS follows several possible courses. The most common is relapsing and remitting. The disease is marked by relapses and remissions that might not return the client to his or her previous baseline level of function. Over time, the client can eventually progress to the point of quadriplegia.

MS is a chronic disease with no known cure that progresses in severity over time. Initial findings can be so vague that diagnosis is not made for several years.

Some forms of MS are aggressive and can shorten the lifespan. In most cases, life expectancy is not adversely affected by this disease.

ASSESSMENT

RISK FACTORS

- The onset of MS is typically between 20 and 40 years of age. MS occurs twice as often in women. The etiology of MS is unknown. There is a family history (first-degree relative) of MS in many cases.
- Research shows association with the interleukin (IL)-7 and IL-2 receptor genes.
- Because MS is an autoimmune disease, there are factors that trigger relapses.
  - Viruses and infectious agents
  - Living in a cold climate
  - Physical injury
  - Emotional stress
  - Pregnancy
  - Fatigue
  - Overexertion
  - Temperature extremes
  - Hot shower/bath

EXPECTED FINDINGS

- Fatigue, especially of the lower extremities
- Pain or paresthesia
- Diplopia, changes in peripheral vision, decreased visual acuity
- Uhthoff's sign (a temporary worsening of vision and other neurological functions commonly seen in clients who have or are predisposed to MS, just after exertion or in situations where they are exposed to heat)
- Tinnitus, vertigo, decreased hearing acuity
- Dysphagia
- Dysarthria (slurred and nasal speech)
- Muscle spasticity
- Ataxia or muscle weakness
- Nystagmus
- Bowel dysfunction (constipation, fecal incontinence)
- Bladder dysfunction (areflexia, urgency, nocturia)
- Cognitive changes (memory loss, impaired judgment)
- Sexual dysfunction

LABORATORY TESTS

Cerebrospinal fluid analysis reveals elevated protein level and a slight increase in WBCs.

DIAGNOSTIC PROCEDURES

Magnetic resonance imaging (MRI) reveals plaques of the brain and spine, which is most diagnostic.

PATIENT-CENTERED CARE

NURSING CARE

- Monitoring of
  - Visual acuity
  - Speech patterns: fatigue with talking
  - Swallowing
  - Activity tolerance
  - Skin integrity
- MS is a potentially debilitating condition. Discuss coping mechanisms and sources of support (family, friends, spiritual figures, support groups).
- Encourage fluid intake and other measures to decrease the risk of developing a urinary tract infection. Assist the client with bladder elimination: intermittent self-catheterization, bladder pacemaker, Credé's maneuver (placing manual pressure on abdomen over the bladder to expel urine).
- Monitor cognitive changes and plan interventions to promote cognitive function. (Reorient the client. Place objects used daily in routine places.)
- Facilitate effective communication for dysarthria using a communication board.
- Apply eye patches to treat diplopia. Alternate between eyes every few hours. Teach scanning techniques. Instruct the client to visually scan his environment by moving his head from side to side.
- Exercise and stretch involved muscles. (Avoid fatigue and overheating.)
- Promote energy conservation by grouping care and planning rest periods.
- Promote and maintain safe home and hospital environment to reduce the risk of injury (walking with wide base of support, assistive devices, skin precautions). Qs

MEDICATIONS

Azathioprine and cyclosporine

Immunosuppressive agents are used to reduce the frequency of relapses.

NURSING CONSIDERATIONS
- Monitor for long-term effects.
- Be alert for manifestations of infection.
- Assess for hypertension.
- Assess for kidney dysfunction.

Prednisone

- Corticosteroids are used to reduce inflammation in acute exacerbations.
- NURSING CONSIDERATIONS: Monitor for increased risk of infection, hypervolemia, hypernatremia, hypokalemia, hyperglycemia, gastrointestinal bleeding, and personality changes.

Dantrolene, tizanidine, baclofen, and diazepam

- Antispasmodics are used to treat muscle spasticity.
- Intrathecal baclofen can be used for severe cases of MS.

NURSING CONSIDERATIONS
- Observe for increased weakness.
- Monitor for liver damage with tizanidine or dantrolene.

CLIENT EDUCATION
- Report increased weakness and jaundice to the provider.
- Avoid stopping baclofen abruptly.

Interferon beta

Immunomodulators are used to prevent or treat relapses.

Carbamazepine

Anticonvulsants are used for paresthesia.

Docusate sodium

Stool softeners are used for constipation.

Propantheline

Anticholinergics are used for bladder dysfunction.

Propranolol and clonazepam

A beta blocker and a benzodiazepine used for tremors.

INTERPROFESSIONAL CARE

- Plan for disease progression. Provide community resources and respite services for the client and family.
- Consider referral to occupational and physical therapy for home environment assessment to determine safety and ease of mobility. Use adaptive devices to assist with activities of daily living.
- Refer to speech language therapist for dysarthria and dysphagia.
- Emphasize need to avoid overexertion, stress, extremes of temperatures, humidity, and people who have infections.

Application Exercises

1. A nurse is caring for a client who has multiple sclerosis. Which of the following findings should the nurse expect?

   A. Fluctuations in blood pressure

   B. Loss of cognitive function

   C. Ineffective cough

   D. Drooping eye lids

2. A nurse is beginning a physical assessment of a client who has a new diagnosis of multiple sclerosis. Which of the following findings should the nurse expect? (Select all that apply.)

   A. Areas of paresthesia

   B. Involuntary eye movements

   C. Alopecia

   D. Increased salivation

   E. Ataxia

3. A nurse is teaching a client who has multiple sclerosis and a new prescription for baclofen. Which of the following statements should the nurse include in the teaching?

   A. "This medication will help you with your tremors."

   B. "This medication will help you with your bladder function."

   C. "This medication may cause your skin to bruise easily."

   D. "This medication may cause you to experience weakness."

PRACTICE Active Learning Scenario

A nurse is providing education to family members of a client who has a new diagnosis of multiple sclerosis. What should be included in the teaching? Use the ATI Active Learning Template: System Disorder to complete this item.

ALTERATION IN HEALTH (DIAGNOSIS)

LABORATORY TESTS

DIAGNOSTIC PROCEDURES

MEDICATIONS: Describe four medications and one teaching point for each.

Application Exercises Key

1. A. Fluctuations in blood pressure is a manifestation associated with amyotrophic lateral sclerosis.

   B. **CORRECT:** Loss of cognitive function is a manifestation associated with MS.

   C. Ineffective cough is a manifestation associated with amyotrophic lateral sclerosis.

   D. Drooping eyelids is a manifestation associated with myasthenia gravis.

   Ⓝ *NCLEX® Connection: Physiological Adaptation, Alterations in Body Systems*

2. A. **CORRECT:** Areas of loss of skin sensation are a finding in a client who has MS.

   B. **CORRECT:** Nystagmus is a finding in a client who has MS.

   C. Hair loss is not a finding in a client who has MS.

   D. Dysphagia, swallowing difficulty, is a finding in a client who has MS.

   E. **CORRECT:** Ataxia occurs in the client who has MS as muscle weakness develops and there is loss of coordination.

   Ⓝ *NCLEX® Connection: Pharmacological and Parenteral Therapies, Adverse Effects/Contraindications/Side Effects/Interactions*

3. A. Propranolol is a beta blocker and clonazepam is a benzodiazepine given to clients who have MS to treat tremors.

   B. Propantheline is an anticholinergic medication that is given to clients who have MS to treat bladder dysfunction.

   C. Prednisone is a corticosteroid medication that is given to clients who have MS to treat inflammation. An adverse effect of this medication is bruising of the skin.

   D. **CORRECT:** Baclofen is an antispasmodic medication that is given to clients who have MS to treat muscle spasms. An adverse effect of this medication is weakness, as well as dizziness. The nurse should instruct the client to monitor for these findings, as they can lead to impaired safety. The client should be instructed not to discontinue baclofen abruptly.

   Ⓝ *NCLEX® Connection: Physiological Adaptation, Pathophysiology*

PRACTICE Answer

Using the ATI Active Learning Template: System Disorder

ALTERATION IN HEALTH (DIAGNOSIS): MS is an autoimmune disorder characterized by the development of plaque in the white matter of the central nervous system. Plaque damages the myelin sheath and interferes with impulse transmission between the CNS and the body.

LABORATORY TESTS:
Cerebrospinal fluid analysis

DIAGNOSTIC PROCEDURES:
MRI of the brain and spine

MEDICATIONS
- Immunosuppressive agents such as azathioprine and cyclosporine: Long-term effects include increased risk for infection, hypertension, and kidney dysfunction.
- Corticosteroids such as prednisone: Increased risk for infection, hypervolemia, hypernatremia, hypokalemia, GI bleeding, and personality changes.
- Antispasmodics such as dantrolene, tizanidine, baclofen, and diazepam are used to treat muscle spasticity. Report increased weakness and jaundice to provider. Avoid stopping baclofen abruptly.
- Immunomodulators such as interferon beta are used to prevent and treat relapses.
- Anticonvulsants such as carbamazepine are used for paresthesia.
- Stool softeners such as docusate sodium are used for constipation.
- Anticholinergics such as propantheline are used for bladder dysfunction.
- Propranolol and clonazepam, a beta blocker and a benzodiazepine, are used for tremors.

Ⓝ *NCLEX® Connection: Physiological Adaptation, Alterations in Body Systems*

UNIT 2   NURSING CARE OF CLIENTS WHO HAVE
NEUROSENSORY DISORDERS
SECTION: CENTRAL NERVOUS SYSTEM DISORDERS

CHAPTER 11 *Headaches*

Headaches can be acute or chronic, temporary, or life-threatening.

Headaches are a common occurrence and affect individuals of all ages. Headaches are associated with other conditions such as colds, allergies, and stress or muscle tension.

Primary headaches have no identifiable organic cause. They include migraine headaches, tension-like, and cluster headaches. They can be managed in the primary care setting.

Secondary headaches are associated with an organic cause, such as a brain tumor or aneurysm, and warrant further investigation and medical management.

This chapter includes migraine headaches and cluster headaches.

HEALTH PROMOTION AND DISEASE PREVENTION

- Promote stress management strategies and recognition of triggers of the onset of a headache.
- Recommend use of a headache diary to help identify type of headache and response to interventions.
- Promote hand hygiene to prevent the spread of viruses that produce cold-like symptoms.
- Review pain management to include over-the-counter medications and herbal remedies.
- Review risk factors (triggers) for both migraine and cluster headaches.
  ○ Alcohol or environmental allergies
  ○ Intense odors, bright lights, overuse of some medications
  ○ Fatigue, sleep deprivation, depression, emotional or physical stress, anxiety
  ○ Menstrual cycles and oral contraceptive use
  ○ Foods containing tyramine, monosodium glutamate (MSG), nitrites, or milk products

Migraine headaches

ASSESSMENT

EXPECTED FINDINGS

- Photophobia and phonophobia (sensitivity to sounds)
- Nausea and vomiting
- Stress and anxiety
- Unilateral pain, often behind one eye or ear
- Health history and family history for headache patterns
- Alterations in ADLs for 4 to 72 hr
- Manifestations that are similar with each headache

Classified by categories and stages

With aura (classic migraine)
- Prodromal stage includes awareness of findings for hours to days before onset: irritability, depression, food cravings, diarrhea/constipation, and frequent urination.
- Aura stage develops over minutes to an hour to include neurologic findings: numbness and tingling of mouth, lips, face, or hands; acute confusional state; visual disturbances (light flashes, bright spots).
- Second stage: severe, incapacitating, throbbing headache that intensifies over several hours and is accompanied by nausea, vomiting, drowsiness, and vertigo.
- Third stage (4 to 72 hr): headache is dull. Older adults can continue with aura, and pain subsides (visual migraine).
- Recovery with pain and aura subsiding. Muscle aches and contraction of head and neck muscles are common. Physical activity worsens pain, and client might sleep.

Without aura (common migraine)
- Pain is aggravated by physical activity.
- Unilateral, pulsating pain.
- One or more manifestations present: photophobia, phonophobia, nausea, and/or vomiting.
- Persists for 4 to 72 hr. Often occurs in early morning, during periods of stress, or with premenstrual tension or fluid retention.

Atypical
- Status migrainous: Headache lasts longer than 72 hr.
- Migrainous infarction: Neurologic manifestations persist for 7 days; neuroimaging can indicate ischemic infarct.
- Unclassified: Does not fit other criteria.

DIAGNOSTIC PROCEDURES

Neuroimaging if neurologic findings present or client is older with a new onset of headaches.

PATIENT-CENTERED CARE

Nursing care focus during headache is pain management.
- Maintain a cool, dark, quiet environment.
- Elevate the head of the bed to 30°.
- Administer medications as prescribed.

MEDICATIONS

- **Abortive therapy** to alleviate pain during aura or soon after start of headache
  - For mild migraines: NSAIDs (ibuprofen, naproxen), acetaminophen, and over-the-counter anti-inflammatory medications in formulations for migraines
  - Antiemetics (metoclopramide) to relieve nausea and vomiting.
  - Severe migraines
    - Triptan preparations (zolmitriptan sumatriptan, eletriptan) to produce a vasoconstrictive effect
    - Ergotamine preparations with caffeine (dihydroergotamine) to narrow blood vessels and reduce inflammation
    - Isometheptene in combination formulations when other medications do not work
- **Preventive therapy** for frequent headaches or when other therapies are ineffective
  - NSAIDs with beta-blocker (propranolol), calcium channel blocker, beta-adrenergic blocker or antiepileptic medications (divalproex, topiramate).
  - Client is instructed to check pulse when taking beta-adrenergic blockers and calcium channel blockers.
  - OnabotulinumtoxinA is approved for adults for chronic migraines. Injected into specific areas of the head and neck up to five treatment cycles.

CLIENT EDUCATION

- Keep a diary to record headache patterns and triggers.
- Report changes in headache intensity, or new visual or neurological disturbances.
- Remain in a cool, dark, quiet environment.
- Elevate the head of the bed as desired.
- Educate women over age 50 about risk factors for cardiovascular disease and stroke. Ⓖ
- Review trigger avoidance and management. Qᴘᴄᴄ
  - Educate about foods with tyramine (pickles, caffeine, beer, wine, aged cheese, artificial sweeteners) and foods with MSG or preservatives.
  - Review current medications for those known to induce migraines: ranitidine, estrogen, nitroglycerin, and nifedipine.
  - Discuss anger issues and handling conflict.
  - Reinforce the need for adequate rest and sleep.
  - Review travel involving a change in altitude.
  - Reinforce the need to avoid light glare or flickering lights.
  - Review the client's menstrual cycle pattern and hormone fluctuations.
  - Discuss avoiding intense environmental odors, perfumes, and tobacco smoke.

- Educate the client about complementary and alternative therapies. Qᴘᴄᴄ
  - Provide referral to community centers offering yoga, meditation, tai chi, exercise, biofeedback, and massage for relaxation and to alleviate muscle tension.
  - Provide referral to acupuncture and acupressure therapy, which can be helpful for pain management.
  - Herbal remedies and nutrition supplements should be reviewed with the provider because there is insufficient evidence to support their use in management of migraines. Qᴇʙᴘ

Cluster headaches

ASSESSMENT

EXPECTED FINDINGS

- Brief episode of intense, unilateral, nonthrobbing pain lasting 30 min to 2 hr that can radiate to forehead, temple, or cheek
  - Occurring daily at about the same time for 4 to 12 weeks
  - Followed by period of remission for up to 9 to 12 months
- More frequent during spring and fall
- No warning signs
- Less common than migraines
- Men between 20 to 50 years of age
- Tearing of the eye with runny nose and nasal congestion
- Facial sweating
- Drooping eyelid and eyelid edema
- Miosis (pupil constriction)
- Facial pallor or flushing
- Bradycardia
- Nausea and vomiting
- Pacing, walking, or sitting and rocking activities

PATIENT-CENTERED CARE

MEDICATIONS

(See medications for migraine headaches.)
- Triptans
- Ergotamine preparations
- Antiepileptic medications
- Calcium channel blockers
- Corticosteroids
- Over-the-counter capsaicin
- Melatonin
- Glucosamine

THERAPEUTIC PROCEDURES

Home oxygen therapy at 12 L/min for 15 to 20 min at onset of headache can provide relief within 15 min.

CLIENT EDUCATION

- Remain in a cool, dark, quiet environment with head elevated.
- Remain in sitting position when using oxygen, and maintain safety precautions when using oxygen in the home. Qs
- Review prevention strategies.
  - Wear sunglasses to reduce light and glare.
  - Obtain adequate rest and sleep, exercise, and relaxation.
- Review use of complementary and alternative therapies to promote relaxation.
- Avoid foods containing tyramine, MSG, and nitrites (preservatives).
- Review of risk factors (triggers) for headaches.
  - Anger outburst
  - Anxiety and prolonged anticipation, or periods of stress
  - Excessive physical activity, fatigue
  - Altered sleep–wake cycles

> ### PRACTICE Active Learning Scenario
>
> A nurse in a clinic is caring for a client who has migraine headaches and a new prescription for sumatriptan nasal spray 5 mg. Using the ATI Active Learning Template: Medication and the ATI Pharmacology Review Module to complete this item.
>
> EXPECTED PHARMACOLOGICAL ACTION
>
> THERAPEUTIC USES
>
> COMPLICATIONS
>
> NURSING INTERVENTIONS
>
> INTERACTIONS
>
> CLIENT EDUCATION
>
> MEDICATION ADMINISTRATION
>
> EVALUATION OF MEDICATION EFFECTIVENESS

Application Exercises

1. A nurse in a clinic is caring for a client who has frequent migraine headaches. The client asks about foods that can cause headaches. The nurse should recommend that the client avoid which of the following foods?

   A. Baked salmon

   B. Salted cashews

   C. Frozen strawberries

   D. Fresh asparagus

2. A nurse in a clinic is teaching a client who has a history of migraine headaches about a new prescription for zolmitriptan. Which of the following statements by the client indicates understanding of the teaching?

   A. "This medication will relieve my symptoms by causing my blood vessels to dilate."

   B. "I should take this medication daily to prevent the headache from occurring."

   C. "I should expect facial flushing when I take this medication."

   D. "This medication will lower my sensitivity to food triggers."

3. A nurse in a provider's office is obtaining a health history from a client who has cluster headaches. Which of the following are expected findings? (Select all that apply.)

   A. Pain is bilateral across the posterior occipital area.

   B. Client experiences altered sleep-wake cycle.

   C. Headache occurs at approximately the same time of the day.

   D. Client describes headache pain as dull and throbbing.

   E. Nasal congestion and drainage occur.

4. A nurse is providing discharge instructions to a client who has a new diagnosis of migraine headaches. Which of the following instructions should the nurse include?

   A. Use music therapy for relaxation with the onset of the headache.

   B. Increase physical activity when a headache is present.

   C. Drink beverages that contain artificial sweeteners to prevent headaches.

   D. Apply a cool cloth to the face during a headache.

5. A nurse is obtaining a health history from a client who is being evaluated for the cause of frequent headaches. Which of the following questions should the nurse ask to identify the findings of migraine headaches?

   A. "Do the headaches occur at the same time each day?"

   B. "Is your headache accompanied by profuse facial sweating?"

   C. "Does your headache occur on one side of your head?"

   D. "Is there a pattern of headaches among family members?"

Application Exercises Key

1. A. The client should avoid fish that is smoked because it contains tyramine. Baked salmon does not contain tyramine and is not a trigger for migraine headaches.

   B. **CORRECT:** Nuts contain tyramine, which can trigger migraine headaches.

   C. Fruits are not a source of tyramine.

   D. Vegetables are not a source of tyramine.

   Ⓝ *NCLEX® Connection: Basic Care and Comfort, Nutrition and Oral Hydration*

2. A. Zolmitriptan causes cranial arteries, the basilar arteries, and blood vessels in the dura mater to constrict.

   B. Zolmitriptan is used for abortive therapy in treating migraine headaches. It is not used for headache prevention.

   C. **CORRECT:** Zolmitriptan can cause facial flushing, tingling, and warmth.

   D. Zolmitriptan is used as a component of abortive therapy for treatment of migraine headaches and does not affect a client's sensitivity to food triggers.

   Ⓝ *NCLEX® Connection: Pharmacological and Parenteral Therapies, Medication Administration*

3. A. Cluster headaches typically cause pain on one side of the head and radiate to the forehead, temple, or cheek.

   B. **CORRECT:** Cluster headaches can be due to a lack of continuity in the sleep-wake cycle.

   C. **CORRECT:** Cluster headaches occur at about the same time of day for 4 to 12 weeks.

   D. Cluster headaches are described as unilateral, intense, and nonthrobbing.

   E. **CORRECT:** A client can have a runny nose and nasal congestion with a cluster headache.

   Ⓝ *NCLEX® Connection: Physiological Adaptation, Pathophysiology*

4. A. A quiet, dark environment can provide comfort during a migraine headache.

   B. Increasing physical activity during a migraine headache can worsen the pain.

   C. Artificial sweeteners contain tyramine, which can trigger a migraine headache.

   D. **CORRECT:** A cool cloth placed over the client's eyes provides comfort and can relieve pain.

   Ⓝ *NCLEX® Connection: Basic Care and Comfort, Non-Pharmacological Comfort Interventions*

5. A. Cluster headaches typically occur at the same time each day.

   B. Profuse facial sweating is typical in the presence of cluster headaches.

   C. Unilateral headaches are associated with cluster headaches.

   D. **CORRECT:** A familial pattern of headaches is a common finding with migraines.

   Ⓝ *NCLEX® Connection: Health Promotion and Maintenance, Health Promotion/Disease Prevention*

PRACTICE Answer

Using the ATI Active Learning Template: Medication

EXPECTED PHARMACOLOGICAL ACTION: Vasoconstriction of cranial carotid arteries

THERAPEUTIC USES: Abortive treatment of acute migraine attacks with or without aura and cluster headaches

COMPLICATIONS: Chest pressure and tightness; mild vertigo, malaise, fatigue and tingling sensations; coronary vasospasm (rare)

NURSING INTERVENTIONS: Report chest pressure and tightness to provider if does not resolve quickly. Do not take medication during pregnancy or if trying to become pregnant, as medication can have teratogenic effects.

INTERACTIONS: Do not use concurrent with ergot alkaloids, monoamine oxidase inhibitors, selective serotonin reuptake inhibitors, or serotonin/norepinephrine reuptake inhibitors.

CLIENT EDUCATION: Avoid use of St. John's wort when taking this medication.

MEDICATION ADMINISTRATION: Administer one unit-dose nasal spray in one nostril. May be repeated in 2 hr if headache remains but not to exceed 40 mg in 24 hr.

EVALUATION OF MEDICATION EFFECTIVENESS: Relief of headache pain should be noted within 15 min after administration, with complete relief anticipated within 2 hr. Relief of photophobia, phonophobia, nausea and vomiting associated with migraine attack.

Ⓝ *NCLEX® Connection: Pharmacological and Parenteral Therapies, Adverse Effects/Contraindications/Side Effects/Interactions*

CHAPTER 12   Disorders of the Eye

Disorders of the eye can be caused by injury, disease processes, and the aging process.

Disorders of the eye that nurses should be knowledgeable about include macular degeneration, cataracts, and glaucoma.

Macular degeneration

Macular degeneration, often called age-related macular degeneration (AMD), is the central loss of vision that affects the macula of the eye.
- There is no cure for macular degeneration.
- AMD is a common cause of vision loss in older adults. ⓒ

Two types of macular degeneration

Dry macular degeneration is the most common and is caused by a gradual blockage in retinal capillary arteries, which results in the macula becoming ischemic and necrotic due to the lack of retinal cells.

Wet macular degeneration is a less common form and is caused by the new growth of blood vessels that have thin walls that leak blood and fluid.

ASSESSMENT

RISK FACTORS

Dry macular degeneration
- Smoking
- Hypertension
- Female
- Short body stature
- Family history
- Diet lacking carotene and vitamin E

Wet macular degeneration can occur at any age

EXPECTED FINDINGS

- Lack of depth perception
- Objects appear distorted
- Blurred vision
- Loss of central vision
- Blindness

DIAGNOSTIC PROCEDURES

Ophthalmoscopy: An ophthalmoscope is used to examine the back part of the eyeball (fundus), including the retina, optic disc, macula, and blood vessels.

Visual acuity tests: Snellen and Rosenbaum eye charts.

PATIENT-CENTERED CARE

Wet macular degeneration

- Laser therapy to seal leaking blood vessels
- Ocular injections to inhibit blood vessel growth

CLIENT EDUCATION
- Encourage clients to consume foods high in antioxidants, carotene, and vitamins E and B_{12}. The provider may prescribe a daily supplement high in carotene and vitamin E. Qpcc
- As loss of vision progresses, clients will be challenged with the ability to eat, drive, write, and read, as well as other activities of daily living.
- Refer clients to community organizations that can assist with transportation, reading devices, and large-print books.

Cataracts

A cataract is an opacity in the lens of an eye that impairs vision. **(12.1)**

Common causes of cataracts

Age-related: Drying of lens due to water loss; increase in lens density due to lens fiber compaction

Traumatic: Blunt or penetrating injury or foreign body in the eye, exposure to radiation or ultra violet light

Toxic: Long term use of corticosteroids, phenothiazine derivatives, beta blockers, or miotic medications

Associated: Diabetes mellitus, hypoparathyroidism, down syndrome, chronic sunlight exposure

Complicated: Intraocular disease such as retinitis pigmentosa, glaucoma, or retinal detachment

HEALTH PROMOTION AND DISEASE PREVENTION

- Teach clients to wear sunglasses while outside.
- Educate clients to wear protective eyewear while playing sports and performing hazardous activities, such as welding and yard work. Qs
- Encourage annual eye examinations and good eye health, especially in adults over the age of 40. ⓒ

ASSESSMENT

RISK FACTORS

- Advanced age Ⓖ
- Diabetes
- Heredity
- Smoking
- Eye trauma
- Excessive exposure to the sun
- Chronic corticosteroid use

EXPECTED FINDINGS

- Decreased visual acuity (prescription changes, reduced night vision, decreased color perception)
- Blurred vision
- Diplopia (double vision)

PHYSICAL ASSESSMENT FINDINGS
- Progressive and painless loss of vision
- Visible opacity
- Absent red reflex

DIAGNOSTIC PROCEDURES

Cataracts can be determined upon examination of the lens using an ophthalmoscope.

PATIENT-CENTERED CARE

NURSING CARE

- Check visual acuity using the Snellen chart.
- Examine external and internal eye structures using an ophthalmoscope.
- Determine the client's functional capacity due to decreased vision.
- Increase the amount of light in a room. Qs
- Provide adaptive devices that accommodate for reduced vision.
  - Magnifying lens and large print books/newspapers
  - Talking devices, such as clocks

MEDICATIONS

Anticholinergic agents (atropine 1% ophthalmic solution): This medication prevents pupil constriction for prolonged periods of time (mydriasis) and relaxes muscles in the eye (cycloplegia). It is used to dilate the eye preoperatively and for visualization of the eye's internal structures.

NURSING CONSIDERATIONS: The medication has a long duration, but a fast onset.

CLIENT EDUCATION
- Remind the client that the effects of the medication can last 7 to 12 days.
- The medication can cause photosensitivity, so remind the client to wear sunglasses to protect the eyes. Qpcc

INTERPROFESSIONAL CARE

Consult with an ophthalmologist (eye surgeon) for cataract surgery.

THERAPEUTIC PROCEDURES

Surgical removal of the lens

A small incision is made, and the lens is either removed in one piece, or in several pieces, after being broken up using sound waves. The posterior capsule is retained. A replacement or intraocular lens is inserted. Replacement lenses can correct refractive errors, resulting in improved vision.

NURSING ACTIONS
Postoperative care should focus on:
- Preventing an increase in intraocular pressure.
- Preventing infection.
- Administering ophthalmic medications.
- Providing pain relief.
- Teaching the client about self-care at home and fall prevention. Qs

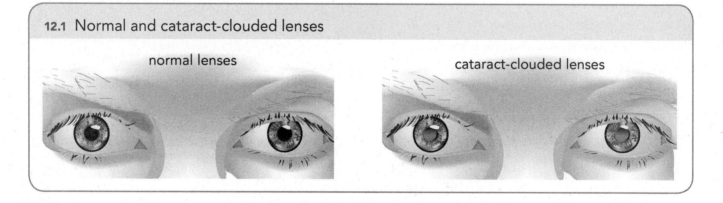

12.1 Normal and cataract-clouded lenses

normal lenses

cataract-clouded lenses

CLIENT EDUCATION
- Wear sunglasses while outside or in brightly lit areas.
- Report signs of infection, such as yellow or green drainage.
- Avoid activities that increase IOP.
  - Bending over at the waist
  - Sneezing
  - Coughing
  - Straining
  - Head hyperflexion
  - Restrictive clothing, such as tight shirt collars
  - Sexual intercourse
- Limit activities.
  - Tilting the head back to wash hair
  - Cooking and housekeeping
  - Rapid, jerky movements, such as vacuuming
  - Driving and operating machinery
  - Playing sports
- Report pain with nausea/vomiting (indications of increased IOP or hemorrhage).
- Best vision is not expected until 4 to 6 weeks following the surgery.
- The client should report if any changes occur, such as lid swelling, decreased vision, bleeding or discharge, sharp sudden eye pain, flashes of light, or floating shapes.

COMPLICATIONS

Infection

- Infection can occur after surgery.
- CLIENT EDUCATION: Manifestations of infection that the client should report include yellow or green drainage, increased redness or pain, reduction in visual acuity, increased tear production, and photophobia. Qᴘᴄᴄ

Bleeding

Bleeding is a potential risk several days following surgery.

CLIENT EDUCATION: Clients should immediately report any sudden change in visual acuity or an increase in pain. Qᴘᴄᴄ

Glaucoma

Glaucoma is a disturbance of the functional or structural integrity of the optic nerve. Decreased fluid drainage or increased fluid secretion increases intraocular pressure (IOP) and can cause atrophic changes of the optic nerve and visual defects. The expected reference range for IOP is 10 to 21 mm/Hg.

- There are two primary types of glaucoma.
  - **Primary open-angle glaucoma (POAG):** more common form. Open-angle refers to the angle between the iris and sclera. The aqueous humor outflow is decreased due to blockages in the eye's drainage system (Canal of Schlemm and trabecular meshwork), causing a gradual rise in IOP.
  - **Primary angle-closure glaucoma:** IOP rises suddenly. The angle between the iris and the sclera suddenly closes, causing a corresponding increase in IOP. The onset is sudden and requires immediate treatment.
- Glaucoma is a frequent cause of blindness. Early diagnosis and treatment is essential in preventing vision loss from glaucoma.

HEALTH PROMOTION AND DISEASE PREVENTION

- Encourage annual eye examinations and good eye health, especially adults over the age of 40. Ⓖ
- Educate clients about the disease process and early indications of glaucoma, such as reduced vision and mild eye pain.

ASSESSMENT

RISK FACTORS

- Age
- Infection
- Tumors
- Diabetes mellitus
- Genetic predisposition
- Hypertension
- Eye trauma

EXPECTED FINDINGS

Primary open-angle glaucoma

- Headache
- Mild eye pain
- Loss of peripheral vision
- Decreased accommodation
- Halos seen around lights
- Elevated IOP (greater than 21 mm Hg: usually 22 to 32)

Primary angle-closure glaucoma

- Rapid onset of elevated IOP (30 mm Hg or higher)
- Decreased or blurred vision
- Colored halos seen around lights
- Pupils nonreactive to light
- Severe pain and nausea
- Photophobia

DIAGNOSTIC PROCEDURES

Visual assessments: Measures decrease in visual acuity and peripheral vision

Tonometry: Measures IOP (expected reference range is 10 to 21 mm Hg). IOP is elevated with glaucoma, especially angle-closure.

Gonioscopy: Used to determine the drainage angle of the anterior chamber of the eyes.

PATIENT-CENTERED CARE

NURSING CARE

- Monitor for increased IOP (greater than 21 mm Hg).
- Monitor for decreased vision and light sensitivity.
- Assess for aching or discomfort around the eye.
- Explain the disease process and allow clients to express their feelings.
- Treat severe pain and nausea that accompanies angle-closure glaucoma with analgesics and antiemetics.

MEDICATIONS

The priority intervention for treating glaucoma is medication therapy.

CLIENT TEACHING

- Prescribed eye medication is beneficial if used every 12 hr.
- Instill one drop in each eye twice daily.
- Wait 5 to 10 min between eye drops if more than one is prescribed to prevent one medication from diluting another.
- Avoid touching the tip of the application bottle to the eye.
- Always wash hands before and after use.
- Once eye drop is instilled, apply pressure using the punctal occlusion technique (placing pressure on the inner corner of the eye).

Pilocarpine ophthalmic solution

Pilocarpine is a miotic medication, which constricts the pupil and allows for improved circulation and outflow of the aqueous humor. Miotics can cause blurred vision. Pilocarpine is considered a second-line drug for POAG.

Beta-blockers (timolol)

Beta-blockers are first-line drug therapy for glaucoma, and decrease IOP by reducing aqueous humor production.

NURSING CONSIDERATIONS: Can be absorbed systemically and cause bronchoconstriction and hypoglycemia. Use with caution in clients who have asthma, COPD, and diabetes mellitus. Can potentiate systemic effects of oral beta-blockers and cause bradycardia and hypotension.

Carbonic anhydrase inhibitors (acetazolamide, dorzolamide, and brinzolamide)

Decrease IOP by reducing aqueous humor production.

NURSING CONSIDERATIONS: Ask clients whether they are allergic to sulfa. Carbonic anhydrase inhibitors are sulfa-based.

IV mannitol

IV mannitol is an osmotic diuretic used in the emergency treatment for primary angle-closure glaucoma to quickly decrease IOP.

THERAPEUTIC PROCEDURES

Glaucoma surgery

Laser trabeculectomy, iridotomy, or the placement of a shunt are procedures used to improve the flow of the aqueous humor by opening a channel out of the anterior chamber of the eye.

NURSING ACTIONS: Educate clients about the disease and importance of adhering to the medication schedule to treat IOP.

CLIENT EDUCATION
- Wear sunglasses while outside or in brightly lit areas.
- Report signs of infection, such as yellow or green drainage.
- Avoid activities that increase IOP.
  - Bending over at the waist
  - Sneezing
  - Coughing
  - Straining
  - Head hyperflexion
  - Restrictive clothing, such as tight shirt collars
  - Sexual intercourse
- Clients should not lie on the operative side and should report severe pain or nausea (possible hemorrhage).
- Clients should report if any changes occur, such as lid swelling, decreased vision, bleeding or discharge, a sharp, sudden pain in the eye and/or flashes of light or floating shapes.
- Limit activities.
  - Tilting head back to wash hair
  - Cooking and housekeeping
  - Rapid, jerky movements, such as vacuuming
  - Driving and operating machinery
  - Playing sports
- Report pain with nausea/vomiting (indications of increased IOP or hemorrhage).
- Final best vision is not expected until 4 to 6 weeks after surgery.

INTERPROFESSIONAL CARE

Refer to an ophthalmologist if surgery is necessary.

CLIENT EDUCATION

Set up services such as community outreach programs, meals on wheels, and services for the blind. Qs

COMPLICATIONS

Blindness

Blindness is a potential consequence of untreated glaucoma.

CLIENT EDUCATION: Encourage adults 40 or older to have an annual examination, including a measurement of IOP. ©

Application Exercises

1. A nurse is caring for an older adult client who has diabetes mellitus and reports a gradual loss of peripheral vision. The nurse should recognize this as a manifestation of which of the following diseases?

   A. Cataracts

   B. Open-angle glaucoma

   C. Macular degeneration

   D. Angle-closure glaucoma

2. A nurse is providing postoperative teaching to a client following cataract surgery. Which of the following statements should the nurse include in the teaching?

   A. "You can resume playing golf in 2 days."

   B. "You need to tilt your head back when washing your hair."

   C. "You can get water in your eyes in 1 day."

   D. "You need to limit your housekeeping activities."

3. A nurse is caring for a male older adult client who has a new diagnosis of glaucoma. Which of the following should the nurse recognize as risk factors associated with this disease? (Select all that apply.)

   A. Gender

   B. Genetic predisposition

   C. Hypertension

   D. Age

   E. Diabetes mellitus

4. A nurse is caring for a client who has a new diagnosis of cataracts. Which of the following manifestations should the nurse expect? (Select all that apply.)

   A. Eye pain

   B. Floating spots

   C. Blurred vision

   D. White pupils

   E. Bilateral red reflexes

5. A nurse is providing teaching for a client who has a new diagnosis of dry macular degeneration. Which of the following instructions should the nurse include in the teaching?

   A. Increase intake of deep yellow and orange vegetables.

   B. Administer eye drops twice daily.

   C. Avoid bending at the waist.

   D. Wear an eye patch at night.

Application Exercises Key

1. A. A client who has cataracts experiences a decrease in peripheral and central vision due to opacity of the lens.

   B. **CORRECT:** This is a manifestation of open-angle glaucoma. A gradual loss of peripheral vision is a manifestation associated with this diagnosis.

   C. A client who has macular degeneration experiences a loss of central vision.

   D. A client who has angle-closure glaucoma experiences sudden nausea and severe pain and halos around lights.

   Ⓝ *NCLEX® Connection: Health Promotion and Maintenance, Health Screening*

2. A. The nurse should not instruct the client to resume playing golf for several weeks. This could cause a rise in intraocular pressure (IOP) or possible injury to the eye.

   B. The nurse should not instruct the client to tilt his head back when washing his hair. This could cause a rise in IOP or possible injury to the eye.

   C. The client should not get water in his eyes for 3 to 7 days following cataract surgery to reduce the risk for infection and promote healing.

   D. **CORRECT:** The nurse should instruct the client to limit housekeeping activities following cataract surgery. This activity could cause a rise in IOP or injury to the eye.

   Ⓝ *NCLEX® Connection: Reduction of Risk Potential, Therapeutic Procedures*

3. A. Gender is not a risk factor associated with glaucoma.

   B. **CORRECT:** Genetic predisposition is a risk factor associated with glaucoma.

   C. **CORRECT:** Hypertension is a risk factor associated with glaucoma.

   D. **CORRECT:** Age is a risk factor associated with glaucoma.

   E. **CORRECT:** Diabetes mellitus is a risk factor associated with glaucoma.

   Ⓝ *NCLEX® Connection: Health Promotion and Maintenance, Health Promotion/Disease Prevention*

4. A. Eye pain is manifestation associated with primary angle-closure glaucoma.

   B. Floating spots are a manifestation associated with retinal detachment.

   C. **CORRECT:** Blurred vision is a manifestation associated with cataracts.

   D. **CORRECT:** White pupils are a manifestation associated with cataracts.

   E. Bilateral red reflexes are absent in a client who has cataracts.

   Ⓝ *NCLEX® Connection: Physiological Adaptation, Pathophysiology*

5. A. **CORRECT:** The nurse should instruct the client to increase dietary intake of carotenoids and antioxidants to slow the progression of the macular degeneration.

   B. A client who has primary open-angle glaucoma should administer eye drops twice daily.

   C. A client who is at risk for increased intraocular pressure, such as following cataract surgery, should avoid bending at the waist.

   D. A client who has had eye surgery, such as cataract surgery, should wear an eye patch at night to protect the eye from injury.

   Ⓝ *NCLEX® Connection: Physiological Adaptation, Unexpected Response to Therapies*

PRACTICE Answer

Using ATI Active Learning Template: Medication

COMPLICATIONS

- CNS: Lethargy, fatigue, anxiety, headache, somnolence, depression
- CV: Bradycardia, palpitations, syncope, hypotension, AV conduction disturbances, CHF
- Specific senses: Eye stinging, tearing, photophobia, eye irritation
- GI: Nausea, dry mouth
- Respiratory: Difficulty breathing, bronchospasm
- Metabolic: Hypoglycemia

Ⓝ *NCLEX® Connection: Pharmacological and Parenteral Therapies, Adverse Effects/Contraindications/Side Effects/Interactions*

UNIT 2   NURSING CARE OF CLIENTS WHO HAVE NEUROSENSORY DISORDERS
SECTION: SENSORY DISORDERS

CHAPTER 13   *Middle and Inner Ear Disorders*

The ear is a sensory organ with two functions: hearing and balance.

The middle ear consists of the tympanic membrane (eardrum) and the three smallest bones (ossicles) of the body (malleus, incus, and stapes), and connects to the nasopharynx via the Eustachian tube.

The inner ear is located deep within the temporal bone, separated from the middle ear by the oval window. It consists of the cochlea (hearing organ) and semicircular canals (responsible for balance). Cranial nerves VII (facial nerve) and VIII (vestibulocochlear nerve) are part of the inner ear anatomy.

Visual, vestibular, and proprioceptive systems provide the brain with input regarding balance. Problems within any of these systems pose a risk for loss of balance. Qs

Nurses should be knowledgeable about the types of middle- and inner-ear disorders, including infection, tumors, and issues with balance and coordination.

TYPES OF EAR DISORDERS

Hearing loss

- Environmental or workplace exposure to noise can lead to hearing loss.
- Conductive hearing loss is caused by factors such as otitis media, otosclerosis, and presence of a foreign body (such as impacted cerumen).
- Color of cerumen and external ear canal varies depending on client's race and skin tone. Normal variations should be recognized during assessment. Qpcc
- Sensorineural hearing loss is caused by damage to cranial nerve VIII.
- Combined hearing loss is caused by a mixture of conductive and sensorineural problems.
- Changes in the middle and inner ear related to aging include thickening of the tympanic membrane (loss of elasticity), loss of sensory hair cells in the organ of Corti, and limitations to movement of the ossicles. Ⓖ

Conditions of the middle ear

- Conditions of the middle ear can be caused by injury, disease, and the aging process.
- Acute otitis media is a viral or bacterial infection of the middle ear.
- Manifestations include ear pain, pressure, fever, headache, conductive hearing loss, and purulent or bloody drainage if perforation of the eardrum occurs.
- Otoscopic exam can show redness, bulging tympanic membrane, and inability to visualize usual landmarks.
- Medical management includes systemic antibiotic therapy, analgesics and application of heat for pain, and decongestants.
- Surgical management includes myringotomy and placement of a grommet to equalize pressure.
- Refer to **RN NURSING CARE OF CHILDREN REVIEW MODULE: CHAPTER 37: ACUTE OTITIS MEDIA**.

Conditions of the inner ear

- Vertigo occurs when the client has the sensation that he or his surroundings are in motion.
- Benign paroxysmal positional vertigo occurs in response to a change in position. It is thought to be caused by the disruption of the debris located within the semicircular canal (small crystals of calcium carbonate). Onset is sudden and can last for a few weeks or years. Bed rest is prescribed along with short course of meclizine.
- Ménière's disease is characterized by episodic vertigo, tinnitus (ringing in the ears), and fluctuating sensorineural hearing loss.
- Labyrinthitis is an inflammation of the labyrinth in the inner ear, often secondary to otitis media. It is characterized by the sudden onset of severe vertigo, nausea, vomiting, and possible hearing loss and tinnitus. Manifestations are treated with bed rest in a darkened environment. Meclizine or dimenhydrinate is prescribed for nausea and vertigo. Systemic antibiotic therapy can also be prescribed.

ASSESSMENT

RISK FACTORS

Middle ear disorders
- Recurrent colds and otitis media
- Enlarged adenoids
- Trauma
- Changes in air pressure (scuba diving, flying)

Inner ear disorders
- Viral or bacterial infection
- Damage due to ototoxic medications

EXPECTED FINDINGS

Middle ear disorders
- Hearing loss
- Feeling of fullness and/or pain in the ear
- Red, inflamed ear canal and tympanic membrane (TM)
- Bulging TM
- Fluid and/or bubbles behind TM
- Diffuse appearance of or inability to visualize normal light reflex
- Fever

Inner ear disorders
- Hearing loss
- Tinnitus
- Dizziness or vertigo
- Vomiting
- Nystagmus
- Alterations in balance

DIAGNOSTIC PROCEDURES

Audiometry

Audiometry is a noninvasive test of hearing ability, including frequency, pitch, and intensity. The client indicates when a tone is heard through earphones. Nurses might collaborate with an audiologist for this and other diagnostic procedures. **Qᴛᴄ**

Tympanogram

Tympanogram measures the mobility of the TM and middle ear structures relative to sound (effective in diagnosing middle ear disease).

Weber and Rinne tests

Weber and Rinne tests use tuning forks to determine whether hearing loss is present.

Otoscopy

An otoscope is used to examine the external auditory canal, TM, and malleus bone visible through the TM.

NURSING ACTIONS
- Otoscopic examination is done if audiometry results indicate possible impairment or if a client reports ear pain.
- After selection of a properly sized speculum, an otoscope is introduced into the external ear.
- If the ear canal curves, pull up and back on the auricle of adults, and down and back on the auricle of children, to straighten out the canal and enhance visualization.
- The TM should be a pearly gray color and intact. It should provide complete structural separation of the outer and middle ear structures.
- The light reflex should be visible from the center of the TM anteriorly (5 o'clock right ear; 7 o'clock left ear). **(13.1)**
- In the presence of fluid or infection in the middle ear, the TM becomes inflamed and can bulge from the pressure of the exudate. This also displaces the light reflex, causing it to look diffuse or completely obscured, a significant diagnostic finding.
- Avoid touching the lining of the ear canal, which causes pain due to sensitivity.

CLIENT EDUCATION: Warn the client that to see the TM clearly, the auricle might need to be firmly pulled.

Electronystagmography (ENG)

ENG detects involuntary eye movements (nystagmus) in order to assess for disease of the vestibular system of the ear. Electrodes are taped near the eyes, and movements of the eyes are recorded when the ear canal is stimulated with cold water instillation or injection of air. Recording of eye movements can be interpreted by a specialist as either normal or abnormal.

NURSING ACTIONS
- Intraprocedure, the nurse should ask simple questions (name recall, math problems) to ensure the client remains alert.
- The client should be maintained on bed rest and NPO postprocedure until vertigo subsides. **Qₛ**

CLIENT EDUCATION
- The client's preparation includes fasting immediately before the procedure, and restricting caffeine, alcohol, sedatives, and antihistamines for several days prior to the test.
- This test is not performed on clients who have a pacemaker. (Pacemaker signals inhibit sensitivity of ENG.)

Caloric testing

- Caloric testing can be done concurrently with ENG.
- Water (warmer or cooler than body temperature) is instilled in the ear in an effort to induce nystagmus.
- The eyes' response to the instillation of cold and warm water is diagnostic of vestibular disorders.

NURSING ACTIONS: The client should follow the same restrictions as those for an ENG.

CLIENT EDUCATION: Inform the client of the above restrictions.

PATIENT-CENTERED CARE

NURSING CARE

- Monitor functional ability and balance. Take fall risk precautions as necessary. Qs
- Evaluate the client's home situation. Collaborate with home health to assess home safety and falls risks, as needed.
- Encourage a client who has balance or functional limitations to rise slowly and use assistance and assistive devices as needed.
- Ototoxic medications can cause tinnitus and sensorineural hearing loss, especially at high doses or with prolonged treatment. Monitor blood levels of ototoxic medication, and teach clients about adverse effects. Routine audiometry is indicated with use of ototoxic IV antibiotics. Ototoxic medications include the following.
  - Antibiotics: gentamicin, erythromycin
  - Diuretics: furosemide, ethacrynic acid
  - NSAIDs: aspirin, ibuprofen
  - Chemotherapeutic agents: cisplatin
- Assist with ENG and caloric testing as needed.
- Administer antivertigo and antiemetic medications as needed.

MEDICATIONS

Meclizine

- Meclizine has antihistamine and anticholinergic effects and is used to treat the vertigo that accompanies inner ear problems.
- NURSING CONSIDERATIONS: Observe for sedation, and take appropriate precautions to ensure safe ambulation. Qs
- CLIENT EDUCATION: Warn the client about the sedative effects of meclizine. (Avoid driving or operating heavy machinery.)

Antiemetics

Ondansetron is one of several antiemetics used to treat nausea and vomiting associated with vertigo.

NURSING CONSIDERATIONS
- Instruct the client to report dizziness or rash.
- Contraindicated for clients who have certain cardiac rhythm disorders. Qs

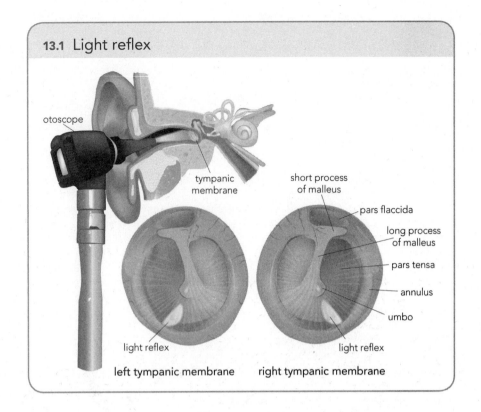

13.1 Light reflex

otoscope

tympanic membrane

short process of malleus

pars flaccida

long process of malleus

pars tensa

annulus

umbo

light reflex

light reflex

left tympanic membrane   right tympanic membrane

Diphenhydramine and dimenhydrinate

Antihistamines are effective in the treatment of vertigo and nausea that accompany inner ear problems.

NURSING CONSIDERATIONS
- Observe for urinary retention.
- Observe for sedation, and take appropriate precautions to ensure safe ambulation. Qs

CLIENT EDUCATION
- Warn the client about the sedative effects. (Avoid driving or operating heavy machinery.)
- Inform the client that dry mouth is expected.

Scopolamine

- Anticholinergics, such as scopolamine, are effective in the treatment of nausea that accompanies inner ear problems.
- It is available transdermally and is used for motion sickness.

NURSING CONSIDERATIONS
- Observe for urinary retention.
- Observe for sedation, and take appropriate precautions to ensure safe ambulation. Qs
- Monitor clients who have open-angle glaucoma for increasing eye pressure. Contraindicated in clients who have angle-closure glaucoma.

CLIENT EDUCATION
- Warn the client about the sedative effects. (Avoid driving or operating heavy machinery.)
- Inform client that dry mouth is expected.

Diazepam

Diazepam is a benzodiazepine that has antivertigo effects.

NURSING CONSIDERATIONS
- Observe for sedation, and take appropriate precautions to ensure safe ambulation. Qs
- Restrict use in clients who have closed-angle glaucoma.
- For older adult clients, use the smallest effective dose (prevent oversedation, ataxia). Ⓖ

CLIENT EDUCATION
- Warn the client about the sedative effects of diazepam. (Avoid driving or operating heavy machinery.)
- Inform the client of diazepam's addictive properties and appropriate use of the medication.

INTERPROFESSIONAL CARE

Vestibular rehabilitation is an option for clients who experience frequent episodes of vertigo or are incapacitated due to vertigo. A team of providers treats the cause and teaches the client exercises that can help him adapt to and minimize the effects of vertigo. A combination of biofeedback, physical therapy, and stress management may be used. Postural education can teach the client positions to avoid and positional exercises that can terminate an attack of vertigo. Qтс

THERAPEUTIC PROCEDURES

Vertigo-reducing activities

CLIENT EDUCATION
- Teach the client how to prevent stimulation/exacerbation of vertigo.
- Teach the client to restrict movement of the head and to change positions slowly.
- Have the client avoid caffeine and alcohol.
- Encourage the client to rest in a quiet, darkened environment when vertigo is severe.
- Have the client use assistive devices (cane, walker) as needed for safe ambulation to assist with balance. Qs
- Encourage the client to maintain a safe environment free of clutter.
- Instruct the client to take a diuretic, if prescribed, to decrease the amount of fluid in semicircular canals.
- Tell the client to space intake of fluids evenly throughout the day.
- Teach the client to decrease intake of salt and sodium-containing foods (processed meats, MSG).
- Remind the client to resume these precautions if vertigo returns.

SURGICAL INTERVENTIONS
- **Pressure point treatment** involves inserting a tympanostomy tube, which applies micropulses at intervals to relieve the vertigo of Ménière's disease by displacing fluid of the inner ear. QEBP
- **Myringotomy** is an incision to the tympanic membrane to drain fluid from the middle ear to prevent ear drum perforation in otitis media. For persistent otitis media, a pressure-equalizing tube or grommet can be inserted to temporarily take the place of the Eustachian tube. It stays in place for 6 to 18 months.

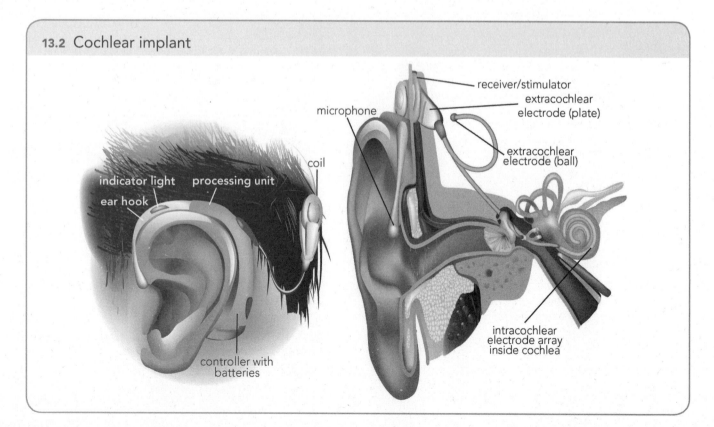

13.2 Cochlear implant

indicator light
processing unit
ear hook
coil
controller with batteries

microphone
receiver/stimulator
extracochlear electrode (plate)
extracochlear electrode (ball)
intracochlear electrode array inside cochlea

Stapedectomy

A stapedectomy is a surgical procedure of the middle ear in which the stapes is removed and replaced with a prosthesis.
- The procedure is done through the external ear canal and TM.
- The TM is repaired, and sterile ear packing is placed postoperatively.
- The procedure is done when otosclerosis has developed and the bones of the middle ear fuse together.
- Otosclerosis is one of the causes of conductive hearing loss in older adults. ©

NURSING ACTIONS
- Assess for facial nerve damage.
- Intervene for vertigo, nausea, and vomiting (common findings following the procedure).

Cochlear implant for sensorineural hearing loss

- Cochlear implants consist of a microphone that picks up sound, a speech processor, a transmitter and receiver that convert sounds into electric impulses, and electrodes that are attached to the auditory nerve. **(13.2)**
- The implant's transmitter is located outside the head behind the ear and connects via a magnet to the receiver located immediately below it, under the skin.
- Young children and adults who lost their hearing after speech development adapt to cochlear implants more quickly than those who were born totally deaf.
- Intensive and prolonged language training is necessary for individuals who did not develop speech.
- NURSING ACTIONS: Follow pre-, intra- and postoperative outpatient surgery guidelines.

CLIENT EDUCATION
- Inform the client that immediately after surgery, the unit is not turned on.
- The external unit is applied and the speech processor is programmed 2 to 6 weeks after surgery.
- Instruct the client on precautions to prevent infection.
- Instruct the client to avoid MRIs.

Labyrinthectomy

A labyrinthectomy is a surgical treatment for vertigo that involves removal of the labyrinthine portion of the inner ear.

NURSING ACTIONS: Client will have severe nausea and vertigo postoperatively. Take appropriate safety precautions and give antiemetics as needed. Q EBP

CLIENT EDUCATION: Inform the client that hearing loss is to be expected in the affected ear.

CLIENT EDUCATION FOLLOWING MIDDLE EAR SURGERY

- Avoid air travel for 2 to 3 weeks.
- Avoid straining or coughing, and blow nose gently with the mouth open for 2 to 3 weeks following surgery.
- Keep ear canal clean and dry. Avoid washing hair or showering for several days to 1 week.
- When able to shower, loosely place a cotton ball with petroleum jelly into the ear canal to prevent water from entering.
- Expect some temporary hearing loss in the affected ear due to presence of fluid or packing.
- Drainage from the ear canal should be reported to the provider.

Application Exercises

1. A nurse is performing an otoscopic examination of a client. Which of the following is an unexpected finding?

   A. Pearly, gray tympanic membrane (TM)

   B. Malleus visible behind the TM

   C. Presence of soft cerumen in the external canal

   D. Fluid bubble seen behind the TM

2. A nurse is reviewing the health record of a client who has severe otitis media. Which of the following are expected findings? (Select all that apply.)

   A. Enlarged adenoids

   B. Report of recent colds

   C. Client prescription for daily furosemide

   D. Light reflex visible on otoscopic exam in the affected ear

   E. Ear pain relieved by meclizine

3. A nurse in a clinic is caring for a client who has been experiencing mild to moderate vertigo due to benign paroxysmal vertigo for several weeks. Which of the following actions should the nurse recommend to help control the vertigo? (Select all that apply.)

   A. Reduce exposure to bright lighting.

   B. Move head slowly when changing positions.

   C. Do not eat fruit high in potassium.

   D. Plan evenly spaced daily fluid intake.

   E. Avoid fluids containing caffeine.

4. A nurse is caring for a client who has suspected Ménière's disease. Which of the following is an expected finding?

   A. Presence of a purulent lesion in the external ear canal

   B. Feeling of pressure in the ear

   C. Bulging, red bilateral tympanic membranes

   D. Unilateral hearing loss

5. A nurse is completing discharge teaching to a client following middle ear surgery. Which of the following statements by the client indicates understanding of the teaching?

   A. "I should restrict rapid movements and avoid bending from the waist for several weeks."

   B. "I should wait until the day after surgery to wash my hair."

   C. "I will remove the dressing behind my ear in 7 days."

   D. "My hearing should be back to normal right after my surgery."

Application Exercises Key

1. A. A pearly, gray TM is an expected finding during an otoscopic examination.

   B. Visualization of the malleus behind the TM is an expected finding during an otoscopic examination.

   C. Cerumen of various colors, depending on the client's skin color or ethnic background, is an expected finding in the external ear canal.

   D. **CORRECT:** Fluid behind the TM indicates the possibility of otitis media and is not an expected finding.

   Ⓝ *NCLEX® Connection: Reduction of Risk Potential, Potential for Complications of Diagnostic Tests/Treatments/Procedures*

2. A. **CORRECT:** Enlarged tonsils and adenoids are a finding associated with a middle ear infection.

   B. **CORRECT:** Frequent colds are findings associated with a middle ear infection.

   C. Furosemide is an ototoxic medication and can cause sensorineural hearing loss, but taking furosemide does not cause a middle ear disorder.

   D. Light reflexes are absent or in altered positions in a client who has a middle ear disorder.

   E. **CORRECT:** Meclizine is prescribed to relieve vertigo for inner ear disorders, but does not relieve the pain of a middle ear infection.

   Ⓝ *NCLEX® Connection: Physiological Adaptation, Pathophysiology*

3. A. **CORRECT:** Remaining in a darkened, quiet environment can reduce vertigo, particularly when it is severe.

   B. **CORRECT:** Moving slowly when standing or changing positions can reduce vertigo.

   C. The client who has vertigo should be instructed to avoid foods containing high levels of sodium to reduce fluid retention, which can cause vertigo.

   D. **CORRECT:** Fluid intake should be planned so that it is evenly spaced throughout the day to prevent excess fluid accumulation in the semicircular canals.

   E. **CORRECT:** The client should avoid fluids containing caffeine or alcohol to minimize vertigo.

   Ⓝ *NCLEX® Connection: Physiological Adaptation, Alterations in Body Systems*

4. A. Ménière's disease is an inner ear disorder. A purulent lesion in the external ear canal is not an expected finding.

   B. A feeling of pressure in the ear can occur with otitis media, but is not an expected finding in Ménière's

   C. Ménière's disease is an inner ear disorder. Bulging, red bilateral tympanic membranes is a finding associated with a middle ear infection.

   D. **CORRECT:** Unilateral sensorineural hearing loss is an expected finding in Ménière's disease.

   Ⓝ *NCLEX® Connection: Physiological Adaptation, Illness Management*

5. A. **CORRECT:** Rapid movements and bending from the waist should be avoided for 3 weeks following ear surgery.

   B. The client should avoid showering and washing hair for at least several days up to 1 week following ear surgery. The ear must remain dry during this time.

   C. Middle ear surgery is performed through the tympanic membrane, and the client will have a dry dressing within the ear canal. There is no external excision.

   D. Decreased hearing is expected following middle ear surgery due to presence of a dressing within the ear canal and possible drainage.

   Ⓝ *NCLEX® Connection: Reduction of Risk Potential, Therapeutic Procedures*

PRACTICE Active Learning Scenario

A nurse in a clinic is completing preoperative teaching for an adult client who will receive a cochlear implant. What should the nurse include in the teaching? Use the ATI Active Learning Template: Therapeutic Procedure to complete this item.

DESCRIPTION OF PROCEDURE: Describe a cochlear implant.

INDICATIONS: Describe the indication for a cochlear implant.

NURSING INTERVENTIONS: List at least four.

PRACTICE Answer

Using the ATI Active Learning Template: Therapeutic Procedure

DESCRIPTION OF PROCEDURE: A cochlear implant consists of a microphone to pick up sound, a speech processor, a transmitter and receiver to convert sounds into electrical impulses, and electrodes that are attached to the auditory nerve. The implant's transmitter is placed outside the head, behind the ear, via a magnet that attaches to the receiver located under the skin below it.

INDICATIONS: A cochlear implant is performed for sensorineural hearing loss.

NURSING INTERVENTIONS

• Pre- and postoperative teaching is completed.
• Intraoperative care is provided in an outpatient setting.
• Client education includes:
• The unit is not turned on immediately after surgery.
• The external unit is applied and the speech processor is programmed 2 to 6 weeks after surgery.
• The client is instructed to prevent infection.
• MRIs should be avoided by clients who have a cochlear implant.

Ⓝ *NCLEX® Connection: Reduction of Risk Potential, Therapeutic Procedures*

UNIT 2   NURSING CARE OF CLIENTS WHO HAVE NEUROSENSORY DISORDERS

SECTION: NEUROLOGIC EMERGENCIES

CHAPTER 14   *Head Injury*

Head injuries are classified as open or closed. In an open head injury, the integrity of the skull is compromised by either a penetrating object or blunt force trauma. A closed head injury occurs from blunt trauma that causes acceleration of the head and then deceleration or hits a stationary object. Head injuries are also classified as mild, moderate, or severe, depending upon Glasgow Coma Scale ratings and the length of time the client was unconscious.

TYPES OF BRAIN INJURY

- Types of brain injury include concussion, contusion, diffuse axonal injury, and intracranial hemorrhage.
  - **A concussion, or mild traumatic brain injury**, occurs after head trauma that result in a change in the client's neurological function but no identified brain damage and usually resolves within 72 hr. Post-concussion syndrome includes persistence of cognitive and physical manifestations for an unknown period of time.
  - **A contusion** occurs when the brain is bruised and the client has a period of unconsciousness associated with stupor and or confusion,
  - **Diffuse axonal injury** is a widespread injury to the brain that results in coma and is seen in severe head trauma.
  - **Intracranial hemorrhage** can occur in the epidural, subdural, or intracerebral space. It is a collection of blood following head trauma. There can be a delay of weeks to months in presenting manifestations for a subacute or chronic subdural hematoma.
- Open-head injuries pose a high risk for infection. Scalp injuries often result in profuse bleeding due to the poor vasoconstriction of the blood vessels of the scalp.
- Skull fractures can occur following forceful head injury. The brain might be damaged as a result. The client can have localized pain at the site of the fracture, and swelling can occur. The nurse should be alert for drainage from the ears or eyes (cerebral spinal fluid [CSF]).
- A cervical spine injury should always be suspected when a head injury occurs. A cervical spine injury must be ruled out prior to removing any devices used to stabilize the cervical spine. Qs

HEALTH PROMOTION AND DISEASE PREVENTION

- Wear helmets when skateboarding, riding a bike or motorcycle, skiing, and playing football or any other sport that could cause a head injury.
- Wear seat belts when driving or riding in a car.
- Avoid dangerous activities (speeding, driving under the influence of alcohol or drugs).
- Owners of firearms should lock all firearms.
- Avoid riding in the back of a pick-up truck.
- Promote programs directed at older adults to prevent falls, which are a major cause of neurological injury in adults ages 65 to 75. Older adults who sustain head injuries are at greater risk for complications, such as hematomas due to increased adherence of dura mater to skull and because of higher rates of anticoagulants prescribed to the older population. ⊙

ASSESSMENT

RISK FACTORS

- Motor vehicle or motorcycle crashes
- Drug and alcohol use
- Sports injuries
- Assault
- Gunshot wounds
- Falls

EXPECTED FINDINGS

- Presence of alcohol or illicit drugs at time of injury.
- Amnesia (loss of memory) before or after the injury.
- Loss of consciousness: Length of time the client is unconscious is significant.
- CSF leakage from the nose and ears can indicate a basilar skull fracture. Test for the presence of glucose by assessing for the presence of a "halo sign" indicated by a clear or yellow-tinted ring surrounding a drop of blood when drainage is placed on a piece of gauze.
- Manifestations of increased intracranial pressure
  - Severe headache, nausea, vomiting
  - Deteriorating level of consciousness, restlessness, irritability
  - Dilated or pinpoint nonreactive pupils
  - Cranial nerve dysfunction
  - Alteration in breathing pattern (Cheyne-Stokes respirations, central neurogenic hyperventilation, apnea)
  - Deterioration in motor function, abnormal posturing (decerebrate, decorticate, flaccidity)
  - Cushing's triad is a late finding characterized by severe hypertension with a widening pulse pressure (systolic – diastolic) and bradycardia.
  - Seizures

LABORATORY TESTS

- ABGs
- CBC with differential
- Blood glucose level
- Electrolyte levels
- Serum and urine osmolarity
- Toxicology screen and electrocardiogram (ECG)
- Monitor anti-seizure medication blood levels

DIAGNOSTIC PROCEDURES

- Cervical spine films to diagnose a cervical spine injury
- Computerized tomography (CT) and/or a magnetic resonance imaging (MRI) of the head and/or neck (with and without contrast if indicated)
- Calculation of cerebral perfusion using the ICP monitor, if it is in place

PATIENT-CENTERED CARE

NURSING CARE

- Support of the family following head injury is of great importance. Effective coping can be very difficult to achieve without support from providers and community members. The Brain Injury Association of America provides families and clients with information needed to cope with this potentially devastating injury. Qpcc
- The family can face difficult decisions following head injury. If brain death has occurred, the family needs support when deciding whether to donate organs.

Assess/monitor the client at regularly scheduled intervals

Respiratory status (the priority assessment): The brain is dependent upon oxygen to maintain function and has little reserve available if oxygen is deprived. Untreated hypoxia leads to brain injury or death if the brain has been denied adequate oxygenation for 3 to 5 min. Changes in level of consciousness, using the Glasgow Coma Scale (GCS), provide the earliest indication of neurological deterioration.

Cranial nerve function: Eye blink response, gag reflex, tongue and shoulder movement

Assess pupils for size, equality, and reaction to light: Pupils that are equal, round, and react to light and accommodation (PERRLA) are a normal finding.

Bilateral sensory and motor responses

Increased intracranial pressure (ICP)

Monitored by placing a screw, catheter or sensor through a burr hole into the ventricle, subarachnoid, epidural, or subdural space. Expected reference range is 10 to 15 mm Hg.

- ICP can be increased by
  - Hypercarbia, which leads to cerebral vasodilation
  - Endotracheal or oral tracheal suctioning
  - Coughing
  - Extreme neck or hip flexion/extension
  - Maintaining the head of the bed at an angle less than 30°
  - Increasing intra-abdominal pressure (restrictive clothing, Valsalva maneuver)
- Implement actions that decrease ICP.
  - Elevate head at least 30° to reduce ICP and to promote venous drainage.
  - Avoid extreme flexion, extension, or rotation of the head, and maintain the body in a midline neutral position.
  - Maintain a patent airway. Provide mechanical ventilation as indicated.
  - Administer oxygen as indicated to maintain PaO_2 greater than 60 mm Hg.
  - The client can be hyperventilated on mechanical ventilation to decrease ICP. The client should receive stool softeners and avoid the Valsalva maneuver with increased ICP.
  - Maintain cervical spine stability until cleared by an x-ray.
  - Report presence of CSF from nose or ears to the provider.
  - Provide a calm, restful environment. (Limit visitors. Minimize noise.)
  - Implement measures to prevent complications of immobility (turn every 2 hr, footboard, and splints). Specialty beds can be used.
  - Monitor fluid and electrolyte values and osmolality to detect changes in sodium regulation, onset of diabetes insipidus, or severe hypovolemia.
  - Provide adequate fluids to maintain cerebral perfusion and to minimize cerebral edema. When a large amount of IV fluids are prescribed, monitor for excess fluid volume which could increase ICP.
  - Brief periods of hyperventilation for the intubated client can be used after the first 24 hr following injury to help lower ICP. During the first 24 hr, hyperventilation can cause cerebral vasoconstriction, which can cause ischemia.
  - Maintain safety and seizure precautions (side rails up, padded side rails, call light within the client's reach). Qs
  - Even if the level of consciousness is decreased, explain to the client the actions being taken and why. (Hearing is the last sense affected by a head injury.)

MEDICATIONS

Mannitol

Mannitol is an osmotic diuretic used to treat cerebral edema. When used for increased ICP, the medication draws fluid from the brain into the blood.

NURSING CONSIDERATIONS
- Administer IV to treat acute cerebral edema.
- Insert indwelling urinary catheter to monitor fluid and renal status. Monitor urine osmolality.
- Monitor serum electrolytes and osmolality closely.

Barbiturates

Client may be placed in coma (barbiturate coma) to decrease cellular metabolic demand until ICP can be decreased.
- Commonly used medications include pentobarbital and thiopental.
- When barbiturate coma is used, the ability to assess neurological function is made more difficult.
- Medication dosage is adjusted to keep the client completely unresponsive.
- Mechanical ventilation, cardiac and hemodynamic monitoring, and ICP monitoring are required.

Phenytoin

Phenytoin is used prophylactically to prevent or treat seizures. It was the first medication used to suppress seizure that did not depress the entire CNS.

NURSING CONSIDERATIONS
- Dosing for this medication is client-specific and based on therapeutic blood levels.
- Check for medication interactions.

Morphine

Morphine is an analgesic used to control pain and restlessness.

NURSING CONSIDERATIONS
- Calm and reassure clients, clarifying misconceptions (brain surgery can be an extremely fearful procedure).
- Avoid opioid use with clients who are not mechanically ventilated due to CNS depressant effects.
  - Prevents accurate assessment of neurological system
  - Can cause respiratory depression

THERAPEUTIC PROCEDURES

Craniotomy

A craniotomy is the removal of nonviable brain tissue that allows for expansion and/or removal of epidural or subdural hematomas. It is also used to decrease ICP and remove brain tumors. It involves drilling a burr hole or creating a bone flap to permit access to the affected area.
- Treatment of intracranial hemorrhages requires surgical evacuation. There are three surgical approaches: supratentorial (above the tentorial), infratentorial (below the tentorial, brain stem), and transsphenoidal (through the mouth and nasal sinuses).
- Burr holes are circular openings through the skull. The burr hole is used to assess cerebral swelling, injury, size, and position of the ventricles.
- This is a life-saving procedure, and is associated with many potential complications, such as severe neurological impairment, infection, persistent seizures, neurological deficiencies, and death.

NURSING ACTIONS
- The goal is to decrease cerebral edema. Medications such as mannitol and dexamethasone can be administered every 6 hr for 24 to 72 hr postoperatively.
- Phenytoin or diazepam can be used to prevent seizure activity.
- Monitor ICP. Follow written protocols to assess for changes in ICP.
- For supratentorial surgery, maintain HOB at least 30° with body positioning to prevent increased ICP.
- For infratentorial craniotomy, keep client flat and on either side for 24 to 48 hr to prevent pressure on neck incision site.

INTERPROFESSIONAL CARE
- Care should include professionals from other disciplines as indicated. This can include physical, occupational, recreational, and/or speech therapists due to neurological deficits that can occur secondary to the area of the brain damaged.
- Contact social services or case manager to provide links to social service agencies and schools.
- Rehabilitation facilities are frequently used to compress the time required to recover from a head injury and support re-emergence into society.

COMPLICATIONS

Brain herniation

- A brain herniation is the downward shift of brain tissue due to cerebral edema.
- The brain consists of brain tissue, cerebrospinal fluid, and blood. Due to the limited space within the skull, an alteration of any one of the components of the brain results in a compromise in the other components. When trauma creates a shift in these components, and the other components are unable to accommodate, the brain shifts from the cranial vault, or herniates. This can result in brain tissue moving downward, through the foramen magnum.
- Findings include fixed dilated pupils, deteriorating level of consciousness, Cheyne-Stokes respirations, hemodynamic instability, and abnormal posturing.
- Recovery after this occurrence is rare, and urgent medical treatment (mannitol) and/or surgical (debulking) treatment is indicated.
- With treatment, severe neurological impairment usually persists.

NURSING ACTIONS
- This situation should be prevented before treatment is needed.
- Close monitoring of the client's vital signs and neurological status allows early reporting of changes in the GCS score, an increase in the blood pressure, and an alteration in respiratory pattern and effort. Qs

CLIENT EDUCATION
- Frequently update family members on the health status of the client. Frequent updates and repeating medical information is often necessary to ensure comprehension among family members.
- The decision to surgically treat brain herniation is made in the presence of a critical situation.
- Social service workers and/or pastoral personnel can be helpful to support the family, while reinforcing the medical situation. Qtc

Hematoma and intracranial hemorrhage

- Monitor for severe headache, rapid decline in level of consciousness, worsening neurological function and herniation, and changes in ICP.
- Surgery is required to remove subdural and epidural hematoma.
- Intracranial hemorrhage is treated with osmotic diuretics.

Pulmonary edema

- Findings mimic acute pulmonary edema without cardiac involvement.
- This is a life-threatening emergency. Immediate, aggressive treatment is used. Survival is rare.

Diabetes insipidus or syndrome of inappropriate antidiuretic hormone

Diabetes insipidus or syndrome of inappropriate antidiuretic hormone (SIADH) is a possible complication.

Cerebral salt wasting

- Cerebral salt wasting (CSW) is caused by effects of atrial natriuretic factor (ANF) located in the hypothalamus.
- Increased ANF production decreases sodium retention in the kidneys. ANF also can prevent renin and aldosterone release.
- CSW causes decreased serum osmolality and hyponatremia. CSW is the primary cause of hyponatremia following neurosurgery.
- CSW causes hypovolemia, compared with increased extracellular fluid in clients who have SIADH.

NURSING ACTIONS
- Monitor serum electrolytes and osmolality daily.
- Document strict intake and output.
- Weigh client daily.
- Treat electrolyte and fluid imbalance, as prescribed.
- Monitor for dehydration or fluid overload during treatment.

Application Exercises

1. A nurse is caring for a client who was recently admitted to the emergency department following a head-on motor vehicle crash. The client is unresponsive, has spontaneous respirations of 22/min, and has a laceration on his forehead that is bleeding. Which of the following is the priority nursing action at this time?

   A. Keep neck stabilized.

   B. Insert nasogastric tube.

   C. Monitor pulse and blood pressure frequently.

   D. Establish IV access and start fluid replacement.

2. A nurse is caring for a client who has just been admitted following surgical evacuation of a subdural hematoma. Which of the following is the priority assessment?

   A. Glasgow Coma Scale

   B. Cranial nerve function

   C. Oxygen saturation

   D. Pupillary response

3. A nursing is caring for a client who has a closed-head injury with ICP readings ranging from 16 to 22 mm Hg. Which of the following actions should the nurse take to decrease the potential for raising the client's ICP? (Select all that apply.)

   A. Suction the endotracheal tube frequently.

   B. Decrease the noise level in the client's room

   C. Elevate the client's head on two pillows.

   D. Administer a stool softener.

   E. Keep the client well hydrated.

4. A nurse in the critical care unit is completing an admission assessment of a client who has a gunshot wound to the head. Which of the following assessment findings are indicative of increased ICP? (Select all that apply.)

   A. Headache

   B. Dilated pupils

   C. Tachycardia

   D. Decorticate posturing

   E. Hypotension

5. A nurse is caring for a client who has increased ICP and a new prescription for mannitol. For which of the following adverse effects should the nurse monitor?

   A. Hyperglycemia

   B. Hyponatremia

   C. Hypervolemia

   D. Oliguria

PRACTICE Active Learning Scenario

A nurse is reviewing the plan of care for a client who has a head injury. What should be included in the plan of care? Use the ATI Active Learning Template: System Disorder to complete this item.

DIAGNOSTIC PROCEDURES
- Identify the priority nursing assessment and describe why this is important.
- Identify the nursing assessment that will provide the earliest indication of neurological deterioration.

NURSING CARE: Describe three additional nursing actions.

CLIENT EDUCATION: Describe two activities the nurse should instruct the client to avoid that will increase ICP.

Application Exercises Key

1. A. **CORRECT:** The greatest risk to the client is permanent damage to the spinal cord if a cervical injury does exist. The priority nursing intervention is to keep the neck immobile until damage to the cervical spine can be ruled out.

   B. Insertion of a nasogastric tube is not the priority nursing action at this time.

   C. Frequent monitoring of pulse and blood pressure is important but not the priority nursing action at this time.

   D. Establishing IV access for fluid replacement is important but not the priority nursing action at this time.

   Ⓝ *NCLEX® Connection: Reduction of Risk Potential, Potential for Complications of Diagnostic Tests/Treatments/Procedures*

2. A. The Glasgow Coma Scale is important. However, another assessment is the priority.

   B. Assessment of cranial nerve function is important. However, another assessment is the priority.

   C. **CORRECT:** Using the airway, breathing, and circulation (ABC) priority-setting framework, assessment of oxygen saturation is the priority action. Brain tissue can only survive for 3 min before permanent damage occurs.

   D. Assessment of pupillary response is important. However, another assessment is the priority.

   Ⓝ *NCLEX® Connection: Physiological Adaptation, Unexpected Response to Therapies*

3. A. Suctioning increases ICP and should be performed only when indicated.

   B. **CORRECT:** Decreasing the noise level and restricting the number of people in the client's room can help prevent increases in ICP.

   C. Hyperflexion of the client's neck with pillows carries the risk of increasing ICP and should be avoided. The head of the bed should be raised to at least 30°, but the head should be maintained in an upright, neutral position.

   D. **CORRECT:** Administration of a stool softener will decrease the need to bear down (Valsalva maneuver) during bowel movements, which can increase ICP.

   E. Overhydration carries the risk of increasing ICP and should be avoided. The nurse should monitor fluid and electrolyte levels closely for the client who has increased ICP.

   Ⓝ *NCLEX® Connection: Reduction of Risk Potential, Diagnostic Tests*

4. A. **CORRECT:** Headache is a finding associated with increased ICP.

   B. **CORRECT:** Dilated pupils is a finding associated with increased ICP.

   C. Bradycardia, not tachycardia, is a finding associated with increased ICP.

   D. **CORRECT:** Decorticate or decerebrate posturing is a finding associated with increased ICP.

   E. Hypertension, not hypotension, is a finding associated with increased ICP.

   Ⓝ *NCLEX® Connection: Physiological Adaptation, Alterations in Body Systems*

5. A. Hyperglycemia is not an adverse effect of mannitol.

   B. **CORRECT:** Mannitol is a powerful osmotic diuretic. Adverse effects include electrolyte imbalances, such as hyponatremia.

   C. Hypovolemia is an adverse effect of mannitol and should be monitored.

   D. Polyuria is an adverse of mannitol and should be monitored.

   Ⓝ *NCLEX® Connection: Physiological Adaptation, Fluid and Electrolyte Imbalances*

PRACTICE Answer

Using the ATI Active Learning Template: System Disorder

DIAGNOSTIC PROCEDURES

- The priority nursing assessment is respiratory status. The brain is dependent on oxygen to maintain function and has minimal reserve if oxygen is not available. Brain function begins to diminish after 3 min of oxygen deprivation.
- The assessment indication of early neurological deterioration is changes in level of consciousness.

NURSING CARE

- Elevate the head to at least 30°.
- Maintain patent airway.
- Administer oxygen to keep oxygen saturation greater than 92%.
- Maintain cervical spine stability until cleared by x-ray.
- Report presence of cerebrospinal fluid from nose or ears to the provider.
- Provide a calm, restful environment. (Limit visitors. Minimize noise.)

- Implement measures to prevent complications of immobility. (Turn every 2 hr. Use footboard and splints.) Provide a specialty bed.
- Monitor fluid and electrolyte values and osmolarity.
- Provide adequate fluids but do not overhydrate. Monitor IV fluids.
- Maintain safety and seizure precautions (side rails up, padded side rails, call light within client's reach).
- Explain all nursing actions to the client and family.

CLIENT EDUCATION: Coughing and blowing the nose forcefully.

Ⓝ *NCLEX® Connection: Physiological Adaptation, Pathophysiology*

UNIT 2 · NURSING CARE OF CLIENTS WHO HAVE NEUROSENSORY DISORDERS
SECTION: NEUROLOGIC EMERGENCIES

CHAPTER 15 · *Stroke*

Strokes, also known as cerebrovascular accidents or brain attacks, involve a disruption in the cerebral blood flow secondary to ischemia, hemorrhage, brain attack, or embolism.

Classifications of strokes are hemorrhagic and ischemic. (Ischemic strokes are thrombotic or embolic.)

Hemorrhagic occur secondary to a ruptured artery or aneurysm. The prognosis for a client who has experienced a hemorrhagic stroke is poor due to the amount of ischemia and increased ICP caused by the expanding collection of blood. If it is caught early and evacuation of the clot can be done with cessation of the active bleed, the prognosis of a hemorrhagic stroke improves significantly. **(15.1)**

Thrombotic is an ischemic stroke that occurs secondary to the development of a blood clot on an atherosclerotic plaque in a cerebral artery that gradually shuts off the artery and causes ischemia distal to the occlusion. Manifestations of a thrombotic stroke evolve over a period of several hours to days. **(15.2)**

Embolic is an ischemic stroke caused by an embolus traveling from another part of the body to a cerebral artery. Blood to the brain distal to the occlusion is immediately shut off causing neurologic deficits or a loss of consciousness to instantly occur. **(15.3)**

Ischemic strokes (thrombotic or embolic) can be reversed with fibrinolytic therapy using alteplase, also known as tissue plasminogen activator (tPA), if given within 3 to 4.5 hr of the initial symptoms (unless contraindicated by factors such as presence of active bleeding).

HEALTH PROMOTION AND DISEASE PREVENTION

- Hypertension, diabetes mellitus, smoking, and other related disorders can increase a client's risk for a stroke. Q EBP
- Early treatment of hypertension, maintenance of blood glucose within expected range, and refraining from smoking will decrease these risk factors.
- Maintaining a healthy weight and getting regular exercise can also decrease the risk of a stroke.

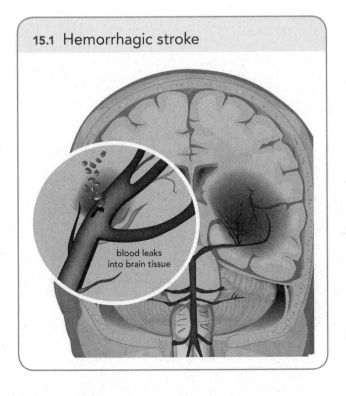

15.1 Hemorrhagic stroke

blood leaks into brain tissue

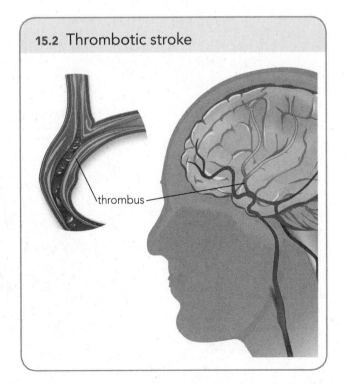

15.2 Thrombotic stroke

thrombus

ASSESSMENT

RISK FACTORS

- Cerebral aneurysm
- Arteriovenous malformation (AV)
- Diabetes mellitus
- Obesity
- Hypertension
- Atherosclerosis
- Hyperlipidemia
- Hypercoagulability
- Atrial fibrillation
- Use of oral contraceptives
- Smoking
- Cocaine use

EXPECTED FINDINGS

Some clients report transient manifestations, such as visual disturbances, dizziness, slurred speech, and a weak extremity.

- These manifestations can indicate a transient ischemic attack (TIA), which can be a warning of an impending stroke.
- Antithrombotic medication and/or surgical removal of atherosclerotic plaques in the carotid artery can prevent the subsequent occurrence of a stroke.

PHYSICAL ASSESSMENT FINDINGS

Manifestations vary based on the area of the brain that is deprived of oxygenated blood.

- **The left cerebral hemisphere** is responsible for language, mathematics skills, and analytic thinking.
  - Expressive and receptive aphasia (inability to speak and understand language)
  - Agnosia (unable to recognize familiar objects)
  - Alexia (reading difficulty)
  - Agraphia (writing difficulty)
  - Right extremity hemiplegia (paralysis) or hemiparesis (weakness)
  - Slow, cautious behavior
  - Depression, anger, and quick to become frustrated
  - Visual changes, such as hemianopsia (loss of visual field in one or both eyes)
- **The right cerebral hemisphere** is responsible for visual and spatial awareness and proprioception. **Qs**
  - Altered perception of deficits (overestimation of abilities)
  - Unilateral neglect syndrome (ignore left side of the body: cannot see, feel, or move affected side, so client unaware of its existence). Can occur with left-hemispheric strokes, but is more common with right-hemispheric strokes.
  - Loss of depth perception
  - Poor impulse control and judgment
  - Left hemiplegia or hemiparesis
  - Visual changes, such as hemianopsia

DIAGNOSTIC PROCEDURES

A magnetic resonance imaging (MRI), computed tomography (CT) imaging, and/or a computed axial tomography (CAT) scan can be used to identify edema, ischemia, and necrosis.

A magnetic resonance angiography or a cerebral angiography are used to identify the presence of a cerebral hemorrhage, abnormal vessel structures (AV malformation, aneurysms), vessel ruptures, and regional perfusion of blood flow in the carotid arteries and brain.

A lumbar puncture is used to assess for the presence of blood in the cerebrospinal fluid. A positive finding is consistent with a cerebral hemorrhage or ruptured aneurysm.

The Glasgow Coma Scale is used when the client has a decreased level of consciousness or orientation. The risk for increased intracranial pressure (ICP) exists related to the swelling of the brain that can occur secondary to ischemic insult.

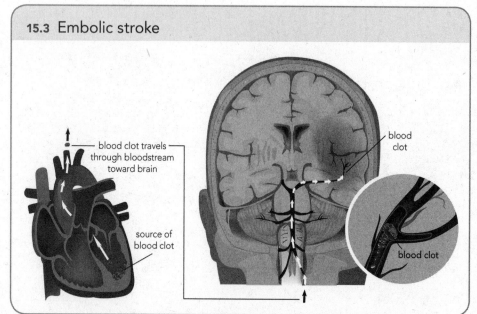

15.3 Embolic stroke

blood clot travels through bloodstream toward brain

source of blood clot

blood clot

blood clot

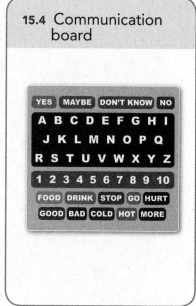

15.4 Communication board

| YES | MAYBE | DON'T KNOW | NO |

A B C D E F G H I
J K L M N O P Q
R S T U V W X Y Z

1 2 3 4 5 6 7 8 9 10

FOOD DRINK STOP GO HURT
GOOD BAD COLD HOT MORE

PATIENT-CENTERED CARE

NURSING CARE

- Monitor vital signs every 1 to 2 hr. Notify the provider immediately if blood pressure exceeds a systolic greater than 180 mm Hg or a diastolic greater than 110 mm Hg. This can indicate the client is experiencing an ischemic stroke. Qs
- Monitor the client's temperature. A fever can cause an increase in intracranial pressure.
- Provide oxygen therapy to maintain oxygen saturation level greater than 92%, or if the client's level of consciousness is decreased.
- Place the client on a cardiac monitor to detect arrhythmias.
- Conduct a cardiac assessment, and auscultate apical heart rate to detect murmurs or irregularity.
- Monitor for changes in level of consciousness (increased ICP sign).
- Monitor vital signs, electrocardiogram.
- Elevate the head of the bed approximately 30° to reduce ICP and to promote venous drainage. Avoid extreme flexion or extension of the neck, and maintain the client's head in the midline neutral position. QEBP
- Institute seizure precautions.
- Assist with the client's communication skills if speech is impaired. **(15.4)**
  - Assess the ability to understand speech by asking the client to follow simple commands.
  - Observe for consistently affirmative answers when the client actually does not comprehend what is being said.
  - Assess accuracy of yes/no responses in relation to closed-ended questions.
  - Supply the client with a picture board of commonly requested items/needs.
  - For expressive and receptive aphasia speak slowly and clearly, use one-step commands.
- Assist with safe feeding. Qs
  - Assess swallowing and gag reflexes before feeding. The speech-language pathologist (SLP) may request a swallowing study that can involve swallowing a barium substrate and radiography of the peristaltic activity of the esophagus.
  - Four liquid consistencies have been identified by a collaborative group of specialists for clients who have dysphagia: thin (water, juice), nectar-like (cream soups, nectars), honey-like (honey, yogurt), and spoon-thick (pudding, cooked cereals). Food levels for dysphagia include pureed, mechanically altered, advanced/mechanically soft, and regular. Use the appropriate consistency and food type as recommended by the SLP to minimize choking.
  - Have the client eat in an upright position and swallow with the head and neck flexed slightly forward.
  - Place food in the back of the mouth on the unaffected side.
  - Have suction on standby.
  - Maintain a distraction-free environment during meals.
  - Collaborate with dietitian to ensure appropriate caloric intake, because weight loss is common following stroke. QTc

- Prevent complications of immobility, such as atelectasis, pneumonia, pressure sores, and deep-vein thrombosis (DVT). Clients who have experienced strokes are ambulated as soon as possible to prevent complications. However, during periods of inactivity, preventive measures related to complications of immobility should be implemented.
- Maintain skin integrity.
  - Reposition the client frequently and use padding.
  - Monitor bony prominences, paying particular attention to the affected extremities.
  - If the client has one-sided neglect, teach him to protect and care for the affected extremity to avoid injuring it in the wheel of the wheelchair or hitting/smashing it against a doorway.
- Encourage passive range of motion every 2 hr to the affected extremities and active range of motion every 2 hr to the unaffected extremities. Teach the client how to use the unaffected side to exercise the affected side of the body.
- Elevate affected extremities to promote venous return and reduce swelling. An elastic glove can be placed on the affected hand if swelling is severe. Teach the client to massage the affected hand by stroking it in a distal to proximal manner, encouraging fluid in the hand to move back into the wrist and arm.
- Maintain a safe environment to reduce the risk of falls. Assistive devices, such as transfer belts and sliding boards, should be used during transfers. Sit-to-stand lifts can also facilitate transfers and reduce strain on the care provider's body. Qs
- If the client has homonymous hemianopsia (loss of the same visual field in both eyes), instruct him to use a scanning technique (turning head from the direction of the unaffected side to the affected side) when eating and ambulating.
- To prevent DVT, provide preventive measures such as sequential compression stockings, frequent position changes, and mobilization.
- Provide assistance with ADLs as needed. Instruct the client to dress the affected side first and sit in a supportive chair that aids in balance. Have occupational therapy assess the client for adaptive aids, such as a plate guard, utensils with built-up handles, a reaching tool to pick things up, and shirts and shoes that have hook and loop fasteners or tape instead of buttons and ties.
- Clients who have experienced strokes have decreased endurance and impaired balance due to paralysis on one side of the body. Provide frequent rest periods from sitting in the wheelchair by returning the client to bed after therapies and meals. When sitting the client up in bed or in the wheelchair, leaning to the affected side typically occurs and should be countered with some manner of support.
- Shoulder subluxation can occur if the affected arm is not supported. The weight of the arm is such that it can cause a painful dislocation of the shoulder from its socket. Support the arm while in bed, the wheelchair, or during ambulation with an arm sling or strategically placed pillows.
- Support the client during periods of emotional lability and depression. QPCC

MEDICATIONS

Anticoagulants (heparin sodium, enoxaparin, warfarin): Use of anticoagulants is controversial and not recommended due to the high risk of intracerebral bleeding.

Antiplatelets (aspirin)
- Low-dose aspirin is given within 24 to 48 hr following a stroke to prevent further clot formation.
- Other antiplatelets, such as clopidogrel, are not recommended.

Thrombolytic medications reteplase recombinant: Give within 4.5 hr of initial symptoms.

Antiepileptic medications (phenytoin, gabapentin)
- These medications are not commonly given following a stroke unless the client develops seizures.
- Gabapentin can be given for paresthetic pain in an affected extremity.

THERAPEUTIC PROCEDURES

Systemic or catheter-directed thrombolytic therapy restores cerebral blood flow. It must be administered within 6 hr of the onset of symptoms. It is contraindicated for treatment of a hemorrhagic stroke and for clients who have an increased risk of bleeding due to anticoagulant therapy or other bleeding anomaly. Possibility of hemorrhagic stroke is ruled out with an MRI prior to the initiation of thrombolytic therapy.

- Carotid artery angioplasty with stenting (CAS) involves inserting a catheter in the femoral artery and placing a distal/embolic protection device to catch clot debris during the procedure while a stent is being placed in the carotid artery to open a blockage. CAS is less invasive, blood loss is decreased, and length of hospitalization is shorter. Postoperative care is the same as carotid endarterectomy.
- Carotid endarterectomy is performed to open the artery by removing atherosclerotic plaque. This procedure is performed when the carotid artery is blocked or when the client is experiencing TIAs.
- Assess for increased headache, neck swelling, and hoarseness of the throat.
- Extracranial-intracranial bypass is a craniotomy performed to improve cerebral perfusion following a stroke or for clients who have had a TIA that is likely to progress to a stroke. It increases blood flow around blocked artery and can help restore blood flow to affected areas of the brain.

INTERPROFESSIONAL CARE

- Speech and language therapists can be consulted for language therapy and swallowing exercises.
- Physical therapy can be consulted for assistance with reestablishment of ambulation with or without assistive devices (single or quad cane, walker) or wheelchair support. Wheelchair adaptations, such as an extended brake handle on the client's affected side of the wheelchair, can be necessary. Safety features, such as placing the brakes on when preparing to transfer and the use of a cushion on the seat, may also be initiated by physical therapy.
- Occupational therapy can be consulted for assistance with reestablishment of partial or full function of the affected hand and arm. If function does not return to the extremity, measures such as massage and elastic gloves will be prescribed by occupational therapy to prevent swelling of the extremity.
- Social services can be consulted to make arrangements for rehabilitation services and temporary placement on a skilled rehabilitation unit or extended-care facility during provision of these services. Prior to discharge, the social worker may make a home visit with selected therapists and nurses to evaluate the need for environmental alterations in the home and adaptive equipment needed for ADLs.

COMPLICATIONS

Dysphagia and aspiration

- Dysphagia can result from neurological involvement of the cranial nerves that innervate the face, tongue, soft palate, and throat. As a result, the client's risk of aspiration is great. Qs
- Not all clients who have experienced a stroke have dysphagia, but all should be evaluated prior to reestablishing oral nutrition and hydration.

NURSING ACTIONS
- Assess gag reflex. If the gag reflex is present, give the client a small sip of water to determine if choking occurs.
- If the client exhibits difficulty managing food or fluids, a swallowing evaluation should be done by an SLP. Qtc
- Keep the client completely NPO until evaluated by the SLP.
- Begin the client with the prescribed liquid-consistency regimen from the National Dysphagia Diet and observe closely for choking. Have suction equipment available, but feed with care because nasotracheal suctioning increases ICP. Qebp
- Initial feedings should be done by an RN, so appropriate interventions can be taken if choking occurs. Some clients require an eating environment without distractions to prevent choking.

CLIENT EDUCATION
- Teach the client's family strategies for eating and give instructions regarding prescribed consistency of liquids and solid foods.
- Instruct the client to sit upright and to flex his head forward when swallowing to decrease the risk of choking. Qs

Unilateral neglect

Unilateral neglect is the loss of awareness of the side affected by the stroke. The client cannot see, feel, or move the affected side of his body; therefore, he forgets that it exists. This lack of awareness poses a great risk for injury to the neglected extremities and creates a self-care deficit.

NURSING ACTIONS
- Observe affected extremities for injury (bruises and abrasions of the affected hand and arm, hyperflexion of the foot from it falling off of the wheelchair during transport).
- Apply an arm sling if the client is unable to remember to care for the affected extremity.
- Ensure that the foot rest is on the wheelchair and that an ankle brace is on the affected foot.

CLIENT EDUCATION
- Instruct the client to dress the affected side first. Qpcc
- Teach the client how to care for the affected side.
- Use the unaffected hand to pull the affected extremity to midline and out of danger from the wheel of the wheelchair or from hitting or smashing it against a doorway.
- Teach the client to look over the affected side periodically.

PRACTICE Active Learning Scenario

A nurse is caring for a client who has dysphagia. Use the ATI Active Learning Template: Nursing Skill to complete this item.

NURSING INTERVENTIONS: List three nursing actions the nurse should include while caring for this client.

Application Exercises

1. A nurse is caring for a client who has experienced a right-hemispheric stroke. Which of the following are expected findings? (Select all that apply.)
    A. Impulse control difficulty
    B. Left hemiplegia
    C. Loss of depth perception
    D. Aphasia
    E. Lack of situational awareness

2. A nurse is caring for a client who has left homonymous hemianopsia. Which of the following is an appropriate nursing intervention?
    A. Teach the client to scan to the right to see objects on the right side of her body.
    B. Place the bedside table on the right side of the bed.
    C. Orient the client to the food on her plate using the clock method.
    D. Place the wheelchair on the client's left side.

3. A nurse is planning care for a client who has dysphagia and a new dietary prescription. Which of the following should the nurse include in the plan of care? (Select all that apply.)
    A. Have suction equipment available for use.
    B. Feed the client thickened liquids.
    C. Place food on the unaffected side of the client's mouth.
    D. Assign an assistive personnel to feed the client slowly.
    E. Teach the client to swallow with her neck flexed.

4. A nurse is caring for a client who has global aphasia (both receptive and expressive). Which of the following should the nurse include in the client's plan of care? (Select all that apply.)
    A. Speak to the client at a slower rate.
    B. Assist the client to use flash cards with pictures.
    C. Speak to the client in a loud voice.
    D. Complete sentences that the client cannot finish.
    E. Give instructions one step at a time.

5. A nurse is assessing a client who has experienced a left-hemispheric stroke. Which of the following is an expected finding?
    A. Impulse control difficulty
    B. Poor judgment
    C. Inability to recognize familiar objects
    D. Loss of depth perception

Application Exercises Key

1. A. **CORRECT:** A client who has experienced a right-hemispheric stroke will exhibit impulse control difficulty, such as the urgency to use the restroom.

    B. **CORRECT:** A client who has experienced a right-hemispheric stroke will exhibit left-sided hemiplegia.

    C. **CORRECT:** A client who has experienced a right-hemispheric stroke will experience a loss in depth perception.

    D. A client who has experienced a left-hemispheric stroke will experience aphasia.

    E. **CORRECT:** A client who has experienced a right-hemispheric stroke will demonstrate a lack of awareness of surroundings.

    Ⓝ *NCLEX® Connection: Physiological Adaptation, Pathophysiology*

2. A. A client who has left homonymous hemianopsia has lost the left visual field of both eyes. The client should be taught to turn his head to the left to visualize the entire field of vision.

    B. **CORRECT:** The client is unable to visualize to the left midline of her body. Placing the bedside table on the right side of the client's bed will permit visualization of items on the table.

    C. Using the clock method of food placement will be ineffective because only half of the plate can be seen.

    D. The wheelchair should be placed to the client's right or unaffected side.

    Ⓝ *NCLEX® Connection: Physiological Adaptation, Illness Management*

3. A. **CORRECT:** Suction equipment should be available in case of choking and aspiration.

    B. **CORRECT:** The client should be given liquids that are thicker than water to prevent aspiration.

    C. **CORRECT:** Placing food on the unaffected side of the client's mouth will allow her to have better control of the food and reduce the risk of aspiration.

    D. Due to the risk of aspiration, assistive personnel should not be assigned to feed the client because the client's swallowing ability should be assessed, and suctioning can be needed if choking occurs.

    E. **CORRECT:** The client should be taught to flex her neck, tucking the chin down and under to close the epiglottis during swallowing.

    Ⓝ *NCLEX® Connection: Reduction of Risk Potential, Potential for Alterations in Body Systems*

4. A. **CORRECT:** Clients who have global aphasia have difficulty with speaking and understanding speech. One strategy that can enhance client understanding is speaking to the client at a slower rate.

    B. **CORRECT:** One strategy that can enhance understanding is the use of alternative forms of communication, such as flash cards with pictures or a computer.

    C. For the client who has aphasia, speaking in a loud voice is unnecessary and can be interpreted as patronizing.

    D. The nurse should allow the client adequate time to finish sentences and not complete the sentences for him.

    E. **CORRECT:** One strategy that can enhance understanding is giving instructions one step at a time.

    Ⓝ *NCLEX® Connection: Physiological Adaptation, Alterations in Body Systems*

5. A. A client who has experienced a right-hemispheric stroke will experience difficulty with impulse control.

    B. A client who has experienced a right-hemispheric stroke will experience poor judgment.

    C. **CORRECT:** A client who experienced a left-hemispheric stroke will demonstrate the inability to recognize familiar objects, known as agnosia.

    D. A client who experienced a right-hemispheric stroke will experience a loss of depth perception.

    Ⓝ *NCLEX® Connection: Physiological Adaptation, Pathophysiology*

PRACTICE Answer

Using the ATI Active Learning Template: Nursing Skill

NURSING INTERVENTIONS

- Assess gag reflex. If the gag reflex is present, give the client a small sip of water to determine if choking occurs.
- If the client exhibits difficulty managing food or fluids, a speech therapist should do a swallowing evaluation.
- Begin the client with a prescribed diet and observe closely for choking. Have suction equipment available. Initial feedings should be done by an RN, so appropriate interventions can be taken if choking occurs.
- Thicker liquids are usually tolerated better than thin liquids. Collaborate with the speech-language pathologist and dietitian to find the proper consistency and type of diet.

Ⓝ *NCLEX® Connection: Physiological Adaptation, Illness Management*

CHAPTER 16 *Spinal Cord Injury*

Spinal cord injuries (SCIs) involve the loss of motor function, sensory function, reflexes, and control of elimination. Injuries in the cervical region result in quadriplegia: paralysis/paresis of all four extremities and trunk. Injuries below T1 result in paraplegia: paralysis/paresis of the lower extremities. Truncal instability also results if the lesion is in the upper thoracic region.

The level of cord involved dictates the consequences of spinal cord injury. For example, an injury at C4 or above poses a great risk for impaired spontaneous ventilation due to the involvement of the phrenic nerve. **(16.1)**

Not all fractures of the vertebrae cause SCIs. Direct injury to the spinal cord secondary to the trauma or bone fragments in the spinal canal must occur for the spinal cord itself to become damaged.

SCIs range from contusions or incomplete lesions of the spinal cord to complete lesions caused by a lesion that extends across the entire diameter of the cord, or an actual transection of the spinal cord. Complete lesions result in the loss of all voluntary movement and sensation below the level of the injury. Incomplete lesions result in varying losses of voluntary movement and sensation below the level of the injury.

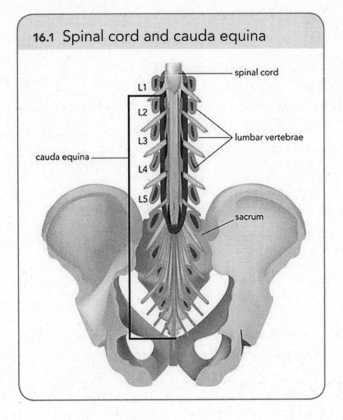

16.1 Spinal cord and cauda equina

spinal cord

L1
L2
L3
L4
L5

lumbar vertebrae

cauda equina

sacrum

HEALTH PROMOTION AND DISEASE PREVENTION

- Causes of most SCIs are trauma (such as motor vehicle accidents), diving accidents, and gunshot wounds.
- Hyperflexion injuries are caused by acceleration injuries that cause sharp forward flexion of the spine (head-on collision, fall, or diving). Hyperextension injuries are caused by a backward snap of the spine (rear-end collision or a downward fall onto the chin).

ASSESSMENT

RISK FACTORS

- Male clients age 16 to 30
- High-risk activities (extreme sports or high-speed driving) Qs
- Participation in impact sports (football or diving)
- Acts of violence (gunshot and knife wounds)
- Alcohol or drug use
- Disease (metastatic cancer or arthritis of the spine)
- Falls, especially in older adults Ⓖ

EXPECTED FINDINGS

- Report of lack of sensation of dermatomes below the level of the lesion
- Report of neck or back pain

PHYSICAL ASSESSMENT FINDINGS

- Inability to feel light touch when touched by a cotton ball, inability to discriminate between sharp and dull when touched with a safety pin or other sharp objects, and inability to discriminate between hot and cold when touched with containers of hot and cold water.
- Absent deep tendon reflexes.
- Flaccidity of muscles.
- Hypotension that is more severe when the client is in sitting in an upright position.
- Shallow respirations.
- Spinal shock, a complication of spinal cord injury, causes a total but temporary loss of all reflexive and autonomic function below the level of injury, lasting for a period of days to weeks.

LABORATORY TESTS

Urinalysis, hemoglobin, ABGs, CBCs (for evaluation of platelets and WBCs): Used to monitor for undiagnosed internal bleeding (the client might not feel pain from internal injuries) and impaired respiratory exchange (due to phrenic nerve involvement and/or inability to voluntarily increase depth and rate of respirations). Qc

DIAGNOSTIC PROCEDURES

X-rays, magnetic resonance imaging (MRI), and computed tomography (CT) imaging/computed axial tomography (CAT) scan can be used to assess the extent of the damage and the location of blood and bone fragments.

PATIENT-CENTERED CARE

NURSING CARE

Respiratory status

- Monitoring respiratory status is the first priority. Involuntary respirations can be affected due to a lesion at or above the phrenic nerve or swelling from a lesion immediately below C4. Lesions in the cervical or upper thoracic area will also impair voluntary movement of muscles used in respiration (increase in depth or rate).
- Provide oxygen and suction as needed.
- Assist with intubation and mechanical ventilation if necessary.
- Assist the client to cough by applying abdominal pressure when attempting to cough.
- Teach the client about incentive spirometer use, and encourage the client to perform coughing and deep breathing regularly.

Tissue perfusion

Neurogenic shock, which is a complication of spinal trauma, causes a sudden loss of communication within the sympathetic nervous system that maintains the normal muscle tone in blood vessel walls. Neurogenic shock can occur within 24 hr of a SCI, resulting in peripheral vasodilation that leads to venous pooling in the extremities, a drop in cardiac output and heart rate, and a life-threatening decrease in blood pressure. This complication can last for a several days to weeks.

- Monitor for hypotension, dependent edema, and loss of temperature regulation, which are common manifestations.
- When in an upright position, clients who are in neurogenic shock will experience postural hypotension. Transferring the client to a wheelchair should occur in stages.
  - Raise the head of the bed and be ready to lower the angle if the client reports dizziness.
  - Transfer the client into a reclining wheelchair with the back of the wheelchair reclined.
  - Be ready to lock and lean the wheelchair back onto the knee to a fully reclined position if the client reports dizziness after the transfer. Do not attempt to return the client to the bed.
  - Monitor for manifestations of thrombophlebitis (swelling of extremity, absent/decreased pulses, and areas of warmth and/or tenderness). The client might be on anticoagulants to prevent development of lower extremity thrombi.

Intake and output

The client might be NPO for several days. Regulation of fluid balance and nutritional support is necessary. Maintain an adequate fluid intake for the client. Fluid will aid in preventing urinary calculi and bladder infections, and will maintain soft stools.

Neurological status

After determining the baseline, monitor for an increasing loss of neurological function.

Muscle strength and tone

After determining the baseline, monitor for an increasing loss of muscle strength in the affected extremities.
- Clients who have upper motor neuron injuries (above L1 and L2) will convert to a spastic muscle tone after neurogenic shock.
- Clients who have lower motor neuron injuries (below L1 and L2) will convert to a flaccid type of paralysis.
- Because most lower motor neuron lesions involve the cauda equina, the motor and sensory deficits can be patchy, with some areas of innervation and others without.
- Encourage active range-of-motion (ROM) exercises when possible, and assist with passive ROM if the client lacks all motor function.

Mobility

Clients who have complete injuries will not regain mobility. Clients who have incomplete injuries can regain some function that will allow mobility with various types of braces. However, functional mobility can still be best attained through the use of a wheelchair.

Sensation

Varying degrees of loss of sensation will be experienced depending on whether the lesion is complete or incomplete. Take care to prevent skin breakdown in both the bed and wheelchair. Various types of foam and air mattresses are available for beds and wheelchairs. Qs

Bowel and bladder function

- **Spastic neurogenic bladder:** Clients who have upper motor neuron injuries develop spastic bladder after the neurogenic shock resolves. Bladder management options for male clients include condom catheters and stimulation of the micturition reflex by tugging on the pubic hair. Female clients need to use an indwelling urinary catheter due to the unpredictably of the release of urine.
- **Flaccid neurogenic bladder:** Clients who have lower motor neuron injuries develop a flaccid bladder. Bladder management options for males and females include intermittent catheterization and Credé's method (downward pressure placed on the bladder to manually express the urine).
- Neurogenic bowel functioning does not differ much between upper and lower motor neuron injuries. Daily use of stool softeners or bulk-forming laxatives is recommended to keep the stool soft. A bowel movement can be stimulated daily or every other day by administration of a bisacodyl suppository or digital stimulation (stimulation of the rectal sphincter with a gloved and lubricated finger) only if requested by the provider. Digital stimulation should be used cautiously to avoid provoking a vagal response, which can result in bradycardia and syncope.
- Development of a schedule as part of bladder and bowel training is critical in preventing complications related to immobility and promoting adequate nutrition and fluid balance.

Gastrointestinal function

An ileus can develop immediately after injury. Monitor for bowel sounds.

Skin integrity

Changing the client's position every 2 hr (every 1 hr when in a wheelchair) is critical. Clients who have a SCI can neither move nor feel pain from prolonged pressure. Pressure-relief devices in both the bed and the wheelchair must be consistently used.

Sexual function

Teach the client about alterations in sexual function and possible adaptive strategies. Clients who have quadriplegia and other clients who have upper motor neuron lesions are usually capable of reflexogenic erections (erections secondary to manual manipulation). Ejaculation coordinated with emission might not occur. Clients who have lower motor neuron injuries are less able to have reflexogenic erections, but clients who have incomplete injuries might be able to have a combination of reflexogenic and psychogenic erections (erections stimulated by sexual thoughts and images). Administer medications as prescribed. Qpcc

MEDICATIONS

Glucocorticoids

Adrenocortical steroids, such as methylprednisolone, aid in decreasing edema of the spinal cord (spinal shock), which can cause spinal cord compression and areas of ischemia.

Vasopressors

Norepinephrine and dopamine are administered to treat hypotension, particularly during neurogenic shock.

Antimuscarinic

Atropine may be used to treat bradycardia.

Plasma expanders

Dextran, a volume expander, is used to treat hypotension secondary to spinal shock.

NURSING ACTIONS: Observe for manifestations of fluid overload.

Muscle relaxants

Baclofen and dantrolene: Administered to clients who have severe muscle spasticity. Spasticity can be so severe that clients develop pressure ulcers, which can make sitting in a wheelchair very difficult.
- Monitor for drowsiness and muscle weakness.
- Baclofen may be administered intrathecally to reduce the sedative effects.

Cholinergics

Bethanechol: Decreases spasticity of the bladder, allowing for easier bladder training and fewer accidents.

NURSING ACTIONS: Observe for urinary retention. Measure residual periodically.

Analgesics

Opioids, nonopioids, and NSAIDs are administered for pain. Clients might not be able to feel pain from spinal cord injury. Clients who have muscle spasticity can report feeling discomfort from the muscle spasms.

Anticoagulants

Heparin or low-molecular-weight heparins are used for DVT prophylaxis.

NURSING CONSIDERATIONS
- Monitor INR, PT, and aPTT for therapeutic levels of anticoagulation.
- Observe for manifestations of gastrointestinal bleeding or bleeding secondary to unrecognized injury.

Stool softeners and bulk-forming laxatives

Docusate sodium or polycarbophil prevent constipation and keep the stool soft.

Vasodilators

- **Hydralazine and nitroglycerin:** Use PRN to treat episodes of hypertension during automatic dysreflexia.
- NURSING ACTIONS: Monitor blood pressure frequently.

THERAPEUTIC PROCEDURES

Application of immobilization devices and traction

Clients who have cervical fractures may be placed in a halo fixation device or cervical tongs. The purpose is to provide traction and/or immobilize the spinal column.

NURSING ACTIONS
- Maintain body alignment and ensure cervical tong weights hang freely.
- Monitor skin integrity by providing pin care and assessing the skin under the halo fixation vest as appropriate.
- Do not use the halo device to turn or move a client.

CLIENT EDUCATION
- If the client goes home with a halo fixation device on, provide instruction on pin and vest care.
- Teach the client signs of infection and skin breakdown.

Spinal surgery

- Spinal fusion is commonly performed when a spinal fracture creates an area of instability of the spine.
- Spinal fusions in the cervical area usually are performed using an anterior approach through the front of the neck.
- Spinal fusions in the thoracic or lumbar areas are performed using a posterior approach and can be combined with a decompressive laminectomy.
- A decompressive laminectomy is performed by removing a section of lamina; accessing the spinal canal; and removing bone fragments, foreign bodies, or hematomas that can place pressure on the spinal cord.
- Donor bone often is obtained from the iliac crest and used to fuse together the vertebrae that are unstable.
- Application of paravertebral rods can be used to mechanically immobilize several vertebral levels.

NURSING ACTIONS
- In clients who have undergone an anterior cervical fusion, monitor for possible airway compromise from swelling or hemorrhage. Observe for deviation of the trachea.
- Assess neurological status and vital signs every hour for the first 4 hr following spinal fusion.

CLIENT EDUCATION
- Inform the client that an area of decreased range of motion will always exist in the area of fusion or paravertebral rods.
- Rods are usually not removed unless they cause pain. Removal can be done after the spine has restabilized.

INTERPROFESSIONAL CARE

- The client needs intensive occupational and physical therapy to learn how to perform ADLs and reestablish mobility using a manual or electric wheelchair, or braces and crutches. The client also will be fitted for splints to prevent contractures and provide wrist support for eating and manipulating the joystick on an electric wheelchair.
- Social services needs to determine the client's financial resources, home care needs, and adaptations needed in the home prior to discharge.
- Referral of the client to an SCI support group can aid in emotionally adapting to changes in body image and role.

CLIENT EDUCATION

- Clients who have experienced SCI with subsequent loss of function will need varying levels of support upon discharge.
- Clients who have quadriplegia require a lengthy and extensive rehabilitative experience, which can occur on an outpatient or in-home basis.
- Family members need to be instructed on all aspects of clients' personal needs.
- With the assistance of social services, referrals are made for a home health nurse, home health aide, and in-home physical and occupational therapists. Q℟ᴄ
- Many adaptations might also need to be made to the home to make it wheelchair accessible.
- Although clients who have paraplegia will require less intensive therapy, all of the referrals and accommodations necessary for clients who have quadriplegia are also needed for clients who have paraplegia.
- Clients and family members will need to be taught all aspects of clients' care (ADLs, transfers, and medication regimen).

COMPLICATIONS

Orthostatic hypotension

Occurs when clients change position due to the interruption in functioning of the automatic nervous system and pooling of blood in lower extremities when in an upright position.

NURSING ACTIONS

- Change the client's positioning slowly and place the client in a wheelchair that reclines.
- Use thigh-high elastic hose or elastic wraps to increase venous return. Elastic wraps might need to extend all the way up the client's legs and include the client's abdomen.

Spinal shock

- Spinal shock is the spinal cord's response to the inflammation caused by the injury.
- Manifestations include flaccid paralysis, loss of reflex activity below level of injury, and paralytic ileus due to the loss of autonomic function.

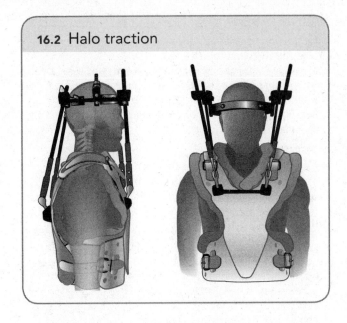

16.2 Halo traction

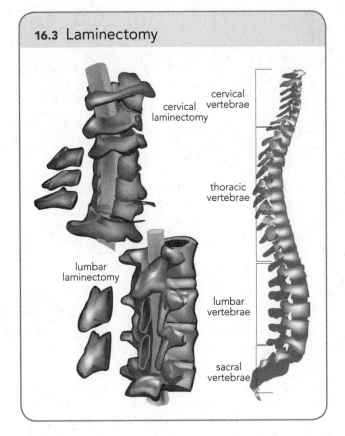

16.3 Laminectomy

cervical laminectomy

cervical vertebrae

thoracic vertebrae

lumbar laminectomy

lumbar vertebrae

sacral vertebrae

Neurogenic shock

- Neurogenic shock is a common response of the spinal cord following an injury.
- Manifestations of bradycardia, hypotension, dependent edema, and loss of temperature regulation are caused by a sudden loss of communication within the sympathetic nervous system that maintains the normal muscle tone in blood vessel walls.

NURSING ACTIONS
- Monitor vital signs for hypotension and bradycardia.
- Treat symptoms with appropriate medications (vasopressors or atropine) and IV fluids.

Autonomic dysreflexia

- Occurs secondary to the stimulation of the sympathetic nervous system and inadequate compensatory response by the parasympathetic nervous system. Clients who have lesions below T6 do not experience dysreflexia because the parasympathetic nervous system is able to neutralize the sympathetic response.
- Sympathetic stimulation is usually caused by a triggering stimulus in the lower part of the body (see Nursing Actions).
- Stimulation of the sympathetic nervous system causes extreme hypertension, sudden severe headache, pallor below the level of the spinal cord's lesion dermatome, blurred vision, diaphoresis, restlessness, nausea, and piloerection (goose bumps).
- Stimulation of the parasympathetic nervous system causes bradycardia, flushing above the corresponding dermatome to the spinal cord lesion (flushed face and neck), and nasal stuffiness.

NURSING ACTIONS
- Sit the client up to decrease blood pressure secondary to postural hypotension.
- Notify the provider.
- Determine the cause.
  - Distended bladder: most common cause (kinked or blocked urinary catheter, urinary retention, or urinary calculi)
  - Fecal impaction
  - Cold stress or drafts on lower part of the body
  - Tight clothing
  - Undiagnosed injury or illness (kidney infection or stone, lower extremity fracture)
- Treat the cause. Q EBP
  - Relieve the kink in the catheter or irrigate to remove blockage.
  - Catheterize the client. (Use anesthetic ointment on the tip of the catheter.)
  - Remove the impaction. (Use anesthetic ointment prior to removal.)
  - Adjust the room temperature and block drafts.
  - Remove tight clothing.
  - Assess for injury, such as lower extremity fracture or kidney/bladder infection.
- Monitor vital signs for severe hypertension and bradycardia.
- Administer antihypertensives (nitrates or hydralazine).

CLIENT EDUCATION
- Provide client education regarding potential causes of dysreflexia.
- Instruct the client to space out fluid intake and increase frequency of intermittent catheterizations if fluid intake is temporarily increased.
- Provide a list of possible actions to pursue if an episode of dysreflexia occurs.

Application Exercises

1. A nurse is planning care for a client who has a spinal cord injury (SCI) involving a T12 fracture 1 week ago. The client has no muscle control of the lower limbs, bowel, or bladder. Which of the following should be the nurse's highest priority?

   A. Prevention of further damage to the spinal cord

   B. Prevention of contractures of the lower extremities

   C. Prevention of skin breakdown of areas that lack sensation

   D. Prevention of postural hypotension when placing the client in a wheelchair

2. A nurse is caring for a client who has a spinal cord injury who reports a severe headache and is sweating profusely. Vital signs include blood pressure 220/110 mm Hg and apical heart rate 54/min. Which of the following actions should the nurse take first?

   A. Notify the provider.

   B. Sit the client upright in bed.

   C. Check the urinary catheter for blockage.

   D. Administer antihypertensive medication.

3. A nurse is caring for a client who has a C4 spinal cord injury. The nurse should recognize the client is at greatest risk for which of the following complications?

   A. Neurogenic shock

   B. Paralytic ileus

   C. Stress ulcer

   D. Respiratory compromise

4. A nurse is caring for a client who experienced a cervical spine injury 24 hr ago. Which of the following types of prescribed medications should the nurse clarify with the provider?

   A. Glucocorticoids

   B. Plasma expanders

   C. H_2 antagonists

   D. Muscle relaxants

5. A nurse is caring for a client who experienced a cervical spine injury 3 months ago. The nurse should plan to implement which of the following types of bladder management methods?

   A. Condom catheter

   B. Intermittent urinary catheterization

   C. Credé's method

   D. Indwelling urinary catheter

PRACTICE Active Learning Scenario

A nurse is assessing a client who has a spinal cord injury. Use the ATI Active Learning Template: System Disorder to complete this item.

EXPECTED FINDINGS: List three physical assessment findings the nurse should look for.

Application Exercises Key

1. A. **CORRECT:** The greatest risk to the client during the acute phase of an SCI is further damage to the spinal cord. When planning care, the priority intervention the nurse should take is to prevent further damage to the spinal cord by administration of corticosteroids, minimizing movement of the client until spinal stabilization is accomplished through either traction or surgery, and adequate oxygenation of the client to decrease ischemia of the spinal cord.

   B. The nurse should implement ROM exercise to prevent contractures. However, another action is the priority.

   C. The nurse should implement a turning schedule to prevent skin breakdown. However, another action is the priority.

   D. The nurse should slowly move the client to an upright position to prevent postural hypotension. However, another action is the priority.

   Ⓝ NCLEX® Connection: Physiological Adaptation, Illness Management

2. A. The nurse should notify the provider. However, another action is the priority.

   B. **CORRECT:** The greatest risk to the client is experiencing a cerebrovascular accident (stroke) secondary to elevated blood pressure caused by autonomic dysreflexia. The first action the nurse should take is to elevate the head of the bed until the client is in an upright position, which should lower the blood pressure secondary to postural hypotension.

   C. The nurse should check the client's catheter for blockage. However, another action is the priority.

   D. The nurse should administer an antihypertensive medication if indicated. However, another action is the priority.

   Ⓝ NCLEX® Connection: Reduction of Risk Potential, Changes/Abnormalities in Vital Signs

3. A. The nurse should monitor for neurogenic shock, which is a response of the sympathetic nervous system of a client who has a SCI. However, another complication is the priority.

   B. The nurse should monitor for a paralytic ileus, which is a complication immediately following a SCI. However, another complication is the priority.

   C. The nurse should monitor for a stress ulcer, which is a response to changes caused from the SCI. However, another complication is the priority.

   D. **CORRECT:** When using the airway, breathing, and circulation (ABC) approach to client care, the priority complication is respiratory compromise secondary to involvement of the phrenic nerve. Maintenance of an airway and provision of ventilatory support as needed is the priority intervention.

   Ⓝ NCLEX® Connection: Physiological Adaptation, Pathophysiology

4. A. The nurse should administer glucocorticoids to decrease edema of the spinal cord.

   B. The nurse should administer plasma expanders to treat hypotension caused by the SCI.

   C. The nurse should administer H2 antagonists to decrease the complication of developing a gastric ulcer from stress.

   D. **CORRECT:** The nurse should clarify with the provider the need for the client to receive muscle relaxants. The client will not experience muscle spasms until after the spinal shock has resolved, making muscle relaxants unnecessary at this time.

   Ⓝ NCLEX® Connection: Pharmacological and Parenteral Therapies, Medication Administration

5. A. **CORRECT:** The nurse should implement the noninvasive use of a condom catheter, because the bladder will empty on its own due to the client having an upper motor neuron injury, which is manifested by a spastic bladder.

   B. The nurse should implement intermittent urinary catheterization method for a client who has a flaccid bladder.

   C. The nurse should implement the Credé's method for a client who has a flaccid bladder.

   D. An indwelling urinary catheter is an invasive procedure. The nurse should not implement this bladder management method for the client.

   Ⓝ NCLEX® Connection: Basic Care and Comfort, Elimination

PRACTICE Answer

Using the ATI Active Learning Template: System Disorder

EXPECTED FINDINGS

- Inability to feel light touch when touched by a cotton ball, inability to discriminate between sharp and dull when touched with a safety pin or other sharp objects, and an inability to discriminate between hot and cold when touched with containers of hot and cold water
- Absent deep tendon reflexes
- Flaccidity of muscles
- Hypotension that is more severe when the client is in sitting in an upright position
- Shallow respirations
- Dependent edema
- Neurogenic shock, which accompanies spinal trauma and causes a total loss of all reflexive and autonomic function below the level of the injury for a period of several days to weeks
- Loss of temperature regulation: hyperthermia or hypothermia

Ⓝ NCLEX® Connection: Reduction of Risk Potential, System Specific Assessments

When reviewing the following chapters, keep in mind the relevant topics and tasks of the NCLEX outline, in particular:

Client Needs: Pharmacological and Parenteral Therapies

ADVERSE EFFECTS/CONTRAINDICATIONS/SIDE EFFECTS/ INTERACTIONS: Assess the client for actual or potential side effects and adverse effects of medications.

EXPECTED ACTIONS/OUTCOMES: Evaluate client response to medication.

MEDICATION ADMINISTRATION: Educate the client on medication self-administration procedures.

Client Needs: Reduction of Risk Potential

LABORATORY VALUES: Identify laboratory values for ABGs, BUN, cholesterol, glucose, hematocrit, hemoglobin, glycosylated hemoglobin, platelets, potassium, sodium, WBC, creatinine, PT, PTT & APTT, INR.

POTENTIAL FOR COMPLICATIONS OF DIAGNOSTIC TESTS/ TREATMENTS/PROCEDURES: Maintain tube patency.

THERAPEUTIC PROCEDURES: Educate client about home management of care.

Client Needs: Physiological Adaptation

ALTERATIONS IN BODY SYSTEMS: Monitor and care for clients on a ventilator.

MEDICAL EMERGENCIES: Apply knowledge of nursing procedures and psychomotor skills when caring for a client experiencing a medical emergency.

PATHOPHYSIOLOGY
Identify pathophysiology related to an acute or chronic condition.

Understand general principles of pathophysiology.

CHAPTER 17 *Respiratory Diagnostic Procedures*

Respiratory diagnostic procedures are used to evaluate a client's respiratory status by checking indicators such as the oxygenation of the blood, lung functioning, and the integrity of the airway.

Respiratory diagnostic procedures nurses should be knowledgeable about include pulmonary function tests, arterial blood gases, bronchoscopy, and thoracentesis.

Pulmonary function tests

Pulmonary function tests (PFTs) determine lung function and breathing difficulties.
- PFTs measure lung volumes and capacities, diffusion capacity, gas exchange, flow rates, and airway resistance, along with distribution of ventilation.
- Helpful in identifying clients who have lung disease.
- Commonly performed for clients who have dyspnea.
- Can be performed before surgical procedures to identify clients who have respiratory risks.
- If client is smoker, instruct client not to smoke 6 to 8 hr prior to testing.
- If a client uses inhalers, withhold 4 to 6 hr prior to testing. (This can vary according to facility policy.)

Arterial blood gases

An arterial blood gas (ABG) sample reports the status of oxygenation and acid–base balance of the blood.
- An ABG measures the following.
  - **pH:** amount of free hydrogen ions in the arterial blood (H+)
  - **PaO$_2$:** partial pressure of oxygen
  - **PaCO$_2$:** partial pressure of carbon dioxide
  - **HCO$_3^-$:** concentration of bicarbonate in arterial blood
  - **SaO$_2$:** percentage of oxygen bound to Hgb as compared with the total amount that can be possibly carried
- ABGs can be obtained by an arterial puncture or through an arterial line.

INDICATIONS

POTENTIAL DIAGNOSES
- Blood pH levels can be affected by a number of disease processes (respiratory, renal, malnutrition, electrolyte imbalance, endocrine, or neurologic).
- These assessments are helpful in monitoring the effectiveness of various treatments (such as acidosis interventions), in guiding oxygen therapy, and in evaluating client responses to weaning from mechanical ventilation.

CONSIDERATIONS

Arterial puncture

PREPROCEDURE

NURSING ACTIONS
- Obtain a heparinized syringe for the sample collection.
- Perform an Allen's test prior to arterial puncture to verify patent radial and ulnar circulation. Compress the ulnar and radial arteries simultaneously while instructing the client to form a fist. Then instruct the client to relax his hand while assessing the palm and fingers for blanching. Next, release pressure on the ulnar artery while observing the hand for flushing caused by capillary refilling. The client's hand should turn pink within 15 seconds, indicating patency of the ulnar artery and an ability to use the radial artery to obtain arterial blood gases. **(17.1)**

CLIENT EDUCATION: Explain and reinforce the procedure with the client. Clients often experience pain with repeated ABG level checks and are often unaware of the purpose of the puncture. Q**PCC**

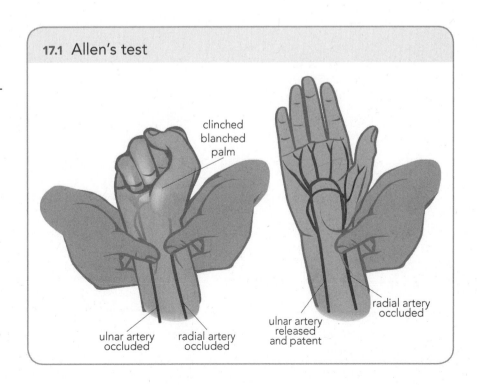

17.1 Allen's test

clinched blanched palm

radial artery occluded

ulnar artery released and patent

ulnar artery occluded

radial artery occluded

INTRAPROCEDURE

NURSING ACTIONS

- Perform an arterial puncture using surgical aseptic technique, and collect a specimen into a heparinized syringe.
- Place the collected and capped specimen into a basin of ice and water to preserve pH levels and oxygen pressure. The specimen should be transported to the laboratory immediately.
- Accessing the radial artery for sampling can be more difficult with older adult clients due to impaired peripheral vasculature. Ⓖ

POSTPROCEDURE

NURSING ACTIONS

- Immediately after an arterial puncture, hold direct pressure over the site for at least 5 min. Pressure must be maintained for at least 20 min if the client is receiving anticoagulant therapy. Ensure that bleeding has stopped prior to removing direct pressure. Qᴘᴄᴄ
- Monitor the ABG sampling site for bleeding, loss of pulse, swelling, and changes in temperature and color.
- Document all interventions and client response.
- Report results to the provider as soon as they are available.
- Administer oxygen. Change ventilator settings as prescribed, or notify a respiratory therapist.

  ! Note: Arterial puncture is frequently done by a respiratory therapist in hospital settings.

INTERPRETATION OF FINDINGS

Blood pH levels less than 7.35 reflect acidosis, and levels greater than 7.45 reflect alkalosis. **(17.2)**

17.2 ABG measures and expected reference ranges

ABG MEASURE	EXPECTED REFERENCE RANGE
pH	7.35 to 7.45
PAO$_2$	80 to 100 mm Hg
PACO$_2$	35 to 45 mm Hg
HCO$_3^-$	21 to 28 mEq/L
SAO$_2$	95% to 100%

COMPLICATIONS

Hematoma, arterial occlusion

A hematoma occurs when blood accumulates under the skin at the IV site.

NURSING ACTIONS

- Observe for changes in temperature, swelling, color, loss of pulse, or pain.
- Notify the provider immediately if manifestations persist. Qᴛᴄ
- Apply pressure to the hematoma site.

Air embolism

Air enters the arterial system during catheter insertion.

NURSING ACTIONS

- Place the client on his left side in the Trendelenburg position.
- Monitor for sudden onset of shortness of breath, decrease in SaO$_2$ levels, chest pain, anxiety, and air hunger.
- Notify the provider immediately if symptoms occur, administer oxygen therapy, and obtain ABGs. Continue to assess the client's respiratory status for any deterioration.

Bronchoscopy

Bronchoscopy permits visualization of the larynx, trachea, and bronchi through either a flexible fiber-optic or rigid bronchoscope.

- Bronchoscopy can be performed as an outpatient procedure, in a surgical suite under general anesthesia, or at the bedside under local anesthesia and moderate (conscious) sedation.
- Bronchoscopy can also be performed on clients who are receiving mechanical ventilation by inserting the scope through the client's endotracheal tube.

INDICATIONS

POTENTIAL DIAGNOSES

- Visualization of abnormalities such as tumors, inflammation, and strictures
- Biopsy of suspicious tissue (lung cancer)
  - Clients undergoing a bronchoscopy with biopsy have additional risks for bleeding and/or perforation.
- Aspiration of deep sputum or lung abscesses for culture and sensitivity or cytology (pneumonia)

  ! Bronchoscopy is also performed for therapeutic reasons, such as removal of foreign bodies and secretions from the tracheobronchial tree, treating postoperative atelectasis, and to destroy and excise lesions.

CONSIDERATIONS

PREPROCEDURE

NURSING ACTIONS

- Assess for allergies to anesthetic agents or routine use of anticoagulants.
- Ensure that a consent form is signed by the client prior to the procedure.
- Remove the client's dentures, if applicable, prior to the procedure.
- Maintain the client on NPO status prior to the procedure, usually 4 to 8 hr, to reduce the risk of aspiration when the cough reflex is blocked by anesthesia.
- Administer preprocedure medications, such as an anxiolytic, atropine, viscous lidocaine, or local anesthetic throat spray.

INTRAPROCEDURE

NURSING ACTIONS

- Position the client in a sitting or supine position.
- Assist in collecting and labeling specimens. Ensure prompt delivery to the laboratory.
- Monitor vital signs, respiratory pattern, and oxygenation status throughout the procedure.
- Sedation given to older adult clients who have respiratory insufficiency can precipitate respiratory arrest. Ⓖ

POSTPROCEDURE

NURSING ACTIONS

- Continuously monitor respirations, blood pressure, pulse oximetry, heart rate, and level of consciousness during the recovery period.
  - Assess level of consciousness while recognizing that older adult clients can develop confusion or lethargy due to the effects of medications given during the bronchoscopy.
- Assess level of consciousness, presence of gag reflex, and ability to swallow prior to resuming oral intake.
  - Allow adequate time for the cough and gag reflex to return prior to resuming oral intake. The gag reflex can be slower to return in older adult clients receiving local anesthesia due to impaired laryngeal reflex.
  - Once the gag reflex returns, the nurse can offer ice chips to the client and eventually fluids.
- Monitor for development of significant fever (mild fever for less than 24 hr is not uncommon), productive cough, significant hemoptysis indicative of hemorrhage (a small amount of blood-tinged sputum is expected), and hypoxemia.
- Be prepared to intervene for unexpected responses, aspiration, and laryngospasm.
- Provide oral hygiene.
- Evaluate and document the client's response to the procedure (stable vital signs, return of gag reflex).
- For older adult clients, encourage coughing and deep breathing every 2 hr. There is an increased risk of respiratory infection and pneumonia in older adult clients due to decreased cough effectiveness and decreased secretion clearance. Respiratory infections can be more severe and last longer in older adult clients. Ⓖ
- The client is not discharged from the recovery room until adequate cough reflex and respiratory effort are present.

CLIENT EDUCATION: Instruct clients that gargling with salt water or using throat lozenges can provide comfort for soreness of the throat.

COMPLICATIONS

Laryngospasm

- Laryngospasm is uncontrolled muscle contractions of the laryngeal cords (vocal cords) that impede the ability to inhale.
- Continuously monitor for signs of respiratory distress.

Pneumothorax

- Pneumothorax can occur following a rigid bronchoscopy.
- Assess breath sounds and oxygen saturation, and obtain a follow-up chest x-ray.

Aspiration

Aspiration can occur if the client chokes on oral or gastric secretions.

NURSING ACTIONS

- Prevent aspiration by withholding oral fluids or food until the gag reflex returns (usually 2 hr). Qs
- Perform suctioning as needed.

Thoracentesis

Thoracentesis is the surgical perforation of the chest wall and pleural space with a large-bore needle. It is performed to obtain specimens for diagnostic evaluation, instill medication into the pleural space, and remove fluid (effusion) or air from the pleural space for therapeutic relief of pleural pressure.

- Thoracentesis is performed under local anesthesia by a provider at the client's bedside, in a procedure room, or in a provider's office.
- Use of an ultrasound for guidance decreases the risk of complications.

INDICATIONS

POTENTIAL DIAGNOSES

- Transudates (heart failure, cirrhosis, nephritic syndrome, hypoproteinemia)
- Exudates (inflammatory, infectious, neoplastic conditions)
- Empyema
- Pneumonia
- Blunt, crushing, or penetrating chest injuries/trauma, or invasive thoracic procedures, such as lung or cardiac surgery

CLIENT PRESENTATION

- Large amounts of fluid in the pleural space compress lung tissue and can cause pain, shortness of breath, cough, and other manifestations of pleural pressure.
- Assessment of the effusion area can reveal abnormal breath sounds, dull percussion sounds, and decreased chest wall expansion. Pain can occur due to inflammatory process.

INTERPRETATION OF FINDINGS

Aspirated fluid is analyzed for general appearance, cell counts, protein and glucose content, the presence of enzymes such as lactate dehydrogenase (LDH) and amylase, abnormal cells, and culture.

CONSIDERATIONS

PREPROCEDURE

Percussion, auscultation, radiography, or sonography is used to locate the effusion and needle insertion site.
It can be necessary for the nurse to assist the older adult client to maintain an appropriate position for the thoracentesis. Arthritis, tremors, or weakness can make it difficult for the client to remain still in the required position for the procedure. ©

NURSING ACTIONS
- Ensure that the client has signed the informed consent form.
- Gather all needed supplies.
- Obtain preprocedure x-ray to locate pleural effusion and to determine needle insertion site.
- Position the client sitting upright with his arms and shoulders raised and supported on pillows and/or on an overbed table and with his feet and legs well-supported.

CLIENT EDUCATION
Instruct the client to remain absolutely still (risk of accidental needle damage) during the procedure and to not cough or talk unless instructed by the provider.

INTRAPROCEDURE

NURSING ACTIONS
- Assist the provider with the procedure (strict surgical aseptic technique). QTc
- Prepare the client for a feeling of pressure with needle insertion and fluid removal.
- Monitor vital signs, skin color, and oxygen saturation throughout the procedure.
- Measure and record the amount of fluid removed from the chest.
- Label specimens at the bedside, and promptly send them to the laboratory.

> ! The amount of fluid removed is limited to 1 L at a time to prevent re-expansion pulmonary edema.

POSTPROCEDURE

NURSING ACTIONS
- Apply a dressing over the puncture site, and assess dressing for bleeding or drainage.
- Monitor vital signs and respiratory status (respiratory rate and rhythm, breath sounds, oxygenation status) hourly for the first several hours after the thoracentesis.
- Auscultate lungs for reduced breath sounds on side of thoracentesis.
- Encourage the client to deep breathe to assist with lung expansion.
- Obtain a postprocedure chest x-ray (check resolution of effusions, rule out pneumothorax).

COMPLICATIONS

Mediastinal shift

Shift of thoracic structures to one side of the body.

NURSING ACTIONS
- Monitor vital signs.
- Auscultate lungs for a decrease in or absence of breath sounds.

Pneumothorax

Pneumothorax is a collapsed lung. It can occur due to injury to the lung during the procedure.

NURSING ACTIONS
- Monitor for manifestations of pneumothorax, such as diminished breath sounds, distended neck veins, asymmetry of the chest wall, respiratory distress, and cyanosis.
- Monitor postprocedure chest x-ray results.
- Educate the client on indications of a pneumothorax, which can develop during the first 24 hr following a thoracentesis. Indications include deviated trachea, pain on the affected side that worsens at the end of inhalation and exhalation, affected side not moving in and out upon inhalation and exhalation, increased heart rate, rapid shallow respirations, nagging cough, or feeling of air hunger.

Bleeding

Bleeding can occur if the client is moved during the procedure or is at an increased risk for bleeding.

NURSING ACTIONS
- Monitor for coughing and hemoptysis.
- Monitor vital signs and laboratory results for evidence of bleeding (hypotension, reduced Hgb level).
- Assess thoracentesis site for bleeding.

Infection

Infection can occur due to the introduction of bacteria with the needle puncture.

NURSING ACTIONS
- Ensure that sterile technique is maintained.
- Monitor the client's temperature following the procedure.

Application Exercises

1. A nurse is caring for a client who is scheduled for a thoracentesis. Prior to the procedure, which of the following actions should the nurse take?

   A. Position the client in an upright position, leaning over the bedside table.

   B. Explain the procedure.

   C. Obtain ABGs.

   D. Administer benzocaine spray.

2. A nurse is reviewing ABG laboratory results of a client who is in respiratory distress. The results are pH 7.47, $PaCO_2$ 32 mm Hg, HCO_3 22 mm Hg. The nurse should recognize that the client is experiencing which of the following acid-base imbalances?

   A. Respiratory acidosis

   B. Respiratory alkalosis

   C. Metabolic acidosis

   D. Metabolic alkalosis

3. A nurse is assessing a client following a bronchoscopy. Which of the following findings should the nurse report to the provider?

   A. Blood-tinged sputum

   B. Dry, nonproductive cough

   C. Sore throat

   D. Bronchospasms

4. A nurse is caring for a client who is scheduled for a thoracentesis. Which of the following supplies should the nurse ensure are in the client's room? (Select all that apply.)

   A. Oxygen equipment

   B. Incentive spirometer

   C. Pulse oximeter

   D. Sterile dressing

   E. Suture removal kit

5. A nurse is caring for a client following a thoracentesis. Which of the following manifestations should the nurse recognize as risks for complications? (Select all that apply.)

   A. Dyspnea

   B. Localized bloody drainage on the dressing

   C. Fever

   D. Hypotension

   E. Report of pain at the puncture site

PRACTICE Active Learning Scenario

A nurse is assessing a client following a thoracentesis. Use the ATI Active Learning Template: Therapeutic Procedure to complete this item.

NURSING INTERVENTIONS (PRE, INTRA, POST): List three postprocedure nursing actions the nurse should take while caring for this client.

Application Exercises Key

1. A. **CORRECT:** Positioning the client in an upright position and bent over the bedside table widens the intercostal space for the provider to access the pleural fluid.

   B. It is the responsibility of the provider, not the nurse, to explain the procedure to the client.

   C. It is not indicated that the client needs ABGs drawn.

   D. Benzocaine spray is administered for a bronchoscopy, not a thoracentesis.

   Ⓝ *NCLEX® Connection: Reduction of Risk Potential, Diagnostic Tests*

2. A. A client who is experiencing respiratory acidosis will have a decreased pH and an increased $PaCO_2$.

   B. **CORRECT:** A client who is experiencing respiratory alkalosis will have an increased pH and a decreased $PaCO_2$. Possible causes of respiratory alkalosis include hyperventilation, fever, and respiratory infections.

   C. A client who is experiencing metabolic acidosis will have a decreased pH and a decreased HCO_3.

   D. A client who is experiencing metabolic alkalosis will have an increased pH and an increased HCO_3.

   Ⓝ *NCLEX® Connection: Reduction of Risk Potential, Diagnostic Tests*

3. A. Blood-tinged sputum is an expecting finding following a bronchoscopy.

   B. A dry, nonproductive cough is an expected finding following a bronchoscopy.

   C. A sore throat is an expected finding following a bronchoscopy.

   D. **CORRECT:** Bronchospams can indicate the client is having difficulty maintaining a patent airway. The nurse should notify the provider immediately.

   Ⓝ *NCLEX® Connection: Reduction of Risk Potential, Diagnostic Tests*

4. A. **CORRECT:** Oxygen equipment is necessary to have in the client's room if the client becomes short of breath following the procedure.

   B. An incentive spirometer is indicated for a client following thoracic surgery to promote improved oxygenation and pulmonary function.

   C. **CORRECT:** Pulse oximetry is necessary to monitor oxygen saturation level during the procedure.

   D. **CORRECT:** A sterile dressing is necessary to apply to the puncture site following the procedure.

   E. A suture removal kit is needed to remove sutures following surgery.

   Ⓝ *NCLEX® Connection: Reduction of Risk Potential, Diagnostic Tests*

5. A. **CORRECT:** Dyspnea can indicate a pneumothorax or a reaccumulation of fluid. The nurse should notify the provider immediately.

   B. Localized bloody drainage contained on a dressing is an expected finding following a thoracentesis.

   C. **CORRECT:** Fever can indicate an infection. The nurse should notify the provider immediately.

   D. **CORRECT:** Hypotension can indicate intrathoracic bleeding. The nurse should notify the provider immediately.

   E. The client's report of pain at the puncture site is an expected finding following a thoracentesis.

   Ⓝ *NCLEX® Connection: Reduction of Risk Potential, Potential for Complications of Diagnostic Tests/Treatments/Procedures*

PRACTICE Answer

Using the ATI Active Learning Template: Therapeutic Procedure

NURSING INTERVENTIONS (PRE, INTRA, POST)

- Apply a dressing over the puncture site, and assess dressing for bleeding or drainage.
- Monitor vital signs and respiratory status (respiratory rate and rhythm, breath sounds, oxygenation status) hourly for the first several hours after the thoracentesis.
- Auscultate lungs for reduced breath sounds on side of thoracentesis.
- Encourage the client to deep breathe to assist with lung expansion.

Ⓝ *NCLEX® Connection: Reduction of Risk Potential, Diagnostic Tests*

UNIT 3   NURSING CARE OF CLIENTS WHO HAVE RESPIRATORY DISORDERS
SECTION: DIAGNOSTIC AND THERAPEUTIC PROCEDURES

CHAPTER 18   # Chest Tube Insertion and Monitoring

Chest tubes are inserted into the pleural space to drain fluid, blood, or air; reestablish a negative pressure; facilitate lung expansion; and restore normal intrapleural pressure.

Chest tubes can be inserted in the emergency department, at the bedside, or in the operating room through a thoracotomy incision.

Chest tubes are removed when the lungs have re-expanded or there is no more fluid drainage.

Chest tube systems

A disposable three-chamber drainage system is most often used.
- First chamber: drainage collection
- Second chamber: water seal
- Third chamber: suction control (can be wet or dry)

Water seals are created by adding sterile fluid to a chamber up to the 2 cm line. While this is the minimum amount required for functioning, recommended amounts can vary by manufacturer. The water seal allows air to exit from the pleural space on exhalation and stops air from entering with inhalation.
- To maintain the water seal, keep the chamber upright and below the chest tube insertion site at all times. Routinely monitor the water level due to the possibility of evaporation. Add fluid as needed to maintain the manufacturer's recommended water seal level.
- **Wet suction:** The height of the sterile fluid in the suction control chamber determines the amount of suction transmitted to the pleural space. A suction pressure of –20 cm H_2O is commonly prescribed. The prescribed amount of suction is applied by setting the regulator on the chest tube drainage device. The application of suction results in continuous bubbling in the suction chamber. Monitor the fluid level and add fluid as needed to maintain the prescribed level of suctioning.
- **Dry suction:** When a dry suction control device is used, the provider prescribes a level of suction for the device, typically –20 cm H_2O. When connected to wall suction, the regulator on the chest tube drainage system is set to the manufacturer's recommendation.

- Tidaling (movement of the fluid level with respiration) is expected in the water seal chamber. With spontaneous respirations, the fluid level will rise with inspiration (increase in negative pressure in lung) and will fall with expiration. With positive-pressure mechanical ventilation, the fluid level will rise with expiration and fall with inspiration.
- Cessation of tidaling in the water seal chamber signals lung re-expansion or an obstruction within the system.
- Continuous bubbling in the water seal chamber indicates an air leak in the system.

Chest tube insertion

INDICATIONS

POTENTIAL DIAGNOSES

Pneumothorax: partial to complete collapse of the lung due to accumulation of air in the pleural space

Hemothorax: partial to complete collapse of the lung due to accumulation of blood in the pleural space

Postoperative chest drainage: thoracotomy or open-heart surgery

Pleural effusion: abnormal accumulation of fluid in the pleural space

Pulmonary empyema: accumulation of pus in the pleural space due to pulmonary infection, lung abscess, or infected pleural effusion

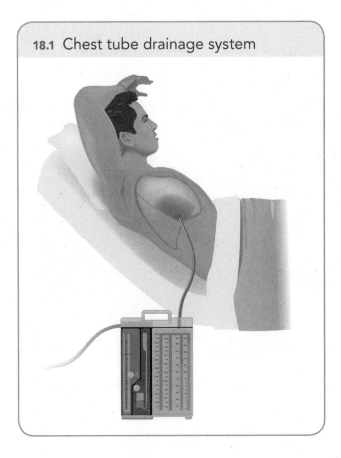

18.1 Chest tube drainage system

CLIENT PRESENTATION

- Dyspnea
- Distended neck veins
- Hemodynamic instability
- Pleuritic chest pain
- Cough
- Absent or reduced breath sounds on the affected side
- Hyperresonance on percussion of affected side (pneumothorax)
- Dullness or flatness on percussion of the affected side (hemothorax, pleural effusion)
- Asymmetrical chest wall motion

CONSIDERATIONS

PREPROCEDURE

- Verify that the consent form is signed.
- Reinforce client teaching. Breathing will improve when the chest tube is in place. Qpcc
- Assess for allergies to local anesthetics.
- Assist the client into the desired position (supine or semi-Fowler's).
- Prepare the chest drainage system prior to the chest tube insertion per the facility's protocol. (Fill the water seal chamber.)
- Administer pain and sedation medications as prescribed.
- Prep the insertion site with povidone-iodine or other facility-approved agent.

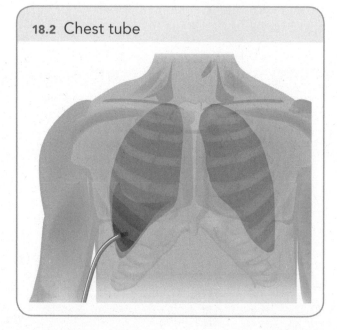

18.2 Chest tube

INTRAPROCEDURE

- Assist the provider with insertion of the chest tube, application of a dressing to the insertion site, and set-up of the drainage system. Qtc
  - Place the chest tube drainage system below the client's chest level with the tubing coiled on the bed. Ensure that the tubing from the bed to the drainage system is straight to promote drainage via gravity.
- The nurse should continually monitor vital signs and response to the procedure.

POSTPROCEDURE

- Assess vital signs, breath sounds, SaO_2, color, and respiratory effort as indicated by the status of the client and at least every 4 hr.
- Encourage coughing and deep breathing every 2 hr.
- Keep the drainage system below the client's chest level, including during ambulation.
- Monitor chest tube placement and function.
  - Check the water seal level every 2 hr, and add fluid as needed. The fluid level should fluctuate with respiratory effort.
  - Document the amount and color of drainage hourly for the first 24 hr and then at least every 8 hr. Mark the date, hour, and drainage level on the container at the end of each shift. Report excessive drainage (greater than 70 mL/hr) or drainage that is cloudy or red to the provider. Drainage often increases with position changes or coughing.
  - Monitor the fluid in the suction control chamber, and maintain the prescribed fluid level.
  - Ensure the regulator dial on the dry suction device is at the prescribed level.
  - Check for expected findings of tidaling in the water seal chamber and continuous bubbling only in the suction chamber.
- Routinely monitor tubing for kinks, occlusions, or loose connections.
- Monitor the chest tube insertion site for redness, pain, infection, and crepitus (air leakage in subcutaneous tissue).
- Tape all connections between the chest tube and chest tube drainage system.
- Position the client in the semi-to high-Fowler's position to promote optimal lung expansion and drainage of fluid from the lungs.
- Administer pain medications as prescribed. Qpcc
- Obtain a chest x-ray to verify the chest tube's placement.
- Keep two enclosed hemostats, sterile water, and an occlusive dressing located at the bedside at all times.
- Due to the risk of causing a tension pneumothorax, chest tubes are clamped only when prescribed in specific circumstances, such as in the case of an air leak, during drainage system change, accidental disconnection of tubing, or damage to the drainage system.
- Do not strip or milk tubing; only perform this action when prescribed. Stripping creates a high negative pressure and can damage lung tissue.

COMPLICATIONS

Air leaks

Air leaks can result if a connection is not taped securely.

NURSING ACTIONS
- Monitor the water seal chamber for continuous bubbling (air leak finding). If observed, locate the source of the air leak, and intervene accordingly (tighten the connection, replace drainage system).
- Check all connections.
- Notify the provider if an air leak is noted. If prescribed, gently apply a padded clamp to determine the location of the air leak. Remove the clamp immediately following assessment. Qtc

Accidental disconnection, system breakage, or removal

These complications can occur at any time.

NURSING ACTIONS
- If the tubing separates, instruct the client to exhale as much as possible and to cough to remove as much air as possible from the pleural space.
- If the chest tube drainage system is compromised, immerse the end of the chest tube in sterile water to restore the water seal.
- If a chest tube is accidentally removed, dress the area with dry, sterile gauze.

Tension pneumothorax

- Sucking chest wounds, prolonged clamping of the tubing, kinks or obstruction in the tubing, or mechanical ventilation with high levels of positive end expiratory pressure (PEEP) can cause a tension pneumothorax.
- Assessment findings include tracheal deviation, absent breath sounds on one side, distended neck veins, respiratory distress, asymmetry of the chest, and cyanosis.

Chest tube removal

- Provide pain medication 30 min before removing chest tubes. QEBP
- Assist the provider with sutures and chest tube removal.
- Instruct the client to take a deep breath, exhale, and bear down (Valsalva maneuver) or to take a deep breath and hold it (increases intrathoracic pressure and reduces risk of air emboli) during chest tube removal.
- Apply airtight sterile petroleum jelly gauze dressing. Secure in place with a heavyweight stretch tape.
- Obtain chest x-rays as prescribed. This is performed to verify continued resolution of the pneumothorax, hemothorax, or pleural effusion.
- Monitor for excessive wound drainage, signs of infection, or recurrent pneumothorax.

Application Exercises

1. A nurse is preparing to care for a client following chest tube placement. Which of the following items should be available in the client's room? (Select all that apply.)
   - A. Oxygen
   - B. Sterile water
   - C. Enclosed hemostat clamps
   - D. Indwelling urinary catheter
   - E. Occlusive dressing

2. A nurse is caring for a client who has a chest tube and drainage system in place. The nurse observes that the chest tube was accidentally removed. Which of the following actions should the nurse take first?
   - A. Obtain a chest x-ray.
   - B. Apply sterile gauze to the insertion site.
   - C. Place tape around the insertion site.
   - D. Assess respiratory status.

3. A nurse is assessing a client who has a chest tube and drainage system in place. Which of the following are expected findings? (Select all that apply.)
   - A. Continuous bubbling in the water seal chamber
   - B. Gentle constant bubbling in the suction control chamber
   - C. Rise and fall in the level of water in the water seal chamber with inspiration and expiration
   - D. Exposed sutures without dressing
   - E. Drainage system upright at chest level

4. A nurse is assisting a provider with the removal of a chest tube. Which of the following should the nurse instruct the client to do?
   - A. Lie on his left side.
   - B. Use the incentive spirometer.
   - C. Cough at regular intervals.
   - D. Perform the Valsalva maneuver.

5. A nurse is planning care for a client following the insertion of a chest tube and drainage system. Which of the following should be included in the plan of care? (Select all that apply.)
   - A. Encourage the client to cough every 2 hr.
   - B. Check for continuous bubbling in the suction chamber.
   - C. Strip the drainage tubing every 4 hr.
   - D. Clamp the tube once a day.
   - E. Obtain a chest x-ray.

Application Exercises Key

1. A. **CORRECT:** Oxygen should be readily available in case the client develops respiratory distress following chest tube placement. The nurse should monitor respiration, oxygen saturation, and lung sounds.

B. **CORRECT:** If the chest tubing becomes disconnected, the end of the tubing should be placed in sterile water to restore the water seal.

C. **CORRECT:** Hemostat clamps should be available for the nurse to use to check for air leaks.

D. An indwelling urinary catheter is not indicated for a client who has a chest tube.

E. **CORRECT:** If the chest tubing becomes disconnected, the nurse should immediately place a gauze dressing over the site. An occlusive dressing can also be necessary to prevent the redevelopment of a pneumothorax.

Ⓝ *NCLEX® Connection: Reduction of Risk Potential, Therapeutic Procedures*

2. A. Obtaining a chest x-ray determines if the lung is inflated or if the client has a pneumothorax after the chest tube was accidentally pulled out is an appropriate action, but it is not the first action the nurse should take.

B. **CORRECT:** Using the airway, breathing, and circulation (ABC) priority-setting framework, application of a sterile gauze to the site should be the first action for the nurse to take. This allows air to escape and reduces the risk for development of a tension pneumothorax.

C. Placing tape around the insertion site ensures that the sterile gauze remains intact and is an appropriate action, but it is not the first action.

D. Assessing respiratory status is an appropriate action, but it is not the first action.

Ⓝ *NCLEX® Connection: Reduction of Risk Potential, Potential for Complications of Diagnostic Tests/Treatments/Procedures*

3. A. Continuous bubbling in the water seal chamber indicates an air leak.

B. **CORRECT:** Gentle bubbling in the suction control chamber is an expected finding as air is being removed.

C. **CORRECT:** A rise and fall of the fluid level in the water seal chamber upon inspiration and expiration indicates that the drainage system is functioning properly.

D. The nurse should cover the sutures at the insertion site with an airtight dressing.

E. The drainage system should be maintained in an upright position below the level of the client's chest.

Ⓝ *NCLEX® Connection: Physiological Adaptation, Alterations in Body Systems*

4. A. The position the client should assume during removal of a chest tube depends upon the location of the insertion site.

B. Use of an incentive spirometer is not indicated during chest tube removal.

C. The client is instructed to breathe normally and remain calm during the procedure.

D. **CORRECT:** The client should be instructed to take a deep breath, exhale, and bear down (Valsalva maneuver) as the chest tube is being removed. This increases intrathoracic pressure and reduces the risk of an air embolism.

Ⓝ *NCLEX® Connection: Reduction of Risk Potential, Therapeutic Procedures*

5. A. **CORRECT:** The nurse should instruct the client to cough every 2 hr. This promotes oxygenation and lung reexpansion.

B. **CORRECT:** The nurse should check for continuous bubbling in the suction chamber to verify that suction is being maintained at an appropriate level.

C. The nurse should not milk or strip the drainage tubing to check for kinks. This action is only to be done when prescribed. Stripping creates negative high pressure and can damage lung tissue.

D. The nurse should not clamp the tubing unless indicated by the provider. This is done to verify for the presence of an air leak or if the tubing accidentally has been disconnected. Clamping can cause a tension pneumothorax.

E. **CORRECT:** A chest x-ray is obtained following the procedure to verify chest tube placement.

Ⓝ *NCLEX® Connection: Reduction of Risk Potential, Therapeutic Procedures*

UNIT 3 NURSING CARE OF CLIENTS WHO HAVE RESPIRATORY DISORDERS
SECTION: DIAGNOSTIC AND THERAPEUTIC PROCEDURES

CHAPTER 19 # Respiratory Management and Mechanical Ventilation

Oxygen is a tasteless and colorless gas that accounts for 21% of atmospheric air.

Oxygen is used to maintain adequate cellular oxygenation. It is used in the treatment of many acute and chronic respiratory problems.

Oxygen is administered in an attempt to maintain an SaO_2 of 95% to 100% by using the lowest amount of oxygen without putting the client at risk for complications.

Clients who cannot spontaneously breathe on their own require mechanical ventilation. This can include clients who need respiratory assistance due to severe respiratory disease, general anesthesia, trauma, or other illnesses.

Oxygen delivery devices

Supplemental oxygen can be delivered by a variety of methods based on the client's particular circumstances. The percentage of oxygen delivered is expressed as the fraction of inspired oxygen (FiO_2).

LOW-FLOW OXYGEN DELIVERY SYSTEMS

These deliver varying amounts of oxygen based on the method and the client's breathing pattern.

Nasal cannula

- A length of tubing with two small prongs for insertion into the nares **(19.1)**
- FiO_2 24% to 44% at flow rates of 1 to 6 L/min

ADVANTAGES
- Safe, easy to apply, comfortable, and well tolerated.
- The client is able to eat, talk, and ambulate.

DISADVANTAGES
- FiO_2 varies with the flow rate, and the client's rate and depth of breathing.
- Extended use can lead to skin breakdown and drying of the mucous membranes.
- Tubing is easily dislodged.

NURSING ACTIONS
- Assess patency of the nares.
- Ensure that the prongs fit in the nares properly.
- Use water-soluble gel to prevent dry nares.
- Provide humidification for flow rates of 4 L/min and greater.

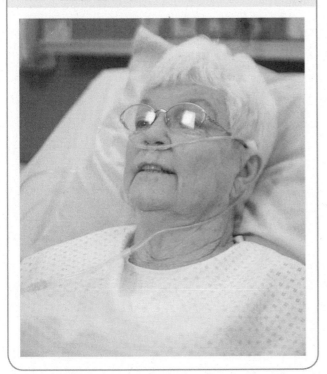

19.1 Nasal cannula

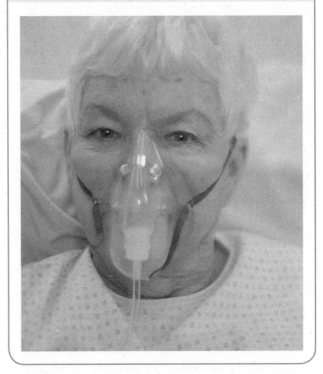

19.2 Simple face mask

Simple face mask

- Covers the client's nose and mouth. **(19.2)**
- FiO_2 40% to 60% at flow rates of 5 to 8 L/min. (The minimum flow rate is 5 L/min to ensure flushing of CO_2 from the mask.)

ADVANTAGES: A face mask is easy to apply and can be more comfortable than a nasal cannula.

DISADVANTAGES
- Flow rates of less than 5 L/min can result in rebreathing of CO_2.
- Device is poorly tolerated by clients who have anxiety or claustrophobia.
- Eating, drinking, and talking are impaired.
- Use caution with clients who have a high risk of aspiration or airway obstruction. Qs
- Moisture and pressure can collect under the mask and cause skin breakdown.

NURSING ACTIONS
- Assess proper fit to ensure a secure seal over the nose and mouth.
- Ensure that the client wears a nasal cannula during meals.

Partial rebreather mask

- Covers the client's nose and mouth
- FiO_2 40% to 75% at flow rates of 6 to 11 L/min

ADVANTAGES: The mask has a reservoir bag attached with no valve, which allows the client to rebreathe up to one third of exhaled air together with room air.

DISADVANTAGES
- Complete deflation of the reservoir bag during inspiration causes CO_2 buildup.
- FiO_2 varies with the client's breathing pattern.
- Mask is poorly tolerated by clients who have anxiety or claustrophobia.
- Eating, drinking, and talking are impaired.
- Use with caution for clients who have a high risk of aspiration or airway obstruction. Qs

NURSING ACTIONS
- Keep the reservoir bag from deflating by adjusting the oxygen flow rate to keep it inflated.
- Assess proper fit to ensure a secure seal over the nose and mouth.
- Assess for skin breakdown beneath the edges of the mask and bridge of nose.
- Ensure that the client uses a nasal cannula during meals.

Nonrebreather mask

- Covers the client's nose and mouth **(19.3)**
- FiO_2 80% to 95% at flow rates of 10 to 15 L/min to keep the reservoir bag two-thirds full during inspiration and expiration

ADVANTAGES
- Delivers the highest O_2 concentration possible (except for intubation).
- A one-way valve situated between the mask and reservoir allows the client to inhale maximum O_2 from the reservoir bag. The two exhalation ports have flaps covering them that prevent room air from entering the mask.

DISADVANTAGES
- The valve and flap on the mask must be intact and functional during each breath.
- Poorly tolerated by clients who have anxiety or claustrophobia.
- Eating, drinking, and talking are impaired.
- Use with caution for clients who have a high risk of aspiration or airway obstruction. Qs

NURSING ACTIONS
- Perform an hourly assessment of the valve and flap.
- Assess proper fit to ensure a secure seal over the nose and mouth.
- Assess for skin breakdown beneath the edges of the mask and bridge of nose.
- Ensure that the client uses a nasal cannula during meals.

HIGH-FLOW OXYGEN DELIVERY SYSTEMS

These deliver precise amounts of oxygen when properly fitted.

Venturi mask

- Covers the client's nose and mouth **(19.4)**
- FiO_2 24% to 50% at flow rates of 4 to 10 L/min via different sizes of adapters, which allow specific amounts of air to mix with oxygen

ADVANTAGES
- Delivers the most precise oxygen concentration.
- Humidification is not required.
- Best suited for clients who have chronic lung disease.

DISADVANTAGES: Use of a Venturi mask is expensive.

NURSING ACTIONS
- Assess frequently to ensure an accurate flow rate.
- Make sure the tubing is free of kinks. Qs
- Assess for skin breakdown beneath the edges of the mask, particularly on the nares.
- Ensure that the client wears a nasal cannula during meals.

19.3 Nonrebreather mask

19.4 Venturi mask

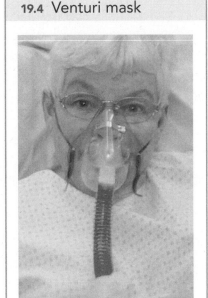

19.5 Face tent

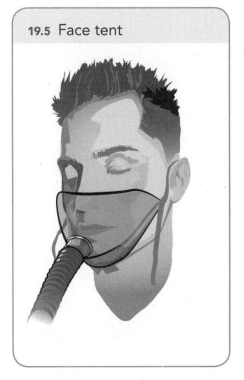

Aerosol mask, face tent, and tracheostomy collar

- Face tent fits loosely around the face and neck. **(19.5)**
- Tracheostomy collar is a small mask that covers a surgically created opening in the trachea.
- FiO₂ 24% to 100% at flow rates of at least 10 L/min. (Provide high humidification with oxygen delivery.)

ADVANTAGES
- Good for clients who do not tolerate masks well.
- Useful for clients who have facial trauma, burns, or thick secretions.

DISADVANTAGES: High humidification requires frequent monitoring.

NURSING ACTIONS
- Empty condensation from the tubing often.
- Ensure that there is adequate water in the humidification canister.
- Ensure that the aerosol mist leaves from the vents during inspiration and expiration.
- Make sure the tubing does not pull on the tracheostomy.

T-piece

FiO₂ 24% to 100% at flow rates of at least 10 L/min

ADVANTAGES: Can be used for clients who have tracheostomies, laryngectomies, or endotracheal tubes (ET).

DISADVANTAGES: High humidification requires frequent monitoring.

NURSING ACTIONS
- Ensure that the exhalation port is open and uncovered.
- Ensure that the T-piece does not pull on the tracheostomy or ET tube.
- Ensure that the mist is evident during inspiration and expiration.

Oxygen therapy

INDICATIONS

POTENTIAL DIAGNOSES

Hypoxemia and hypoxia: Hypoxemia is an inadequate level of oxygen in the blood. Hypovolemia, hypoventilation, and interruption of arterial flow can lead to hypoxemia.

CLIENT PRESENTATION

Early findings

- Tachypnea
- Tachycardia
- Restlessness
- Pale skin and mucous membranes
- Elevated blood pressure
- Symptoms of respiratory distress (use of accessory muscles, nasal flaring, tracheal tugging, and adventitious lung sounds)

Late findings

- Confusion and stupor
- Cyanotic skin and mucous membranes
- Bradypnea
- Bradycardia
- Hypotension
- Cardiac dysrhythmias

CONSIDERATIONS

PREPARATION OF THE CLIENT

- Explain all procedures to the client.
- Place the client in semi-Fowler's or Fowler's position to facilitate breathing and promote chest expansion.
- Ensure that all equipment is working properly.

ONGOING CARE

- Provide oxygen therapy at the lowest flow that will correct hypoxemia.
- Assess/monitor respiratory rate, rhythm and effort, and lung sounds to determine the client's need for supplemental oxygen.
  - Manifestations of hypoxemia are shortness of breath, anxiety, tachypnea, tachycardia, restlessness, pallor or cyanosis of the skin or mucous membranes, adventitious breath sounds, and confusion.
  - Manifestations of hypercarbia (elevated levels of CO_2) are restlessness, hypertension, and headache.
- Assess/monitor oxygenation status with pulse oximetry and ABGs.
- Apply the oxygen delivery device as prescribed. Assess the fit of the mask to ensure a secure seal over the client's nose and mouth.
- Promote good oral hygiene, and provide as needed.
- Promote turning, coughing, deep breathing, use of incentive spirometer, and suctioning.
- Promote rest, and decrease environmental stimuli. Qpcc
- Provide emotional support for clients who appear anxious.
- Assess nutritional status. Provide supplements as prescribed.
- Assess/monitor skin integrity. Provide moisture and pressure-relief devices as indicated.
- Assess/monitor and document the client's response to oxygen therapy.
- Titrate oxygen to maintain prescribed oxygen saturation.
- Discontinue supplemental oxygen gradually.

INTERVENTIONS

Monitor for manifestations of respiratory depression, such as decreased respiratory rate and decreased level of consciousness. Notify the provider if findings are present.

Respiratory distress
- Position the client for maximum ventilation (Fowler's or semi-Fowler's position).
- Complete a focused respiratory assessment.
- Promote deep breathing, and use supplemental oxygen as prescribed.
- Stay with the client, and provide emotional support to decrease anxiety.
- Promote airway clearance by encouraging coughing and oral/oropharyngeal suctioning if necessary.

COMPLICATIONS

Oxygen toxicity

- Oxygen toxicity can result from high concentrations of oxygen (typically above 50%), long durations of oxygen therapy (typically more than 24 to 48 hr), and the client's degree of lung disease.
- Manifestations include a nonproductive cough, substernal pain, nasal stuffiness, nausea, vomiting, fatigue, headache, sore throat, and hypoventilation.

NURSING ACTIONS
- Use the lowest level of oxygen necessary to maintain an adequate SaO_2.
- Monitor ABGs. Notify the provider if PaO_2 levels are outside the expected reference range of 90 mm Hg.
- Use an oxygen mask with continuous positive airway pressure (CPAP) or bi-level positive airway pressure (BiPAP) if prescribed to help decrease the amount of oxygen needed.
- Use positive end expiratory pressure (PEEP) as prescribed while the client is on a mechanical ventilator to help decrease the amount of needed oxygen.

Oxygen-induced hypoventilation

Oxygen-induced hypoventilation can develop in clients who have COPD and chronic hypoxemia with hypercarbia.

NURSING ACTIONS
- Monitor respiratory rate and pattern, level of consciousness, and SaO_2.
- Provide oxygen therapy at the lowest flow rate that manages hypoxemia.
- If the client tolerates it, use a Venturi mask to deliver precise oxygen levels.
- Notify the provider of impending respiratory depression, such as a decreased respiratory rate and a decreased level of consciousness.

Combustion

Oxygen is combustible.

NURSING ACTIONS
- Post "No Smoking" or "Oxygen in Use" signs to alert others of a fire hazard. Qs
- Know where the closest fire extinguisher is located.
- Educate the client and others about the fire hazard of smoking during oxygen use.
- Have the client wear a cotton gown because synthetic or wool fabrics can generate static electricity.
- Ensure that all electric devices (razors, hearing aids, radios) are working well.
- Ensure electric machinery (monitors, suction machines) are well-grounded.
- Do not use volatile, flammable materials (alcohol or acetone) near clients who are receiving oxygen.

Noninvasive positive pressure ventilation

Continuous positive airway pressure

Provides positive pressure using a leak-proof mask via noninvasive positive-pressure ventilation device.
- The device is to keep the airways throughout the respiratory cycle open and improve gas exchange in the alveoli.
- Most effective treatment for sleep apnea because the positive pressure acts as a splint to keep the upper airway and trachea open during sleep

Bi-level positive airway pressure

Machine cycles to provide a set positive inspiratory pressure when inspiration takes place and then during expiration to deliver a lower set end expiratory pressure
- Requires wearing a leak-proof mask.
- Most often used for clients who have COPD and who require ventilatory assistance.

NURSING ACTIONS
- Assess skin around the masks for breakdown as a tight seal is required.
- Check the percentage of oxygen on the machine (both) for both the inspiratory pressure and expiratory pressure when the client is on BiPAP.

Transtracheal oxygen therapy

Delivers oxygen directly in to the lungs per a small, flexible catheter that is passed through trachea via a small incision.
- The oxygen delivery is reduced by 55% for a client at rest and 30% for a client who is active.
- The catheter is less visible and avoids irritation that occurs from the use of nasal prongs.

Endotracheal tube and endotracheal intubation

INDICATIONS
- A tube is inserted through the client's nose or mouth into the trachea. This allows for emergency airway management of the client.
- Mouth intubation is the easiest and quickest form of intubation and is often performed in the emergency department.
- Nasal intubation is performed when the client has facial or oral trauma. This route is not used if the client has a clotting problem.

PLACEMENT
- Intubation is typically performed by a nurse anesthetist, anesthesiologist, or pulmonologist.
- A chest x-ray verifies correct placement of the endotracheal (ET) tube.
- ET tubes can be cuffed or uncuffed. The cuff on the tracheal end of an ET tube is inflated to ensure proper placement and the formation of a seal between the cuff and the tracheal wall. This prevents air from leaking around the ET tube.
- The seal ensures that an adequate amount of tidal volume is delivered by the mechanical ventilator when attached to the external end of the ET tube.
- The client is unable to talk when the cuff is inflated.

NURSING ACTIONS
- Have resuscitation equipment to include a manual resuscitation bag with a face mask at the bedside at all times.
- Ensure the intubation attempts last no longer than 30 seconds and then reoxygenate before another attempt to intubate.
- Monitor vital signs, and check tube placement.
- Auscultate for breath sounds bilaterally after intubation.
- Observe for symmetric chest movement.
- Stabilize the endotracheal tube with a tube holding device or secure with tape.
- Monitor for hypoxemia, dysrhythmias, and aspiration.

Mechanical ventilation

Mechanical ventilation provides breathing support until lung function is restored, delivering warm (body temperature 37° C [98.6° F]), 100% humidified oxygen at FiO_2 levels between 21% to 100%.

- Positive–pressure ventilators deliver air to the lungs under pressure throughout inspiration and/or expiration to keep the alveoli open during inspiration and to prevent alveolar collapse during expiration. Benefits include the following.
  - Forced/enhanced lung expansion
  - Improved gas exchange (oxygenation)
  - Decreased work of breathing
- Mechanical ventilation can be delivered via:
  - ET tube.
  - Tracheostomy tube.
- Mechanical ventilators can be cycled based on pressure, volume, time, and/or flow. **(19.6)**

INDICATIONS

To maintain a patent airway and adequate oxygen saturation of 95% or greater.

POTENTIAL DIAGNOSES

- Hypoxemia, hypoventilation with respiratory acidosis
  - Airway trauma
  - Exacerbation of COPD
  - Acute pulmonary edema due to myocardial infarction or heart failure
  - Asthma attack
  - Head injuries, cerebrovascular accident, or coma
  - Neurological disorders (multiple sclerosis, myasthenia gravis, Guillain–Barré)
  - Obstructive sleep apnea
- Respiratory support following surgery (decrease workload)
- Respiratory support while under general anesthesia or heavy sedation

---

19.6 Common modes of ventilation, adjunctive therapy, and weaning modalities

Mode of ventilation

ASSIST-CONTROL (AC)
- Preset rate and tidal volume. Client initiates breath and ventilator takes over for the intubated client.
- Hyperventilation can result in respiratory alkalosis.
- Client can require sedation to decrease respiratory rate.

SYNCHRONIZED INTERMITTENT MANDATORY VENTILATION (SIMV)
- Preset rate and tidal volume for machine breaths.
- Client initiates breath and tidal volume will depend upon client's effort.
- Ventilator initiated breaths are synchronized to reduce competition between ventilator and client.
- Used as a regular mode of ventilation or a weaning mode (rate decreased to allow more spontaneous ventilation) for the intubated client.
- Can increase work of breathing, causing respiratory muscle fatigue.

INVERSE RATIO VENTILATION (IRV)
- Lengthens inspiratory phase to maximize oxygenation in the intubated client.
- Used for hypoxemia refractory to PEEP.
- Uncomfortable for clients and requires sedation and/or neuromuscular blocking agents.
- High risk of volutrauma and decreased cardiac output due to air trapping.

AIRWAY PRESSURE RELEASE VENTILATION (APRV)
- Allows alveolar gas to be expelled by the lungs own natural recoil
- Time-triggered and pressure-limited
- Breaths can be initiated spontaneously or by the ventilator
- Causes less ventilator-induced lung injury and fewer adverse effects on the cardiovascular system

INDEPENDENT LUNG VENTILATION (ILV)
- Double-lumen ET tube allows ventilation of each lung separately.
- Used for clients who have unilateral lung disease.
- Requires two ventilators, sedation and/or use of neuromuscular blocking agents.

HIGH-FREQUENCY VENTILATION
- Delivers small amount of gas at rates of 60 to 3,000 cycles/min.
- High frequency ventilation often used in children.
- Client must be sedated and/or receiving neuromuscular blocking agents.
- Breath sounds difficult to assess.

Adjunctive therapy

POSITIVE END EXPIRATORY PRESSURE (PEEP)
- Preset pressure delivered during expiration.
- Added to prescribed ventilator settings to treat persistent hypoxemia.
- Improves oxygenation by enhancing gas exchange and preventing atelectasis.
- Amount of PEEP added is typically 5 to 15 cm H_2O.

Weaning modality

PRESSURE SUPPORT VENTILATION (PSV)
- Works to keep the alveoli from collapsing during expiration.
- Allows for greater oxygenation and makes the work of breathing easier.
- Allows for lower levels of FiO_2 to be used.
- Can be used with IMV or AC modes to treat or prevent atelectasis.
- Settings 5 to 20 cm H_2O (greater than 20 cm H_2O can cause lung damage).

CONTINUOUS POSITIVE AIRWAY PRESSURE (CPAP)
- Positive pressure supplied during spontaneous breathing. No ventilator breaths delivered unless in conjunction with SIMV.
- Risks include volutrauma, decreased cardiac output and ICP.

CONSIDERATIONS

PREPARATION OF THE CLIENT

- Explain the procedure to the client.
- Establish a method for the client to communicate, such as asking yes/no questions, providing writing materials, using a dry-erase and/or picture communication board, or lip reading. Qpcc

ONGOING CARE

- Maintain a patent airway.
  - Assess the position and placement of tube.
  - Document tube placement in centimeters at the client's teeth or lips.
  - Use two staff members for repositioning and to resecuring the tube.
  - Apply protective barriers (soft wrist restraints) according to hospital protocol to prevent self-extubation.
  - Use caution when moving the client. Qs
  - Suction oral and tracheal secretions to maintain tube patency.
  - Support ventilator tubing to prevent mucosal erosion and displacement.
  - Have a resuscitation bag with a face mask available at the bedside at all times in case of ventilator malfunction or accidental extubation.
- Assess respiratory status every 1 to 2 hr: breath sounds equal bilaterally, presence of reduced or absent breath sounds, respiratory effort, or spontaneous breaths.
- Suction the tracheal tube to clear secretions from the airway.
- Monitor and document ventilator settings hourly.
  - Rate, FiO_2, and tidal volume
  - Mode of ventilation
  - Use of adjuncts (PEEP, CPAP)
  - Plateau or peak inspiratory pressure (PIP)
  - Alarm settings
- Monitor ventilator alarms, which signal if the client is not receiving the correct ventilation.
  - Never turn off ventilator alarms.
  - There are three types of ventilator alarms.
    - **Volume (low pressure) alarms** indicate a low exhaled volume due to a disconnection, cuff leak, and/or tube displacement.
    - **Pressure (high pressure) alarms** indicate excess secretions, client biting the tubing, kinks in the tubing, client coughing, pulmonary edema, bronchospasm, or pneumothorax.
    - **Apnea alarms** indicate that the ventilator does not detect spontaneous respiration in a preset time period.
- Maintain adequate (but not excessive) volume in the cuff of the endotracheal tube.
  - Assess the cuff pressure at least every 8 hr. Maintain the cuff pressure below 20 mm Hg (or 20 to 30 cm H_2O) to reduce the risk of tracheal necrosis.
  - Assess for an air leak around the cuff (client speaking, air hissing, or decreasing SaO_2). Inadequate cuff pressure can result in inadequate oxygenation and/or accidental extubation.

- Administer medications as prescribed.
  - **Analgesics:** morphine and fentanyl
  - **Sedatives:** propofol, diazepam, lorazepam, midazolam, and haloperidol
    - Clients receiving mechanical ventilation can require sedation or paralytic agents to prevent competition between extrinsic and intrinsic breathing and the resulting effects of hyperventilation. Qpcc
  - **Neuromuscular blocking agents:** pancuronium, atracurium, and vecuronium are infrequently used in the clinical setting due to the their long half-life.
    - Neuromuscular blocking agents paralyze muscles, but do not sedate or relieve pain. The use of a sedative or analgesic agent in conjunction with a neuromuscular blocking agent is typically prescribed.
  - **Ulcer-preventing agents:** famotidine or lansoprazole
  - **Antibiotics** for established infections
- Reposition the oral endotracheal tube every 24 hr or according to protocol. Assess for skin breakdown.
  - Older adult clients have fragile skin and are more prone to skin and mucous membrane breakdown. Older adult clients have decreased oral secretions. They require frequent, gentle skin and oral care. Ⓖ
- Provide adequate nutrition.
  - Assess gastrointestinal functioning every 8 hr.
  - Monitor bowel habits.
  - Administer enteral or parenteral feedings as prescribed.
- Continually monitor the client during the weaning process and watch for signs of weaning intolerance.
  - Respirations greater than 30/min or less than 8/min
  - Blood pressure or heart rate changes more than 20% of baseline
  - SaO_2 less than 90%
  - Dysrhythmias, elevated ST segment
  - Significant decrease in tidal volume
  - Labored respirations, increased use of accessory muscles, and diaphoresis
  - Restlessness, anxiety, and decreased level of consciousness
- Have a manual resuscitation bag with a face mask and oxygen readily available at the client's bedside.
- Have reintubation equipment at bedside.
- Suction the oropharynx and trachea.
- Deflate the cuff on the endotracheal tube, and remove the tube during peak inspiration.
- Following extubation, monitor for signs of respiratory distress or airway obstruction, such as ineffective cough, dyspnea, and stridor.
- Assess SpO_2 and vital signs every 5 min.
- Encourage coughing, deep breathing, and use of the incentive spirometer.
- Reposition the client to promote mobility of secretions.
- Older adult clients have decreased respiratory muscle strength and chest wall compliance, which makes them more susceptible to aspiration, atelectasis, and pulmonary infections. Older adult clients require more frequent position changes to promote mobility of secretions. Ⓖ

COMPLICATIONS

Trauma

Barotrauma (damage to the lungs by positive pressure) can occur due to a pneumothorax, subcutaneous emphysema or pneumomediastinum.

Volutrauma (damage to the lungs by volume delivered from one lung to the other).

Fluid retention

Fluid retention in clients who are receiving mechanical ventilation is due to decreased cardiac output, activation of renin-angiotensin-aldosterone system, and/or ventilator humidification.

NURSING ACTIONS: Monitor intake and output, weight, breath sounds, and endotracheal secretions.

Oxygen toxicity

Oxygen toxicity can result from high concentrations of oxygen (typically greater than 50%), long durations of oxygen therapy (typically more than 24 to 48 hr), and/or the client's degree of lung disease.

NURSING ACTIONS: Monitor for fatigue, restlessness, severe dyspnea, tachycardia, tachypnea, crackles, and cyanosis.

Hemodynamic compromise

Mechanical ventilation has a risk of increased thoracic pressure (positive pressure), which can result in decreased venous return.

NURSING ACTIONS: Monitor for tachycardia, hypotension, urine output less than or equal to 30 mL/hr, cool, clammy extremities, decreased peripheral pulses, and a decreased level of consciousness.

Aspiration

Keep the head of the bed elevated 30° at all times to decrease the risk of aspiration. Q EBP

NURSING ACTIONS: Check residuals every 4 hr if the client is receiving enteral feedings to decrease the risk of aspiration.

Gastrointestinal ulceration (stress ulcer)

Gastric ulcers can be evident in clients receiving mechanical ventilation.

NURSING ACTIONS
- Monitor gastrointestinal drainage and stools for occult blood.
- Administer ulcer prevention medications (sucralfate and $histamine_2$ blockers).

Application Exercises

1. A nurse is orienting a newly licensed nurse who is caring for a client who is receiving mechanical ventilation and is on pressure support ventilation (PSV) mode. Which of the following statements by the newly licensed nurse indicates an understanding of PSV?

   A. "It keeps the alveoli open and prevents atelectasis."

   B. "It allows preset pressure delivered during spontaneous ventilation."

   C. "It guarantees minimal minute ventilator."

   D. "It delivers a preset ventilatory rate and tidal volume to the client."

2. A nurse is caring for a client who is experiencing respiratory distress. Which of the following early manifestations of hypoxemia should the nurse recognize? (Select all that apply.)

   A. Confusion

   B. Pale skin

   C. Bradycardia

   D. Hypotension

   E. Elevated blood pressure

3. A nurse is orienting a newly licensed nurse on performing routine assessment of a client who is receiving mechanical ventilation via an endotracheal tube. Which of the following information should the nurse include in the teaching?

   A. Apply a vest restraint if self-extubation is attempted.

   B. Monitor ventilator settings every 8 hr.

   C. Document tube placement in centimeters at the angle of jaw.

   D. Assess breath sounds every 1 to 2 hr.

4. A nurse is caring for a client who has dyspnea and will receive oxygen continuously. Which of the following oxygen devices should the nurse use to deliver a precise amount of oxygen to the client?

   A. Nonrebreather mask

   B. Venturi mask

   C. Nasal cannula

   D. Simple face mask

5. A nurse is planning care for a client who is receiving mechanical ventilation. Which of the following modes of ventilation that increases the effort of the client's respiratory muscles should the nurse include in the plan of care? (Select all that apply.)

   A. Assist-control

   B. Synchronized intermittent mandatory ventilation

   C. Continuous positive airway pressure

   D. Pressure support ventilation

   E. Independent lung ventilation

PRACTICE Active Learning Scenario

A nurse is planning care for a client who is receiving mechanical ventilation. What nursing actions should be included to maintain the client's airway? Use the ATI Active Learning Template: Therapeutic Procedure to complete this item.

NURSING INTERVENTIONS: Describe three nursing actions to maintain the client's airway.

Application Exercises Key

1. A. PEEP maintains pressure in the lungs to keep alveoli open or prevent atelectasis.

    B. **CORRECT:** PSV allows preset pressure delivered during spontaneous ventilation to decrease the work of breathing.

    C. PSV does not guarantee minimal minute ventilation because no ventilator breaths are delivered.

    D. Assist-control (AC) mode delivers a preset ventilatory rate and tidal volume to the client.

    Ⓝ *NCLEX® Connection: Reduction of Risk Potential, Therapeutic Procedures*

2. A. Confusion is a late manifestation of hypoxemia.

    B. **CORRECT:** Pale skin is an early manifestation of hypoxemia.

    C. Bradycardia is a late manifestation of hypoxemia.

    D. Hypotension is a late manifestation of hypoxemia.

    E. **CORRECT:** Elevated blood pressure is an early manifestation of hypoxemia.

    Ⓝ *NCLEX® Connection: Physiological Adaptation, Illness Management*

3. A. The nurse should apply soft wrist restraints to prevent self-extubation or according to facility policy.

    B. The nurse should monitor ventilator settings hourly.

    C. The nurse should document tube placement in centimeters at the client's teeth or lips.

    D. **CORRECT:** The nurse should assess the breath sounds of a client on mechanical ventilation every 1 to 2 hr.

    Ⓝ *NCLEX® Connection: Physiological Adaptation, Alterations in Body Systems*

4. A. A nonrebreather mask delivers an approximated amount of oxygen.

    B. **CORRECT:** A venturi mask incorporates an adapter that allows a precise amount of oxygen to be delivered.

    C. A nasal cannula delivers an approximated amount of oxygen.

    D. A simple face mask delivers an approximated amount of oxygen.

    Ⓝ *NCLEX® Connection: Physiological Adaptation, Illness Management*

5. A. Assist-control mode takes over the work of breathing.

    B. **CORRECT:** Synchronized intermittent mandatory ventilation requires that the client generate force to take spontaneous breaths.

    C. **CORRECT:** Continuous positive airway pressure requires that the client generate force to take spontaneous breaths.

    D. **CORRECT:** Pressure support ventilation requires that the client generate force to take spontaneous breaths.

    E. Independent lung ventilation mode is used for unilateral lung disease to ventilate the lung individually.

    Ⓝ *NCLEX® Connection: Physiological Adaptation, Alterations in Body Systems*

PRACTICE Answer

Using ATI Active Learning Template: Therapeutic Procedure

NURSING INTERVENTIONS

- Maintain a patent airway.
- Assess the position and placement of the tube.
- Document tube placement in centimeters at the client's teeth or lips.
- Use two staff members for repositioning and resecuring the tube.
- Apply protective barriers (soft wrist restraints) according to hospital protocol to prevent self-extubation.
- Use caution when moving the client.
- Suction oral and tracheal secretions to maintain tube patency.
- Support ventilator tubing to prevent mucosal erosion and displacement.
- Have a resuscitation bag with a face mask available at the bedside at all times in case of ventilator malfunction or accidental extubation.

Ⓝ *NCLEX® Connection: Physiological Adaptation, Alterations in Body Systems*

UNIT 3 NURSING CARE OF CLIENTS WHO HAVE RESPIRATORY DISORDERS
SECTION: RESPIRATORY SYSTEM DISORDERS

CHAPTER 20 *Acute Respiratory Disorders*

The airway structures permit air to enter and provide for adequate oxygenation and tissue perfusion. Common acute and chronic disorders affect these airway structures.

A nursing priority for clients who have acute respiratory disorders is to maintain a patent airway to promote oxygenation.

Acute respiratory disorders include rhinitis, sinusitis, influenza, and pneumonia.

Pneumonia is an inflammatory process in the lungs that produces excess fluid. Pneumonia is triggered by infectious organisms or by the aspiration of an irritant, such as fluid or a foreign object. The inflammatory process in the lung parenchyma results in edema and exudate that fills the alveoli. Pneumonia can be a primary disease or a complication of another disease or condition. It affects people of all ages, but young clients, older adult clients, and clients who are immunocompromised are more susceptible. Immobility is a contributing factor in the development of pneumonia. Ⓖ

There are two types of pneumonia. Community-acquired pneumonia (CAP) is the most common type and often occurs as a complication of influenza. Health care-associated pneumonia (HAP) has a higher mortality rate and is more likely to be resistant to antibiotics. It usually takes 24 to 48 hr from the time the client is exposed to acquire HAP.

Older adult clients are more susceptible to infections and have decreased pulmonary reserves due to normal lung changes, including decreased lung elasticity and thickening alveoli.

HEALTH PROMOTION AND DISEASE PREVENTION

- Perform hand hygiene to prevent the spread of infection by bacteria and viruses.
- Encourage immunizations that prevent respiratory disorders, especially immunizations for influenza and pneumonia to younger children and older adults, and people who have chronic illnesses or who are immunocompromised. Ⓖ
- Limit exposure to airborne allergens, which trigger a hypersensitivity reaction.
- Promote smoking cessation.

RISK FACTORS

- Extremely young or advanced age Ⓖ
- Recent exposure to viral, bacterial, or influenza infections
- Lack of current immunization status (pneumonia, influenza)
- Exposure to plant pollen, molds, animal dander, foods, medications, and environmental contaminants
- Tobacco smoke
- Substance use (alcohol, cocaine)
- Chronic lung disease (asthma, emphysema)
- Immunocompromised status
- Presence of a foreign body
- Conditions that increase the risk of aspiration (dysphagia)
- Impaired ability to mobilize secretions (decreased level of consciousness, immobility, recent abdominal or thoracic surgery)
- Inactivity and immobility
- Mechanical ventilation (ventilator-acquired pneumonia)

Rhinitis

Rhinitis is an inflammation of the nasal mucosa and often the mucosa in the sinuses that can be caused by infection (viral or bacterial) or allergens.

- The common cold (coryza) is caused by viruses spread from person to person in droplets from sneezing and coughing, or by direct contact.
- This disorder often coexists with other disorders, such as asthma and allergies, and can be acute or chronic, nonallergic or allergic (seasonal or perennial).
- The presence of an allergen causes histamine release and other mediators from WBCs in the nasal mucosa. The mediators bind to blood vessel receptors causing capillary leakage, which leads to local edema and swelling.

ASSESSMENT

EXPECTED FINDINGS

- Excessive nasal drainage, runny nose (rhinorrhea), and nasal congestion
- Purulent nasal discharge
- Sneezing and pruritus of the nose, throat, and ears
- Itchy, watery eyes
- Sore, dry throat
- Red, inflamed, swollen nasal mucosa
- Low-grade fever
- Diagnostic testing can include allergy tests to identify possible allergens.

PATIENT-CENTERED CARE

NURSING CARE

- Encourage rest (8 to 10 hr/day) and increased fluid intake (at least 2,000 mL/day).
- Encourage the use of a home humidifier or breathing steamy air after running hot shower water.
- Promote proper disposal of tissues and use of cough etiquette (sneeze or cough into tissue, elbow or shoulder and not the hands).

MEDICATIONS

Antihistamines, such as brompheniramine/pseudoephedrine; **leukotriene inhibitors**, such as montelukast; and **mast cell stabilizers**, such as cromolyn, are used to block the release of chemicals from WBCs that bind with receptors in nasal tissues, which prevent edema and itching.

NURSING CONSIDERATIONS: Older adults should be aware of adverse effects such as vertigo, hypertension, and urinary retention. Ⓖ

Decongestants, such as phenylephrine, constrict blood vessels and decrease edema.

NURSING CONSIDERATIONS: Encourage clients to use as prescribed for 3 to 4 days to avoid rebound nasal congestion.

Intranasal glucocorticoid sprays are the most effective for prevention and treatment of seasonal and perennial rhinitis.

Antipyretics are used if fever is present.

Antibiotics are given if a bacterial infection can be identified.

CLIENT EDUCATION

- Review hand hygiene as a measure to prevent transmission.
- Complementary therapies such as echinacea, large doses of vitamin C, and zinc preparations (lozenges and nasal sprays) can be useful in promoting improved immune response. ⓆEBP
- Limiting exposure to others will prevent and reduce transmission. This is especially important for vulnerable populations such as the very young, older adults, and people who are immunosuppressed. Ⓖ

Sinusitis

Sinusitis, often called rhinosinusitis, is an inflammation of the mucous membranes of one or more of the sinuses, usually the maxillary or frontal sinus. Swelling of the mucosa can block the drainage of secretions, which can cause a sinus infection.

- Sinusitis often occurs after rhinitis and can be associated with a deviated nasal septum, nasal polyps, inhaled air pollutants or cocaine, facial trauma, dental infections, or loss of immune function.
- The infection is commonly caused by *Streptococcus pneumoniae*, *Haemophilus influenzae*, diplococcus, and bacteroides.

ASSESSMENT

EXPECTED FINDINGS

- Nasal congestion
- Headache
- Facial pressure or pain (worse when head is tilted forward)
- Cough
- Bloody or purulent nasal drainage
- Tenderness to palpation of forehead, orbital, and facial areas
- Low-grade fever

DIAGNOSTIC PROCEDURES

- CT scan or sinus x-rays confirm the diagnosis, which is typically based upon findings and physical assessment.
- Endoscopic sinus cavity lavage or surgery to relieve the obstruction and promote drainage of secretions may be done.

PATIENT-CENTERED CARE

NURSING CARE

- Encourage the use of steam humidification, sinus irrigation, saline nasal sprays, and hot and wet packs to relieve sinus congestion and pain.
- Teach the client to increase fluid intake and rest.
- Discourage air travel, swimming, and diving.
- Encourage cessation of tobacco use in any form.
- Instruct the client on correct technique for sinus irrigation and self-administration of nasal sprays.

MEDICATIONS

Nasal decongestants, such as phenylephrine, are used to reduce swelling of the mucosa.

NURSING CONSIDERATIONS
- Clients should be encouraged to begin over-the-counter decongestant use at the first manifestation of sinusitis.
- Signs of rebound nasal congestion may occur if decongestants are used for more than 3 to 4 days.

Broad-spectrum antibiotics, such as amoxicillin, are used on a limited basis for a confirmed causative bacterial pathogen.

Pain relief medications include NSAIDs, acetaminophen, and aspirin.

CLIENT EDUCATION

- Sinus irrigation and saline nasal sprays are an effective alternative to antibiotics for relieving nasal congestion.
- Contact the provider for manifestations of a severe headache, neck stiffness (nuchal rigidity), and high fever, which can indicate possible complications.

COMPLICATIONS

Meningitis and encephalitis can occur if pathogens enter the bloodstream from the sinus cavity.

Influenza

Seasonal influenza, or "flu," occurs as an epidemic, usually in the fall and winter months.
- It is a highly contagious acute viral infection that occurs in children and adults of all ages.
- Influenza can be caused by one of several virus families, and this can vary yearly. Adults are contagious from 24 hr before manifestations develop and up to 5 days after they begin.

Pandemic influenza refers to a viral infection among animals or birds that has mutated and is becoming highly infectious to humans. The resulting viral infection has the potential to spread globally, such as H1N1 ("swine flu") and H5N1 ("avian flu").

ASSESSMENT

EXPECTED FINDINGS

- Severe headache and muscle aches
- Chills
- Fatigue, weakness
- Severe diarrhea and cough (avian flu)
- Fever
- Hypoxia (avian flu)

DIAGNOSTIC PROCEDURES

AV Avantage A/H5N1 Flu Test

PATIENT-CENTERED CARE

NURSING CARE

- Maintain droplet and contact precautions for hospitalized clients who have pandemic influenza.
- Provide saline gargles.
- Monitor hydration status, intake, and output.
- Administer fluid therapy as prescribed.
- Monitor respiratory status.

MEDICATIONS

Antivirals

- Amantadine, rimantadine, and ribavirin may be prescribed for treatment and prevention of influenza.
- Duration of the influenza infection can be shortened by antivirals such as the oral inhalant zanamivir and the oral tablet oseltamivir. In cases of pandemic influenza, these medications may be distributed widely among the population.
- CLIENT EDUCATION: Encourage clients to begin antiviral medications within 24 to 48 hr after the onset of manifestations.

Influenza vaccines

- Trivalent vaccines are prepared yearly depending upon the suspected strain of influenza expected to appear. They include an IM injection of Fluvirin or Fluzone and a live attenuated influenza vaccine by intranasal spray.
  - Vaccination is encouraged for everyone older than 6 months of age.
  - Clients who have a history of pneumonia, chronic medical conditions, and those over age 65, pregnant women, and health care providers are at higher risk and require vaccination.
- H1N1 vaccine is available for the general population.
- H5N1 vaccine is stockpiled for distribution if a pandemic occurs.

INTERPROFESSIONAL CARE

- Respiratory services should be consulted for respiratory support.
- Community health officials are notified of influenza outbreaks.
- State and federal public health officials are consulted for containment and prevention directives during pandemic influenza.

CLIENT EDUCATION

- Encourage annual influenza vaccination when vaccines become available.
- Reduce the risk for spreading viruses by thoroughly washing hands and following cough etiquette.
- Avoid places where people gather. Avoid close personal contact (handshaking, kissing and hugging).
- If flu manifestations develop, increase fluid intake, rest and stay home from work or school.
- Avoid travel to areas where pandemic influenza is identified.
- Be aware of public health announcements and activation of the early warning system by public health officials in case of pandemic influenza.

COMPLICATIONS

Pneumonia is a complication of influenza and affects older adults and clients who are debilitated or immunocompromised. Ⓖ

Pneumonia

ASSESSMENT

EXPECTED FINDINGS

- Anxiety
- Fatigue
- Weakness
- Chest discomfort due to coughing
- Confusion from hypoxia is the most common manifestation of pneumonia in older adult clients. Ⓖ

PHYSICAL ASSESSMENT FINDINGS
- Fever
- Chills
- Flushed face
- Diaphoresis
- Shortness of breath or difficulty breathing
- Tachypnea
- Pleuritic chest pain (sharp)
- Sputum production (yellow-tinged)
- Crackles and wheezes
- Coughing
- Dull chest percussion over areas of consolidation
- Decreased oxygen saturation levels (expected reference range is 95% to 100%)
- Purulent, blood-tinged or rust-colored sputum, which may not always be present

LABORATORY TESTS

Sputum culture and sensitivity
- Obtain specimen before starting antibiotic therapy.
- Obtain specimen by suctioning if the client is unable to cough.
- Older adult clients have a weak cough reflex and decreased muscle strength. Therefore, older adult clients have trouble expectorating, which can lead to difficulty in breathing and make specimen retrieval more difficult. Ⓖ

CBC: Elevated WBC count (might not be present in older adult clients)

ABGs: Hypoxemia (decreased PaO2 less than 80 mm Hg)

Blood culture: To rule out organisms in the blood

Serum electrolytes: To identify causes of dehydration

DIAGNOSTIC PROCEDURES

Chest x-ray

- A chest x-ray will show consolidation (solidification, density) of lung tissue. **(20.1)**
- Chest x-ray might not indicate pneumonia for a few days after manifestations.
- A chest x-ray is an important diagnostic tool because the early manifestations of pneumonia are often vague in older adult clients. Ⓖ

Pulse oximetry

Clients who have pneumonia usually have oximetry levels less than the expected reference range of 95% to 100%.

PATIENT-CENTERED CARE

NURSING CARE

- Position the client to maximize ventilation (high-Fowler's = 90%) unless contraindicated.
- Encourage coughing or suction to remove secretions.
- Administer breathing treatments and medications.
- Administer oxygen therapy.
- Monitor for skin breakdown around the nose and mouth from the oxygen device.
- Encourage deep breathing with an incentive spirometer to prevent alveolar collapse.
- Determine the client's physical limitations and structure activity to include periods of rest. Ⓠpcc
- Promote adequate nutrition and fluid intake.
  - The increased work of breathing requires additional calories.
  - Proper nutrition aids in the prevention of secondary respiratory infections.
  - Encourage fluid intake of 2 to 3 L/day to promote hydration and thinning of secretions, unless contraindicated due to another condition.
- Provide rest periods for clients who have dyspnea.
- Reassure the client who is experiencing respiratory distress.

MEDICATIONS

Antibiotics

- Antibiotics are given to destroy infectious pathogens. Commonly used antibiotics include penicillins and cephalosporins.
- Antibiotics are often initially given via IV and then switched to an oral form as the condition improves.
- It is important to obtain any culture specimens prior to giving the first dose of an antibiotic. Once the specimen has been obtained, the antibiotics can be given while waiting for the results of the prescribed culture.

NURSING CONSIDERATIONS

- Observe clients taking cephalosporins for frequent stools.
- Monitor kidney function, especially older adults who are taking penicillins and cephalosporins. Ⓖ

CLIENT EDUCATION: Encourage clients to take penicillins and cephalosporins with food. Some penicillins should be taken 1 hr before meals or 2 hr after.

Bronchodilators

- Bronchodilators are given to reduce bronchospasms and reduce irritation.
- Short-acting beta$_2$ agonists, such as albuterol, provide rapid relief.
- Cholinergic antagonists (anticholinergic medications), such as ipratropium, block the parasympathetic nervous system, allowing for increased bronchodilation and decreased pulmonary secretions.
- Methylxanthines, such as theophylline, require close monitoring of serum medication levels due to the narrow therapeutic range.

NURSING CONSIDERATIONS

- Monitor serum medication levels for toxicity for clients taking theophylline. Adverse effects will include tachycardia, nausea, and diarrhea.
- Watch for tremors and tachycardia for clients taking albuterol.
- Observe for dry mouth in clients taking ipratropium, and monitor heart rate. Adverse effects can include headache, blurred vision, and palpitations, which can indicate toxicity.

CLIENT EDUCATION

- Encourage clients to suck on hard candies to moisten dry mouth while taking ipratropium. Ⓠebp
- Encourage increased fluid intake unless contraindicated.

20.1 Pneumonia

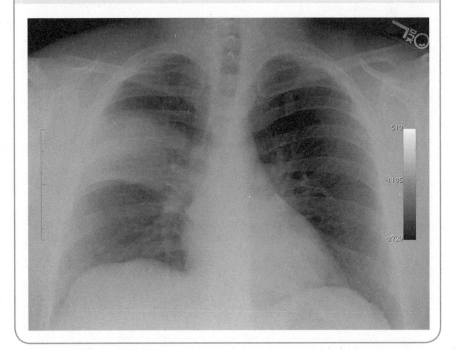

Anti-inflammatories

- Anti-inflammatories decrease airway inflammation.
- Glucocorticosteroids, such as fluticasone and prednisone, are prescribed to reduce inflammation. Monitor for immunosuppression, fluid retention, hyperglycemia, hypokalemia, and poor wound healing.

NURSING CONSIDERATIONS

- Monitor for decreased immunity function.
- Monitor for hyperglycemia.
- Advise the client to report black, tarry stools.
- Observe for fluid retention and weight gain. This can be common.
- Monitor the throat and mouth for aphthous lesions (canker sores).

CLIENT EDUCATION

- Encourage the client to drink plenty of fluids to promote hydration.
- Encourage the client to take glucocorticosteroids with food.
- Encourage the client to avoid discontinuing glucocorticosteroids without consulting the provider.

INTERPROFESSIONAL CARE

- Respiratory services should be consulted for inhalers, breathing treatments, and suctioning for airway management.
- Nutritional services can be contacted for weight loss or gain related to medications or diagnosis.
- Rehabilitation care can be consulted if the client has prolonged weakness and needs assistance with increasing level of activity.

CLIENT EDUCATION

- Educate the client on the importance of continuing medications for treatment of pneumonia. Qᴘᴄᴄ
- Encourage rest periods as needed.
- Encourage the client to maintain hand hygiene to prevent infection.
- Encourage the client to avoid crowded areas to reduce the risk of infection. Qᴇʙᴘ
- Remind the client that treatment and recovery from pneumonia can take time.
- Encourage immunizations for influenza and pneumonia.
- Promote smoking cessation if needed.

COMPLICATIONS

Atelectasis

- Airway inflammation and edema lead to alveolar collapse and increase the risk of hypoxemia.
- The client reports shortness of breath and exhibits findings of hypoxemia.
- The client has diminished or absent breath sounds over the affected area.
- A chest x-ray shows an area of density.

Bacteremia (sepsis): This occurs if pathogens enter the bloodstream from the infection in the lungs.

Acute respiratory distress syndrome

- Hypoxemia persists despite oxygen therapy.
- Dyspnea worsens as bilateral pulmonary edema develops that is noncardiac related.
- A chest x-ray shows an area of density with a ground-glass appearance.
- Blood gas findings demonstrate high arterial blood levels of carbon dioxide (hypercarbia) even though pulse oximetry shows decreased saturation.

Application Exercises

1. A nurse is monitoring a group of clients for increased risk for developing pneumonia. Which of the following clients should the nurse expect to be at risk? (Select all that apply.)

   A. Client who has dysphagia

   B. Client who has AIDS

   C. Client who was vaccinated for pneumococcus and influenza 6 months ago

   D. Client who is postoperative and has received local anesthesia

   E. Client who has a closed head injury and is receiving ventilation

   F. Client who has myasthenia gravis

2. A nurse in a clinic is caring for a client whose partner states the client woke up this morning, did not recognize him, and did not know where she was. The client reports chills and chest pain that is worse upon inspiration. Which of the following actions is the nursing priority?

   A. Obtain baseline vital signs and oxygen saturation.

   B. Obtain a sputum culture.

   C. Obtain a complete history from the client.

   D. Provide a pneumococcal vaccine.

3. A nurse is caring for a client who has pneumonia. Assessment findings include temperature 37.8° C (100° F), respirations 30/min, blood pressure 130/76, heart rate 100/min, and SaO2 91% on room air. Prioritize the following nursing interventions.

   A. Administer antibiotics.

   B. Administer oxygen therapy.

   C. Perform a sputum culture.

   D. Administer an antipyretic medication to promote client comfort.

4. A nurse in a clinic is assessing a client who has sinusitis. Which of the following techniques should the nurse use to identify manifestations of this disorder?

   A. Percussion of posterior lobes of lungs

   B. Auscultation of the trachea

   C. Inspection of the conjunctiva

   D. Palpation of the orbital areas

5. A nurse is teaching a group of clients about influenza. Which of the following client statements indicates an understanding of the teaching?

   A. "I should wash my hands after blowing my nose to prevent spreading the virus."

   B. "I need to avoid drinking fluids if I develop symptoms."

   C. "I need a flu shot every 2 years because of the different flu strains."

   D. "I should cover my mouth with my hand when I sneeze."

PRACTICE Active Learning Scenario

A nurse in a clinic is discussing health promotion and disease management with a client who has rhinitis. What should the nurse include in this discussion? Use the ATI Active Learning Template: System Disorder to complete this item.

RISK FACTORS: Identify three risk factors for rhinitis.

EXPECTED FINDINGS: Describe at least four.

CLIENT EDUCATION: Describe two client self-care activities.

MEDICATIONS: Identify two over-the-counter medications the client can use.

Application Exercises Key

1. A. **CORRECT:** The client who has difficulty swallowing is at increased risk for pneumonia due to aspiration.

   B. **CORRECT:** The client who has AIDS is immunocompromised, which increases the risk of opportunistic infections, such as pneumonia.

   C. The client who has recently been vaccinated in the past few months has a decreased risk to acquire pneumonia.

   D. A client who is postoperative and has received local anesthesia has a decreased risk to acquire pneumonia.

   E. **CORRECT:** Mechanical ventilation is invasive and increases the risk of pneumonia.

   F. **CORRECT:** A client who has myasthenia gravis has generalized weakness and can have difficulty clearing airway secretions, which increases the risk of pneumonia.

   Ⓝ *NCLEX® Connection: Health Promotion and Maintenance, Health Promotion/Disease Prevention*

2. A. **CORRECT:** The first action the nurse should take using the nursing process is to assess the client, which is essential in planning client-centered care.

   B. The nurse should obtain a sputum culture to determine sensitivity for antibiotic therapy. However, there is another action the nurse should take first.

   C. The nurse should obtain a complete history from the client to determine the plan of care. However, there is another action the nurse should take first.

   D. The nurse should provide for a pneumococcal vaccination to decrease the risk of pneumonia in the future. However, there is another action the nurse should take first.

   Ⓝ *NCLEX® Connection: Physiological Adaptation, Alterations in Body Systems*

3. Correct order

   B. The client's respiratory and heart rates are elevated, and her oxygen saturation is 91% on room air. Using the ABC priority framework, providing oxygen is the first intervention.

   C. Obtaining a sputum culture is the second nursing intervention. It should be done prior to administering oral medications to obtain an appropriate and adequate specimen.

   A. Administration of antibiotics is the third action the nurse should take. The sputum culture should be obtained prior to antibiotic administration.

   D. Administering an antipyretic medication is the fourth nursing intervention.

   Ⓝ *NCLEX® Connection: Physiological Adaptation, Illness Management*

4. A. Lung percussion is not an appropriate technique to identify manifestations of sinusitis; it is appropriate for a client who has pneumonia.

   B. Auscultation of the trachea is not an appropriate technique to identify manifestations of sinusitis; it is appropriate for a client who has bronchitis.

   C. Inspection of the conjunctiva is not an appropriate technique to identify manifestations of sinusitis; it is appropriate for a client who has anemia.

   D. **CORRECT:** Palpation of the orbital, frontal, and facial areas will elicit a report of tenderness, which is a manifestation in a client who has sinusitis.

   Ⓝ *NCLEX® Connection: Reduction of Risk Potential, Therapeutic Procedures*

5. A. **CORRECT:** Hand hygiene decreases the risk of the client spreading influenza viruses.

   B. Fluid intake should be increased if findings develop to maintain hydration and effectiveness of expectoration of mucous.

   C. Influenza vaccines are administered yearly. The client should receive a vaccination yearly.

   D. Cough etiquette includes the client to sneeze into the shoulder or elbow rather than the hands.

   Ⓝ *NCLEX® Connection: Physiological Adaptation, Illness Management*

PRACTICE Answer

Using the ATI Active Learning Template: System Disorder

RISK FACTORS
- Recent exposure to viral, bacterial or influenza infections
- Lack of current immunization status (pneumonia, influenza)
- Exposure to plant pollen, molds, animal dander, foods, medications, and environmental contaminants
- Tobacco smoke
- Substance use (alcohol, cocaine)
- Presence of a foreign body
- Inactivity and immobility

EXPECTED FINDINGS
- Excessive nasal drainage, runny nose (rhinorrhea), nasal congestion
- Purulent nasal drainage
- Sneezing and pruritus of the nose, throat, and ears
- Itchy, watery eyes
- Sore, dry throat
- Red, inflamed, swollen nasal mucosa
- Low-grade fever

CLIENT EDUCATION
- Rest (8 to 10 hr/day), increased fluid intake (at least 2,000 mL/day)
- Use of a home humidifier or breathing steamy air after running hot shower water
- Proper disposal of tissues and use of cough etiquette

MEDICATIONS: Brompheniramine/pseudoephedrine, cromolyn sodium, phenylephrine, antipyretics

Ⓝ *NCLEX® Connection: Health Promotion and Maintenance, Health Promotion/Disease Prevention*

UNIT 3 NURSING CARE OF CLIENTS WHO
HAVE RESPIRATORY DISORDERS
SECTION: RESPIRATORY SYSTEM DISORDERS

CHAPTER 21 *Asthma*

Asthma is a chronic inflammatory disorder of the airways that results in intermittent and reversible airflow obstruction of the bronchioles. The obstruction occurs either by inflammation or airway hyperresponsiveness.

Asthma can occur at any age. The cause is unknown.

Manifestations of asthma include mucosal edema, bronchoconstriction, and excessive mucus production.

HEALTH PROMOTION AND DISEASE PREVENTION

- If the client smokes, promote smoking cessation.
- Advise the client to use protective equipment (mask) and ensure proper ventilation while working in environments that contain carcinogens or particles in the air. **Q**s
- Encourage influenza and pneumonia vaccinations for older adults and all clients who have asthma. **©**
- Instruct the client how to recognize and avoid triggering agents.
  - Environmental factors, such as changes in temperature (especially warm to cold) and humidity
  - Air pollutants
  - Strong odors (perfume)
  - Seasonal allergens (grass, tree, and weed pollens) and perennial allergens (mold, feathers, dust, roaches, animal dander, foods treated with sulfites)
  - Stress and emotional distress
  - Medications (aspirin, NSAIDs, beta-blockers, cholinergics)
  - Enzymes, including those in laundry detergents
  - Chemicals (household cleaners)
  - Sinusitis with postnasal drip
  - Viral respiratory tract infection
- Teach the client how to self-administer medications (nebulizers and inhalers).
- Educate the client regarding infection prevention techniques.
- Encourage regular exercise as part of asthma therapy.
  - Promotes ventilation and perfusion.
  - Maintains cardiac health.
  - Enhances skeletal muscle strength.
  - Clients can require pre-medication.
- Instruct the client to use hot water to eliminate dust mites in bed linens.

ASSESSMENT

Diagnosis is based on symptoms and classified into one of the following four categories.
- **Mild intermittent:** Symptoms occur less than twice a week.
- **Mild persistent:** Symptoms arise more than twice a week but not daily.
- **Moderate persistent:** Daily symptoms occur in conjunction with exacerbations twice a week.
- **Severe persistent:** Symptoms occur continually, along with frequent exacerbations that limit physical activity and quality of life.

RISK FACTORS

- Older adult clients have decreased pulmonary reserves due to physiologic lung changes that occur with the aging process. **©**
  - Older adult clients are more susceptible to infections.
  - The sensitivity of beta-adrenergic receptors decreases with age. As the beta receptors age and lose sensitivity, they are less able to respond to agonists, which relax smooth muscle and can result in bronchospasms.
- Family history of asthma
- Smoking
- Secondhand smoke exposure
- Environmental allergies
- Exposure to chemical irritants or dust
- Gastroesophageal reflux disease (GERD)

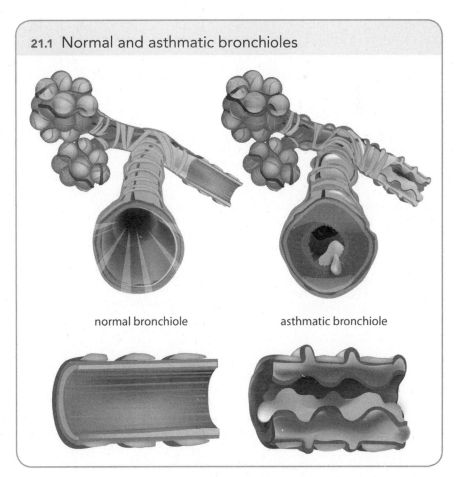

21.1 Normal and asthmatic bronchioles

normal bronchiole   asthmatic bronchiole

EXPECTED FINDINGS

- Dyspnea
- Chest tightness
- Anxiety or stress

PHYSICAL ASSESSMENT FINDINGS
- Coughing
- Wheezing
- Mucus production
- Use of accessory muscles
- Prolonged exhalation
- Poor oxygen saturation (low SaO_2)
- Barrel chest or increased chest diameter

Obtain history regarding current and previous asthma exacerbations. Qpcc
- Onset and duration
- Precipitating factors (stress, exercise, exposure to irritant)
- Changes in medication regimen
- Medications that relieve symptoms
- Other medications taken
- Self-care methods used to relieve symptoms

LABORATORY TESTS

Arterial blood gases

Hypoxemia (decreased PaO_2 less than 80 mm Hg)

Hypocarbia (decreased $PaCO_2$ less than 35 mm Hg: early in attack)

Hypercarbia (increased $PaCO_2$ greater than 45 mm Hg: later in attack)

Sputum cultures

Bacteria can indicate infection. QL

DIAGNOSTIC PROCEDURES

- Pulmonary function tests (PFTs) are the most accurate tests for diagnosing asthma and its severity.
  - Forced vital capacity (FVC) is the volume of air exhaled from full inhalation to full exhalation.
  - Forced expiratory volume in the first second (FEV1) is the volume of air blown out as hard and fast as possible during the first second of the most forceful exhalation after the greatest full inhalation.
  - Peak expiratory flow is the fastest airflow rate reached during exhalation.
  - A decrease in FEV1 by 15% to 20% below the expected value is common in clients who have asthma. An increase in these values by 12% following the administration of bronchodilators is diagnostic for asthma.
- A chest x-ray is used to diagnose changes in chest structure over time.

PATIENT-CENTERED CARE

NURSING CARE

- Position the client to maximize ventilation (high-Fowler's). QEBP
- Administer oxygen therapy as prescribed.
- Monitor cardiac rate and rhythm for changes during an acute attack (can be irregular, tachycardic, or with PVCs).
- Initiate and maintain IV access.
- Maintain a calm and reassuring demeanor.
- Provide rest periods for older adult clients who have dyspnea. Design room and walkways with opportunities for rest. Incorporate rest into ADLs. Ⓖ
- Encourage prompt medical attention for infections and appropriate vaccinations.
- Administer medications as prescribed.

MEDICATIONS

Bronchodilators (inhalers)

- **Short-acting beta₂ agonists**, such as albuterol, provide rapid relief of acute symptoms and prevent exercise-induced asthma.
- **Anticholinergic medications**, such as ipratropium, block the parasympathetic nervous system. This allows for the sympathetic nervous system effects of increased bronchodilation and decreased pulmonary secretions. These medications are long-acting and used to prevent bronchospasms.
- **Methylxanthines**, such as theophylline, require close monitoring of serum medication levels due to a narrow therapeutic range. Use only when other treatments are ineffective.
- **Long-acting beta₂ agonists**, such as salmeterol, primarily are used for asthma attack prevention.

NURSING CONSIDERATIONS
- Albuterol: Watch for tremors and tachycardia.
- Ipratropium: Observe for dry mouth.
- Theophylline: Monitor serum levels for toxicity. Side effects include tachycardia, nausea, and diarrhea.

CLIENT EDUCATION
- Ipratropium: Advise the client to suck on hard candies to help relieve dry mouth; increase fluid intake; and report headache, blurred vision, or palpitations, which can indicate toxicity of ipratropium. Monitor heart rate.
- Salmeterol: Advise the client to use to prevent an asthma attack and not at the onset of an attack.

Anti-inflammatory agents

These medications are for prophylaxis and are used to decrease airway inflammation.
- **Corticosteroids**, such as fluticasone and prednisone
- **Leukotriene antagonists**, such as montelukast
- **Mast cell stabilizers**, such as cromolyn
- **Monoclonal antibodies**, such as omalizumab

NURSING CONSIDERATIONS

- Watch for decreased immunity function.
- Monitor for hyperglycemia.
- Advise the client to report black, tarry stools.
- Observe for fluid retention and weight gain. This can be common.
- Monitor the throat and mouth for aphthous lesions (canker sores).
- Omalizumab can cause anaphylaxis.

CLIENT EDUCATION

- Encourage the client to drink plenty of fluids to promote hydration.
- Encourage the client to take prednisone with food.
- Advise the client to use this medication to prevent asthma, not for the onset of an attack.
- Encourage the client to avoid people who have respiratory infections.
- Remind the client to use good mouth care.
- Warn the client to not discontinue this type of medication suddenly.

Combination agents (bronchodilator and anti-inflammatory)

If prescribed separately for inhalation administration at the same time, administer the bronchodilator first in order to increase the absorption of the anti-inflammatory agent.
- Ipratropium and albuterol
- Fluticasone and salmeterol

INTERPROFESSIONAL CARE

- Respiratory services should be consulted for inhalers and breathing treatments for airway management.
- Nutritional services can be contacted for weight loss or gain related to medications or diagnosis.
- Rehabilitation care can be consulted if the client has prolonged weakness and needs assistance with increasing level of activity.

COMPLICATIONS

Respiratory failure

Persistent hypoxemia related to asthma can lead to respiratory failure.

NURSING ACTIONS

- Monitor oxygenation levels and acid–base balance.
- Prepare for intubation and mechanical ventilation.

Status asthmaticus

This is a life-threatening episode of airway obstruction that is often unresponsive to common treatment. It involves extreme wheezing, labored breathing, use of accessory muscles, distended neck veins, and creates a risk for cardiac and/or respiratory arrest.

NURSING ACTIONS

- Prepare for emergency intubation.
- Administer IV fluids, oxygen, bronchodilators, and epinephrine. Initiate systemic steroid therapy.

Application Exercises

1. A nurse in the emergency department is caring for a client who is having an acute asthma attack. Which of the following assessments indicates that the respiratory status is declining? (Select all that apply.)

   A. SaO_2 95%

   B. Wheezing

   C. Retraction of sternal muscles

   D. Pink mucous membranes

   E. Premature ventricular complexes (PVCs)

2. A nurse is caring for a client 2 hr after admission. The client has an SaO_2 of 91%, exhibits audible wheezes, and is using accessory muscles when breathing. Which of the following classes of medications should the nurse expect to administer?

   A. Antibiotic

   B. Beta-blocker

   C. Antiviral

   D. Beta$_2$ agonist

3. A nurse is providing discharge teaching to a client who has a new prescription for prednisone for asthma. Which of the following client statements indicates an understanding of the teaching?

   A. "I will decrease my fluid intake while taking this medication."

   B. "I will expect to have black, tarry stools."

   C. "I will take my medication with meals."

   D. "I will monitor for weight loss while on this medication."

4. A nurse is assessing a client who has a history of asthma. Which of the following factors should the nurse identify as a risk for asthma?

   A. Gender

   B. Environmental allergies

   C. Alcohol use

   D. Race

5. A nurse is reinforcing teaching with a client on the purpose of taking a bronchodilator. Which of the following client statements indicates an understanding of the teaching?

   A. "This medication can decrease my immune response."

   B. "I take this medication to prevent asthma attacks."

   C. "I need to take this medication with food."

   D. "This medication has a slow onset to treat my symptoms."

Application Exercises Key

1. A. Oxygen saturation 95% is an expected finding within the respiratory system and exhibits no signs of distress.

   B. **CORRECT:** Wheezing is a manifestation indicating the client's respiratory status is declining.

   C. **CORRECT:** Retraction of sternal muscles is a manifestation that the client's respiratory status is declining.

   D. Pink mucous membranes is an expected finding within the respiratory system and exhibits no signs of distress.

   E. **CORRECT:** PVCs are a manifestation that the client's respiratory status is declining.

   Ⓝ *NCLEX® Connection: Physiological Adaptation, Illness Management*

2. A. An antibiotic typically is given for a bacterial infection.

   B. A beta-blocker typically is given for dysrhythmias, heart disease, or hypertension.

   C. An antiviral typically is given for a virus.

   D. **CORRECT:** The nurse should administer a beta₂ agonist, which causes dilation of the bronchioles to relieve symptoms.

   Ⓝ *NCLEX® Connection: Pharmacological and Parenteral Therapies, Medication Administration*

3. A. The client should drink plenty of fluids while taking this prednisone. This medication can cause the client to have a dry mouth or to become thirsty.

   B. The client should inform the provider of any black, tarry stools. This medication can increase bleeding tendency. Black stools can be an indication of blood in the stool.

   C. **CORRECT:** The client should take this medication with food. Taking prednisone on an empty stomach can cause gastrointestinal distress.

   D. The client should monitor the mouth for canker sores. This medication can cause bleeding of the gums and soreness in the mouth. It also decreases immune function.

   Ⓝ *NCLEX® Connection: Pharmacological and Parenteral Therapies, Adverse Effects/Contraindications/Side Effects/Interactions*

4. A. Gender is not a risk factor associated with asthma.

   B. **CORRECT:** Environmental allergies are a risk factor associated with asthma. A client who has environmental allergies typically has other allergic problems, such as rhinitis or a skin rash.

   C. Alcohol use is not a risk factor associated with asthma.

   D. Race is not a risk factor associate with asthma.

   Ⓝ *NCLEX® Connection: Health Promotion and Maintenance, Health Promotion/Disease Prevention*

5. A. A bronchodilator does not decrease the body's immune response. However, an anti-inflammatory medication can cause this effect.

   B. **CORRECT:** A bronchodilator can prevent asthma attacks from occurring.

   C. An oral bronchodilator does not need to be taken with food. However, an anti-inflammatory medication can cause gastrointestinal distress and needs to be to be given with food.

   D. A bronchodilator has a fast onset to relieve asthma attack symptoms.

   Ⓝ *NCLEX® Connection: Pharmacological and Parenteral Therapies, Medication Administration*

PRACTICE Active Learning Scenario

A nurse is caring for a client who has asthma and a prescription for prednisone. Use the ATI Active Learning Template: Medication to complete this item.

NURSING INTERVENTIONS: Include at least three.

PRACTICE Answer

Using the ATI Active Use the ATI Active Learning Template: Medication

NURSING INTERVENTIONS

• Watch for decreased immune function.
• Monitor for hyperglycemia.
• Advise the client to report black, tarry stools.
• Observe for fluid retention and weight gain.
• Monitor the throat and mouth for aphthous lesions (canker sores).
• Omalizumab can cause anaphylaxis.

Ⓝ *NCLEX® Connection: Pharmacological and Parenteral Therapies, Medication Administration*

UNIT 3   NURSING CARE OF CLIENTS WHO
HAVE RESPIRATORY DISORDERS
SECTION: RESPIRATORY SYSTEM DISORDERS

CHAPTER 22   *Chronic Obstructive Pulmonary Disease*

Chronic obstructive pulmonary disease (COPD) encompasses two diseases: emphysema and chronic bronchitis. Most clients who have emphysema also have chronic bronchitis. COPD is irreversible.

Emphysema is characterized by the loss of lung elasticity and hyperinflation of lung tissue. Emphysema causes destruction of the alveoli, leading to a decreased surface area for gas exchange, carbon dioxide retention, and respiratory acidosis.

Chronic bronchitis is an inflammation of the bronchi and bronchioles due to chronic exposure to irritants.

COPD typically affects middle-age to older adults. Ⓖ

HEALTH PROMOTION AND DISEASE PREVENTION

- Promote smoking cessation.
- Avoid exposure to secondhand smoke.
- Use protective equipment, such as a mask, and ensure proper ventilation while working in environments that contain carcinogens or particles in the air.
- Influenza and pneumonia vaccinations are important for all clients who have COPD, but especially for older adults. Ⓖ

ASSESSMENT

RISK FACTORS

- Advanced age: Older adult clients have a decreased pulmonary reserve due to normal lung changes.
- Cigarette smoking is the primary risk factor for the development of COPD.
- Alpha$_1$–antitrypsin (AAT) deficiency
- Exposure to environmental factors (air pollution)

EXPECTED FINDINGS

Chronic dyspnea

PHYSICAL ASSESSMENT FINDINGS
- Dyspnea upon exertion
- Productive cough that is most severe upon rising in the morning
- Hypoxemia
- Crackles and wheezes
- Rapid and shallow respirations
- Use of accessory muscles
- Barrel chest or increased chest diameter (with emphysema) **(22.1)**
- Hyperresonance on percussion due to "trapped air" (with emphysema)
- Irregular breathing pattern
- Thin extremities and enlarged neck muscles
- Dependent edema secondary to right-sided heart failure
- Clubbing of fingers and toes (late stages of the disease)
- Pallor and cyanosis of nail beds and mucous membranes (late stages of the disease)
- Decreased oxygen saturation levels (expected reference range is 95% to 100%)
- In older adults or clients who have dark-colored skin, oxygen saturation levels can be slightly lower. Ⓖ

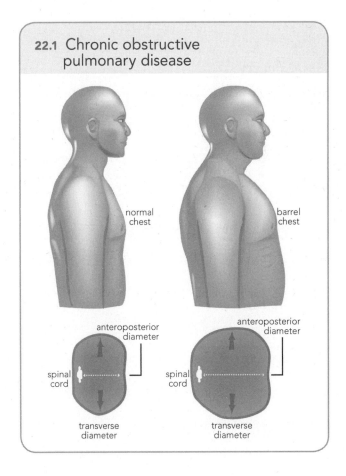

22.1 Chronic obstructive pulmonary disease

normal chest

barrel chest

anteroposterior diameter

spinal cord

transverse diameter

anteroposterior diameter

spinal cord

transverse diameter

LABORATORY TESTS

- Increased hematocrit level is due to low oxygenation levels.
- Use sputum cultures and WBC counts to diagnose acute respiratory infections.
- Arterial blood gases (ABGs)
  - Hypoxemia (decreased PaO_2 less than 80 mm Hg)
  - Hypercarbia (increased $PaCO_2$ greater than 45 mm Hg)
- Serum electrolytes

DIAGNOSTIC PROCEDURES

Pulmonary function tests

These tests are used for diagnosis, as well as determining the effectiveness of therapy.
- Comparisons of forced expiratory volume (FEV) to forced vital capacity (FVC) are used to classify COPD as mild to very severe.
- As COPD advances, the FEV-to-FVC ratio decreases. The expected reference range is 100%. For mild COPD, the FEV/FVC ratio is decreased to less than 70%. As the disease progresses to moderate and severe, the ratio decreases to less than 50%.

Chest x-ray

- Reveals hyperinflation of alveoli and flattened diaphragm in the late stages of emphysema. **(22.2)**
- It is often not useful for the diagnosis of early or moderate disease.

Pulse oximetry

Clients who have COPD usually have oxygen levels less than the expected reference range of 95% to 100%

Alpha₁ antitrypsin levels

Used to assess for deficiency in AAT, an enzyme produced by the liver that helps regulate other enzymes (which help break down pollutants) from attacking lung tissue.

PATIENT-CENTERED CARE

NURSING CARE

- Position the client to maximize ventilation (high-Fowler's). **QEBP**
- Encourage effective coughing, or suction to remove secretions.
- Encourage deep breathing and use of an incentive spirometer.
- Administer breathing treatments and medications.
- Administer oxygen as prescribed.
- Monitor for skin breakdown around the nose and mouth from the oxygen device.

- Promote adequate nutrition.
  - Increased work of breathing increases caloric demands.
  - Proper nutrition aids in the prevention of infection.
  - Encourage fluids to promote adequate hydration.
  - Dyspnea decreases energy available for eating, so soft, high-calorie foods should be encouraged.
- Monitor weight and note any changes.
- Instruct the client to practice breathing techniques to control dyspneic episodes. **QEBP**
  - For diaphragmatic (abdominal) breathing, instruct the client to:
    - Take breaths deep from the diaphragm.
    - Lie on back with knees bent.
    - Rest a hand over the abdomen to create resistance.
    - If the client's hand rises and lowers upon inhalation and exhalation, the breathing is being performed correctly.
  - For pursed-lip breathing, instruct the client to:
    - Form the mouth as if preparing to whistle.
    - Take a breath in through the nose and out through the lips/mouth.
    - Not puff the cheeks.
    - Take breaths deep and slow.
- Clients who have COPD can need 2 to 4 L/min of oxygen via nasal cannula or up to 40% via Venturi mask.
  - Clients who have chronically increased $PaCO_2$ levels usually require 1 to 2 L/min of oxygen via nasal cannula.
  - In COPD, low arterial levels of oxygen serve as the primary drive for breathing.
  - **Positive expiratory pressure device**
    - Assists client to remove airway secretions.
    - Client inhales deeply and exhales through device.
    - While exhaling, a ball inside the device moves, causing a vibration that results in loosening secretions.
  - **Exercise conditioning**
    - Includes improving pulmonary status by strengthening the condition of the lungs by exercise.
    - The client walks daily at a self-paced rate until symptoms of dyspnea occur allowing rest periods and then resuming walking.
    - The client walks 20 min daily 2 to 3 times weekly.
    - Determine the client's physical limitations, and structure activity to include periods of rest.
    - Provide rest periods for older adult clients who have dyspnea. Design the room and walkways with opportunities for relaxation. **Ⓖ**
- Provide support to the client and family. Talk about disease and lifestyle changes, including home care services such as portable oxygen.
- Encourage verbalization of feelings. **QPCC**
- Increase fluid intake. Encourage the client to drink 2 to 3 L/day to liquefy mucus.

Incentive spirometry

Incentive spirometry is used to monitor optimal lung expansion.

NURSING ACTIONS: Show the client how to use the incentive spirometry machine.

CLIENT EDUCATION: Instruct the client to keep a tight mouth seal around mouthpiece and to inhale and hold breath for 3 to 5 seconds. As the client inhales, the needle of the spirometry machine will rise. This promotes lung expansion.

MEDICATIONS

Bronchodilators (inhalers)

Short-acting beta₂ agonists, such as albuterol, provide rapid relief.

Cholinergic antagonists (anticholinergic medications), such as ipratropium, block the parasympathetic nervous system. This allows for the sympathetic nervous system effects of increased bronchodilation and decreased pulmonary secretions. These medications are long-acting and are used to prevent bronchospasms.

Methylxanthines, such as theophylline, relax smooth muscles of the bronchi. These medications require close monitoring of serum medication levels due to narrow therapeutic ranges. Use only when other treatments are ineffective.

NURSING CONSIDERATIONS
- Monitor serum levels for toxicity when taking theophylline. Adverse effects include tachycardia, nausea, and diarrhea.
- Watch for tremors and tachycardia when taking albuterol.
- Observe for dry mouth when taking ipratropium.

CLIENT EDUCATION
- Encourage the client to suck on hard candies to help moisten dry mouth while taking ipratropium.
- Encourage the client to increase fluid intake, report headaches, or blurred vision.
- Monitor heart rate. Palpitations can occur, which can indicate toxicity of ipratropium.

Anti-inflammatory agents

These medications decrease airway inflammation.
- If **corticosteroids**, such as fluticasone and prednisone, are given systemically, monitor for serious adverse effects (immunosuppression, fluid retention, hyperglycemia, hypokalemia, poor wound healing).
- **Leukotriene antagonists**, such as montelukast; **mast cell stabilizers**, such as cromolyn; and **monoclonal antibodies**, such as omalizumab, can be used.

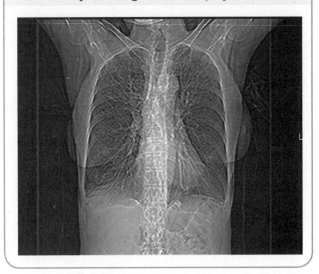

22.2 X-ray of lungs with emphysema

NURSING CONSIDERATIONS
- Watch for a decrease in immunity function.
- Monitor for hyperglycemia.
- Advise the client to report black, tarry stools.
- Observe for fluid retention and weight gain. This is common.
- Check the throat and mouth for aphthous lesions (canker sores).
- Omalizumab can cause anaphylaxis.

CLIENT EDUCATION
- Encourage the client to drink plenty of fluids to promote hydration.
- Encourage the client to take glucocorticoids with food.
- Advise the client to use medication to prevent and control bronchospasms.
- Advise the client to avoid people who have respiratory infections.
- Remind the client to use good mouth care.
- Tell the client to use medication as a prophylactic prevention of COPD symptoms.
- Instruct the client to not discontinue medication suddenly.

Mucolytic agents

These agents help thin secretions, making them easier for the client to expel.
- Nebulizer treatments include acetylcysteine and dornase alfa.
- Guaifenesin is an oral agent that can be taken.
- A combination of guaifenesin and dextromethorphan also can be taken orally to loosen secretions.

THERAPEUTIC PROCEDURES

- Chest physiotherapy uses percussion and vibration to mobilize secretions.
- Raising the foot of the bed slightly higher than the head can facilitate optimal drainage and removal of secretions by gravity.

INTERPROFESSIONAL CARE

- Consult respiratory services for inhalers, breathing treatments, and suctioning for airway management.
- Contact nutritional services for weight loss or gain related to medications or diagnosis.
- Consult rehabilitative care if the client has prolonged weakness and needs assistance with increasing activity level.

CLIENT EDUCATION

- COPD is debilitating for older adult clients. Referrals to assistance programs, such as food delivery services, can be indicated. Ⓖ
- Set up referral services, including home care services such as portable oxygen.
- Encourage the client to eat high-calorie foods to promote energy. Qᴘᴄᴄ
- Encourage rest periods as needed.
- Promote hand hygiene to prevent infection.
- Reinforce the importance of taking medications (inhalers, oral medications) as prescribed.
- Promote smoking cessation if needed.
- Encourage immunizations, such as influenza and pneumonia, to decrease the risk of infection.
- Clients should use oxygen as prescribed. Inform other caregivers not to smoke around the oxygen due to flammability.
- Provide support to the client and family.

COMPLICATIONS

Respiratory infection

Respiratory infections result from increased mucus production and poor oxygenation levels.

NURSING ACTIONS
- Administer oxygen therapy.
- Monitor oxygenation levels.
- Administer antibiotics and other medications.
- Advise the client to avoid crowds and people who have respiratory infections.
- Encourage the client to obtain pneumonia and influenza immunizations.

Right-sided heart failure (cor pulmonale)

- Air trapping, airway collapse, and stiff alveoli lead to increased pulmonary pressures.
- Blood flow through the lung tissue is difficult. This increased workload leads to enlargement and thickening of the right atrium and ventricle.

MANIFESTATIONS
- Low oxygenation levels
- Cyanotic lips
- Enlarged and tender liver
- Distended neck veins
- Dependent edema

NURSING ACTIONS
- Monitor respiratory status and administer oxygen therapy.
- Monitor heart rate and rhythm.
- Administer medications as prescribed.
- Administer IV fluids and diuretics to maintain fluid balance.

Application Exercises

1. A nurse is providing discharge teaching to a client who has COPD and a new prescription for albuterol. Which of the following statements by the client indicates an understanding of the teaching?

   A. "This medication can increase my blood sugar levels."

   B. "This medication can decrease my immune response."

   C. "I can have an increase in my heart rate while taking this medication."

   D. "I can have mouth sores while taking this medication."

2. A nurse is preparing to administer a dose of a new prescription of prednisone to a client who has COPD. The nurse should monitor for which of the following adverse effects of this medication? (Select all that apply.)

   A. Hypokalemia

   B. Tachycardia

   C. Fluid retention

   D. Nausea

   E. Black, tarry stools

3. A nurse is discharging a client who has COPD. Upon discharge, the client is concerned that he will never be able to leave his house now that he is on continuous oxygen. Which of the following is an appropriate response by the nurse?

   A. "There are portable oxygen delivery systems that you can take with you."

   B. "When you go out, you can remove the oxygen and then reapply it when you get home."

   C. "You probably will not be able to go out as much as you used to."

   D. "Home health services will come to you so you will not need to get out."

4. A nurse is instructing a client on the use of an incentive spirometer. Which of the following statements by the client indicates an understanding of the teaching?

   A. "I will place the adapter on my finger to read my blood oxygen saturation level."

   B. "I will lie on my back with my knees bent."

   C. "I will rest my hand over my abdomen to create resistance."

   D. "I will take in a deep breath and hold it before exhaling."

5. A nurse is planning to instruct a client on how to perform pursed-lip breathing. Which of the following should the nurse include in the plan of care?

   A. Take quick breaths upon inhalation.

   B. Place your hand over your stomach.

   C. Take a deep breath in through your nose.

   D. Puff your cheeks upon exhalation.

PRACTICE Active Learning Scenario

A nurse is reviewing discharge instructions for a client who has a new prescription for ipratropium. Use the ATI Active Learning Template: Medication to complete this item.

NURSING INTERVENTIONS: List at least three.

Application Exercises Key

1. A. Anti-inflammatory agents, such as corticosteroids, can cause hyperglycemia.

   B. Anti-inflammatory agents can decrease the immune response.

   C. **CORRECT:** Bronchodilators, such as albuterol, can cause tachycardia.

   D. Anti-inflammatory agents can cause mouth sores.

   Ⓝ *NCLEX® Connection: Pharmacological and Parenteral Therapies, Medication Administration*

2. A. **CORRECT:** The nurse should observe for hypokalemia. This is an adverse effect of prednisone.

   B. Tachycardia is an adverse effect of a bronchodilator.

   C. **CORRECT:** The nurse should observe for fluid retention. This is an adverse effect of prednisone.

   D. Nausea is an adverse effect of a bronchodilator.

   E. **CORRECT:** The nurse should monitor for black, tarry stools. This is an adverse effect of prednisone.

   Ⓝ *NCLEX® Connection: Pharmacological and Parenteral Therapies, Expected Actions/Outcomes*

3. A. **CORRECT:** The nurse should inform the client that there are portable oxygen systems that he can use to leave the house. This should alleviate the client's anxiety.

   B. The nurse should tell the client use oxygen at all times to prevent becoming hypoxic.

   C. The nurse should encourage the client to return to his daily routine, but include periods of rest.

   D. The nurse should encourage the client to return to his daily routine. Home health services promote a client's independence.

   Ⓝ *NCLEX® Connection: Physiological Adaptation, Illness Management*

4. A. The client should place an adapter on her finger to read the blood oxygen saturation level while performing a pulse oximetry reading.

   B. The client who practices diaphragmatic or abdominal breathing should lie on her back with knees bent.

   C. The client who practices diaphragmatic or abdominal breathing should rest her hand over her abdomen to determine if the breathing is done correctly.

   D. **CORRECT:** The client who is using the spirometer should take in a deep breath and hold it for 3 to 5 seconds before exhaling. As the client exhales, the needle of the spirometer rises. This promotes lung expansion.

   Ⓝ *NCLEX® Connection: Reduction of Risk Potential, Diagnostic Tests*

5. A. The client should take a slow deep breath upon inhalation. This improves breathing and allows oxygen into lungs.

   B. The client should place her hand on her stomach while performing diaphragmatic or abdominal breathing. This allows resistance to be met and serves as a guide that the client is inhaling and exhaling correctly.

   C. **CORRECT:** The client should take a deep breath in through her nose while performing pursed-lip breathing. This controls the client's breathing.

   D. The client should not puff her cheeks upon exhalation. This does not allow the client to optimally exhale the carbon dioxide from her lungs.

   Ⓝ *NCLEX® Connection: Physiological Adaptation, Alterations in Body Systems*

PRACTICE Answer

Using ATI Active Learning Template: Medication

NURSING INTERVENTIONS

- Observe the client for dry mouth when taking this medication.
- Encourage the client to suck on hard candies to help moisten dry mouth while taking ipratropium.
- Encourage the client to increase fluid intake, and to report headaches or blurred vision.
- Monitor heart rate. Palpitations can occur, which can indicate toxicity of ipratropium.

Ⓝ *NCLEX® Connection: Pharmacological and Parenteral Therapies, Medication Administration*

UNIT 3 NURSING CARE OF CLIENTS WHO
HAVE RESPIRATORY DISORDERS
SECTION: RESPIRATORY SYSTEM DISORDERS

CHAPTER 23 *Tuberculosis*

Tuberculosis (TB) is an infectious disease caused by *Mycobacterium tuberculosis*. TB is transmitted through aerosolization (airborne route).

Once inside the lung, the body encases the TB bacillus with collagen and other cells. This can appear as a Ghon tubercle on a chest x-ray.

Only a small percentage of people infected with TB actually develop an active form of the infection. The TB bacillus can lie dormant for many years before producing the disease.

TB primarily affects the lungs but can spread to any organ in the blood. The risk of transmission decreases after 2 to 3 weeks of antituberculin therapy.

HEALTH PROMOTION AND DISEASE PREVENTION

- Clients who live in high-risk areas for tuberculosis should be screened on a yearly basis.
- Family members of clients who have tuberculosis should be screened.
- Early detection and treatment are vital. TB has a slow onset, and the client might not be aware until the symptoms and disease are advanced. TB diagnosis should be considered for any client who has a persistent cough, chest pain, weakness, weight loss, anorexia, hemoptysis, dyspnea, fever, night sweats, or chills.
- Increasing the percentage of clients who complete treatment for TB should be a goal.
- Individuals who have been exposed to TB but have not developed the disease can have latent TB. This means that *Mycobacterium tuberculosis* is in the body, but the body has been able to fight off the infection. If not treated, it can lie dormant for several years and then become active as the individual becomes older or immunocompromised. Ⓖ

ASSESSMENT

RISK FACTORS

- Frequent and close contact with an untreated individual
- Lower socioeconomic status and homelessness
- Immunocompromised status (HIV, chemotherapy, kidney disease, diabetes mellitus, Crohn's disease)
- Poorly ventilated, crowded environments (prisons, long-term care facilities)
- Advanced age
- Recent travel outside of the United States to areas where TB is endemic
- Immigration (especially from Mexico, Philippines, Vietnam, China, Japan, and Eastern Mediterranean countries)
- Substance use
- Health care occupation that involves performance of high-risk activities (respiratory treatments, suctioning, coughing procedures)

EXPECTED FINDINGS

- Persistent cough lasting longer than 3 weeks
- Purulent sputum, possibly blood-streaked
- Fatigue and lethargy
- Weight loss and anorexia
- Night sweats and low-grade fever in the afternoon

PHYSICAL ASSESSMENT FINDINGS: Older adult clients often present with atypical symptoms of the disease (altered mentation or unusual behavior, fever, anorexia, weight loss). Ⓖ

LABORATORY TESTS

A client will have a positive intradermal TB test within 2 to 10 weeks of exposure to the infection.

QuantiFERON-TB Gold

Blood test that detects release of interferon-gamma (IFN-g) in fresh heparinized whole blood from sensitized people
- Diagnostic for infection, whether active or latent.
- Results are available within 24 hr.

DIAGNOSTIC PROCEDURES

Mantoux test (23.1)

- Should be read in 48 to 72 hr.
- An intradermal injection of an extract of the tubercle bacillus is made.
- An induration (palpable, raised, hardened area) of 10 mm or greater in diameter indicates a positive skin test.
- An induration of 5 mm is considered a positive test for immunocompromised clients.
- A positive Mantoux test indicates that the client has developed an immune response to TB. It does not confirm that active disease is present. Clients who have been treated for TB can retain a positive reaction. Q EBP
- Individuals who have latent TB can have a positive Mantoux test and can receive treatment to prevent development of an active form of the disease.
- Clients who have received a Bacillus Calmette-Guerin vaccine within the past 10 years can have a false-positive Mantoux test. These clients need a chest x-ray or QuantiFERON-TB Gold test to evaluate the presence of active TB infection.
- Clients who are immunocompromised (such as those who have HIV) and older adult clients should be tested for TB. Clients starting immunosuppressive therapy (such as tumor necrosis factor antagonists) should be tested for TB prior to starting treatment.

CLIENT EDUCATION: Reinforce the importance of returning for a reading of the injection site by a health care personnel within 48 to 72 hr.

Chest x-ray

Can be prescribed to detect active lesions in the lungs.

Acid-fast bacilli smear and culture

- A positive acid-fast test suggests an active infection.
- The diagnosis is confirmed by a positive culture for *Mycobacterium tuberculosis*.

NURSING ACTIONS
- Obtain three early-morning sputum samples.
- Wear personal protective equipment when obtaining specimens.
- Samples should also be obtained in a negative airflow room.

PATIENT-CENTERED CARE

NURSING CARE

- Administer heated and humidified oxygen therapy as prescribed.
- Prevent infection transmission.
  - Wear a N95 HEPA filter or powered air purifying respirator when caring for clients who are hospitalized with TB. (23.2)
  - Place the client in a negative-airflow room, and implement airborne precautions.
  - Use barrier protection when the risk of hand or clothing contamination exists.
  - Have the client wear a surgical mask if transportation to another department is necessary. The client should be transported using the shortest and least busy route.
  - Teach the client to cough and expectorate sputum into tissues that are disposed of by the client into provided plastic bags or no-touch receptacles.
- Administer prescribed medications.
- Promote adequate nutrition.
  - Encourage fluid intake and a well-balanced diet for adequate caloric intake.
  - Encourage foods that are rich in protein, iron, and vitamins C and B.
- Provide emotional support.

23.1 Mantoux test

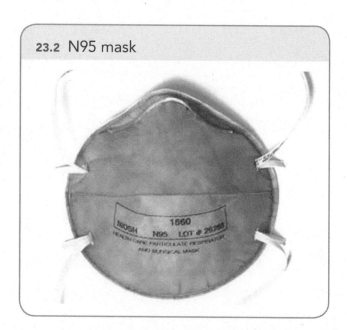

23.2 N95 mask

MEDICATIONS

Due to the resistance that is developing against the antituberculin medications, combination therapy of two or more medications at a time is recommended.

- Because these medications must be taken for 6 to 12 months, medication noncompliance is a significant contributing factor in the development of resistant strains of TB.
- The current four-medication regimen includes isoniazid, rifampin, pyrazinamide, and ethambutol.

CLIENT EDUCATION: Instruct the client to complete a series of prescribed medication.

Isoniazid

Isoniazid, commonly referred to as INH, is bactericidal and inhibits growth of mycobacteria by preventing synthesis of mycolic acid in the cell wall.

NURSING CONSIDERATIONS

- This medication should be taken on an empty stomach.
- Monitor for hepatotoxicity (jaundice, anorexia, malaise, fatigue, and nausea) and neurotoxicity (such as tingling of the hands and feet).
- Vitamin B_6 (pyridoxine) is used to prevent neurotoxicity from isoniazid.
- Liver function testing should be completed prior to and monthly after starting INH.

CLIENT EDUCATION

- Advise the client not to drink alcohol while taking isoniazid because it can increase the risk for hepatotoxicity. Qs
- Advise the client to report any manifestations of hepatotoxicity.

Rifampin

Rifampin, commonly referred to as RIF, is a bacteriostatic and bactericidal antibiotic that inhibits DNA-dependent RNA polymerase activity in susceptible cells.

NURSING CONSIDERATIONS

- Observe for hepatotoxicity.
- Liver function testing should be completed prior to and at least monthly after starting RIF.

CLIENT EDUCATION

- Inform the client that urine and other secretions will be orange.
- Advise the client to immediately report yellowing of the skin, pain or swelling of joints, loss of appetite, or malaise.
- Inform the client this medication can interfere with the efficacy of oral contraceptives.

Pyrazinamide

Pyrazinamide, commonly referred to as PZA, is a bacteriostatic and bactericidal. Its exact mechanism of action is unknown.

NURSING CONSIDERATIONS

- Observe for hepatotoxicity.
- Assess for history of gout, as the medication will cause an adverse effect of nongouty polyarthralgias.
- Liver enzymes should be completed baseline and every 2 weeks after starting PZA.

CLIENT EDUCATION

- Instruct the client to drink a glass of water with each dose and increase fluids during the day to help prevent gout and kidney problems.
- Advise the client to immediately report yellowing of the skin, pain or swelling of joints, loss of appetite, or malaise.
- Advise the client to avoid using alcohol while taking pyrazinamide.

Ethambutol

Ethambutol, commonly referred to as EMB, is a bacteriostatic and works by suppressing RNA synthesis, subsequently inhibiting protein synthesis.

NURSING CONSIDERATIONS

- Obtain baseline visual acuity tests, and complete monthly after starting treatment.
- Determine color discrimination ability.
- This medication should not be given to children younger than 8 years of age.
- Stop medication immediately if ocular toxicity occurs.

CLIENT EDUCATION: Instruct the client to report changes in vision immediately. QEBP

Streptomycin sulfate

Streptomycin sulfate is an aminoglycoside antibiotic. It potentiates the efficacy of macrophages during phagocytosis.

NURSING CONSIDERATIONS

- Due to its high level of toxicity, this medication should be used only in clients who have multidrug-resistant TB (MDR-TB).
- Streptomycin can cause ototoxicity, so monitor hearing function and tolerance often.
- Report significant changes in urine output and renal function studies.

CLIENT EDUCATION

- Advise the client to drink at least 2 L of fluid daily.
- Advise the client to notify the provider if hearing declines.

INTERPROFESSIONAL CARE

- Contact social services if the client will need assistance in obtaining prescribed medications.
- Refer the client to a community clinic as needed for follow-up appointments to monitor medication regimen and status of disease.

CLIENT EDUCATION

- Provide the client and family education because TB is often treated in the home setting. Qpcc
- Airborne precautions are not needed in the home setting because family members have already been exposed.
- Exposed family members should be tested for TB.
- Educate the client and family to continue medication therapy for its full duration of 6 to 12 months, even up to 2 years for multidrug-resistant TB. Emphasize that failure to take the medications can lead to a resistant strain of TB.
- Instruct the client to continue with follow-up care for 1 full year.
- Inform the client that sputum samples are needed every 2 to 4 weeks to monitor therapy effectiveness. Clients are no longer considered infectious after three consecutive negative sputum cultures, and may return to former employment.
- Encourage proper hand hygiene.
- Instruct the client to cover mouth and nose when coughing or sneezing.
- Inform the client that contaminated tissues should be disposed of in plastic bags.
- Advise clients who have active TB to wear a mask when in public places or in contact with crowds.

COMPLICATIONS

Miliary TB

The organism invades the bloodstream and can spread to multiple body organs with complications including the following.

- Headaches, neck stiffness, and drowsiness (can be life-threatening)
- Pericarditis: Dyspnea, swollen neck veins, pleuritic pain, and hypotension due to an accumulation of fluid in pericardial sac that inhibits the heart's ability to pump effectively

NURSING ACTIONS: Treatment is the same as for pulmonary TB.

Application Exercises

1. A home health nurse is teaching a client who has active tuberculosis. The provider has prescribed the following medication regimen: isoniazid 250 mg PO daily, rifampin 500 mg PO daily, pyrazinamide 750 mg PO daily, and ethambutol 1 mg PO daily. Which of the following client statements indicate the client understands the teaching? (Select all that apply.)

   A. "I can substitute one medication for another if I run out because they all fight infection."

   B. "I will wash my hands each time I cough."

   C. "I will wear a mask when I am in a public area."

   D. "I am glad I don't have to have any more sputum specimens."

   E. "I don't need to worry where I go once I start taking my medications."

2. A nurse is teaching a client who has tuberculosis. Which of the following statements should the nurse include in the teaching?

   A. "You will need to continue to take the multimedication regimen for 4 months."

   B. "You will need to provide sputum samples every 4 weeks to monitor the effectiveness of the medication."

   C. "You will need to remain hospitalized for treatment."

   D. "You will need to wear a mask at all times."

3. A nurse is caring for a client who has a new diagnosis of tuberculosis and has been placed on a multimedication regimen. Which of the following instructions should the nurse give the client related to ethambutol?

   A. "Your urine can turn a dark orange."

   B. "Watch for a change in the sclera of your eyes."

   C. "Watch for any changes in vision."

   D. "Take vitamin B_6 daily."

4. A nurse is preparing to administer a new prescription for isoniazid (INH) to a client who has tuberculosis. The nurse should instruct the client to report which of the following findings as an adverse effect of the medication?

   A. "You might notice yellowing of your skin."

   B. "You might experience pain in your joints."

   C. "You might notice tingling of your hands."

   D. "You might experience a loss of appetite."

5. A nurse is providing information about tuberculosis to a group of clients at a local community center. Which of the following manifestations should the nurse include in the teaching? (Select all that apply.)

   A. Persistent cough

   B. Weight gain

   C. Fatigue

   D. Night sweats

   E. Purulent sputum

PRACTICE Active Learning Scenario

A nurse is caring for a client who has tuberculosis. Use the ATI Active Learning Template: System Disorder to complete this item.

PATHOPHYSIOLOGY RELATED TO CLIENT PROBLEM

NURSING CARE: Include three nursing interventions.

COMPLICATIONS: Identify one potential complication.

Application Exercises Key

1. A. Medications should not be replaced for one another. It is important that the client adhere to the multimedication regimen prescribed to treat tuberculosis.

   B. **CORRECT:** The client should wash her hands each time she coughs to prevent spreading the infection.

   C. **CORRECT:** The client should wear a mask while in public areas to prevent spreading the infection. The client has active TB, which is transmitted through the airborne route.

   D. The client will need to collect sputum cultures every 2 to 4 weeks until three consecutive sputum cultures have come back negative.

   E. The client should continue to avoid crowded areas if possible and take preventative measures, such as wearing a mask when going out.

   Ⓝ *NCLEX® Connection: Pharmacological and Parenteral Therapies, Medication Administration*

2. A. The client who has tuberculosis needs to continue taking the multimedication regimen for 6 to 12 months.

   B. **CORRECT:** The client who has tuberculosis needs to provide sputum samples every 2 to 4 weeks to monitor the effectiveness of the medication.

   C. The client who has tuberculosis is often treated in the home setting.

   D. The client who has tuberculosis needs to wear a mask when in public areas.

   Ⓝ *NCLEX® Connection: Reduction of Risk Potential, Laboratory Values*

3. A. The client who is receiving rifampin should expect to see his urine turn a dark orange.

   B. The client who is taking ethambutol does not have an adverse effect resulting in changes to the sclera of the eyes.

   C. **CORRECT:** The client who is receiving ethambutol will need to watch for visual changes due to optic neuritis, which can result from taking this medication.

   D. The client who is taking isoniazid should take vitamin B$_6$ daily and observe for signs of hepatotoxicity.

   Ⓝ *NCLEX® Connection: Pharmacological and Parenteral Therapies, Medication Administration*

4. A. Yellowing of the skin is an adverse effect of rifampin or pyrazinamide.

   B. Experiencing pain in the joints is an adverse effect of rifampin.

   C. **CORRECT:** Tingling of the hands is an adverse effect of isoniazid.

   D. Loss of appetite is an adverse effect of rifampin.

   Ⓝ *NCLEX® Connection: Pharmacological and Parenteral Therapies, Adverse Effects/Contraindications/Side Effects/Interactions*

5. A. **CORRECT:** The nurse should include in the teaching that a persistent cough is a manifestation of tuberculosis.

   B. The nurse should include in the teaching that weight loss is a manifestation of tuberculosis.

   C. **CORRECT:** The nurse should include in the teaching that fatigue is a manifestation of tuberculosis.

   D. **CORRECT:** The nurse should include in the teaching that night sweats is a manifestation of tuberculosis.

   E. **CORRECT:** The nurse should include in the teaching that purulent sputum is a manifestation of tuberculosis.

   Ⓝ *NCLEX® Connection: Physiological Adaptation, Alterations in Body Systems*

PRACTICE Answer

Using the ATI Active Learning Template: System Disorder

PATHOPHYSIOLOGY RELATED TO CLIENT PROBLEM:
Tuberculosis (TB) is an infectious disease caused by *Mycobacterium tuberculosis*. TB is transmitted through aerosolization (airborne route). Once inside the lung, the body encases the TB bacillus with collagen and other cells. This can appear as a Ghon tubercle on a chest x-ray. Only a small percentage of people infected with TB actually develop an active form of the infection. The TB bacillus can lie dormant for many years before producing the disease. TB primarily affects the lungs but can spread to any organ in the blood.

NURSING CARE
Nursing Interventions
- Administer heated and humidified oxygen therapy as prescribed.
- Prevent infection transmission.
- Wear an N95 or HEPA respirator when caring for clients who are hospitalized with TB.
- Place the client in a negative airflow room, and implement airborne precautions.
- Use barrier protection when the risk of hand or clothing contamination exists.
- Have the client wear a surgical mask if transportation to another department is necessary.
- Transport the client using the shortest and least busy route.
- Teach the client to cough and expectorate sputum into tissues that are disposed of by the client into provided sacks.
- Administer medications as prescribed.
- Promote adequate nutrition.
- Encourage fluid intake and a well-balanced diet for adequate caloric intake.

COMPLICATIONS
Miliary TB: The organism invades the bloodstream and can spread to multiple body organs with complications including the following:
- Headaches, neck stiffness, and drowsiness (can be life-threatening)
- Pericarditis: dyspnea, swollen neck veins, pleuritic pain, and hypotension due to an accumulation of fluid in the pericardial sac that inhibits the heart's ability to pump effectively
- Nursing Actions: Treatment is the same as for pulmonary TB.

Ⓝ *NCLEX® Connection: Physiological Adaptation, Alterations in Body Systems*

CHAPTER 24 *Pulmonary Embolism*

A pulmonary embolism (PE) occurs when a substance (solid, gaseous, or liquid) enters venous circulation and forms a blockage in the pulmonary vasculature.

Emboli originating from venous thromboembolism, also known as deep-vein thrombosis (DVT), are the most common cause. Tumors, bone marrow, amniotic fluid, air, and foreign matter also can become emboli.

Increased hypoxia to pulmonary tissue and impaired blood flow can result from a large embolus. A PE is a medical emergency.

Prevention, rapid recognition, and treatment of a PE are essential for a positive outcome.

HEALTH PROMOTION AND DISEASE PREVENTION

- Promote smoking cessation.
- Encourage maintenance of appropriate weight for height and body frame.
- Encourage a healthy diet and physical activity.
- Prevent DVT by encouraging clients to do leg exercises, wear compression stockings, and avoid sitting for long periods of time.

ASSESSMENT

RISK FACTORS

- Long-term immobility
- Oral contraceptive use and estrogen therapy
- Pregnancy
- Tobacco use
- Hypercoagulability (elevated platelet count)
- Obesity
- Surgery (especially orthopedic surgery of the lower extremities or pelvis)
- Central venous catheters
- Heart failure or chronic atrial fibrillation
- Autoimmune hemolytic anemia (sickle cell)
- Long bone fractures
- Cancer
- Trauma
- Advanced age ⓒ
  - Older adult clients have decreased pulmonary reserves due to normal lung changes, including decreased lung elasticity and thickening alveoli. Older adult clients can decompensate more quickly.
  - Certain pathological conditions and procedures that predispose clients to DVT formation (peripheral vascular disease, hypertension, hip and knee arthroplasty) are more prevalent in older adults.
  - Many older adult clients experience decreased physical activity levels, thus predisposing them to DVT formation and pulmonary emboli.

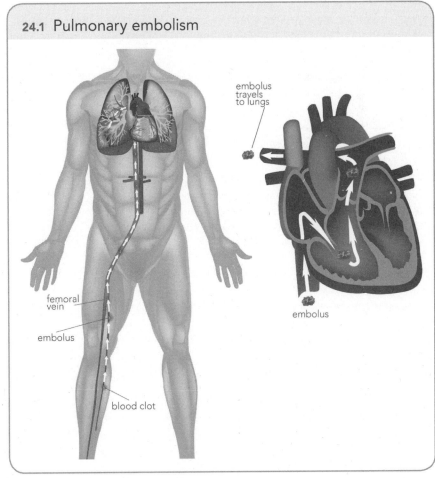

24.1 Pulmonary embolism

embolus travels to lungs

femoral vein

embolus

blood clot

embolus

EXPECTED FINDINGS

- Anxiety
- Feelings of impending doom
- Pressure in chest
- Pain upon inspiration and chest wall tenderness
- Dyspnea and air hunger
- Cough
- Hemoptysis

PHYSICAL ASSESSMENT FINDINGS

- Pleurisy
- Pleural friction rub
- Tachycardia
- Hypotension
- Tachypnea
- Adventitious breath sounds (crackles) and cough
- Heart murmur in S_3 and S_4
- Diaphoresis
- Low-grade fever
- Decreased oxygen saturation levels (expected reference range is 95% to 100%), low SaO_2, cyanosis
- Petechiae (red dots under the skin) over chest and axillae
- Pleural effusion (fluid in the lungs)
- Distended neck veins
- Syncope
- Cyanosis

LABORATORY TESTS

ABG analysis

- $PaCO_2$ levels are low (expected reference range is 35 to 45 mm Hg) due to initial hyperventilation (respiratory alkalosis).
- As hypoxemia progresses, respiratory acidosis occurs.
- Further progression leads to metabolic acidosis due to buildup of lactic acid from tissue hypoxia.

CBC analysis

To monitor hemoglobin and hematocrit

D-dimer

Elevated above expected reference range in response to clot formation and release of fibrin degradation products (expected reference range is less than 0.4 mcg/mL).

DIAGNOSTIC PROCEDURES

Chest x-ray and computed tomography scan

These provide initial identification of a PE. A computed tomography (CT) scan is most commonly used. A chest x-ray can show a large PE.

Ventilation-perfusion scan

Ventilation-perfusion (V/Q) scan images show circulation of air and blood in the lungs and can detect a PE.

Pulmonary angiography

- This is the gold standard and most thorough test to detect a PE, but it is invasive and costly. A catheter is inserted into the vena cava to visually see a PE.
- Pulmonary angiography is a higher risk procedure than a V/Q scan.

NURSING ACTIONS

- Verify that informed consent has been obtained.
- Monitor status (vital signs, SaO_2, anxiety, bleeding with angiography) during and after the procedure.

PATIENT-CENTERED CARE

NURSING CARE

- Administer oxygen therapy to relieve hypoxemia and dyspnea. Position the client to maximize ventilation (high-Fowler's = 90°).
- Initiate and maintain IV access.
- Administer medications as prescribed.
- Assess respiratory status at least every 30 min. Qpcc
  - Auscultate lung sounds.
  - Measure rate, rhythm, and ease of respirations.
  - Inspect skin color and capillary refill.
  - Examine for position of trachea.
- Assess cardiac status. Qpcc
  - Compare blood pressure in both arms.
  - Palpate pulse quality.
  - Check for dysrhythmias on cardiac monitor.
  - Examine the neck for distended neck veins.
  - Inspect the thorax for petechiae.
- Provide emotional support and comfort to control client anxiety.
- Monitor changes in level of consciousness and mental status.

MEDICATIONS

Anticoagulants

Heparin, enoxaparin, warfarin, and fondaparinux are used to prevent clots from getting larger or additional clots from forming.

NURSING CONSIDERATIONS
- Assess for contraindications (active bleeding, peptic ulcer disease, history of stroke, recent trauma).
- Monitor bleeding times: Prothrombin time (PT) and international normalized ratio (INR) for warfarin, partial thromboplastin time (aPTT) for heparin, and complete blood count (CBC). Q_EBP
- Monitor for side effects of anticoagulants (e.g., thrombocytopenia, anemia, hemorrhage).

Direct factor Xa inhibitor

Rivaroxaban binds directly with the active center of factor Xa, which inhibits the production of thrombin.

NURSING CONSIDERATIONS
- Assess for bleeding from any site. (Clients have experienced epidural hematomas, as well as intracranial, retinal, adrenal, and GI bleeds).
- Risk for spinal or epidural hematoma. Should discontinue medication for 18 hr prior to removing an epidural catheter, and wait another 6 hr to restart.

Thrombolytic therapy

- Alteplase, reteplase, and tenecteplase are used to dissolve blood clots and restore pulmonary blood flow.
- Similar side effects and contraindications as anticoagulants.

NURSING CONSIDERATIONS
- Assess for contraindications (known bleeding disorders, uncontrolled hypertension, active bleeding, peptic ulcer disease, history of stroke, recent trauma or surgery, pregnancy).
- Monitor for evidence of bleeding, thrombocytopenia, and anemia.
- Monitor blood pressure, heart rate, respirations, and oxygen saturation per facility protocol before, during, and after administration of medication. Q_S

INTERPROFESSIONAL CARE

- Cardiology and pulmonary services should be consulted to manage a PE and treatment.
- Respiratory services should be consulted for oxygen therapy, breathing treatments, and ABGs.
- Radiology should be consulted for diagnostic studies to determine PE.

THERAPEUTIC PROCEDURES

Embolectomy

Surgical removal of embolus

NURSING ACTIONS
- Prepare the client for the procedure (NPO status, informed consent).
- Monitor postoperatively (vital signs, SaO_2, incision drainage, pain management).

Vena cava filter

Insertion of a filter in the vena cava to prevent further emboli from reaching the pulmonary vasculature

NURSING ACTIONS
- Prepare the client for the procedure (NPO status, informed consent).
- Monitor postoperatively (vital signs, SaO_2, incision drainage, pain management).

CLIENT EDUCATION

- If the client is homebound, set up home care services to perform weekly blood draws.
- Set up referral services to supply portable oxygen for clients who have severe dyspnea.
- Provide education about treatment and prevention of a PE. Q_PCC
  - Promote smoking cessation if the client smokes.
  - Encourage the client to avoid long periods of immobility.
  - Encourage physical activity such as walking.
  - Encourage the client to wear compression stockings to promote circulation.
  - Encourage the client to avoid crossing his legs.
- Advise the client to monitor intake of foods high in vitamin K (green, leafy vegetables) if taking warfarin. Vitamin K can reduce the anticoagulant effects of warfarin.
- Advise the client to adhere to a schedule for monitoring PT and INR, follow instructions regarding medication dosage adjustments (for clients on warfarin), and adhere to weekly blood draws.
- Remind the client of the increased risk for bruising and bleeding.
  - Instruct the client to avoid taking aspirin products, unless specified by the provider.
  - Encourage the client to check his mouth and skin daily for bleeding and bruising.
  - Encourage the client to use electric shavers and soft-bristled toothbrushes.
  - Instruct the client to avoid blowing his nose hard, and to gently apply pressure if nose bleeds occur.
- Encourage clients who travel about measures to prevent PE.
  - Instruct the client to arise from a sitting position for 5 min out of every hour.
  - Advise the client to wear support stockings.
  - Inform the client to remain hydrated by drinking plenty of water.
  - Instruct the client to perform active ROM exercises when sitting.

COMPLICATIONS

Decreased cardiac output

Blood volume is decreased.

NURSING ACTIONS

- Monitor for hypotension, tachycardia, cyanosis, jugular venous distention, and syncope.
- Assess for the presence of S_3 or S_4 heart sounds.
- Initiate and maintain IV access.
- Monitor urinary output (should be 30 mL/hr or more).
- Administer IV fluids (crystalloids) to replace vascular volume.
- Continuously monitor the ECG.
- Monitor pulmonary pressures. IV fluids can contribute to pulmonary hypertension for clients who have right-sided heart failure (cor pulmonale).
- Administer inotropic agents (milrinone, dobutamine), to increase myocardial contractility.
- Vasodilators can be needed if pulmonary artery pressure is high enough to interfere with cardiac contractility.

Hemorrhage

Risk for bleeding increases due to anticoagulant therapy.

NURSING ACTIONS

- Assess for oozing, bleeding, or bruising from injection and surgical sites at least every 2 hr.
- Monitor cardiovascular status (blood pressure, heart rate and rhythm).
- Monitor CBC (hemoglobin, hematocrit, platelets) and bleeding times (PT, aPTT, INR).
- Administer IV fluids and blood products as required.
- Test stools, urine, and vomit for occult blood.
- Monitor for internal bleeding (measure abdominal girth and abdominal or flank pain) at least every 8 hr.

Application Exercises

1. A nurse is caring for a group of clients. Which of the following clients are at risk for a pulmonary embolism? (Select all that apply.)

   A. A client who has a BMI of 30

   B. A female client who is postmenopausal

   C. A client who has a fractured femur

   D. A client who is a marathon runner

   E. A client who has chronic atrial fibrillation

2. A nurse is assessing a client who has a pulmonary embolism. Which of the following manifestations should the nurse expect to find? (Select all that apply.)

   A. Bradypnea

   B. Pleural friction rub

   C. Hypertension

   D. Petechiae

   E. Tachycardia

3. A nurse is reviewing prescriptions for a client who has acute dyspnea and diaphoresis. The client states she is anxious and is unable to get enough air. Vital signs are heart rate 117/min, respirations 38/min, temperature 38.4° C (101.2° F), and blood pressure 100/54 mm Hg. Which of the following nursing actions is the priority?

   A. Notify the provider.

   B. Administer heparin via IV infusion.

   C. Administer oxygen therapy.

   D. Obtain a spiral CT scan.

4. A nurse is caring for a client who has a new prescription for heparin therapy. Which of the following statements by the client should indicate an immediate concern for the nurse?

   A. "I am allergic to morphine."

   B. "I take antacids several times a day."

   C. "I had a blood clot in my leg several years ago."

   D. "It hurts to take a deep breath."

5. A nurse is caring for a client who is to receive thrombolytic therapy. Which of the following factors should the nurse recognize as a contraindication to the therapy?

   A. Hip arthroplasty 2 weeks ago

   B. Elevated sedimentation rate

   C. Incident of exercise-induced asthma 1 week ago

   D. Elevated platelet count

PRACTICE Active Learning Scenario

A nurse is caring for a client who has a pulmonary embolism. Use the ATI Active Learning Template: System Disorder to complete this item.

PATHOPHYSIOLOGY RELATED TO CLIENT PROBLEM

NURSING CARE: Describe three nursing interventions.

MEDICATIONS: Identify two.

Application Exercises Key

1. A. **CORRECT:** The client who has a BMI of 30 is considered obese and is at increased risk for a blood clot.

   B. A woman who is postmenopausal has decreased estrogen levels and is not at risk for developing a pulmonary embolism.

   C. **CORRECT:** The client who has a fractured bone, particularly in a long bone such as the femur, increases the risk of fat emboli.

   D. The client who is a marathon runner has increased blood flow and circulation of his body, which decreases the risk for developing a pulmonary embolism.

   E. **CORRECT:** The client who has turbulent blood flow in the heart, such as with atrial defibrillation, is also at increased risk of a blood clot.

   (N) *NCLEX® Connection: Health Promotion and Maintenance, Health Promotion/Disease Prevention*

2. A. The nurse should expect the client to have tachypnea, which is a manifestation associated with a pulmonary embolism.

   B. **CORRECT:** The nurse should expect the client to have a pleural friction rub, which is a manifestation associated with a pulmonary embolism.

   C. The nurse should expect the client to have hypotension, which is a manifestation associated with a pulmonary embolism.

   D. **CORRECT:** The nurse should expect the client to have petechiae, which is a manifestation associated with a pulmonary embolism.

   E. **CORRECT:** The nurse should expect the client to have tachycardia, which is a manifestation associated with a pulmonary embolism.

   (N) *NCLEX® Connection: Physiological Adaptation, Unexpected Response to Therapies*

3. A. The nurse should notify the provider about the condition. However, another action is the priority.

   B. The nurse should administer IV heparin as a treatment to prevent growth of the existing clot and to prevent additional clots from forming. However, another action is the priority.

   C. **CORRECT:** When using the airway, breathing, circulation (ABC) priority approach to care, the nurse determines that the priority finding is related to the respiratory status. Meeting oxygenation needs by administering oxygen therapy is the priority action.

   D. The nurse should obtain a spiral CT scan to detect the presence and location of the blood clot. However, another action is the priority

   (N) *NCLEX® Connection: Physiological Adaptation, Medical Emergencies*

4. A. The nurse should document the client's allergy to morphine to manage the client's discomfort due to a blood clot. However, another action is the priority.

   B. **CORRECT:** The greatest risk to the client is the possibility of bleeding from a peptic ulcer. The priority intervention is to notify the provider of the finding.

   C. The nurse should know the client's history of a blood clot to provide preventative measures. However, another action is the priority.

   D. The nurse should expect the client to report pain with breathing. However, another action is the priority.

   (N) *NCLEX® Connection: Pharmacological and Parenteral Therapies, Expected Actions/Outcomes*

5. A. **CORRECT:** The client who has undergone a major surgical procedure within the last 3 weeks should not receive thrombolytic therapy because of the risk of hemorrhage from the surgical site.

   B. An elevated sedimentation rate does not place the client at risk for hemorrhage.

   C. An incident of exercise-induced asthma does not place the client at risk for hemorrhage, nor is it contraindicated with this type of medication.

   D. An elevated platelet count does not place the client at risk for hemorrhage when receiving this medication.

   (N) *NCLEX® Connection: Pharmacological and Parenteral Therapies, Adverse Effects/Contraindications/Side Effects/Interactions*

PRACTICE Answer

Using the ATI Active Learning Template: System Disorder

PATHOPHYSIOLOGY RELATED TO CLIENT PROBLEM: A pulmonary embolism (PE) occurs when a substance (solid, gaseous, or liquid) enters venous circulation and forms a blockage in the pulmonary vasculature. Emboli originating from deep-vein thrombosis (DVT) are the most common cause. Tumors, bone marrow, amniotic fluid, and foreign matter can also become emboli.

NURSING CARE
- Administer oxygen therapy as prescribed to relieve hypoxemia and dyspnea.
- Position the client to maximize ventilation (high-Fowler's = 90%).
- Initiate and maintain IV access.
- Administer medications as prescribed.
- Provide emotional support and comfort to control client anxiety.
- Monitor changes in level of consciousness and mental status.

MEDICATIONS
- Anticoagulants: enoxaparin, heparin, and warfarin
- Thrombolytic therapy: alteplase, reteplase, and tenecteplase

(N) *NCLEX® Connection: Physiological Adaptation, Unexpected Response to Therapies*

UNIT 3 NURSING CARE OF CLIENTS WHO
HAVE RESPIRATORY DISORDERS
SECTION: RESPIRATORY EMERGENCIES

CHAPTER 25
Pneumothorax, Hemothorax, and Flail Chest

A **pneumothorax** is the presence of air or gas in the pleural space that causes lung collapse.

A tension pneumothorax occurs when air enters the pleural space during inspiration through a one-way valve and is not able to exit upon expiration. The trapped air causes pressure on the heart and the lung. As a result, the increase in pressure compresses blood vessels and limits venous return, leading to a decrease in cardiac output. Death can result if not treated immediately. As a result of a tension pneumothorax, air and pressure continue to rise in the pleural cavity, which causes a mediastinal shift.

A **hemothorax** is an accumulation of blood in the pleural space.

A spontaneous pneumothorax can occur when there has been no trauma. A small bleb on the lung ruptures and air enters the pleural space.

A **flail chest** occurs when at least two neighboring ribs, usually on one side of the chest, sustain multiple fractures causing instability of the chest wall and paradoxical chest wall movement. This results in significant limitation in chest wall expansion.

Pneumothorax and hemothorax

ASSESSMENT

RISK FACTORS

- Blunt chest trauma
- Penetrating chest wounds
- Closed/occluded chest tube
- Older adult clients have decreased pulmonary reserves due to normal lung changes, including decreased lung elasticity and thickening alveoli. ⓒ
- Chronic obstructive pulmonary disease (COPD)

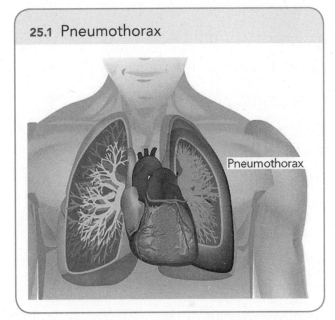

25.1 Pneumothorax

Pneumothorax

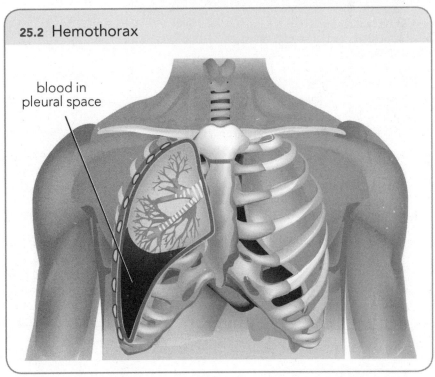

25.2 Hemothorax

blood in pleural space

EXPECTED FINDINGS

- Anxiety
- Pleuritic pain

PHYSICAL ASSESSMENT FINDINGS

- Signs of respiratory distress (tachypnea, tachycardia, hypoxia, cyanosis, dyspnea, and use of accessory muscles)
- Tracheal deviation to the unaffected side (tension pneumothorax)
- Reduced or absent breath sounds on the affected side
- Asymmetrical chest wall movement
- Hyperresonance on percussion due to trapped air (pneumothorax)
- Dull percussion (hemothorax)
- Subcutaneous emphysema (air accumulating in subcutaneous tissue)

LABORATORY TESTS

ABGs: Hypoxemia (PaO_2 less than 80 mm Hg)

DIAGNOSTIC PROCEDURES

Chest x-ray

Used to confirm pneumothorax or hemothorax

Thoracentesis

Thoracentesis can be used to confirm hemothorax. Thoracentesis is the surgical perforation of the chest wall and pleural space with a large-bore needle.

NURSING ACTIONS

- Ensure that informed consent has been obtained.
- Make sure the client understands the importance of remaining still during the procedure (no moving, coughing, or deep breathing).
- Assist with client positioning and specimen transport.
- Monitor status (vital signs, SaO_2, injection site).
- Assist the client to the edge of the bed and to lean over a bedside table.
- Inform the client he will feel discomfort when the local anesthetic solution is injected. When the needle is inserted into the lung, some pressure can be felt, but no pain.

PATIENT-CENTERED CARE

NURSING CARE

- Administer oxygen therapy.
- Auscultate heart and lung sounds and monitor vital signs every 4 hr.
- Document ventilator settings hourly if the client is receiving ventilation.
- Check ABGs, SaO_2, CBC, and chest x-ray results.
- Position the client to maximize ventilation (high-Fowler's = 90°).
- Provide emotional support to the client and family.
- Monitor chest tube drainage. Q EBP
- Administer medications as prescribed.
- Encourage prompt medical attention when evidence of infection occurs.
- Instruct the client to deep breathe to promote lung expansion.

MEDICATIONS

Benzodiazepines (sedatives)

Lorazepam or midazolam can be used to decrease anxiety.

NURSING CONSIDERATIONS

- Monitor vital signs. (Benzodiazepines can cause hypotension and respiratory distress.)
- The medications have amnesiac effect.
- Monitor for paradoxical effects (euphoria, rage).

CLIENT EDUCATION: Remind the client that medications have amnesic effects and cause drowsiness.

Opioid agonists (pain medications)

- Morphine sulfate and fentanyl are opioid agents used to treat moderate to severe pain. These medications act on the mu and kappa receptors that help alleviate pain.
- Activation of these receptors produces analgesia (pain relief), respiratory depression, euphoria, sedation, and decrease in gastrointestinal motility.

NURSING CONSIDERATIONS

- Use cautiously for clients who have asthma or emphysema, due to the risk of respiratory depression.
- Assess pain every 4 hr.
- Remind clients who are receiving a fentanyl patch that the initial patch takes several hours to take effect. A short-acting pain medication is administered for breakthrough pain.
- Monitor clients, especially older adults, for manifestations of respiratory depression. If respirations are 12/min or less, stop the medication and notify provider immediately.
- Monitor vital signs for hypotension and bradypnea.
- Assess for nausea and vomiting.
- Assess level of sedation (drowsiness, level of consciousness).
- Monitor for constipation.
- Encourage fluid intake and activity related to a decrease in gastric motility.
- Monitor intake and output and fluid retention (common in clients who have an enlarged prostate).

- Encourage clients who do not have fluid restrictions due to other conditions to drink plenty of fluids to prevent constipation.
- Teach the client how to use a patient-controlled analgesia (PCA) pump if applicable. The client is the only person who should push the medication administration button. Reassure the client that the safety lockout mechanism on the PCA prevents overdosing of medication.
- If the client is receiving ventilation, the nursing considerations and client education can vary.

INTERPROFESSIONAL CARE

Respiratory services should be consulted for ABGs, breathing treatments, and suctioning for airway management.

Pulmonary services may be consulted for chest tube management and pulmonary care.

Pain management services may be consulted if pain persists or is uncontrolled.

Rehabilitation care may be consulted if the client has prolonged weakness and needs assistance with an increasing level of activity.

THERAPEUTIC PROCEDURES

Chest tube insertion

Chest tubes are inserted in the pleural space to drain fluid, blood, or air; re-establish a negative pressure; facilitate lung expansion; and restore normal intrapleural pressure.

NURSING ACTIONS

- Obtain informed consent, gather supplies, monitor the client's status (vital signs, SaO_2, chest tube drainage), report abnormalities to the provider, and administer pain medications.
- Continually monitor vital signs and the client's response to the procedure.
- Monitor chest tube placement, function, and dressing.

CLIENT EDUCATION

- Set up referral services (home health, respiratory services) to provide portable oxygen if needed. **Qтc**
- Encourage the client to take rest periods as needed.
- Remind the client to use proper hand hygiene to prevent infection.
- Encourage immunizations for influenza and pneumonia.
- Remind the client that recovery from a pneumothorax/hemothorax can be lengthy.
- Educate the client and family about the illness, and encourage them to express their feelings.
- Encourage smoking cessation if the client smokes.
- Stress the importance of follow-up care, and instruct the client to report the following to the provider.
  - Upper respiratory infection
  - Fever
  - Cough
  - Difficulty breathing
  - Sharp chest pain

COMPLICATIONS

Decreased cardiac output

- The amount of blood pumped by the heart decreases as intrathoracic pressure rises.
- Hypotension develops.

NURSING ACTIONS

- Administer IV fluids and blood products as prescribed.
- Monitor heart rate and rhythm.
- Monitor intake and output (chest tube drainage).

Respiratory failure

Inadequate gas exchange due to lung collapse

NURSING ACTIONS

- Prepare for mechanical ventilation.
- Continue respiratory assessment.

Flail chest

Flail chest is the inability of the injured side of the chest to expand adequately upon inhalation and contract upon exhalation. One side of the chest is typically affected due to multiple rib fractures.

ASSESSMENT

RISK FACTORS

Multiple rib fractures from blunt chest trauma (often caused by motor-vehicle crash or as a result of cardiopulmonary resuscitation on older adults)

EXPECTED FINDINGS

- Unequal chest expansion (the unaffected side of the chest will expand, while the affected side can appear to diminish in size or remain stationary)
- Paradoxical chest wall movement (inward movement of segment during inspiration, outward movement of segment during expiration)
- Tachycardia
- Hypotension
- Dyspnea
- Cyanosis
- Anxiety
- Chest pain

PATIENT-CENTERED CARE

NURSING CARE

- Administer humidified oxygen.
- Monitor vital signs and SaO_2.
- Review findings of pulmonary function tests, periodic chest x-rays, and ABGs.
- Assess lung sounds, color, and capillary refill.
- Promote lung expansion by encouraging deep breathing and proper positioning.
- Maintain mechanical ventilation in the event of severe injury to establish adequate gas exchange and stabilize the injury. (Flail chest is usually stabilized by positive-pressure ventilation).
- Suction trachea and endotracheal tube as needed.
- Administer pain medication. Patient-controlled analgesia or an epidural block commonly is used.
- Administer IV fluids as prescribed.
- Monitor intake and output.
- Offer support and reassurance by explaining all procedures.

1. A nurse is assessing a client following a gunshot wound to the chest. For which of the following findings should the nurse monitor to detect a pneumothorax? (Select all that apply.)

   A. Tachypnea

   B. Deviation of the trachea

   C. Bradycardia

   D. Decreased use of accessory muscles

   E. Pleuritic pain

2. A nurse is reviewing the prescriptions for a client who has a pneumothorax. Which of the following actions should the nurse perform first?

   A. Assess the client's pain.

   B. Obtain a large-bore IV needle for decompression.

   C. Administer lorazepam.

   D. Prepare for chest tube insertion.

3. A nurse is reviewing discharge instructions for a client who experienced a pneumothorax. Which of the following statements should the nurse use when teaching the client?

   A. "Notify your provider if you experience weakness."

   B. "You should be able to return to work in 1 week."

   C. "You need to wear a mask when in crowded areas."

   D. "Notify your provider if you experience a productive cough."

4. A nurse in the emergency department is assessing a client who has a suspected flail chest. Which of the following findings should the nurse expect? (Select all that apply.)

   A. Bradycardia

   B. Cyanosis

   C. Hypotension

   D. Dyspnea

   E. Paradoxic chest movement

PRACTICE Active Learning Scenario

A nurse is teaching a newly licensed nurse regarding care for a client who has a hemothorax. What should be included in this review? Use the ATI Active Learning Template: System Disorder to complete this item.

DESCRIPTION OF DISORDER/DISEASE PROCESS

NURSING CARE: Describe three nursing interventions.

MEDICATIONS: Describe two medications used for hemothorax

Application Exercises Key

1. A. **CORRECT:** The client who has a pneumothorax can experience tachypnea related to respiratory distress caused by the injury.

   B. **CORRECT:** The client who has a pneumothorax can experience deviation of the trachea as tension increases within the chest.

   C. The client who has a pneumothorax can experience tachycardia related to respiratory distress and pain.

   D. The client who has a pneumothorax can experience an increase in the use of accessory muscles as respiratory distress occurs.

   E. **CORRECT:** The client who has a pneumothorax can experience pleuritic pain related to the inflammation of the pleura of the lung caused by the injury.

   Ⓝ NCLEX® *Connection: Physiological Adaptation, Medical Emergencies*

2. A. The nurse should assess the client's pain and administer pain medication. However, another action is the priority.

   B. **CORRECT:** The priority action the nurse should take when using the airway, breathing, circulation (ABC) approach to client care is to establish and maintain the client's respiratory function. Obtaining a large-bore IV needle for decompression is the priority action by the nurse.

   C. The nurse can administer benzodiazepine to treat anxiety. However, another action is the priority.

   D. The nurse should gather supplies to prepare for chest tube insertion. However, another action is the priority.

   Ⓝ NCLEX® *Connection: Physiological Adaptation, Pathophysiology*

3. A. Weakness is an expected finding following recovery from a pneumothorax.

   B. The client should expect a lengthy recovery following a pneumothorax.

   C. The client should wear a mask if immunosuppressed.

   D. **CORRECT:** The client should notify the provider of a productive or persistent cough. This can indicate that the client might need treatment of a respiratory infection.

   Ⓝ NCLEX® *Connection: Reduction of Risk Potential, Therapeutic Procedures*

4. A. The client will have tachycardia as a manifestation indicative of flail chest due to inadequate oxygenation.

   B. **CORRECT:** The client can have cyanosis as a manifestation indicative of flail chest due to inadequate oxygenation.

   C. **CORRECT:** The client can have hypotension as a manifestation indicative of flail chest.

   D. **CORRECT:** The client can have dyspnea as a manifestation indicative of flail chest. This is due to injury and the client's inability to effectively inhale and exhale.

   E. **CORRECT:** The client can have paradoxic chest movement as a manifestation indicative of flail chest. This is due to injury to the chest and the inability to inhale and exhale.

   Ⓝ NCLEX® *Connection: Physiological Adaptation, Pathophysiology*

PRACTICE Answer

Using the ATI Active Learning Template: System Disorder

ALTERATION IN HEALTH (DIAGNOSIS): Hemothorax is an accumulation of blood in the pleural space

NURSING CARE
- Administer oxygen therapy.
- Document ventilator settings hourly if the client is receiving ventilation.
- Monitor ABGs, SaO$_2$, CBC, and chest x-ray findings.
- Position the client to maximize ventilation (high-Fowler's = 90°).
- Provide emotional support to the client and family.

- Monitor chest tube drainage.
- Administer medications as prescribed.
- Encourage prompt medical attention when manifestations of infection occur.
- Auscultate heart and lung sounds and monitor vital signs every 4 hr.

MEDICATIONS
- Benzodiazepines (sedatives): Lorazepam or midazolam can be used to decrease anxiety.
- Opioid agonists (pain medications): Morphine sulfate and fentanyl are opioid agents used to treat moderate to severe pain. These medications act on the mu and kappa receptors that help alleviate pain.

Ⓝ NCLEX® *Connection: Physiological Adaptation, Medical Emergencies*

CHAPTER 26 *Respiratory Failure*

Respiratory failure includes acute respiratory failure (ARF), acute respiratory distress syndrome (ARDS), and severe acute respiratory syndrome (SARS). Because older adult clients have decreased pulmonary reserves due to normal lung changes, including decreased lung elasticity and thickening alveoli they can decompensate more quickly. Ⓒ

Acute respiratory failure

ARF is caused by failure to adequately ventilate and/or oxygenate.

- Ventilatory failure is due to a mechanical abnormality of the lungs or chest wall, impaired muscle function (especially the diaphragm), or a malfunction in the respiratory control center of the brain.
- Oxygenation failure can result from a lack of perfusion to the pulmonary capillary bed (pulmonary embolism) or a condition that alters the gas exchange medium (pulmonary edema, pneumonia).
- Both inadequate ventilation and oxygenation can occur in clients who have diseased lungs (asthma, emphysema, or cystic fibrosis). Diseased lung tissue can cause oxygenation failure and increased work of breathing, eventually resulting in respiratory muscle fatigue and ventilatory failure. Combined failure leads to more profound hypoxemia than either ventilatory failure or oxygenation failure alone.
- Criteria for acute respiratory failure are based on ABG values.

Acute respiratory distress syndrome

ARDS is a state of acute respiratory failure with a mortality rate of about 60%.

- A systemic inflammatory response injures the alveolar-capillary membrane. It becomes permeable to large molecules, and the lung space is filled with fluid.
- A reduction in surfactant weakens the alveoli, which causes collapse or filling of fluid, leading to worsening edema.

Severe acute respiratory syndrome

SARS is the result of a viral infection from a mutated strain of the coronaviruses, a group of viruses that also cause the common cold.

- The virus invades the pulmonary tissue, which leads to an inflammatory response.
- The virus is spread easily through airborne droplets from sneezing, coughing, or talking.
- The virus does not spread to the bloodstream because it flourishes at temperatures slightly below normal core body temperature.

ASSESSMENT

RISK FACTORS

Acute respiratory failure

Ventilatory failure
- COPD
- Pulmonary embolism
- Pneumothorax
- Flail chest
- ARDS
- Asthma Ⓠ EBP
- Pulmonary edema
- Fibrosis of lung tissue
- Neuromuscular disorders (multiple sclerosis, Guillain-Barré syndrome), spinal cord injuries, and cerebrovascular accidents that impair the client's rate and depth of respiration
- Elevated intracranial pressure (closed-head injuries, cerebral edema, hemorrhagic stroke)

Oxygenation failure
- Pneumonia
- Hypoventilation
- Hypovolemic shock
- Pulmonary edema
- Pulmonary embolism
- ARDS
- Low hemoglobin
- Low concentrations of oxygen (carbon monoxide poisoning, high altitude, smoke inhalation)

Combined ventilatory and oxygenation failure
- Decreased gas exchange results in poor diffusion of oxygen into arterial blood with carbon dioxide retention
- Hypoventilation (poor respiratory movement)
- Chronic bronchitis
- Asthma attack
- Emphysema

Cardiac failure

Acute respiratory distress syndrome

- Can result from localized lung damage or from the effects of other systemic problems
- Aspiration
- Pulmonary emboli (fat, amniotic fluid)
- Pneumonia and other pulmonary infections
- Sepsis
- Near-drowning accident
- Trauma
- Transfusion
- Damage to the central nervous system
- Smoke or toxic gas inhalation
- Drug ingestion/overdose (heroin, opioids, salicylates)

Severe acute respiratory syndrome

- Exposure to an infected individual
- Immunocompromised individuals (chemotherapy, AIDS)

EXPECTED FINDINGS

- Shortness of breath
- Dyspnea with or without exertion
- Orthopnea (difficulty breathing lying flat)
- Rapid, shallow breathing
- Cyanotic, mottled, dusky skin Qpcc
- Tachycardia
- Hypotension
- Substernal or suprasternal retractions
- Decreased SaO_2 (less than 90%)
- Adventitious breath sounds (wheezing, rales)
- Cardiac arrhythmias
- Confusion
- Lethargy

Acute respiratory failure

- Dyspnea
- Orthopnea
- Cyanosis
- Pallor
- Hypoxemia
- Tachycardia
- Confusion
- Irritability or agitation
- Restlessness
- Hypercarbia (high levels of carbon dioxide in the blood)

Acute respiratory distress syndrome

- Dyspnea
- Bilateral noncardiogenic pulmonary edema
- Reduced lung compliance
- Dense patchy bilateral pulmonary infiltrates
- Severe hypoxemia despite administration of 100% oxygen

LABORATORY TESTS

ABGs to confirm and monitor ARF, ARDS, and SARS
- PaO_2 less 60 mm Hg and oxygen saturation less than 90% on room air (hypoxemia)
- $PaCO_2$ greater than 45 mm Hg and pH less than 7.35 (hypoxemia, hypercarbia)

Acute respiratory failure

ABGs to confirm and monitor combined ventilatory and oxygenation failure
- Room air, PaO_2 less than 60 mm Hg (hypoxemic/oxygenation failure), OR $PaCO_2$ greater than 45 mm Hg in conjunction with a pH less than 7.35 (hypercapnic/ventilatory failure)
- AND SaO_2 less than 90% in both cases

DIAGNOSTIC PROCEDURES

Chest x-ray QEBP

Results can include:
- Pulmonary edema (ARF, ARDS)
- Cardiomegaly (ARF)
- Diffuse infiltrates and white-out or ground-glass appearance (ARDS)
- Infiltrates (SARS)

NURSING ACTIONS
- Assist with client positioning before and after the x-ray.
- Interpret and communicate the results to the appropriate personnel in a timely manner.

Electrocardiogram (ECG)

To rule out cardiac involvement.

Hemodynamic monitoring

Pulmonary capillary wedge pressure with ARDS is usually low or within the expected reference range (4 to 12 mm Hg). Continuous hemodynamic monitoring is important for fluid management.

NURSING ACTIONS
- Monitor the ECG during placement of central venous pressure catheter and hemodynamic monitor.
- Have resuscitation medications and equipment available. Qpcc
- Monitor hemodynamic waveforms and readings.
- Confirm catheter placement using a chest x-ray.

PATIENT-CENTERED CARE

NURSING CARE

- Maintain a patent airway and monitor respiratory status every hour and more often as needed.
- Mechanical ventilation is often required with positive-end expiratory pressure (PEEP) or continuous positive airway pressure (CPAP) to prevent alveolar collapse during expiration. Follow facility protocol for monitoring and documenting ventilator settings.
- Oxygenate before suctioning secretions to prevent further hypoxemia.
- Suction the client as needed.
- Assess and document sputum color, amount, and consistency.
- Assess lung sounds per facility protocol.
- Monitor for pneumothorax (a high PEEP can cause the lungs to collapse).
- Obtain ABGs as prescribed and following each ventilator setting adjustment.
- Maintain continuous ECG monitoring for changes that can indicate increased hypoxemia, especially when repositioning and applying suction.
- Continually monitor vital signs, including SaO_2. Assess pain level.

- Position the client to facilitate ventilation and perfusion.
- Prevent infection.
  - Perform frequent hand hygiene.
  - Use appropriate suctioning technique.
  - Provide oral care every 2 hr and as needed.
  - Wear protective clothing (gown, gloves, mask) when appropriate.
- Promote nutrition.
  - Assess bowel sounds.
  - Monitor elimination patterns.
  - Obtain daily weights. Qs
  - Monitor intake and output.
  - Administer enteral and/or parenteral feedings as prescribed.
  - Prevent aspiration with enteral feedings (elevate the head of the bed 30° to 45°).
  - Confirm nasogastric (NG) tube placement prior to feeding.
- Provide emotional support to the client and family.
  - Encourage verbalization of feelings.
  - Provide alternative communication means (dry erase board, pen and paper).

MEDICATIONS

Benzodiazepines

EXAMPLES
- Lorazepam
- Midazolam

ACTIONS: Reduces anxiety and resistance to ventilation and decreases oxygen consumption

NURSING CONSIDERATIONS
- Monitor respirations on clients who are not ventilated.
- Monitor blood pressure and SaO_2.
- Use cautiously in conjunction with opioid narcotics.

General anesthesia

EXAMPLES: Propofol

ACTIONS
- Induces and maintains anesthesia
- Sedates clients who are to be placed on mechanical ventilation

NURSING CONSIDERATIONS
- Contraindicated for clients who have hyperlipidemia and egg allergies.
- Administer only to clients who are intubated and ventilated.
- Monitor ECG, blood pressure, and sedation levels.
- IV rate must be slowed to assess neurological status. (Follow facility protocol.)
- Monitor for hypotension.
- Titrate to desired sedation.
- No analgesic actions. Monitor pain, and administer analgesics as prescribed

Corticosteroids

EXAMPLES
- Cortisone acetate
- Methylprednisolone sodium succinate
- Dexamethasone sodium phosphate

ACTIONS: Reduces WBC migration, decreases inflammation, and helps stabilize the alveolar–capillary membrane during ARDS

NURSING CONSIDERATIONS
- Discontinue medication gradually.
- Administer with an antiulcer medication to prevent peptic ulcer formation.
- Monitor weight and blood pressure.
- Monitor glucose and electrolytes.
- Advise the client to take oral doses with food and avoid stopping the medication suddenly.

Opioid analgesics

EXAMPLES
- Morphine sulfate
- Fentanyl

ACTIONS: Provides pain management

NURSING CONSIDERATIONS
- Monitor respirations for clients who are not ventilated.
- Monitor blood pressure, heart rate, and SaO_2.
- Monitor ABGs. (Hypercapnia can result from depressed respirations.)
- Use cautiously in conjunction with hypnotic sedatives.
- Assess pain level and response to medication.
- Have naloxone and resuscitation equipment available for severe respiratory depression in clients who are not receiving ventilation.

Neuromuscular blocking agents

EXAMPLES: Vecuronium

ACTIONS
- Facilitates ventilation and decreases oxygen consumption
- Often used with painful ventilatory modes (inverse ratio ventilation and PEEP)

NURSING CONSIDERATIONS
- Administer only to clients who are intubated and ventilated.
- Monitor ECG, blood pressure, and muscle strength.
- Give pain medication and sedatives with neuromuscular blocking agents.
- Neuromuscular blocking agents do not sedate or relieve pain. (Clients can be awake and frightened.)
- Have neostigmine and atropine available to reverse the effects of the neuromuscular blocking agent.
- Have resuscitation equipment available.
- Reassure the client that paralysis is medication induced.
- Explain all procedures.

Antibiotics sensitive to cultured organism(s)

EXAMPLES: Vancomycin

ACTIONS: Treats identified organisms

NURSING CONSIDERATIONS
- Culture sputum prior to administration of first dose.
- Monitor for a hypersensitivity reaction.
- Give IV doses slowly (over at least 60 min) to avoid red man syndrome.
- Monitor the IV site for infiltration.
- Do not give with other medications.
- Monitor coagulopathy and renal function.
- Advise client to take oral doses with food and finish the prescribed dose.

INTERPROFESSIONAL CARE

Respiratory therapy
- The respiratory therapist typically manages the ventilator, adjusts the settings, and provides chest physiotherapy to improve ventilation and chest expansion.
- The respiratory therapist also can suction the endotracheal tube and administer inhalation medications, such as bronchodilators.

Physical therapy for extended ventilatory support and rehabilitation

Nutritional therapy
- Enteral or parenteral feeding
- Nutritional support following extubation

THERAPEUTIC PROCEDURES

Intubation and mechanical ventilation

Artificial airway insertion with mechanical ventilation

NURSING ACTIONS
- Monitor ECG, SaO_2, lung sounds, and color.
- Sedate as needed.
- Provide reassurance to calm the client.
- Have suction equipment, manual resuscitation bag, and face mask available at all times.
- Suction secretions as needed.
- PREINTUBATION
  - Oxygenate with 100% oxygen.
  - Assist ventilation with manual resuscitation bag and face mask.
  - Have emergency resuscitation equipment readily available.
- POSTINTUBATION
  - Assess end-tidal carbon dioxide levels, bilateral lung sounds, symmetrical chest movement, and chest x-ray findings to confirm placement of the endotracheal tube. Qpcc
  - Secure the endotracheal tube per facility guidelines.
  - Assess the balloon cuff for air leaks periodically.
- PEEP
  - Positive pressure is applied at the end of expiration to keep the alveoli expanded.
  - PEEP is added to the ventilator setting to increase oxygenation and improve lung expansion.

CLIENT EDUCATION
- Explain all procedures to the client.
- Reassure and calm the client.
- Explain to the client and family that the client will be unable to speak while the endotracheal tube is in place.

Kinetic therapy

A kinetic bed that rotates laterally alters client positioning to reduce atelectasis and improve ventilation.

NURSING ACTIONS
- Begin slowly and gradually to increase the degree of rotation as tolerated.
- Monitor ECG, SaO_2, breath sounds, and blood pressure.
- Stop rotation if the client becomes distressed.
- Provide routine skin care to prevent breakdown.
- Sedate as needed.

CLIENT EDUCATION: Explain all procedures to the client.

COMPLICATIONS

ENDOTRACHEAL TUBE

Trauma

Trauma during intubation or long-term intubation can cause damage to trachea and vocal cords.

NURSING ACTIONS: Consider a tracheostomy for long-term ventilation.

Altered position of endotracheal tube

NURSING ACTIONS
- Check tube positioning every 1 to 2 hr and as needed.
- Assess lung sounds, SaO_2, and chest movement. Assess lung sounds each time the client is moved, transferred, or turned.
- Secure endotracheal tube per facility guidelines to maintain tube placement.

Aspiration pneumonia

NURSING ACTIONS
- Check the cuff on the endotracheal tube for leaks.
- Assess suction contents for gastric secretions.
- Verify NG tube placement.

Infection

NURSING ACTIONS
- Prevent infection by using proper hand hygiene and suctioning technique.
- Assess color, amount, and consistency of secretions.

Blocked endotracheal tube

Indicated by high-pressure alarm on ventilator

NURSING ACTIONS: Suction secretions to relieve a mucous plug or insert an oral airway to prevent biting on the tube.

MECHANICAL VENTILATION

Increased intrathoracic pressure

- PEEP increases intrathoracic pressure, which can cause a decreased blood return to the heart, decreased cardiac output, and/or hypotension.
- Decreased cardiac output can activate the renin-angiotensin-aldosterone system, leading to fluid retention and/or decreased urine output.

NURSING ACTIONS: Monitor input and output, weight, and hydration status.

CLIENT EDUCATION: Advise the client to avoid using the Valsalva maneuver (straining with bowel movement), because it can further increase intrathoracic pressure.

Barotrauma

Ventilation with positive pressure causes damage to the lungs (pneumothorax, subcutaneous emphysema).

NURSING ACTIONS
- Monitor oxygenation status and chest x-ray.
- Assess for subcutaneous emphysema (crackles and/or air movement felt under skin).
- Document all ventilator changes made.
- A high-pressure ventilator alarm can indicate pneumothorax.

Immobilization

Can result in muscle atrophy, pneumonia, and pressure sores

NURSING ACTIONS
- Reposition and suction every 2 hr and as needed.
- Provide routine skin care.
- Implement range-of-motion exercises to prevent muscle atrophy.

PRACTICE Active Learning Scenario

A nurse is reviewing the plan of care for a client who has acute respiratory distress syndrome (ARDS). What should be included in the plan of care? Use the ATI Active Learning Template: System Disorder to complete this item.

RISK FACTORS: Describe three conditions related to ARDS.

NURSING CARE: Describe three nursing actions to maintain oxygenation.

COMPLICATIONS: Identify two complications of ARDS.

Application Exercises

1. A nurse in the emergency department is assessing a client who was in a motor vehicle crash. Findings include absent breath sounds in the left lower lobe with dyspnea, blood pressure 118/68 mm Hg, heart rate 124/min, respirations 38/min, temperature 38.6° C (101.4° F), and SaO₂ 92% on room air. Which of the following actions should the nurse take first?

    A. Obtain a chest x-ray.
    B. Prepare for chest tube insertion.
    C. Administer oxygen via a high-flow mask.
    D. Initiate IV access.

2. A nurse is orienting a newly licensed nurse on the purpose of administering vecuronium to a client who has acute respiratory distress syndrome (ARDS). Which of the following statements by the newly licensed nurse indicates understanding of the teaching?

    A. "This medication is given to treat infection."
    B. "This medication is given to facilitate ventilation."
    C. "This medication is given to decrease inflammation."
    D. "This medication is given to reduce anxiety."

3. A nurse is reviewing the health records of five clients. Which of the following clients are at risk for developing acute respiratory distress syndrome? (Select all that apply.)

    A. A client who experienced a near-drowning incident
    B. A client following coronary artery bypass graft surgery
    C. A client who has a hemoglobin of 15.1 mg/dL
    D. A client who has dysphagia
    E. A client who experienced a drug overdose

4. A nurse is planning care for a client who has severe acute respiratory distress system (SARS). Which of the following actions should be included in the plan of care for this client? (Select all that apply.)

    A. Administer antibiotics.
    B. Provide supplemental oxygen.
    C. Administer antiviral medications.
    D. Administer of bronchodilators.
    E. Maintain ventilatory support.

5. A nurse is caring for a client who is receiving vecuronium for acute respiratory distress syndrome. Which of the following medications should the nurse anticipate administering with this medication? (Select all that apply.)

    A. Fentanyl
    B. Furosemide
    C. Midazolam
    D. Famotidine
    E. Dexamethasone

Application Exercises Key

1. A. Obtaining a chest x-ray to determine the level of injury to the lungs is important, but is not the priority action at this time.

   B. Preparing the client for chest tube insertion is important to facilitate lung expansion and restore normal intrapleural pressure, but is not the priority action at this time.

   C. **CORRECT:** According to the airway, breathing, and circulation to client care, the nurse should place the priority on administering oxygen via high-flow mask to provide the client oxygen to restore optimal breathing.

   D. Initiating IV access to administer medications is important, but is not the priority action at this time.

   Ⓝ *NCLEX® Connection: Physiological Adaptation, Illness Management*

2. A. Antibiotics are given to treat infection.

   B. **CORRECT:** Vecuronium is a neuromuscular blocking agent given to facilitate ventilation and decrease oxygen consumption.

   C. Corticosteroids are given to treat inflammation.

   D. Benzodiazepines are given to treat anxiety.

   Ⓝ *NCLEX® Connection: Pharmacological and Parenteral Therapies, Expected Actions/Outcomes*

3. A. **CORRECT:** A client who experienced a near-drowning incident is at risk for developing ARDS due to trauma to the lungs and cerebral edema.

   B. **CORRECT:** A client following coronary artery bypass graft surgery is at risk for developing ARDS due to trauma to the chest.

   C. Hemoglobin of 15.1 mg/dL is within the expected reference range. A client who has a low hemoglobin is at risk for developing ARDS.

   D. **CORRECT:** A client who has dysphagia is at risk for developing ARDS due to difficulty swallowing and risk for aspiration.

   E. **CORRECT:** A client who experienced a drug overdose is at risk for developing ARDS due to damage to the central nervous system.

   Ⓝ *NCLEX® Connection: Physiological Adaptation, Alterations in Body Systems*

4. A. Antibiotics are given to treat bacterial infections. This would not be indicated for SARS.

   B. **CORRECT:** Providing supplemental oxygen should be included in the plan of care for SARS. Oxygen is administered given to treat severe hypoxemia.

   C. SARS is caused by the coronavirus. There are no effective antiviral medications to treat this virus.

   D. **CORRECT:** Administration of bronchodilators should be included in the plan of care for SARS. Bronchodilators are used to vasodilate the client's airway.

   E. **CORRECT:** Maintaining ventilatory support should be included in the plan of care for SARS. Intubation can be required to maintain a patent airway.

   Ⓝ *NCLEX® Connection: Physiological Adaptation, Illness Management*

5. A. **CORRECT:** Fentanyl is a pain medication used to treat clients who have ARDS when a neuromuscular blocking agent such as vecuronium is administered.

   B. Furosemide is a diuretic used to release fluid from the body.

   C. **CORRECT:** Midazolam is a sedative medication used to treat clients who have ARDS when a neuromuscular blocking agent such as vecuronium is administered.

   D. Famotidine is an H_2 receptor antagonist given to treat upset stomach and heartburn.

   E. Dexamethasone is a corticosteroid used to treat inflammation such as arthritis or an immune disorder.

   Ⓝ *NCLEX® Connection: Pharmacological and Parenteral Therapies, Medication Administration*

PRACTICE Answer

Using the ATI Active Learning Template: System Disorder

RISK FACTORS

- Can result from localized lung damage or from the effects of other systemic problems
- Aspiration
- Pulmonary emboli (fat, amniotic fluid)
- Pneumonia and other pulmonary infections
- Sepsis
- Near-drowning accident
- Trauma
- Damage to the central nervous system
- Smoke or toxic gas inhalation
- Drug ingestion/overdose (heroin, opioids, salicylates)

NURSING CARE

- Maintain a patent airway and monitor respiratory status every hour as needed.
- Suction the client as needed.
- Assess lung sounds.
- Assess and document sputum color, amount, and consistency.
- Oxygenate before suctioning secretions to prevent further hypoxemia.
- Mechanical ventilation often is required. PEEP often is used to prevent alveolar collapse during expiration.
- Monitor for pneumothorax. (A high PEEP can cause the lungs to collapse.)
- Obtain ABGs as prescribed and following each ventilator setting adjustment.
- Maintain continuous ECG monitoring for changes that can indicate increased hypoxemia, especially when repositioning and applying suction.
- Continually monitor vital signs, including SaO_2.
- Position the client to facilitate ventilation and perfusion.

COMPLICATIONS

- Endotracheal tube
  - Trauma during intubation or long-term intubation
  - Can cause damage to trachea and vocal cords
  - Nursing Actions: Consider a tracheostomy for long-term ventilation.
- Aspiration pneumonia nursing actions
  - Check the cuff on the endotracheal tube for leaks.
  - Assess suction contents for gastric secretions.
  - Verify NG tube placement.
- Infection nursing actions
  - Prevent infection by using proper hand hygiene and suctioning technique.
  - Assess color, amount, and consistency of secretions.
- Blocked endotracheal tube
  - The high-pressure alarm on the ventilator can indicate a blocked endotracheal tube.
  - Nursing Actions: Suction secretions to relieve a mucous plug or insert an oral airway to prevent biting on the tube.
- Altered position of endotracheal tube nursing actions
  - Check tube positioning every 1 to 2 hr and as needed.
  - Assess breath sounds, SaO_2, and chest movement.
  - Secure endotracheal tube per institution's guidelines to maintain tube placement.
- Mechanical ventilation
  - Increased intrathoracic pressure
  - PEEP increases intrathoracic pressure, which can cause a decreased blood return to the heart, decreased cardiac output and/or hypotension.
  - Decreased cardiac output can activate the renin-angiotensin-aldosterone system, leading to fluid retention and/or decreased urine output.
  - Nursing Actions: Monitor input and output, weight, and hydration status.
  - Client Education: Advise the client to avoid using the Valsalva maneuver (straining with bowel movement), because it can further increase intrathoracic pressure.
- Barotrauma: Ventilation with positive pressure causes damage to the lungs (pneumothorax, subcutaneous emphysema).

Ⓝ *NCLEX® Connection: Physiological Adaptation, Alterations in Body Systems*

When reviewing the following chapters, keep in mind the relevant topics and tasks of the NCLEX outline, in particular:

Client Needs: Pharmacological and Parenteral Therapies

ADVERSE EFFECTS/CONTRAINDICATIONS/SIDE EFFECTS/ INTERACTIONS: Identify a contraindication to the administration of a medication to the client.

CENTRAL VENOUS ACCESS DEVICES: Provide care for the client with a central venous access device.

PARENTERAL/INTRAVENOUS THERAPY: Apply knowledge and concepts of mathematics/nursing procedures/psychomotor skills when caring for a client receiving intravenous and parenteral therapy.

Client Needs: Reduction of Risk Potential

CHANGES/ABNORMALITIES IN VITAL SIGNS: Evaluate invasive monitoring data.

DIAGNOSTIC TESTS: Apply knowledge of related nursing procedures and psychomotor skills when caring for clients undergoing diagnostic testing.

SYSTEM SPECIFIC ASSESSMENTS: Assess the client for abnormal peripheral pulses after a procedure or treatment.

Client Needs: Physiological Adaptation

ALTERATIONS IN BODY SYSTEMS: Assist with invasive procedures.

HEMODYNAMICS
Identify cardiac rhythm strip abnormalities.

Intervene to improve client cardiovascular status.

UNEXPECTED RESPONSES TO THERAPIES: Assess the client for unexpected adverse response to therapy.

CHAPTER 27 Cardiovascular Diagnostic and Therapeutic Procedures

Cardiovascular diagnostic procedures evaluate the functioning of the heart by monitoring for enzymes in the blood; using ultrasound to visualize the heart; determining the heart's response to exercise; and using catheters to determine blood volume, perfusion, fluid status, how the heart is pumping, and degree of artery blockage.

Cardiovascular diagnostic procedures that nurses should be familiar with include cardiac enzymes and lipid profile, echocardiogram, stress testing, hemodynamic monitoring, angiography, and vascular access.

Cardiac enzymes and lipid profile

Cardiac enzymes are released into the bloodstream when the heart muscle suffers ischemia. A lipid profile provides information regarding cholesterol levels and is used for early detection of heart disease.

Cardiac enzymes are specific markers in diagnosing a myocardial infarction (MI).

INDICATIONS

- Angina
- MI
- Heart disease
- Hyperlipidemia

CONSIDERATIONS

PREPROCEDURE: Explain the purpose for the test to the client.

INTRAPROCEDURE: Obtain a blood specimen via venipuncture.

POSTPROCEDURE: Discuss lab findings with the provider who will determine the need for treatment.

INTERPRETATION OF FINDINGS

27.1 Cardiac enzymes

EXPECTED REFERENCE RANGE	ELEVATED LEVELS FIRST DETECTABLE FOLLOWING MYOCARDIAL INJURY	EXPECTED DURATION OF ELEVATED LEVELS
Creatine kinase MB isoenzyme more sensitive to myocardium		
0% of total CK (30 to 170 units/L)	3 to 6 hr	2 to 3 days
Troponin T		
Less than 0.1 ng/mL	2 to 3 hr	10 to 14 days
Troponin I		
Less than 0.03 ng/mL	2 to 3 hr	7 to 10 days
Myoglobin		
Less than 90 mcg/L	2 to 3 hr	24 hr

27.2 Cardiac tests

EXPECTED REFERENCE RANGE	PURPOSE
Cholesterol (total)	
Less than 200 mg/dL	Screening for heart disease
LDL	
Less than 130 mg/dL	"Bad" cholesterol Transports cholesterol to the body's cells from the liver
Triglycerides	
MALES: 40 to 160 mg/dL FEMALES: 35 to 135 mg/dL	Evaluates the client's risk for heart disease
HDL	
FEMALES: greater than 55 mg/dL MALES: greater than 45 mg/dL	"Good" cholesterol Protects coronary arteries from heart disease by transporting cholesterol from the body's cells to the liver

Echocardiogram

An echocardiogram is an ultrasound of the heart. It is used to diagnose valve disorders and cardiomyopathy.

INDICATIONS

- Cardiomyopathy
- Heart failure
- Angina
- MI

CONSIDERATIONS

PREPROCEDURE: Explain the reason for the test to the client. This is a noninvasive test and takes up to 1 hr.

INTRAPROCEDURE: Instruct the client to lie on left side and remain still.

POSTPROCEDURE: Provider reviews test results and a plan for follow-up care with the client.

Stress testing

The client exercises the cardiac muscle by walking on a treadmill. This provides information regarding the workload of the heart. The test is discontinued once the heart rate reaches a certain rate.

Clients can become too tired, or be disabled or physically challenged, and be unable to finish the test. The provider can prescribe the test to be done as a pharmacological (chemical) stress test.

INDICATIONS

- Angina
- Heart failure
- MI
- Dysrhythmia

CONSIDERATIONS

PREPROCEDURE

- Assist the provider in obtaining a signed informed consent form.
- Explain to the client that he will be walking on a treadmill, and comfortable athletic shoes and clothing are recommended.
  - If a pharmacological stress test is prescribed, a medication such as dipyridamole, adenosine, or dobutamine is given to stress the heart instead of walking on the treadmill.
- Instruct the client to fast 2 to 4 hr before the procedure according to facility policy and to avoid tobacco, alcohol, and caffeine before the test. Qs
- Instruct the client to get adequate rest the night before the procedure.

INTRAPROCEDURE

- Apply a 12-lead ECG to monitor heart rate during the test. Monitor for dysrhythmias throughout the procedure.
- Instruct the client to report any chest pain, shortness of breath, or dizziness during the procedure.

POSTPROCEDURE

- Monitor the client by 12-lead ECG.
- Check blood pressure frequently until the client is stable.
- The provider reviews findings with the client.

Hemodynamic monitoring

Hemodynamic monitoring involves special indwelling catheters, which provide information about blood volume and perfusion, fluid status, and how well the heart is pumping.
- Hemodynamic status is assessed with several parameters.
  - Central venous pressure (CVP)
  - Pulmonary artery pressure (PAP)
  - Pulmonary artery wedge pressure (PAWP)
  - Cardiac output (CO)
  - Intra-arterial blood pressure
- Mixed venous oxygen saturation (SvO_2) indicates the balance between oxygen supply and demand. It is measured by a pulmonary artery catheter with fiberoptics.
- A hemodynamic monitoring system is used to display a client's hemodynamic data.
  - Pressure transducer
  - Pressure tubing
  - Monitor
  - Pressure bag and flush device
- Arterial lines are placed in the radial (most common), brachial, or femoral artery.
  - Arterial lines provide continuous information about changes in blood pressure and permit the withdrawal of samples of arterial blood. Intra-arterial pressures can differ from cuff pressures.
  - The integrity of the arterial waveform should be assessed to verify the accuracy of blood pressure readings.
  - Monitor circulation in the limb with the arterial line (capillary refill, temperature, color).
  - Arterial lines are not used for IV fluid administration.

Pulmonary artery (PA) catheters

The PA catheter is inserted into a large vein (internal jugular, femoral, subclavian, brachial) and threaded through the right atria and ventricle into a branch of the PA.
- PA catheters have multiple lumens, ports, and components that allow for various hemodynamic measurements, blood sampling, and infusion of IV fluids.
  - Proximal lumen can be used to measure right atrial pressure (CVP), infuse IV fluids, and obtain venous blood samples.
  - Distal lumen can be used to measure PAPs (PA systolic, PA diastolic, mean PA pressure, and PA wedge pressure). This lumen is not used for IV fluid administration.
  - Balloon inflation port is intermittently used for PAWP measurements. When not in use, it should be left deflated and in the locked position.
  - Thermistor measures the temperature differences between the right atrium and the PA in order to determine CO.
  - Additional infusion ports can be available, depending on the brand.

INDICATIONS

- Serious or critical illness
- Heart failure
- Post coronary artery bypass graft (CABG) clients
- ARDS
- Acute kidney injury
- Burn injury
- Trauma injury

CONSIDERATIONS

PREPROCEDURE

Line insertion

NURSING ACTIONS

- Ensure the client's understanding of the procedure prior to obtaining signed informed consent form.
- Assemble the pressure monitoring system. Purge air from the system and maintain sterility of connections.
- Place the client in supine or Trendelenburg position.
- Administer sedation and pain medications as prescribed.
- Level transducer with phlebostatic axis (4th intercostal space, midaxillary line), which corresponds with the right atrium.
- Zero system with atmospheric pressure, because the hemodynamic pressure lines must be calibrated to read zero atmospheric pressure.
- Obtain initial readings as prescribed. Compare arterial blood pressure to noninvasive blood pressure (NIBP).
- Document the client's response.

INTRAPROCEDURE

Monitor for manifestations of altered hemodynamics.

27.3 Manifestations of altered hemodynamics

Preload			Afterload	
RIGHT HEART: CVP **LEFT HEART:** PAWP			**RIGHT HEART:** pulmonary vascular resistance **LEFT HEART:** systemic vascular resistance	
ELEVATED	**DECREASED**	**ELEVATED**	**DECREASED**
Crackles in lungs Jugular vein distention Hepatomegaly Peripheral edema Taut skin turgor	Poor skin turgor Dry mucous membranes	Cool extremities Weak peripheral pulses	Warm extremities Bounding peripheral pulses

POSTPROCEDURE

NURSING ACTIONS

- Obtain chest x-ray to confirm catheter placement. Q**EBP**
- Continually monitor respiratory and cardiac status (vital signs, heart rhythm, SaO₂).
  - Observe respiratory pattern and effort.
  - Compare noninvasive blood pressure (NIBP) to arterial blood pressure.
- Maintain line placement and integrity.
  - Observe and document waveforms. Report changes in waveforms to the provider, as this can indicate catheter migration or displacement.
  - Document catheter placement each shift and as needed (after movement for transport).
  - Monitor and secure connections between pressure tubing, transducers, and catheter ports.

- Obtain readings from hemodynamic catheter.
  - Place the client in supine position prior to recording hemodynamic values. Head of bed can be elevated 15° to 30°.
  - Level the transducer at the phlebostatic axis before readings and with all position changes.
  - Zero system to atmospheric pressure.
  - Compare hemodynamic findings to physical assessment.
  - Monitor trends in values obtained over time.

INTERPRETATION OF FINDINGS

27.4 Hemodynamic monitoring

27.4 Hemodynamic monitoring	EXPECTED REFERENCE RANGES
CVP	2 to 6 mm Hg
PULMONARY ARTERY SYSTOLIC	15 to 28 mm Hg
PULMONARY ARTERY DIASTOLIC	5 to 16 mm Hg
PAWP	6 to 15 mm Hg
CO	3 to 6 L/min
SVO₂	60% to 80%

The intravascular volume in older adult clients is often reduced. The nurse should anticipate lower hemodynamic values, particularly if dehydration is a complication. Ⓖ

COMPLICATIONS

Infection/Sepsis

Infection at insertion site can occur if aseptic technique is not used.

NURSING ACTIONS

- Change dressings per facility protocol and as needed.
- Use surgical aseptic technique with dressing changes (mask, sterile gloves, maintain sterile field).
- Monitor for evidence of infection (elevated WBC count or temperature).
- Perform thorough hand hygiene.
- Collect specimens (blood cultures, catheter tip cultures) and deliver to the laboratory.
- Administer antibiotic therapy as prescribed.
- Administer IV fluids for intravascular support.
- Administer vasopressors (dopamine) for vasodilation secondary to sepsis.

Embolism

Plaque or a clot can become dislodged during the procedure.

NURSING ACTIONS

- Use 0.9% sodium chloride for flushing system. (Heparin is not used, and heparin-coated catheters are no longer used due to the possibility of heparin-induced thrombocytopenia.) Q**EBP**
- Avoid introduction of air into flushing system to prevent air embolism.
- Recognize the risk of pneumothorax with insertion of the line.
- Recognize the risk of dysrhythmias with insertion/ movement of the line.

Angiography

A coronary angiogram, also called a cardiac catheterization, is an invasive diagnostic procedure used to evaluate the presence and degree of coronary artery blockage.

- Angiography is also done on the lower extremities to determine blood flow and areas of blockage.
- Angiography involves the insertion of a catheter into a femoral (sometimes a brachial) vessel and threading it into the right or left side of the heart. Coronary artery narrowings and/or occlusions are identified by the injection of contrast media under fluoroscopy.

INDICATIONS

- Unstable angina and ECG changes (T wave inversion, ST segment elevation, depression).
- Confirm and determine location and extent of heart disease.

CONSIDERATIONS

PREPROCEDURE

NURSING ACTIONS

- Maintain NPO status for at least 8 hr due to the risk for aspiration when lying flat for the procedure.
- Obtain vital signs, auscultate heart and lung sounds, and assess peripheral pulses.
- Ensure that the consent form is signed.
- Ensure that the client and family understand the procedure.
- Assess for iodine/shellfish allergy (contrast media).
- Assess renal function prior to introduction of contrast dye.
- Administer premedications as prescribed (methylprednisolone, diphenhydramine).

CLIENT EDUCATION: Instruct the client that he is awake and sedated during procedure. A local anesthetic is used. A small incision is made, often in the groin, to insert the catheter. The client can feel warmth and flushed when the dye is inserted. After the procedure, the client must keep the affected leg straight. Pressure (a sandbag) can be placed on the incision to prevent bleeding.

INTRAPROCEDURE

NURSING ACTIONS

- Administer sedatives and analgesia as prescribed.
- Continually monitor vital signs and heart rhythm.
- Be prepared to intervene for dysrhythmias.
- Have resuscitation equipment and emergency medications readily available. Qs

POSTPROCEDURE

NURSING ACTIONS

- Assess vital signs every 15 min × 4, every 30 min × 2, every hour × 4, and then every 4 hr. (Follow facility protocol.)
- Assess the groin site at the same intervals for:
  - Bleeding and hematoma formation.
  - Thrombosis. (Document pedal pulse, color, temperature.)
- Maintain bed rest in supine position with extremity straight for prescribed time.
  - A vascular closure device can be used to hasten hemostasis following catheter removal.
  - Older adult clients can have arthritis, which can make lying in bed for 4 to 6 hr after the procedure painful. The provider can prescribe medication. Ⓖ
- Conduct continuous cardiac monitoring for dysrhythmias. (Reperfusion following angioplasty can cause dysrhythmias.)
- Administer antiplatelet or thrombolytic agents as prescribed to prevent clot formation and restenosis.
  - Aspirin
  - Clopidogrel, ticlopidine
  - Heparin
  - Low molecular weight heparin (enoxaparin)
  - GP IIb/IIIa inhibitors, such as eptifibatide
- Administer anxiolytics and analgesics as needed.
- Monitor urine output and administer IV fluids for hydration.
  - Contrast media acts as an osmotic diuretic.
- Perform/assist with sheath removal from vessel.
  - Apply pressure to arterial/venous sites for the prescribed period of time (varies depending upon the method used for vessel closure).
  - Observe for vagal response (hypotension, bradycardia) from compression of nerves.
  - Apply pressure dressing.

CLIENT EDUCATION

- Instruct the client to do the following.
  - Leave the dressing in place for the first 24 hr following discharge.
  - Avoid strenuous exercise for the prescribed period of time.
  - Immediately report bleeding from the insertion site, chest pain, shortness of breath, and changes in the color or temperature of the extremity.
  - Restrict lifting to less than 10 lb (4.5 kg) for the prescribed period of time.
- Clients who have stent placement will receive anticoagulation therapy for 6 to 8 weeks. Instruct the client to:
  - Take the medication at the same time each day.
  - Have regular laboratory tests to determine therapeutic levels.
  - Avoid activities that could cause bleeding. (Use soft toothbrush. Wear shoes when out of bed.)
- Encourage the client to follow lifestyle guidelines. (Manage weight. Consume a low-fat/low-sodium diet. Exercise regularly. Stop smoking. Decrease alcohol intake.)

COMPLICATIONS

Cardiac tamponade

Cardiac tamponade can result from fluid accumulation in the pericardial sac.

- Manifestations include hypotension, jugular venous distention, muffled heart sounds, and paradoxical pulse (variance of 10 mm Hg or more in systolic blood pressure between expiration and inspiration).
- Hemodynamic monitoring reveals intracardiac and PAPs are similar and elevated (plateau pressures).

NURSING ACTIONS

- Notify the provider immediately.
- Administer IV fluids to combat hypotension.
- Obtain a chest x-ray or echocardiogram to confirm diagnosis.
- Prepare the client for pericardiocentesis. (Verify informed consent. Gather materials. Administer medications as appropriate.)
- Monitor hemodynamic pressures.
- Monitor heart rhythm. Changes indicate improper positioning of the needle.
- Monitor for reoccurrence of manifestations after the procedure.

Hematoma formation

Blood clots can form near the insertion site.

NURSING ACTIONS

- Assess the groin at prescribed intervals and as needed.
- Hold pressure for uncontrolled oozing/bleeding.
- Monitor peripheral circulation.
- Notify the provider.

Restenosis of treated vessel

Clot reformation in the coronary artery can occur immediately or several weeks after procedure.

NURSING ACTIONS

- Assess ECG patterns and for occurrence of chest pain.
- Notify the provider immediately.
- Prepare the client for return to the cardiac catheterization laboratory.

Retroperitoneal bleeding

Bleeding into retroperitoneal space (abdominal cavity behind the peritoneum) can occur due to femoral artery puncture.

NURSING ACTIONS

- Assess for flank pain and hypotension.
- Notify the provider immediately.
- Administer IV fluids and blood products as prescribed.

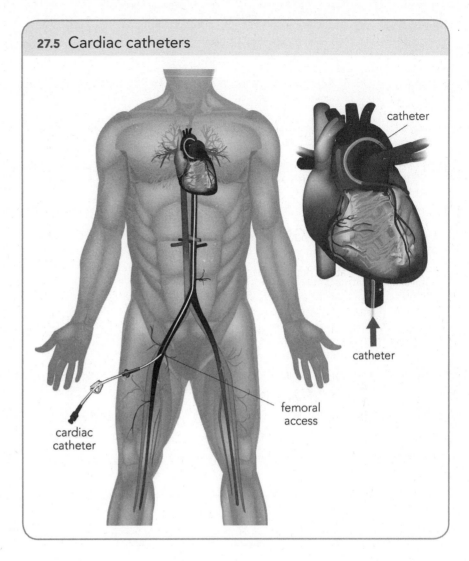

27.5 Cardiac catheters

catheter

catheter

femoral access

cardiac catheter

Vascular access

The site and type of vascular access device (VAD) is determined by the characteristics of the prescribed therapy (medication type, pH and osmolality, length of time for therapy). The goal is to minimize the number of catheter insertions and the risk for adverse reactions.

Central intravenous therapy

- Central IV catheters are appropriate for any fluids due to rapid hemodilution in the superior vena cava (SVC).
- Ensure x-ray verification of tip placement prior to use.
- Central IV catheters are inserted using sterile technique by a provider, physician assistant, or specifically trained nurses. Insertion occurs in the OR, the client's room, or in an outpatient facility.
- Tunneled and implanted catheters require surgical removal.
- Central IV catheter types include nontunneled percutaneous central venous catheters, peripherally inserted central catheters, tunneled central venous catheters (Hickman, Groshong), and implanted ports.

Nontunneled percutaneous central venous catheter (CVC)
- Description: 18 to 25 cm (7 to 10 in) in length with one to five lumens
- Length of use: short-term use only
- Insertion location: subclavian vein, jugular vein; tip in the distal third of the superior vena cava
- Indications: administration of blood, long-term administration of chemotherapeutic agents, antibiotics, and total parenteral nutrition

Peripherally inserted central catheter (PICC)
- Description: 45 to 74 cm (18 to 29 in) with single or multiple lumens
- Length of use: up to 12 months
- Insertion location: basilic or cephalic vein at least one fingerbreadth below or above the antecubital fossa. The catheter should be advanced until the tip is positioned in the lower one-third of the SVC.
- Indications: administration of blood, long-term administration of chemotherapeutic agents, antibiotics, and total parenteral nutrition
- When possible, insert a PICC early in the course of therapy before veins are exposed to repeated venipunctures.

CONSIDERATIONS

PREPROCEDURE
- Cleanse the site with chlorhexidine.
- Ensure sterility of equipment.
- Place a STOP sign on the door to the room to restrict entry during the procedure.

POSTPROCEDURE
- Confirm placement of the PICC with an x-ray.
- Assess the site for redness, swelling, drainage, tenderness, and condition of the dressing.
- Clean the insertion port with alcohol for 15 seconds and allowing it to dry completely prior to accessing it. Valve disinfection caps which contain alcohol are available for single use.
- Use transparent dressing to allow for visualization. Follow facility protocol for dressing changes, usually every 7 days and when indicated (wet, loose, soiled).
- Advise the client not to immerse his arm in water. To shower, cover dressing site to avoid water exposure.
- Educate the client not to have venipuncture or blood pressure taken in arm with PICC line.
- Follow the Infusion Nurses Society (INS) practice recommendations for flushing. Q EBP
  - Use a 10 mL syringe for flushing the PICC line. Do not apply force if resistance is met.
  - Flush with 10 mL 0.9% sodium chloride before, between, and after medications.
  - Flush with 20 mL 0.9% sodium chloride after drawing blood.
  - Flush with 5 mL heparin (10 units/mL) when the PICC is not actively in use. The frequency of the flush depends on the type of PICC.

Tunneled percutaneous central venous catheter
- For long-term use.
- Insertion location: A portion of the catheter lies in a subcutaneous tunnel separating the point where the catheter enters the vein from where it enters the skin with a cuff. Tissue granulates into the cuff to provide a mechanical barrier to organisms and an anchoring for the catheter.
- Indications: Frequent and long-term need for vascular access.
- No dressing is needed because entrance into skin and vein are separate and tissue granulates into catheter cuff, providing a barrier. Groshong catheters have pressure-sensitive valves to prevent blood reflux and do not require a clamp.

Implanted port
- Description: Port is comprised of a small reservoir covered by a thick septum.
- Insertion location: Port is surgically implanted into chest wall pocket. The catheter is inserted into the subclavian vein with the tip in the SVC.
- Indications: Long-term (1 year or more) need for vascular access; commonly used for chemotherapy.
- Only specifically trained personnel wearing a mask and aseptic technique should access implanted ports.
  - Apply topical anesthetic cream to skin if indicated. Palpate skin to locate the port body septum to ensure proper insertion of the needle.
  - Access with a noncoring (Huber) needle.
  - Check for blood return prior to medication administration to confirm patency and placement.
  - Flush with 5 mL heparin 100 units/mL after every use and at least once per month (INS recommendation).

COMPLICATIONS

Phlebitis

Phlebitis is a common complication of PICCs and can be chemical (osmolarity or pH is different, veins too small for substance), bacterial, or mechanical irritation (excess IV manipulation).

NURSING ACTIONS
- Monitor for findings.
  - Erythema at the site (usual initial indication)
  - Pain or burning at the site and the length of the vein
  - Discomfort when the skin over the tip is palpated
  - Warmth over the site
  - Edema at the site
  - Vein indurated (hard), red streak, and/or cordlike
  - Slowing infusion rate
  - Temperature elevation of 1° F or more
  - Infection appearing 7 to 10 days after insertion
- Take preventive measures.
  - Practice hand hygiene before working with a CVC.
  - Observe the site every 2 hr for infection or infiltration.
  - Nontunneled catheters require an intact sterile dressing (tunneled catheters do not).
  - Clean the site with chlorhexidine for 30 seconds and allow to air dry prior to insertion.

Occlusion

Occlusion is a blockage in the central IV catheter that impedes flow. Thrombosis/emboli can coagulate and cause an occlusion.

NURSING ACTIONS
- Flush the line according to INS recommendations or facility policy.
- Do not force fluid if resistance is encountered (can dislodge thrombosis).
- Use a 10 mL to avoid excess pressure per square inch that could cause catheter fracture/rupture.

Mechanical complications

Implanted ports can have the catheter tip and port become dislodged.

NURSING ACTIONS
- Use only a noncoring (Huber) needle to avoid damaging the mesh on implanted ports.
- Teach clients the manifestations of a dislodged port. Report findings to the provider immediately.
  - Swelling a the port site
  - Unrestricted movement of the port
  - Inability to access the port
- Teach clients the manifestations of a dislodged catheter tip. Report findings to the provider immediately.
  - Gurgling or swishing sounds
  - Pain on the affected side in the neck or ear

Application Exercises

1. A nurse is orienting a newly licensed nurse on the care of a client who is to have a line placed for hemodynamic monitoring. Which of the following statements by the newly licensed nurse indicates effectiveness of the teaching?
   - A. "Air should be instilled into the monitoring system prior to the procedure."
   - B. "The client should be positioned on the left side during the procedure."
   - C. "The transducer should be level with the second intercostal space after the line is placed."
   - D. "A chest x-ray is needed to verify placement after the procedure."

2. A nurse is assessing a client who is undergoing hemodynamic monitoring. The client has a CVP of 7 mm Hg and a PAWP of 17 mm Hg. Which of the following findings should the nurse expect? (Select all that apply.)
   - A. Poor skin turgor
   - B. Bilateral crackles in the lungs
   - C. Jugular vein distension
   - D. Dry mucous membranes
   - E. Hepatomegaly

3. A nurse is teaching a client who is scheduled for an angiography. Which of the following statements should the nurse include in the teaching?
   - A. "You should have nothing to eat or drink for 4 hours prior to the procedure."
   - B. "You will be given general anesthesia during the procedure."
   - C. "You should not have this procedure done if you are allergic to eggs."
   - D. "You will need to keep your affected leg straight following the procedure."

4. A nurse at a provider's office is reviewing the laboratory test results for a group of clients. The nurse should identify that which of the following results indicates the client is at risk for heart disease? (Select all that apply.)
   - A. Cholesterol (total) 245 mg/dL
   - B. HDL 90 mg/dL
   - C. LDL 140 mg/dL
   - D. Triglycerides 125 mg/dL
   - E. Troponin I 0.02 ng/mL

5. A nurse planning care for a client who has a PICC line in the right arm. Which of the following interventions should the nurse include in the plan of care? (Select all that apply.)
   - A. Use a 10 mL syringe to flush the PICC line.
   - B. Apply gentle force if resistance is met during injection.
   - C. Cleanse ports with alcohol for 15 seconds prior to use.
   - D. Maintain a transparent dressing over the insertion site.
   - E. Flush with 10 mL heparin before and after medication administration.

Application Exercises Key

1. A. The nurse should purge air from, rather than instill air into, the monitoring system.

   B. The nurse should place the client in the supine or Trendelenburg position.

   C. For hemodynamic monitoring, the nurse should place the transducer level with the 4th intercostal space, which is at the base of the right atrium.

   D. **CORRECT:** The nurse should ensure that a chest x-ray is obtained to confirm proper placement of the lines following placement.

   (N) *NCLEX® Connection: Reduction of Risk Potential, Potential for Complications of Diagnostic Tests/Treatments/Procedures*

2. A. The client's CVP and PAWP are above the expected reference range. The nurse should expect the client to have poor skin turgor for a decreased CVP and PAWP.

   B. **CORRECT:** The nurse should expect the client to have bilateral crackles in the lungs for an increased CVP and PAWP.

   C. **CORRECT:** The nurse should expect the client to have jugular vein distension for an increased CVP and PAWP.

   D. The nurse should expect the client to have dry mucous membranes for a decreased CVP and PAWP.

   E. **CORRECT:** The nurse should expect the client to have hepatomegaly for an increased CVP and PAWP.

   (N) *NCLEX® Connection: Reduction of Risk Potential, Potential for Complications of Diagnostic Tests/Treatments/Procedures*

3. A. The nurse should instruct the client to remain NPO for at least 8 hr prior to the procedure to decrease the risk for aspiration while lying flat during the angiography.

   B. The nurse should instruct the client that he is awake and sedated during the procedure and that a local anesthetic is used at the catheter insertion site.

   C. The nurse should assess the client for an allergy to iodine/shellfish due to the use of contrast dye. An allergy to eggs is not a contraindication to angiography.

   D. **CORRECT:** The nurse should instruct the client of the need to remain on bed rest in the supine position with the affected leg straight for a prescribed amount of time. This positioning decreases the client's risk for bleeding and hematoma formation at the catheter insertion site.

   (N) *NCLEX® Connection: Reduction of Risk Potential, Therapeutic Procedures*

4. A. **CORRECT:** A client who has a total cholesterol level greater than 200 mg/dL is at increased risk for heart disease.

   B. An HDL level greater than 55 mg/dL for a female client or greater than 45 mg/dL for a male client decreases the client's risk for heart disease.

   C. **CORRECT:** A client who has an LDL level greater than 130 mg/dL is at increased risk for heart disease.

   D. A triglyceride level between 35 and 135 mg/dL for a female client or 40 and 160 mg/dL for a male client is within the expected reference range and does not indicate an increased risk for heart disease.

   E. Troponin I level is monitored to detect cardiac injury due to an MI rather than to identify a client's risk for heart disease. A Troponin I level less than 0.03 ng/mL is within the expected reference range.

   (N) *NCLEX® Connection: Reduction of Risk Potential, Laboratory Values*

5. A. **CORRECT:** The nurse should use a 10 mL syringe to flush the PICC line to avoid excess pressure that could cause catheter fracture/rupture.

   B. The nurse should avoid the application of force if resistance is met during injection.

   C. **CORRECT:** The nurse should cleanse insertion ports with alcohol for 15 seconds and allow it to air dry prior to use. This action decreases the risk for bacterial contamination.

   D. **CORRECT:** The nurse should maintain a transparent dressing over the insertion site to decrease the risk for infection and allow for visualization. The nurse should plan to change the dressing at least every 7 days and when wet, loose, or soiled.

   E. The nurse should flush the PICC line with 10 mL 0.9% sodium chloride before, between, and after medications. A flush of 5 mL heparin (10 units/mL) is recommended when the PICC is not actively in use.

   (N) *NCLEX® Connection: Physiological Adaptation, Hemodynamics*

PRACTICE Answer

Using the ATI Active Learning Template: Diagnostic Procedure

DESCRIPTION OF THE PROCEDURE: The cardiac muscle is exercised by walking on a treadmill. This provides information regarding the workload of the heart.

INDICATIONS
- Angina
- Heart failure
- Myocardial infarction
- Dysrhythmia

NURSING ACTIONS (PRE, INTRA, POST)

Preprocedure
- Ensure that a signed informed consent form is obtained.
- Explain to the client that he will walk on a treadmill. Comfortable athletic shoes and clothing are recommended.
- Explain that a pharmacological stress test can be prescribed if the client cannot walk on the treadmill and complete the test. A medication such as dipyridamole, adenosine, or dobutamine is administered to stress the heart instead of walking on the treadmill.
- Instruct the client to fast 2 to 4 hr before the procedure or according to facility policy and to avoid tobacco, alcohol, and caffeine before the test.
- Instruct the client to get adequate rest the night before the test.

Intraprocedure
- Monitor heart rate and rhythm with a 12-lead ECG during the test.
- Instruct the client to report any chest pain, shortness of breath, or dizziness during the test.

(N) *NCLEX® Connection: Reduction of Risk Potential, Therapeutic Procedures*

UNIT 4   NURSING CARE OF CLIENTS WHO HAVE
CARDIOVASCULAR DISORDERS
SECTION: DIAGNOSTIC AND THERAPEUTIC PROCEDURES

CHAPTER 28 *Electrocardiography and Dysrhythmia Monitoring*

Cardiac electrical activity can be monitored by using an electrocardiogram (ECG). The heart's electrical activity can be monitored by a standard 12-lead ECG (resting ECG), ambulatory ECG (Holter monitoring), continuous cardiac monitoring, or by telemetry.

Cardiac monitoring is used to diagnose dysrhythmias, chamber enlargement, myocardial ischemia, injury, or infarction and to monitor the effects of electrolyte imbalances or medication administration.

Cardiac dysrhythmias are heartbeat disturbances (beat formation, beat conduction, or myocardial response to beat).

Nurses should be familiar with cardioversion and defibrillation procedures for treating dysrhythmias. **(28.1)**

28.1 ECG strip

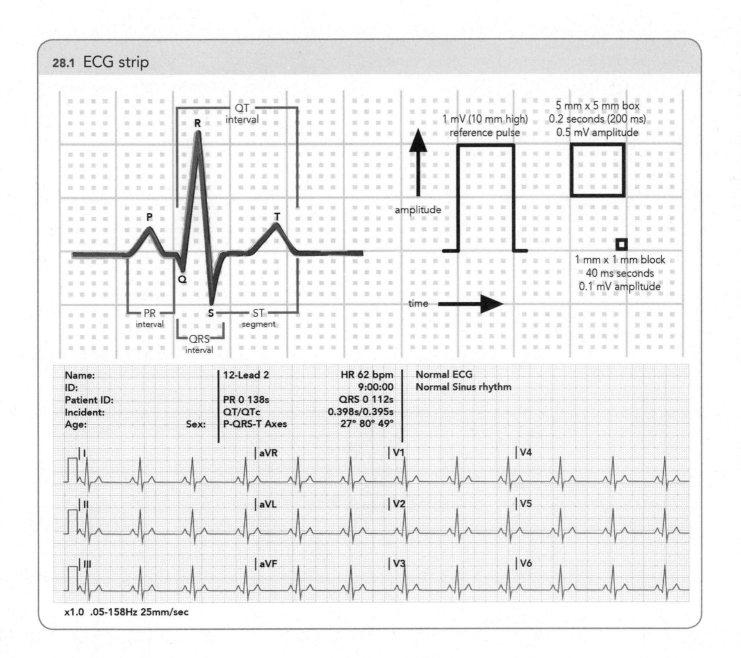

Name:
ID:
Patient ID:
Incident:
Age: Sex:

12-Lead 2
PR 0 138s
QT/QTc
P-QRS-T Axes

HR 62 bpm
9:00:00
QRS 0 112s
0.398s/0.395s
27° 80° 49°

Normal ECG
Normal Sinus rhythm

x1.0 .05-158Hz 25mm/sec

Electrocardiography

Electrocardiography uses an electrocardiograph to record the electrical activity of the heart over time. The electrocardiograph is connected by wires (leads) to skin electrodes placed on the chest and limbs of a client.

- Continuous cardiac monitoring requires the client to be in close proximity to the monitoring system.
- Telemetry allows the client to ambulate while maintaining proximity to the monitoring system.
- Inform clients receiving continuous ECG monitoring that the monitoring will not detect shortness of breath, chest pain, or other manifestations of acute coronary syndrome. The client should be instructed to report new or worsening symptoms. Qs

INDICATIONS

Dysrhythmias
- Sinus bradycardia and tachycardia
- Atrioventricular (AV) blocks
- Atrial fibrillation
- Ventricular asystole
- Premature atrial complexes (PACs) and premature ventricular complexes (PVCs)
- Supraventricular tachycardia
- Ventricular tachycardia
- Ventricular fibrillation

CLIENT PRESENTATION

- Cardiovascular disease
- Myocardial infarction (MI)
- Hypoxia
- Acid-base imbalances
- Electrolyte disturbances
- Kidney failure, liver, or lung disease
- Pericarditis
- Drug or alcohol use
- Hypovolemia
- Shock

CONSIDERATIONS

PREPROCEDURE

NURSING ACTIONS
Prepare the client for a 12-lead ECG, if prescribed. **(28.2)**
- Position the client in a supine position with chest exposed.
- Wash the client's skin to remove oils.
- If the area on which the electrode is to be placed has hair on it, clip — do not shave — the area to provide skin adherence and electrical conduction.
- Attach one electrode to each of the client's extremities by applying electrodes to flat surfaces above the wrists and ankles and the other six electrodes to the chest, avoiding chest hair. (Chest hair might need to be shaved on male clients).

INTRAPROCEDURE

NURSING ACTIONS
- Instruct the client to remain still and breathe normally while the 12-lead ECG is performed.
- Monitor the client for manifestations of dysrhythmia (chest pain, decreased level of consciousness, and shortness of breath) and hypoxia.

POSTPROCEDURE

NURSING ACTIONS
- Remove leads from the client, print the ECG report, and notify the provider.
- Apply a Holter monitor if the client is on a telemetry unit and/or needs continuous cardiac monitoring.
- Continue to monitor the client for dysrhythmia.

Dysrhythmias

- Dysrhythmias are classified by the following:
  - Site of origin: sinoatrial (SA) node, atria, atrioventricular (AV) node, or ventricle
    - Electrophysiological study is performed to determine the area of the heart causing the dysrhythmia. Ablation of the area is possible.
  - Effect on the rate and rhythm of the heart: bradycardia, tachycardia, heart block, premature beat, flutter, fibrillation, or asystole
- Dysrhythmias can be benign or life-threatening.
- The life-threatening effects of dysrhythmias are generally related to decreased cardiac output and ineffective tissue perfusion.
- Cardiac dysrhythmias are a primary cause of death in clients suffering acute MI and other sudden death disorders.

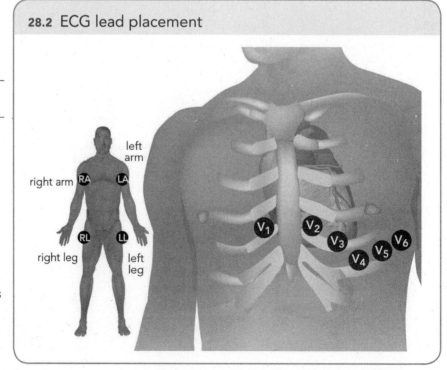

28.2 ECG lead placement

- Rapid recognition and treatment of serious dysrhythmias is essential to preserve life. Treatment is based on the cardiac rhythm, which can require cardioversion, defibrillation or pacemaker insertion, and/or medications. (28.4)
- Symptoms of dysrhythmia in the older adult might be present only with increased activity. ⓖ
- Risks for heart disease, hypertension, dysrhythmias, and atherosclerosis increase with age.
- Treatment of dysrhythmias follows Advanced Cardiac Life Support (ACLS) evidence-based protocols. See **CHAPTER 2: EMERGENCY NURSING PRINCIPLES AND MANAGEMENT** for further information. Ⓠ**EBP**

28.4 Dysrhythmia treatments

	MEDICATION	ELECTRICAL MANAGEMENT
Bradycardia *(any rhythm less than 60/min)* Treat if the client is symptomatic	Atropine and isoproterenol	Pacemaker
Atrial fibrillation *Supraventricular tachycardia* *Ventricular tachycardia with pulse*	Amiodarone, adenosine, and verapamil	Synchronized cardioversion
Ventricular tachycardia without pulse or ventricular fibrillation	Amiodarone, lidocaine, and epinephrine	Defibrillation

28.3 Dysrhythmias

ATRIAL FIBRILLATION

PREMATURE ATRIAL COMPLEXES

PREMATURE VENTRICULAR COMPLEXES

VENTRICULAR TACHYCARDIA

Cardioversion and defibrillation

Cardioversion is the delivery of a direct countershock to the heart synchronized to the QRS complex. Defibrillation is the delivery of an unsynchronized, direct countershock to the heart. Defibrillation stops all electrical activity of the heart, allowing the SA node to take over and reestablish a perfusing rhythm.

INDICATIONS

Cardioversion: Elective treatment of atrial dysrhythmias, supraventricular tachycardia, and ventricular tachycardia with a pulse. Cardioversion is the treatment of choice for clients who are symptomatic.

Defibrillation: Ventricular fibrillation or pulseless ventricular tachycardia.

CONSIDERATIONS

PREPROCEDURE

Clients who have atrial fibrillation of unknown duration must receive adequate anticoagulation for 4 to 6 weeks prior to cardioversion therapy to prevent dislodgement of thrombi into the bloodstream.

NURSING ACTIONS
- Explain the procedure to the client, and obtain consent.
- Administer oxygen.
- Document preprocedure rhythm.
- Have emergency equipment available.
- Digoxin is held for 48 hr prior to elective cardioversion.

INTRAPROCEDURE

NURSING ACTIONS
- Administer sedation as prescribed.
- Ensure proper placement of leads and machine settings, including joules to be delivered.
- Monitor the client in a lead that provides an upright QRS complex.
- All staff must stand clear of the client, equipment connected to the client, and the bed when a shock is delivered.
- Cardioversion requires activation of the synchronizer button in addition to charging the machine. This allows the shock to be in sync with the client's underlying rhythm. Failure to synchronize can lead to development of a lethal dysrhythmia, such as ventricular fibrillation.
- Perform CPR for cardiac asystole or other pulseless rhythms.
- Defibrillate the client immediately for ventricular fibrillation.
- Administer a prescribed antidysrhythmic agent or other prescribed medications.
- Monitor the client for pulmonary or systemic emboli following cardioversion.

POSTPROCEDURE

NURSING ACTIONS
- After cardioversion or defibrillation, monitor vital signs, assess airway patency, and obtain an ECG.
- Provide the client/family with reassurance and emotional support.
- Document the following:
  - Postprocedure rhythm
  - Number of defibrillation or cardioversion attempts, energy settings, time, and response
  - The client's condition and state of consciousness following the procedure
  - Skin condition under the electrodes

CLIENT EDUCATION
- Teach the client and family how to assess pulse.
- Advise the client to report palpitations or irregularities.

COMPLICATIONS

Embolism

Cardioversion can dislodge blood clots, potentially causing:
- A pulmonary embolism (evidenced by dyspnea, chest pain, air hunger, and decreasing SaO_2)
- A cerebrovascular accident (evidenced by decreased level of consciousness, slurred speech, and muscle weakness/paralysis)
- An MI (evidenced by chest pain and ST segment depression or elevation)

NURSING ACTIONS: Provide therapeutic anticoagulation for clients who have dysrhythmias.

Decreased cardiac output and heart failure

Cardioversion might damage heart tissue and impair heart function.

NURSING ACTIONS
- Monitor the client for signs of decreased cardiac output (hypotension, syncope, increased heart rate) and heart failure (dyspnea, productive cough, edema, venous distention).
- Provide medications to increase output (inotropic agents) and to decrease cardiac workload.

Application Exercises

1. A nurse on a cardiac unit is caring for a group of clients. The nurse should recognize which of the following clients as being at risk for the development of a dysrhythmia? (Select all that apply.)

   A. A client who has metabolic alkalosis

   B. A client who has a serum potassium level of 4.3 mEq/L

   C. A client who has an SaO_2 of 96%

   D. A client who has COPD

   E. A client who underwent stent placement in a coronary artery

2. A nurse working on a cardiac unit is admitting a client who is to undergo a cardioversion and is reviewing the health record. Which of the following data requires that the nurse notify the provider to cancel the procedure? (Review the data below for additional client information.)

   MAR
   Ferrous Sulfate 200 mg
      PO 0800 and 2000
   Diazepam 2 mg PO
      0800 and 2000
   Isosorbide 2.5 mg PO
      4 times a day AC and HS

   VITAL SIGNS
   0800
   T 99° F (37.2° C)
   Blood pressure 142/86 mm Hg
   Heart rate 88/min and irregular
   Respirations 20/min

   HISTORY AND PHYSICAL
   Bariatric surgery 10 years ago
   Dyspnea with exertion
      for 3 years
   Atrial fibrillation began
      3 years ago
   Client reports taking the
      following medications
      for the past 6 weeks: iron
      supplement, multivitamin,
      antilipemic, and nitroglycerin

   A. Respiratory history

   B. Vital signs

   C. Medication history

   D. Medications to be administered

3. A nurse is caring for a client who experienced defibrillation. Which of the following should be included in the documentation of this procedure? (Select all that apply.)

   A. Follow-up ECG

   B. Energy settings used

   C. IV fluid intake

   D. Urinary output

   E. Skin condition under electrodes

4. A nurse on a cardiac unit is caring for a client who is on telemetry. The nurse recognizes the client's heart rate is 46/min and notifies the provider. The nurse should anticipate that which of the following management strategies will be used for this client?

   A. Defibrillation

   B. Pacemaker insertion

   C. Synchronized cardioversion

   D. Administration of IV lidocaine

5. A student nurse is observing a cardioversion procedure and hears the team leader call out, "Stand clear." The student should recognize the purpose of this action is to alert personnel that

   A. the cardioverter is being charged to the appropriate setting.

   B. they should initiate CPR due to pulseless electrical activity.

   C. they cannot be in contact with equipment connected to the client.

   D. a time-out is being called to verify correct protocols.

PRACTICE Active Learning Scenario

A nurse educator is reviewing electrocardiography with a group of nurses. What information should be included in this discussion? Use the ATI Active Learning Template: Therapeutic Procedure to complete this item.

DESCRIPTION OF PROCEDURE: Describe electrocardiography and describe the difference between continuous cardiac monitoring and telemetry.

INDICATIONS: List four dysrhythmias that can be identified.

NURSING INTERVENTIONS (PRE, INTRA, POST): Identify at least two preprocedure, one intraprocedure, and two postprocedure.

Application Exercises Key

1. A. **CORRECT:** A client who has an acid-base imbalance such as metabolic alkalosis is at risk for a dysrhythmia.

   B. A serum potassium of 4.3 mEq/L is within the expected reference range and does not increase the risk of a dysrhythmia.

   C. SaO$_2$ of 96% is within the expected reference range and does not increase the risk of a dysrhythmia.

   D. **CORRECT:** A client who has lung disease, such as COPD, is at risk for a dysrhythmia.

   E. **CORRECT:** A client who has cardiac disease and underwent a stent placement is at risk for a dysrhythmia.

   (N) *NCLEX® Connection: Physiological Adaptation, Pathophysiology*

2. A. A client who has a dysrhythmia often has a history of lung disease, which can make him a candidate for cardioversion.

   B. A client who has a dysrhythmia might have an irregular pulse, which can make him a candidate for cardioversion.

   C. **CORRECT:** A client who is to undergo cardioversion needs to be on anticoagulant therapy for 4 to 6 weeks prior to the procedure.

   D. A client who has a dysrhythmia often has a history of cardiac disease and angina, which can make him a candidate for cardioversion.

   (N) *NCLEX® Connection: Reduction of Risk Potential, Potential for Complications of Diagnostic Tests/Treatments/Procedures*

3. A. **CORRECT:** The client's ECG rhythm is documented following the procedure.

   B. **CORRECT:** Energy settings used during the procedure are documented.

   C. IV fluid intake is not documented during defibrillation.

   D. Urinary output is not documented during defibrillation.

   E. **CORRECT:** The condition of the client's skin where electrodes were placed is documented.

   (N) *NCLEX® Connection: Reduction of Risk Potential, Therapeutic Procedures*

4. A. Defibrillation is used when a client has ventricular fibrillation or pulseless ventricular tachycardia.

   B. **CORRECT:** A client who has bradycardia is a candidate for a pacemaker to increase his heart rate.

   C. Synchronized cardioversion is used when a client has a dysrhythmia such as atrial fibrillation, supraventricular tachycardia (SVT), or ventricular tachycardia with pulse.

   D. The administration of IV lidocaine is used in clients who have a pulseless ventricular dysrhythmia to stimulate cardiac electrical function.

   (N) *NCLEX® Connection: Physiological Adaptation, Hemodynamics*

5. A. The cardioverter is charged prior to the delivery of the shock during cardioversion.

   B. The team leader calls out "Initiate CPR" when members of the team are to begin CPR.

   C. **CORRECT:** A safety concern for personnel performing cardioversion is to "stand clear" of the client and equipment connected to the client when a shock is delivered to prevent them from also receiving a shock.

   D. A "time-out" is called by personnel during a procedure to verify that proper protocols are being followed.

   (N) *NCLEX® Connection: Physiological Adaptation, Hemodynamics*

PRACTICE Answer

Using the ATI Active Learning Template: Therapeutic Procedure

DESCRIPTION OF PROCEDURE

- Electrocardiography is the use of an electrocardiograph to record the electrical activity of the heart over time by connecting wires (leads) to skin electrodes placed on the chest and limbs of the client.
- Continuous monitoring requires the client to be in close proximity to the monitoring system. Telemetry allows the client to ambulate.

INDICATIONS

- Sinus bradycardia and tachycardia
- Atrioventricular (AV) blocks
- Atrial fibrillation
- Supraventricular tachycardia
- Ventricular fibrillation
- Ventricular asystole
- Premature ventricular complexes (PVCs)
- Premature atrial complexes (PACs)

NURSING INTERVENTIONS (PRE, INTRA, POST)

Preprocedure
- Position the client in a supine position with chest exposed.
- Wash the skin to remove oils.
- Attach one electrode to each of the client's extremities by applying electrodes to flat surfaces above the wrists and ankles and the other six electrodes to the chest, avoiding chest hair, which might need to be shaved on male clients.

Intraprocedure
- Instruct the client to remain still and breathe normally.
- Monitor for manifestations of dysrhythmia (chest pain, decreased level of consciousness, shortness of breath) and hypoxia.

Postprocedure
- Remove leads, print ECG report, and notify the provider.
- Apply Holter monitor if the client is on the telemetry unit and/or needs continuous monitoring.
- Continue monitoring for manifestations of dysrhythmia and hypoxia.

(N) *NCLEX® Connection: Reduction of Risk Potential, Potential for Complications of Diagnostic Tests/Treatments/Procedures*

CHAPTER 29 *Pacemakers*

An artificial pacemaker is a battery-operated device that electrically stimulates the heart when the natural pacemaker of the heart fails to maintain an acceptable rhythm.

Pacemakers can be temporary or permanent and are composed of two parts. The pulse generator houses the energy source (battery) and the control center. The electrodes are wires that attach to the myocardial muscle on one side and connect to the pulse generator on the other.

Nurses should be familiar with the various types of pacemakers, how they function, and the care involved with their placement/insertion.

Conduction of electrical impulses through the sinoatrial (SA) node can be slowed with aging, causing bradycardia and conduction defects. ©

When a pacing stimulus is delivered to the heart, a pacer spike (or pacemaker artifact) will be seen on a cardiac monitor or ECG strip. The pacer spike, a vertical line, should be followed by a P wave (atrial pacing) or QRS complex (ventricular pacing).

Types of pacemakers

TEMPORARY PACEMAKERS

The energy source is provided by an external battery pack.

External (transcutaneous)

- Pacing energy is delivered transcutaneously through the thoracic musculature to the heart via two electrode patches placed on the skin.
- It requires large amounts of electricity, which can be painful for a client.
- It is used only in emergency resuscitation of a client who does not have pacing wires inserted.

Epicardial

- Pacemaker leads are attached directly to the heart during open-heart surgery. Wires run externally through the chest incision and can be attached to an external impulse generator if needed.
- It is commonly used during and immediately following open-heart surgery.

Endocardial (transvenous)

Pacing wires are threaded through a large central vein (subclavian, jugular, or cephalic) and lodged into the wall of the right ventricle (ventricular pacing), right atrium (atrial pacing), or both chambers (dual chamber pacing).

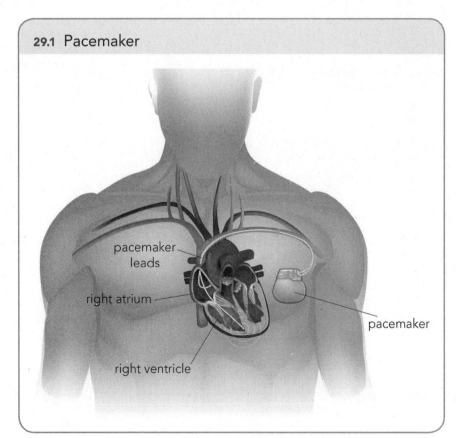

29.1 Pacemaker

pacemaker leads

right atrium

right ventricle

pacemaker

PERMANENT PACEMAKERS

- Contain an internal pacing unit
- Indicated for chronic or recurrent dysrhythmias due to sinus or atrioventricular (AV) node malfunction
- Can be programmed to pace the atrial (A) or ventricular (V) chamber, or both (AV)

PACEMAKER MODES

- **Fixed rate (asynchronous):** Fires at a constant rate without regard for the heart's electrical activity.
- **Demand mode (synchronous):** Detects the heart's electrical impulses and fires at a preset rate only if the heart's intrinsic rate is below a certain level. Pacemaker response modes include the following:
  - **Inhibited:** Pacemaker activity is inhibited/does not fire.
  - **Triggered:** Pacemaker activity is triggered/fires when intrinsic activity is sensed.
- **Tachydysrhythmia function:** Can overpace a tachydysrhythmia and/or deliver an electrical shock.

29.2 Five-letter system to identify pacemaker function

CHAMBER PACED	CHAMBER SENSED	RESPONSE MODE
O: None	O: None	O: None
A: Atria	A: Atria	T: Triggered
V: Ventricle	V: Ventricle	I: Inhibited
D: Dual (AV)	D: Dual (AV)	D: Dual (AV)
PROGRAMMABLE FUNCTIONS	**TACHYDYSRHYTHMIC FUNCTIONS**	
O: None	O: None	
R: Rate Modulation	P: Pacing (anti-tachydysrhythmia)	
	S: Shock	
	D: Dual (P + S)	

Often, the first three letters are used to describe the pacemaker function:

> Example: VVI mode

> Function: Ventricular paced, ventricular sensed, inhibited. If no QRS detected within desired time, pacemaker fires. If QRS detected, pacemaker does not fire.

Pacemaker placement

INDICATIONS

POTENTIAL DIAGNOSES

- Symptomatic bradycardia
- Complete heart block
- Sick sinus syndrome
- Sinus arrest
- Asystole
- Atrial tachydysrhythmias
- Ventricular tachydysrhythmias

CLIENT PRESENTATION

SUBJECTIVE DATA

- Dizziness
- Palpitations (racing heart)
- Chest pain or pressure
- Anxiety
- Fatigue
- Nausea
- Breathing difficulties

OBJECTIVE DATA

- Bradycardia or tachycardia
- Abnormal ECG
- Dyspnea, tachypnea
- Restlessness
- Jugular venous distention
- Vomiting
- Hypotension
- Diaphoresis
- Decreased cardiac output

CONSIDERATIONS

PREPROCEDURE

NURSING ACTIONS

- Assess the client's knowledge of the procedure and need for pacemaker (if nonemergent situation).
- Obtain signed informed consent form from the client.
- Prepare client's skin (clean with soap and water; trim excess hair). Do not shave, rub, or apply alcohol to the skin.

CLIENT EDUCATION: Teach the client about the type of pacemaker that is to be inserted and information about the procedure.

Temporary pacemaker

- Explain that wires and a pacemaker box will be on the client's chest after the procedure.
- Instruct the client not to touch the dials on the pacemaker box.
- The wires and box need to be kept dry. The client will not be able to shower.

Permanent pacemaker

- Explain that a small incision is made using a local anesthetic and IV sedation.
- The pacemaker may be reprogrammed externally after the procedure.
- The pacemaker battery will last about 10 years. The pacemaker pulse generator must be replaced when this occurs.

POSTPROCEDURE

NURSING ACTIONS

- Document the time and date of insertion, model (permanent pacemaker), settings, rhythm strip, presence of adequate pulse and blood pressure, and client response.
- Continually monitor heart rate and rhythm. Compare ECG rhythm to prescribed pacemaker settings. Notify provider of any discrepancies.
- Obtain chest x-ray to assess lead placement and for pneumothorax, hemothorax, or pleural effusion.
- Provide analgesia as prescribed.
- Minimize shoulder movement initially, and provide a sling (if prescribed) to allow leads to anchor.
- Monitor the incision site for bleeding, hematoma formation, or infection.
- Assess for hiccups, which can indicate that the generator is pacing the diaphragm.
- Maintain the client's safety. Following transcutaneous pacing, inspect the skin under the electrodes for thermal burns. Clients who are older, dehydrated, or have had external pacing for an extended period of time are most at risk for thermal burns. Qs
- For a permanent pacemaker: Provide the client with a pacemaker identification card including the manufacturer's name, model number, mode of function, rate parameters, and expected battery life.

CLIENT EDUCATION

- **Temporary pacemakers** are used only in a controlled facility with telemetry for continuous ECG monitoring. If needed, a permanent pacemaker is inserted before discharge to home.
- **Permanent pacemaker discharge teaching**
  - Carry a pacemaker identification card at all times.
  - Prevent wire dislodgement. (Wear sling when out of bed. Do not raise arm above shoulder for 1 to 2 weeks.)
  - Take pulse daily at the same time. Notify the provider if heart rate is less than the pacemaker rate.
  - Report signs of dizziness, fainting, fatigue, weakness, chest pain, hiccupping, palpitations, difficulty breathing, or weight gain.
  - For clients who have pacemaker-defibrillators, when the device delivers a shock, anyone touching the client will feel a slight electrical impulse, but the impulse is not harmful.
  - Follow activity restrictions as prescribed, including no contact sports or heavy lifting for 2 months.
  - Avoid direct blows or injury to the generator site.
  - Resume sexual activity as desired, avoiding positions that put stress on the incision site.
  - Never place items that generate a magnetic field directly over the pacemaker generator. These items can affect function and settings. This includes garage door openers, burglar alarms, strong magnets, generators and other power transmitters, and large stereo speakers. The use of household items is not prohibited. Qs
  - Inform providers and dentists about the pacemaker. Some tests, such as magnetic resonance imaging and therapeutic diathermy (heat therapy), can be contraindicated.
  - Pacemakers set off airport security detectors, and officials should be notified. The airport security device should not affect pacemaker functioning. Airport security personnel should not place wand detection devices directly over the pacemaker.

PACEMAKER INSERTION COMPLICATIONS

Infection or hematoma at insertion site

NURSING ACTIONS

- Assess the incision site for redness, pain, drainage, or swelling.
- Administer antibiotics as prescribed.
- Monitor PT, PTT, and CBC.

Pneumothorax or hemothorax

NURSING ACTIONS

- Assess breath sounds and chest movement.
- Monitor oxygen saturation.
- Obtain a chest x-ray after the procedure.

Arrhythmias

Related to ventricular irritation from pacemaker electrode

NURSING ACTIONS

- Monitor ECG and blood pressure.
- Administer antiarrhythmics as prescribed.
- Have emergency resuscitation equipment and medications readily available.

PACEMAKER COMPLICATIONS

- Pacemaker complications relate to improper sensing or pacing electrical charge being outside the heart. Causes include insufficient pacemaker settings, lead wire placement and function, battery function, myocardial damage, and electrolyte imbalance.
- Complications often are detectable by ECG. **Qs**
  - Monitor ECG to ensure heart rate is within programmed parameters. Pacer spikes should be adequate in number and occur directly before P or QRS complexes.
  - Pacer spikes that occur on the T wave can cause life-threatening arrhythmias.
- Treatment of complications is related to identifying the cause.
- Pacemaker settings should be manipulated only as prescribed.

Application Exercises

1. A nurse is admitting a client who has complete heart block as demonstrated by ECG. The client's heart rate is 34/min and blood pressure is 83/48 mm Hg. The client is lethargic and unable to complete sentences. Which of the following actions should the nurse perform first?

   A. Transport the client to the cardiovascular laboratory.

   B. Prepare the client for insertion of a permanent pacemaker.

   C. Obtain a signed informed consent form for a pacemaker.

   D. Apply transcutaneous pacemaker pads.

2. A nurse is caring for a client following the insertion of a temporary venous pacemaker via the femoral artery that is set as a VVI pacemaker rate of 70/min. Which of the following findings should the nurse report to the provider? (Select all that apply.)

   A. Cool and clammy foot with capillary refill of 5 seconds

   B. Observed pacing spike followed by a QRS complex

   C. Persistent hiccups

   D. Heart rate 84/min

   E. Blood pressure 104/62 mm Hg

3. A nurse is completing discharge teaching with a client who has a permanent pacemaker. Which of the following statements by the client indicates understanding of the teaching?

   A. "I will notify the airport screeners about my pacemaker."

   B. "I will expect to have occasional hiccups."

   C. "I will have to disconnect my garage door opener."

   D. "I will take my pulse every 2 to 3 days."

4. A cardiac nurse educator is reviewing the use of the fixed rate mode pacemaker with a group of newly hired nurses. Which of the following statements by a newly hired nurse indicates understanding of the review?

   A. "This means the pacemaker fires in an asynchronous pattern."

   B. "This means the pacemaker fires only when the heart rate is below a certain rate."

   C. "The pacemaker can automatically adjust to a client's increased activity level."

   D. "The pacemaker activity is triggered by heart muscle activity."

5. A nurse is admitting a client to the coronary care unit following placement of a temporary pacemaker. Which of the following nursing actions should the nurse use to promote client safety? (Select all that apply.)

   A. Wear gloves when handling pacemaker leads.

   B. Ensure electronic equipment has three-pronged grounding plugs.

   C. Minimize the client's shoulder movements.

   D. Hold the lead wires taut when turning the client.

   E. Keep extra pacemaker batteries at least 300 ft away from the client.

PRACTICE Active Learning Scenario

A coronary care nurse is orienting a newly hired nurse and discussing care of a client who has complications related to pacemaker insertion. What should be included in the discussion? Use the ATI Active Learning Template: Therapeutic Procedure to complete this item.

POTENTIAL COMPLICATIONS: Describe two. Describe at least two nursing actions for each complication.

Application Exercises Key

1. A. The nurse should plan to transport the client to the cardiovascular laboratory for placement of a permanent pacemaker to control the client's heart rate; however, there is another action the nurse should take first.

   B. The nurse should plan to prepare the client for insertion of a permanent pacemaker by cleansing the skin and clipping excess hair; however, there is another action the nurse should take first.

   C. The nurse should obtain informed consent for placement of a permanent pacemaker if an individual with authority to make decisions for the client is present; however, there is another action the nurse should take first. Emergency procedures can be performed without consent if the client is not coherent.

   D. **CORRECT:** The greatest risk to this client is injury or death from inadequate tissue perfusion; therefore, the first action the nurse should take is to apply transcutaneous pacemaker pads and begin external pacing of the heart until a permanent pacemaker can be placed.

   Ⓝ *NCLEX® Connection: Physiological Adaptation, Hemodynamics*

2. A. **CORRECT:** A cool, clammy foot can be an indication of a femoral hematoma secondary to insertion of the lead wires and should be reported.

   B. A pacing spike followed by a QRS complex is an expected finding.

   C. **CORRECT:** Persistent hiccups can indicate lead wire perforation and stimulation of the diaphragm and should be reported.

   D. A heart rate of 84/min is an expected finding.

   E. A blood pressure of 104/62 mm Hg is an expected finding.

   Ⓝ *NCLEX® Connection: Physiological Adaptation, Unexpected Response to Therapies*

3. A. **CORRECT:** The client should notify airport screening personnel about a pacemaker.

   B. The client should report hiccups to the provider because they can indicate improper lead placement.

   C. The use of household appliances, such as microwaves and garage door openers, does not affect pacemaker function.

   D. The client should check her pulse at the same time every day to ensure the pacemaker is maintaining the prescribed heart rate.

   Ⓝ *NCLEX® Connection: Physiological Adaptation, Illness Management*

4. A. **CORRECT:** Fixed rate mode is asynchronous, meaning the pacemaker fires without regard for electrical activity in the heart.

   B. Demand mode detects an electrical impulse, and the pacemaker will then fire only if this impulse remains below a certain level.

   C. Fixed rate pacemaker mode means the rate does not change in relation to activity level.

   D. Fixed rate mode means the pacemaker fires without regard for electrical activity in the heart.

   Ⓝ *NCLEX® Connection: Reduction of Risk Potential, Therapeutic Procedures*

5. A. **CORRECT:** The nurse should wear gloves when handling pacemaker leads.

   B. Three-pronged grounding plugs reduce the risk of accidental electrical discharge by equipment being used.

   C. **CORRECT:** The client should wear a sling to minimize shoulder movement and promote secure anchoring of the lead wires.

   D. The nurse should hold the lead wires with some slack in them to prevent dislodging the wires when the client is turned.

   E. The nurse should keep additional batteries at the client's bedside for quick access when needed.

   Ⓝ *NCLEX® Connection: Reduction of Risk Potential, Therapeutic Procedures*

PRACTICE Answer

Using ATI Active Learning Template: Therapeutic Procedure

POTENTIAL COMPLICATIONS

Infection or hematoma
- Assess incision site for redness, pain, drainage, or swelling.
- Administer antibiotics as prescribed.
- Monitor PT, PTT, and CBC.

Pneumothorax or hemothorax
- Monitor breath sounds and chest movement.
- Monitor oxygen saturation.
- Obtain a chest x-ray following the procedure.

Arrhythmias
- Monitor ECG and blood pressure.
- Administer antiarrhythmics as prescribed.
- Have emergency resuscitation equipment and medications readily available.

Ⓝ *NCLEX® Connection: Reduction of Risk Potential, Therapeutic Procedures*

UNIT 4   NURSING CARE OF CLIENTS WHO HAVE
CARDIOVASCULAR DISORDERS
SECTION: DIAGNOSTIC AND THERAPEUTIC PROCEDURES

CHAPTER 30 *Invasive Cardiovascular Procedures*

Cardiovascular procedures include invasive methods used to improve blood flow for occluded arteries and veins.

Invasive cardiovascular procedures are indicated after noninvasive interventions have been tried, such as diet, exercise, and medications.

Invasive cardiovascular procedures that nurses should be knowledgeable about include percutaneous coronary intervention (PCI), coronary artery bypass grafts (CABG), and peripheral bypass grafts.

Percutaneous coronary intervention

PCI is a nonsurgical procedure performed to open coronary arteries through one of the following means:
- **Atherectomy**: Used to break up and remove plaques within cardiac vessels.
- **Stent**: Placement of a mesh-wire device to hold an artery open and prevent restenosis.
- **Percutaneous transluminal coronary angioplasty**: Also referred to simply as angioplasty, this involves inflating a balloon to dilate the arterial lumen and the adhering plaque, thus widening the arterial lumen. This can include stent placement.

INDICATIONS

- Can be performed on an elective basis to treat coronary artery disease when there is occlusion of one to two coronary arteries. The area of occlusion is confined, not scattered, and easy to access (proximal).
- Might reduce ischemia during the occurrence of an acute myocardial infarction (MI) by opening coronary arteries and restoring perfusion. It is usually performed within 3 hours of the onset of symptoms.
- Might be used as an alternative to coronary artery bypass graft.
- Might be used with stent placement to prevent artery reocclusion and to dilate the coronary artery.

CLIENT PRESENTATION

SUBJECTIVE DATA: Chest pain might occur with or without exertion. Pain might radiate to the jaw, left arm, through the back, or to the shoulder. Manifestations might increase in cold weather or with exercise. Other manifestations might include dyspnea, nausea, fatigue, and diaphoresis.

OBJECTIVE DATA: ECG changes might include ST elevation, depression, or nonspecific ST changes. Other findings might include bradycardia, tachycardia, hypotension, elevated blood pressure, vomiting, and mental disorientation.

CONSIDERATIONS

PREPROCEDURE

NURSING ACTIONS
- Ensure that the client signs the consent form.
- Maintain the client on NPO status for at least 8 hr if possible (risk for aspiration when lying flat for the procedure).
- Assess that the client and family understand the procedure.
- Assess the client for an iodine/shellfish allergy (contrast dye used instead of contrast media for consistency).
- Assess renal function prior to introduction of contrast dye.
- Administer premedications as prescribed (antiplatelet medications).

CLIENT EDUCATION: Instruct the client that he might be awake and sedated for the procedure. A local anesthetic might be administered. A small incision is made, often in the groin, to insert the catheter. The client might feel warmth and flushing when the dye is inserted. After the procedure, the client will be asked to keep the affected leg straight. Pressure (a sandbag) might be placed on the incision to prevent bleeding.

INTRAPROCEDURE

NURSING ACTIONS
- Administer sedatives, such as midazolam, and analgesia, such as fentanyl, as prescribed.
- Monitor the client for chest pain.
- Continually monitor vital signs and heart rhythm.
- Have resuscitation equipment and emergency medications readily available. Qs
- Be prepared to intervene for dysrhythmias.

POSTPROCEDURE

NURSING ACTIONS

- Assess the client's vital signs every 15 min × 4, every 30 min × 2, every hour × 4, and then every 4 hr (or per facility protocol).
- Assess the insertion site at the same intervals for bleeding and hematoma formation.
- Assess for signs of thrombosis. Document pedal or radial pulse, capillary refill, color, and temperature of extremity.
- Maintain bed rest in a supine position with leg or arm straight for prescribed time.
  - Older adult clients might have arthritis, which can make lying in bed for 4 to 6 hr after the procedure painful. ⒸⓈ
- Conduct continuous cardiac monitoring for dysrhythmias. (Reperfusion following angioplasty might cause dysrhythmias.)
- Administer antiplatelet or thrombolytic agents as prescribed to prevent clot formation and restenosis.
  - Aspirin
  - Clopidogrel, tirofiban
  - Heparin
  - Enoxaparin
  - Glycoprotein (GP IIb/IIIa) inhibitors (antiplatelet), such as eptifibatide
- Administer anxiolytics and analgesics as needed.
- Monitor urine output and administer IV fluids for hydration.
  - Contrast dye acts as an osmotic diuretic.
- Assist with sheath removal from insertion site (artery or vein).
  - The catheter sheath is a short hollow tube placed inside the artery or vein at the insertion site. It is used as a guide for the balloon catheter. After angioplasty, the catheter sheath might be left in for access, so that the angioplasty might be repeated, if needed (for restenosis or perforation).
  - Apply pressure to arterial/venous sites for prescribed period of time (varies depending upon method used for vessel closure).
  - Observe for vagal response (hypotension, bradycardia) from compression of vagus nerve.
  - Apply a pressure dressing.

CLIENT EDUCATION

- Avoid strenuous exercise for prescribed period of time.
- Immediately report bleeding from insertion site, chest pain, shortness of breath, and changes in color or temperature of the extremity.
- Restrict lifting (less than 5 lb) for prescribed period of time.
- A client who had a stent placement receives anticoagulation therapy for 6 to 8 weeks. Instruct the client to:
  - Take medication at the same time each day.
  - Have regular laboratory tests to determine therapeutic levels.
  - Avoid activities that could cause bleeding (use a soft toothbrush, wear shoes when out of bed, use an electric razor).
- Encourage the client to follow lifestyle guidelines (manage weight, consume a low-fat/low-cholesterol diet, exercise regularly, stop smoking, and decrease alcohol intake).

COMPLICATIONS

Artery dissection

- Perforation of an artery by the catheter might cause cardiac tamponade or require emergency bypass surgery.
- Artery dissection findings include severe hypotension and tachycardia, and might require extended occlusion of perforation with a balloon catheter and reversal of anticoagulants.

Cardiac tamponade

Cardiac tamponade can result from fluid accumulation in the pericardial sac.

- Findings include hypotension, jugular venous distention, muffled heart sounds, and paradoxical pulse (variance of 10 mm Hg or more in systolic blood pressure between expiration and inspiration).
- Hemodynamic monitoring reveals that intracardiac and pulmonary artery pressures are similar and elevated (plateau pressures) and that cardiac output is decreased.

NURSING ACTIONS

- Notify the provider immediately. Ⓠⓢ
- Administer IV fluids to manage hypotension as prescribed.
- Obtain a chest x-ray or echocardiogram to confirm findings.
- Prepare the client for pericardiocentesis or return to surgical suite (informed consent, gather materials, administer medications as appropriate).
  - Monitor hemodynamic pressures and heart rhythm for reoccurrence of findings after the procedure.

Hematoma formation near insertion site

NURSING ACTIONS

- Monitor for sensation, color, capillary refill, and peripheral pulses in the extremity distal to the insertion site.
- Assess groin or wrist for development of a hematoma at prescribed intervals and as needed.
- Hold pressure for uncontrolled oozing/bleeding.
- Notify the provider.

Allergic reaction related to the contrast dye

Manifestations can include chills, fever, rash, wheezing, tachycardia, and bradycardia.

NURSING ACTIONS

- Monitor for an allergic reaction.
- Have resuscitation equipment readily available.
- Administer diphenhydramine or epinephrine if prescribed.

External bleeding at the insertion site

NURSING ACTIONS

- Monitor insertion site for bleeding or swelling.
- Apply pressure to site.
- Keep client's leg or arm straight.

Embolism

Plaque or a clot can become dislodged.

NURSING ACTIONS
- Monitor client for chest pain during and after the procedure.
- Monitor client's vital signs and SaO_2.

Retroperitoneal bleeding

Bleeding in the retroperitoneal space (abdominal cavity behind the peritoneum) can occur due to femoral artery puncture.

NURSING ACTIONS
- Assess for flank pain and hypotension.
- Notify the provider immediately.
- Administer IV fluids and blood products as prescribed.

CLIENT EDUCATION
- Advise the client that pressure will be applied to the insertion site.
- Remind the client to keep his leg straight.
- Advise the client to report chest pain, shortness of breath, cardiac manifestations.

Restenosis of treated vessel

Clot formation can occur in the coronary vessel immediately or several days after the procedure.

NURSING ACTIONS
- Assess ECG patterns and for report of chest pain.
- Notify the provider immediately.
- Prepare the client for return to the cardiac catheterization laboratory.

CLIENT EDUCATION: Advise the client to notify the provider of cardiac manifestations and to take medications as prescribed.

Acute kidney injury

Damage to the kidney can result from use of contrast agent, which is nephrotoxic.

NURSING ACTIONS
- Monitor urine output, BUN, creatinine, and electrolytes.
- Promote adequate hydration (oral and IV).
- Administer acetylcysteine to protect the kidneys before and after the procedure as prescribed.

Coronary artery bypass grafts

- CABG is an invasive surgical procedure that aims to restore vascularization of the myocardium.
  - Performed to bypass an obstruction in one or more of the coronary arteries, CABG does not alter the atherosclerotic process but improves the quality of life for clients restricted by painful coronary artery disease.
  - The procedure is most effective when a client has sufficient ventricular function (ejection fraction greater than 50%).
  - Older adult clients are more likely to experience transient neurological changes, toxic effects from cardiac medications, and dysrhythmias. Ⓖ
- Less invasive revascularization procedures have been developed to reduce risk and improve client outcomes (off-pump coronary artery bypass, robotic heart surgery, minimally invasive direct coronary artery bypass). These procedures have characteristics similar to traditional CABG.

30.1 Bypass graft

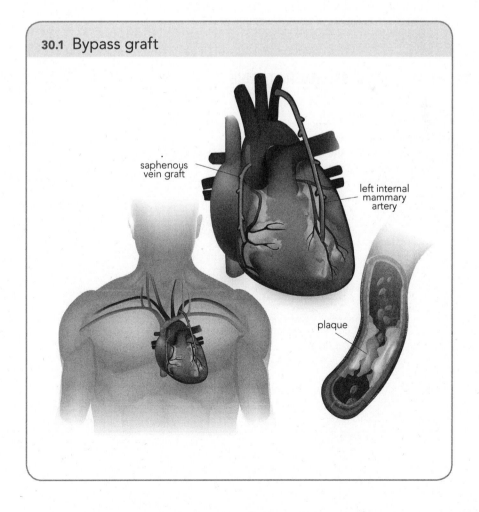

saphenous vein graft

left internal mammary artery

plaque

INDICATIONS

POTENTIAL DIAGNOSES

- Over 50% blockage of left main coronary artery with anginal episodes (blockage inaccessible to angioplasty and stenting)
- Significant two-vessel disease with unstable angina
- Triple-vessel disease with or without angina
- Persistent ischemia or likely MI following coronary angiography, PCI, or stent placement
- Heart failure or cardiogenic shock with acute MI or ischemia (might not be reasonable for clients who have poor ejection fractions)
- Coronary arteries that are unable to be accessed or treated by angioplasty and stent placement (narrow or calcified)
- Coronary artery disease nonresponsive to medical management
- Heart valve disease

CLIENT PRESENTATION

SUBJECTIVE DATA: Chest pain might occur with or without exertion. Pain might radiate to jaw, left arm, through the back, or to the shoulder. Effects might increase in cold weather or with exercise. Other findings can include dyspnea, nausea, fatigue, and diaphoresis.

OBJECTIVE DATA: ECG changes might include ST elevation, depression, or nonspecific ST changes. Other findings might include bradycardia, tachycardia, hypotension, elevated blood pressure, vomiting, and mental disorientation.

CONSIDERATIONS

PREPROCEDURE

NURSING ACTIONS

- A CABG might be an elective procedure or done as an emergency. When planned, preparation begins before the client comes to the facility for the procedure.
- Verify that the client has signed the informed consent form.
- Confirm that recent chest x-ray, ECG, and laboratory reports are available if needed.
- Complete a baseline assessment of the client's cognitive status, identify any health issues that might complicate postoperative recovery (diabetes, hypertension, stroke) and the client's support system.
- Administer preoperative medications as prescribed.
  - Anxiolytics, such as lorazepam and diazepam
  - Prophylactic antibiotics
  - Anticholinergics, such as scopolamine, to reduce secretions
- Provide safe transport of the client to the operating suite. Monitor heart rate and rhythm, oxygenation, and other vital indicators.

CLIENT EDUCATION

- Provide instruction to the client and family about the procedure and postsurgical environment.
- Inform the client of the importance of coughing and deep breathing after the procedure to prevent complications.
- Instruct the client to splint the incision when coughing and deep breathing. Allow the client to provide a return demonstration.
- Instruct the client on arm and leg exercises to prevent complications.
- Instruct the client to report pain to the nursing staff. The majority of pain stems from the harvest site for the vein.
- Inform the client and family to expect the following postoperatively:
  - Endotracheal tube and mechanical ventilator for airway management for several hours following surgery
  - Inability to talk while endotracheal tube is in place
  - Sternal incision and possible leg incision
  - Early ambulation to prevent complications
  - Administration of analgesics for pain control
  - One to two mediastinal chest tubes
  - Indwelling urinary catheter
  - Pacemaker wires
  - Hemodynamic monitoring devices (pulmonary artery catheter, arterial line)
- Instruct the client to alter or discontinue regular medications as prescribed by the provider.
  - Medications frequently discontinued for CABG
    - Diuretics 2 to 3 days before surgery
    - Aspirin and other anticoagulants 1 week before surgery
  - Medications often continued for CABG
    - Potassium supplements
    - Scheduled antidysrhythmics, such as amiodarone
    - Scheduled antihypertensives, such as metoprolol, a beta-blocker, and diltiazem, a calcium-channel blocker
    - Insulin (clients who have diabetes mellitus and are insulin-dependent usually receive half the regular insulin dose)
- Assess the client and family anxiety levels surrounding the procedure. Qpcc
  - Encourage the client to verbalize his feelings.

INTRAPROCEDURE

- An extracardiac vein (saphenous vein), artery (usually the radial or mammary artery), or synthetic graft is used to bypass an obstruction in one or more of the coronary arteries.
- Most often, a median sternotomy incision is made to visualize the heart and the great vessels.
- The client is placed on cardiopulmonary bypass, and the client's core temperature might be lowered to decrease the rate of metabolism and demand for oxygen. A normal core temperature might be maintained during cardiopulmonary bypass to improve postoperative myocardial function and reduce postoperative complications.
- A cardioplegic solution is used to stop the heart. This prevents myocardial ischemia and allows for a motionless operative field.
- The artery or vein to be used is harvested.
- The harvested vessel is anastomosed from the aorta to the affected coronary artery distal to the occlusion.
- Once the bypass is complete, the hypothermic client is rewarmed by heat exchanges on the bypass machine. Grafts are monitored for patency and leakage as the client is weaned from the bypass machine and blood is redirected through coronary vasculature.
- Lastly, pacemaker wires might be sutured into the myocardium, and chest tubes are placed. The incision is closed with wire sutures, and the client is transported to the intensive care unit.

NURSING ACTIONS

- Provide padding to bony prominences to provide comfort and prevent skin breakdown.
- Communicate surgical progress to family members, if appropriate.
- Assist in monitoring urine output and blood loss.
- Document appropriate surgical events.
- Assist in arranging intensive care unit placement and communicate the client's postoperative needs.

POSTPROCEDURE

NURSING ACTIONS

- Maintain patent airway and adequate ventilation.
  - Monitor respiratory rate and effort.
  - Auscultate breath sounds. Report crackles.
  - Monitor SaO_2.
  - Document ventilator settings.
  - Suction as needed.
  - Assist with extubation.
- Encourage the client to splint the incision while deep breathing and coughing.
- Dangle and turn the client from side to side as tolerated within 2 hr following extubation. Assist the client to a chair within 24 hr. Ambulate the client 25 to 100 ft three times a day by first postoperative day.
- Consult respiratory services to aid in recovery and client education.

- Consult case management services to initiate discharge planning: need for home oxygen therapy, transfer to tertiary care facility.
- Continually monitor the client's heart rate and rhythm. Treat dysrhythmias per protocol.
- Maintain an adequate circulating blood volume.
  - Monitor blood pressure.
    - Hypotension might result in graft collapse.
    - Hypertension might result in bleeding from grafts and sutures.
    - Titrate IV drips (dopamine , dobutamine , milrinone, sodium nitroprusside) per protocol to control blood pressure and/or increase cardiac output.
  - Monitor hemodynamic pressures and catheter placement. Observe waveforms and markings on the catheter.
  - Monitor the client's level of consciousness. Assess neurological status every 30 to 60 min until the client awakens from anesthesia, then every 2 to 4 hr, or per facility policy.
  - Notify the surgeon of significant changes in values.
- Monitor chest tube patency and drainage.
  - Measure drainage at least once an hour.
  - Volume exceeding 150 mL/hr could be a sign of possible hemorrhage and should be reported to the surgeon.
  - Avoid dependent loops in tubing to facilitate drainage.
- Assess and control pain.
  - Determine source of pain (angina, incisional pain).
    - Anginal pain often radiates and is unaffected by breathing.
    - Incisional pain is localized, sharp, aching, burning, and often worsens with deep breathing.
- Administer analgesics as prescribed (morphine, fentanyl).
  - Pain will stimulate the sympathetic nervous system, resulting in increased heart rate and systemic vascular resistance.
  - Provide frequent and adequate doses to control pain. Maintain around-the-clock administration.
- Monitor fluid and electrolyte status.
  - Fluid administration is determined by blood pressure, pulmonary artery wedge pressure, right atrial pressure, cardiac output and index, systemic vascular resistance, blood loss, and urine output.
  - Follow provider or unit-specific orders for fluid administration.
  - Monitor the client for electrolyte imbalances, especially for hypokalemia and hyperkalemia.
- Prevent and monitor for infection.
  - Practice proper hand hygiene.
  - Use surgical aseptic technique during procedures such as dressing changes and suctioning.
  - Administer antibiotics.
  - Monitor WBC counts, incisional redness and drainage, and fever.
  - Monitor the client's temperature and provide warming measures if indicated.

CLIENT EDUCATION

- Instruct the client to monitor and report manifestations of infection, such as fever, incisional drainage, and redness.
- Instruct the client to treat angina.
  - Maintain a fresh supply of sublingual nitroglycerin.
  - Store nitroglycerin in a light-resistant container.
  - Discontinue activity and rest with the onset of pain. Follow directions for treating anginal pain.
  - Instruct the older female client that she might show milder symptoms (dyspnea, indigestion). Ⓖ
- Instruct the client to adhere to the pharmacological regimen.
- Instruct the client who has diabetes mellitus to closely monitor blood glucose levels.
- Encourage the client to consume a heart-healthy diet (low fat, low cholesterol, high fiber, low salt).
- Encourage the client to quit smoking if applicable. Provide resources on smoking cessation.
- Encourage physical activity. Consult the cardiac rehabilitation program or a physical therapist to devise a specific program.
- Discuss home environment and social supports. Consult case management to assist with home planning needs.
- Instruct the client to remain home during the first week after surgery and to resume normal activities slowly.
  - Week 2: possible return to work part time, increase in social activities
  - Week 3: lifting of up to 15 lb (avoidance of heavier lifting for 6 to 8 weeks)
- Clients can resume sexual activity based on the advice of the provider.
  - Walking one block or climbing two flights of stairs symptom-free generally indicates that it is safe for the client to resume normal sexual activity.
- Encourage the client to verbalize his feelings.

COMPLICATIONS

Pulmonary complications

These include the primary complication of atelectasis, as well as pneumonia and pulmonary edema.

NURSING ACTIONS

- While the client is intubated, suction every 1 to 2 hr and as needed.
- Turn the client every 2 hr, and advance him out of bed as soon as possible.
- Monitor breath sounds, SaO_2, ABGs, pulmonary artery pressures, cardiac output, and urine output and obtain a chest x-ray as indicated.

CLIENT EDUCATION: Encourage coughing, deep breathing, and use of an incentive spirometer. Explain that increasing activity reduces postoperative complications.

Hypothermia

Hypothermia can cause vasoconstriction, metabolic acidosis, and hypertension.

NURSING ACTIONS

- Monitor temperature, and provide warming measures, such as warm blankets and heat lamps.
- Monitor blood pressure.
- Administer vasodilators if prescribed.

CLIENT EDUCATION: Assure the client that shivering is common following surgery.

Decreased cardiac output

Decreased cardiac output can result from dysrhythmias, cardiac tamponade, hypovolemia, left ventricular failure, or MI.

Cardiac tamponade results from bleeding while chest tubes are occluded, causing fluid to build up in the pericardium. Increased pericardial fluid compresses heart chambers and inhibits effective pumping.

- Indications include a sudden decrease/cessation of chest-tube drainage following heavy drainage, jugular-venous distention with clear lung sounds, and equal pulmonary artery wedge pressure and central venous pressure values.

Hypovolemia might be the result of bleeding, decreased intravascular volume, or vasodilation; hypotension and decreased urine output are the results.

Left ventricular heart failure might occur with an MI or hypervolemia.

NURSING ACTIONS
- Monitor ECG, blood pressure, pulmonary artery pressures, cardiac output, urine output, and bleeding through the chest tube.
- Administer inotropic medications and fluid and blood products as prescribed.
- Treat dysrhythmias as prescribed.
  - Use pacemaker wires if heart block is present.
- Treatment of cardiac tamponade involves volume expansion (fluid administration) and an emergency sternotomy with drainage. Pericardiocentesis is avoided because blood might have clotted.

Electrolyte disturbances

Potassium and magnesium depletion is common.

NURSING ACTIONS
- Always dilute potassium supplements in adequate fluid (40 to 80 mEq in 100 mL of IV solution).
- Administer supplements via infusion pump to control the rate of delivery. The maximum administration rate varies from 10 to 40 mEq/hr.
- Administer supplements through a central catheter.
- Monitor ECG and electrolytes.

Neurologic deficits

Transient hypertension, hypotension, or a blood clot might cause an intraoperative cerebrovascular accident.

NURSING ACTIONS
- Assess neurologic status, including pupils, level of consciousness, and sensory and motor function.
- Maintain the client's blood pressure within prescribed parameters.

CLIENT EDUCATION
- Explain procedures to the client.
- Assure the client that memory loss and neurological deficits might be temporary.

Peripheral bypass grafts

Bypass graft surgery aims to restore adequate blood flow to the areas affected by peripheral artery disease.
- A peripheral bypass graft involves suturing graft material or autogenous saphenous veins proximal and distal to occluded area of an artery. This procedure improves blood supply to the area normally served by the blocked artery.
- If bypass surgery fails to restore circulation, the client might need to undergo amputation of the limb.

INDICATIONS
- Acute circulatory compromise in limb
- Severe pain at rest that interferes with the ability to work

CLIENT PRESENTATION

SUBJECTIVE DATA
- Numbness or burning pain to the lower extremity with exercise; might stop with rest (intermittent claudication)
- Numbness or burning pain to the lower extremity at rest; might wake the client at night; pain might be relieved by lowering the extremity below the level of the heart

OBJECTIVE DATA
- Decreased or absent pulses to feet.
- Dry, hairless, shiny skin on calves.
- Muscles might atrophy with advanced disease.
- Skin might be cold and dark colored.
- Feet and toes might be mottled and dusky, and toenails might be thick.
- Skin might become reddened (rubor) when extremity is dropped to a dependent position.
- Ulcers or lesions might be noted on toes (arterial ulcers) or ankles (venous ulcers).

CONSIDERATIONS

PREPROCEDURE

NURSING ACTIONS
- Assess the client and family's understanding of the procedure.
- Verify that the client has signed the informed consent form.
- Assess for allergies.
- Document baseline vital signs and peripheral pulses.
- Administer prophylactic antibiotic therapy as prescribed.
- Instruct the client to maintain NPO status for at least 8 hr prior to surgery.

CLIENT EDUCATION
- Include information about postoperative pain management and teach deep breathing/incentive spirometer exercises.
- Advise the client not to cross his legs.
- The client might have an arterial line inserted for blood and blood pressure.
- Explain that pedal pulses will be checked frequently.

INTRAPROCEDURE

NURSING ACTIONS

- Provide padding to bony prominences to provide comfort and to prevent skin breakdown.
- Communicate surgical progress to family members, if appropriate.
- Assist in monitoring urine output and blood loss.
- Document appropriate surgical events.
- Communicate the client's postoperative needs to the postanesthesia care unit.

POSTPROCEDURE

NURSING ACTIONS

- Assess and monitor vital signs every 15 min for 1 hr and then hourly after the first hour (or per facility policy).
- Follow standing orders to maintain blood pressure within the prescribed range. Hypotension might reduce blood flow to graft, and hypertension might cause bleeding.
- Assess and monitor the operative limb every 15 min for 1 hr and then hourly after that, paying particular attention to the following:
  - Incision site for bleeding.
  - Peripheral pulses, capillary refill, skin color/temperature, and sensory and motor function for signs of bypass graft occlusion. In clients who have dark skin, assess nail beds and soles of feet to detect early cyanosis.
  - Site is marked with an indelible marker.
- Administer IV fluids as prescribed.
- Assess the type of pain experienced by the client. **Qs**
  - Throbbing pain is experienced due to an increase in blood flow to extremity.
  - Ischemic pain is often difficult to relieve with opioid administration.
- Administer analgesics, such as morphine sulfate and fentanyl.
- Administer antibiotics as prescribed.
- Use surgical aseptic technique for dressing changes.
- Monitor incision sites for evidence of infection, such as erythema, tenderness, and drainage.
- Administer anticoagulant therapy, such as warfarin, heparin, and enoxaparin to prevent reocclusion.
- Administer antiplatelet therapy, such as clopidogrel, tirofiban, and aspirin.
- Help the client turn, cough, and deep breathe every 2 hr.
- Maintain bed rest for 18 to 24 hr. The leg should be kept straight during this time.
- Assist the client to get out of bed and ambulate. Encourage the use of a walker initially.
- Discourage the client from sitting for long periods of time.
- Apply antiembolic stockings to promote venous return.
- Set up a progressive exercise program that includes walking. Consider a physical therapy consult.

CLIENT EDUCATION

- Advise the client to completely abstain from smoking. Suggest smoking-cessation program.
- Reinforce activity restrictions.
- Remind the client to avoid crossing his legs.
- Instruct the client to avoid elevating the legs above heart level.
- Advise the client to avoid risk factors for atherosclerosis (smoking, sedentary lifestyle, uncontrolled diabetes mellitus).
- Teach techniques of foot inspection and care.
  - Keep feet dry and clean.
  - Avoid extreme temperatures.
  - Use lotion.
  - Avoid socks with tight cuffs.
  - Wear clean white cotton socks and always wear shoes.

COMPLICATIONS

Graft occlusion

The graft might occlude due to reduced blood flow and clot formation. Occurs primarily in first 24 hr after the procedure.

NURSING ACTIONS

- Notify the provider immediately for changes in pedal pulse, extremity color, or temperature.
- Prepare the client for thrombectomy or thrombolytic therapy.
- Monitor for bleeding with thrombolytics.
- Monitor coagulation studies.
- Monitor for anaphylaxis.

Compartment syndrome

Pressure from tissue swelling or bleeding within a compartment or a restricted space causes reduced blood flow to the area. Untreated, the affected tissue will become necrotic and die.

NURSING ACTIONS

- Assess for worsening pain, swelling, and tense or taut skin.
- Report unusual findings to the provider immediately.
- Prepare the client for a fasciotomy to relieve compartmental pressure.

Infection

Infection of the surgical site might result in the loss of the graft and increased ischemia.

NURSING ACTIONS

- Assess the wound for increased redness, swelling, and drainage.
- Monitor WBC count and temperature.
- Collect specimens (wound or blood cultures).
- Administer antibiotic therapy.

CLIENT EDUCATION: Advise the client to notify the provider of decreased sensation, increased ischemic pain, redness, or swelling at the incisional site or in the affected limb.

Application Exercises

1. A nurse is caring for a client who is 4 hr postoperative following coronary artery bypass grafting (CABG) surgery. He is able to inspire 200 mL with the incentive spirometer, then refuses to cough because he is tired and it hurts too much. Which of the following actions should the nurse take?

   A. Allow the client to rest, and return in 1 hr.

   B. Administer IV bolus analgesic, and return in 15 min.

   C. Document the 200 mL as an appropriate inspired volume.

   D. Tell the client that he must try to cough if he does not want to get pneumonia.

2. A nurse is caring for a client following peripheral bypass graft surgery of the left lower extremity. Which of the following findings pose an immediate concern? (Select all that apply.)

   A. Trace of bloody drainage on dressing

   B. Capillary refill of affected limb of 6 seconds

   C. Mottled appearance of the limb

   D. Throbbing pain of affected limb that is decreased following IV bolus analgesic

   E. Pulse of 2+ in the affected limb

3. A nurse educator is reviewing the use of cardiopulmonary bypass during surgery for coronary artery bypass grafting with a group of nurses. Which of the following statements should the nurse include in the discussion? (Select all that apply.)

   A. "The client's demand for oxygen is lowered."

   B. "Motion of the heart ceases."

   C. "Rewarming of the client takes place."

   D. "The client's metabolic rate is increased."

   E. "Blood flow to the heart is stopped."

4. A nurse is caring for a client following an angioplasty that was inserted through the femoral artery. While turning the client, the nurse discovers blood underneath the client's lower back. Which of the following findings should the nurse suspect?

   A. Retroperitoneal bleeding

   B. Cardiac tamponade

   C. Bleeding from the incisional site

   D. Heart failure

5. A nurse is completing the admission assessment of a client who will undergo peripheral bypass graft surgery on the left leg. Which of the following findings should the nurse expect?

   A. Rubor of the affected leg when elevated

   B. 3+ dorsal pedal pulse in left foot

   C. Thin, peeling toenails of left foot

   D. Report of intermittent claudication in the affected leg

---

PRACTICE Active Learning Scenario

A nurse is developing the plan of care for a client who is returning to the unit following angioplasty. What should be included in the plan of care? Use the ATI Active Learning Template: Therapeutic Procedure to complete this item.

NURSING INTERVENTIONS: Describe five postprocedure nursing actions.

POTENTIAL COMPLICATIONS:
• Describe at least two.
• Describe at least two actions related to each of these complications.

Application Exercises Key

1. A. Turning, coughing, and deep breathing should be performed every 2 hr to promote oxygenation and circulation.

   B. **CORRECT:** Providing adequate analgesia and returning in 15 min will reduce pain and improve coughing effectiveness.

   C. This is not an adequate inspired air volume to promote effective oxygenation.

   D. This intervention is non-therapeutic communication.

   Ⓝ *NCLEX® Connection: Pharmacological and Parenteral Therapies, Pharmacological Pain Management*

2. A. A trace of bloody drainage on the dressing is an expected finding and does not require immediate concern.

   B. **CORRECT:** Capillary refill greater than 3 seconds is outside the expected reference range and should be reported to the provider.

   C. **CORRECT:** Mottled appearance of the affected extremity is an unexpected finding and should be reported to the provider.

   D. Pain that is decreased following IV bolus analgesia is an expected finding and does not require immediate concern.

   E. Pulse of 2+ in the affected extremity is an expected finding and does not require immediate concern.

   Ⓝ *NCLEX® Connection: Reduction of Risk Potential, Potential for Complications of Diagnostic Tests/Treatments/Procedures*

3. A. **CORRECT:** The use of cardiopulmonary bypass reduces the client's demand for oxygen, which reduces the risk of inadequate oxygenation of vital organs.

   B. **CORRECT:** Motion of the heart ceases during cardiopulmonary bypass to allow for placement of the graft near the affected coronary artery.

   C. **CORRECT:** The core body temperature is lowered for the procedure, and rewarming then occurs through heat exchanges on the cardiopulmonary bypass machine.

   D. The use of cardiopulmonary bypass decreases the rate of metabolism.

   E. Blood flow to the heart is maintained by the action of the cardiopulmonary bypass machine.

   Ⓝ *NCLEX® Connection: Reduction of Risk Potential, Potential for Complications of Diagnostic Tests/Treatments/Procedures*

4. A. Retroperitoneal bleeding is internal bleeding.

   B. Cardiac tamponade includes manifestations of bleeding in the pericardial sac, which is internal.

   C. **CORRECT:** Bleeding is occurring from the incision site and then draining under the client. The nurse should assess the incision for hematoma, apply pressure, monitor the client, and notify the provider.

   D. Heart failure does not including findings of blood underneath the client's lower back.

   Ⓝ *NCLEX® Connection: Reduction of Risk Potential, Potential for Complications of Diagnostic Tests/Treatments/Procedures*

5. A. Reddening (rubor) of a leg affected by peripheral artery disease occurs when it is placed in a dependent position.

   B. Pulses are decreased or absent in the feet in cases of peripheral artery disease.

   C. Toenails are thickened in cases of peripheral artery disease.

   D. **CORRECT:** A client who has peripheral artery disease might report that numbness or burning pain in the extremity ceases with rest (intermittent claudication).

   Ⓝ *NCLEX® Connection: Physiological Adaptation, Alterations in Body Systems*

PRACTICE Answer

Using ATI Active Learning Template: Therapeutic Procedure

NURSING INTERVENTIONS

- Assess vital signs every 15 min × 4, every 30 min × 2, every hour × 4, and then every 4 hr (or per facility protocol).
- Assess the groin site with vital signs.
- Maintain bed rest in supine position with leg straight for prescribed time.
- Conduct continuous cardiac monitoring for dysrhythmia.
- Administer antiplatelet or thrombolytic agents as prescribed.
- Administer anxiolytics and analgesics as prescribed.
- Monitor urine output and administer IV fluids for hydration.
- Assist with sheath removal from insertion site.

POTENTIAL COMPLICATIONS

- Cardiac tamponade: Notify the provider; administer IV fluids to manage hypotension; obtain chest x-ray or echocardiogram; prepare for pericardiocentesis.
- Hematoma formation: Monitor sensation, color, capillary refill, and pulse in extremity distal to insertion site; hold pressure for uncontrolled oozing/bleeding; notify the provider.
- Allergic reaction: Monitor the client; have resuscitation equipment available; administer diphenhydramine or epinephrine as needed.
- External bleeding: Monitor insertion site for bleeding or swelling; apply pressure to insertion site; keep client's leg straight.
- Embolism: Monitor for chest pain; monitor vital signs and SaO₂.
- Retroperitoneal bleeding: Assess for flank pain and hypotension; notify the provider; administer IV fluids and blood products as prescribed.
- Restenosis of vessel: Assess ECG pattern and for report of chest pain; notify the provider; prepare for return to cardiac catheterization laboratory.

Ⓝ *NCLEX® Connection: Physiological Adaptation, Alterations in Body Systems*

UNIT 4 NURSING CARE OF CLIENTS WHO HAVE
CARDIOVASCULAR DISORDERS
SECTION: CARDIAC DISORDERS

CHAPTER 31 *Angina and Myocardial Infarction*

The continuum from angina to myocardial infarction (MI) is acute coronary syndrome. Symptoms of acute coronary syndrome are due to an imbalance between myocardial oxygen supply and demand.

Angina pectoris is a warning sign of an impending acute MI. Women and older adults do not always experience manifestations typically associated with angina or MI. ©

The area of infarction in clients experiencing a myocardial infarction (MI) develops over minutes to hours. Early recognition and treatment of an acute MI is essential to prevent death.

Research shows improved outcomes following an MI in clients treated with aspirin, beta-blockers, and angiotensin-converting enzyme inhibitors or angiotensin receptor blockers.

When blood flow to the heart is compromised, ischemia causes chest pain. Anginal pain is often described as a tight squeezing, heavy pressure, or constricting feeling in the chest. The pain can radiate to the jaw, neck, or arm. Pain unrelieved by rest or nitroglycerin and lasting for more than 15 min differentiates an MI from angina.

An abrupt interruption of oxygen to the heart muscle produces myocardial ischemia. Ischemia can lead to tissue necrosis (infarction) if blood supply and oxygen are not restored. Ischemia is reversible. An infarction results in permanent damage. When the cardiac muscle suffers ischemic injury, cardiac enzymes are released into the bloodstream, providing specific markers of MI.

HEALTH PROMOTION AND DISEASE PREVENTION

- Maintain an exercise routine to remain physically active. Consult with a provider before starting any exercise regimen.
- Have cholesterol level and blood pressure checked regularly.
- Consume a diet low in saturated fats and sodium. Consult with a provider regarding diet restrictions.
- Promote smoking cessation.

ASSESSMENT

Types of angina

Stable (exertional) angina occurs with exercise or emotional stress and is relieved by rest or nitroglycerin.

Unstable (preinfarction) angina occurs with exercise or at rest, but increases in occurrence, severity, and duration over time.

Variant (Prinzmetal's) angina is due to a coronary artery spasm, often occurring during periods of rest.

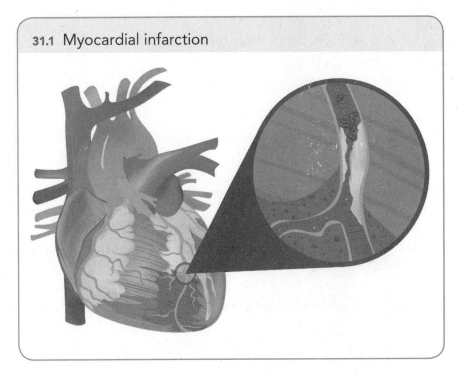

31.1 Myocardial infarction

RISK FACTORS

- Male gender or postmenopausal women
- Ethnic background
- Sedentary lifestyle
- Hypertension
- Tobacco use
- Hyperlipidemia
- Obesity
- Excessive alcohol consumption
- Metabolic disorders (diabetes mellitus, hyperthyroidism)
- Methamphetamine or cocaine use
- Stress (with ineffective coping skills)
- An increased risk of coronary artery disease exists for older adult clients who are physically inactive, have one or more chronic diseases (hypertension, heart failure, and diabetes mellitus), or have lifestyle habits (smoking and diet) that contribute to atherosclerosis. Atherosclerotic changes related to aging predispose the heart to poor blood perfusion and oxygen delivery. ⓒ
- Incidence of cardiac disease increases with age, especially in the presence of hypertension, diabetes mellitus, hypercholesterolemia, elevated homocysteine, and highly sensitive C-reactive protein (HS-CRP).

EXPECTED FINDINGS

- Anxiety, feeling of impending doom
- Chest pain: substernal or precordial
  - Can radiate down the shoulder or arm, or present as jaw pain
  - Can be described as a crushing or aching pressure
- Nausea
- Dizziness

PHYSICAL ASSESSMENT FINDINGS

- Pallor, and cool, clammy skin
- Tachycardia and heart palpitations
- Tachypnea and shortness of breath
- Diaphoresis
- Vomiting
- Decreased level of consciousness

LABORATORY TESTS

Cardiac enzymes released with cardiac muscle injury:

- **Myoglobin:** Earliest marker of injury to cardiac or skeletal muscle. Levels no longer evident after 24 hr.
- **Creatine kinase-MB:** Peaks around 24 hr after onset of chest pain. Levels no longer evident after 3 days.
- **Troponin I or T:** Any positive value indicates damage to cardiac tissue and should be reported.
  - **Troponin I:** Levels no longer evident after 7 to 10 days.
  - **Troponin T:** Levels no longer evident after 10 to 14 days.

DIAGNOSTIC PROCEDURES

Refer to **CHAPTER 27: CARDIOVASCULAR DIAGNOSTIC AND THERAPEUTIC PROCEDURES**.

Electrocardiogram (ECG)

Recording of electrical activity of the heart over time

NURSING ACTIONS

- Assess for changes on serial ECGs.
- Angina: ST depression and/or T-wave inversion indicates presence of ischemia.
- MI: T-wave inversion indicates ischemia; ST-segment elevation indicates injury; abnormal Q-wave indicates necrosis.

31.2 Anginal pain

Possible areas of referred pain:
Jaw, chest, shoulders, neck, arms

31.3 Assessment

Angina	*Myocardial infarction*
Precipitated by exertion or stress	Can occur without cause, often in the morning after rest
Relieved by rest or nitroglycerin	Relieved only by opioids
Symptoms last less than 15 min	Symptoms last more than 30 min
Not associated with nausea, epigastric distress, dyspnea, anxiety, diaphoresis	Associated with nausea, epigastric distress, dyspnea, anxiety, diaphoresis

Stress test

Also known as exercise electrocardiography. Client tolerance of activity is tested using a treadmill, bicycle, or medication to evaluate response to increased heart rate.

Thallium scan

Assesses for ischemia or necrosis. Radioisotopes cannot reach areas with decreased or absent perfusion, and the areas appear as "cold spots."

NURSING ACTIONS: Instruct the client to avoid smoking and consuming caffeinated beverages 4 hr prior to the procedure. These can affect the test.

Cardiac catheterization

- A coronary angiogram, also called a cardiac catheterization, is an invasive diagnostic procedure used to evaluate the presence and degree of coronary artery blockage.
- Angiography involves the insertion of a catheter into a femoral (sometimes a brachial) vessel and threading it into the right or left side of the heart. Coronary artery narrowing and occlusions are identified by the injection of contrast media under fluoroscopy.

NURSING ACTIONS
- Ensure the client understands the procedure prior to signing informed consent. Qᴘᴄᴄ
- Ensure that the client remains NPO 8 hr prior to procedure.
- Ensure that the client and family understand the procedure.
- Assess for iodine/shellfish allergy (contrast media).

MI CLASSIFICATION

MIs are classified based on:
- Affected area of the heart: anterior, lateral, inferior, or posterior
- ECG changes produced: ST elevation myocardial infarction vs. non-ST elevation myocardial infarction
- The time frame within the progression of the infarction: acute, evolving, old

PATIENT-CENTERED CARE

NURSING CARE

- Monitor the following.
  - Vital signs every 5 min until stable, then every hour
  - Serial ECG, continuous cardiac monitoring
  - Location, precipitating factors, severity, quality, and duration of pain
  - Hourly urine output: greater than 30 mL/hr indicates renal perfusion
  - Laboratory data: cardiac enzymes, electrolytes, ABGs
- Administer oxygen: 2 to 4 L/min.
- Obtain and maintain IV access.
- Promote energy conservation. Cluster nursing interventions.

MEDICATIONS

Vasodilators

Nitroglycerin prevents coronary artery vasospasm and reduces preload and afterload, decreasing myocardial oxygen demand.

NURSING CONSIDERATIONS
- Used to treat angina and help control blood pressure.
- Used cautiously with other antihypertensive medications.
- Can cause orthostatic hypotension.

CLIENT EDUCATION FOR CHEST PAIN
- Instruct the client to stop activity and rest.
- Instruct the client to place a nitroglycerin tablet under the tongue to dissolve (quick absorption).
- If pain is unrelieved in 5 min, the client should call 911 or be driven to an emergency department.
- The client can take up to two more doses of nitroglycerin at 5-min intervals.
- Remind the client that a headache is a common side effect of this medication.
- Encourage the client to sit and lie down slowly.

Analgesics

Morphine sulfate is an opioid analgesic used to treat moderate to severe pain. Analgesics act on the mu and kappa receptors that help alleviate pain. Activation of these receptors produces analgesia (pain relief), respiratory depression, euphoria, sedation, and decreases in myocardial oxygen consumption and gastrointestinal (GI) motility.

> ! Use cautiously with clients who have asthma or emphysema due to the risk of respiratory depression.

NURSING CONSIDERATIONS
- For the client having chest pain, assess pain every 5 to 15 min.
- Watch for manifestations of respiratory depression, especially in older adults. If respirations are 12/min or less, stop medication, and notify the provider immediately. ⓖ
- Monitor vital signs for hypotension and decreased respirations.
- Assess for nausea and vomiting.

CLIENT EDUCATION
- If nausea and vomiting persist, advise the client to notify a nurse.
- Teach the client to use the PCA pump, if applicable. The client is the only person who should push the medication administration button. Reassure the client that the safety lockout mechanism on the PCA pump prevents overdosing of the medication.

Beta-blockers

- Metoprolol has antidysrhythmic and antihypertensive properties that decrease the imbalance between myocardial oxygen supply and demand by reducing afterload and slowing heart rate.
- In an acute MI, beta-blockers decrease infarct size and improve short- and long-term survival rates.

NURSING CONSIDERATIONS
- Beta-blockers can cause bradycardia and hypotension. Hold the medication if the apical pulse rate is less than 60/min, and notify the provider. Qs
- Avoid giving to clients who have asthma. Cardioselective beta blockers (which affect only beta$_1$ receptors), such as metoprolol, are preferred because they minimize the effects on the respiratory system.
- Use with caution in clients who have heart failure.
- Monitor for decreased level of consciousness, crackles in the lungs, and chest discomfort.

CLIENT EDUCATION
- Encourage the client to sit and lie down slowly.
- Remind the client to notify the provider immediately of shortness of breath, edema, weight gain, or cough.

Thrombolytic agents

- Alteplase and reteplase are used to break up blood clots.
- Thrombolytic agents have similar side effects and contraindications as anticoagulants.
- For best results, give within 6 hr of infarction.

NURSING CONSIDERATIONS
- Assess for contraindications (active bleeding, peptic ulcer disease, history of stroke, recent trauma).
- Monitor for effects of bleeding (mental status changes, hematuria).
- Monitor bleeding times: PT, aPTT, INR, fibrinogen levels, and CBC.
- Monitor for the same side effects as anticoagulants (thrombocytopenia, anemia, hemorrhage).
- Administer streptokinase slowly to prevent hypotension.

CLIENT EDUCATION: Remind the client of the risk for bruising and bleeding while on this medication.

Antiplatelet agents

- Aspirin and clopidogrel prevent platelets from forming together, which can produce arterial clotting.
- Aspirin prevents vasoconstriction. Due to this and antiplatelet effects, it should be administered with nitroglycerin at the onset of chest pain. QEBP

NURSING CONSIDERATIONS
- Antiplatelet agents can cause GI upset.
- Use cautiously with clients who have a history of GI ulcers.
- Tinnitus (ringing in the ears) can be a sign of aspirin toxicity.

CLIENT EDUCATION
- Remind the client of the risk for bruising and bleeding while on this medication.
- Encourage the client to use aspirin tablets with enteric coating and to take with food.
- Tell the client to report ringing in the ears.

Anticoagulants

Heparin and enoxaparin are used to prevent clots from becoming larger or other clots from forming.

NURSING CONSIDERATIONS
- Assess for contraindications (active bleeding, peptic ulcer disease, history of stroke, recent trauma).
- Monitor platelet levels and bleeding times: PT, aPTT, INR, and CBC.
- Monitor for adverse effects of anticoagulants (thrombocytopenia, anemia, hemorrhage).

CLIENT EDUCATION: Remind the client of the risk for bruising and bleeding while on this medication.

Glycoprotein IIB/IIIA inhibitors

Eptifibatide is used to prevent binding of fibrinogen to platelets, in turn blocking platelet aggregation. In combination with aspirin therapy, IIB/IIA inhibitors are standard therapy.

NURSING CONSIDERATIONS
- This medication can cause active bleeding.
- Monitor platelet levels.

CLIENT EDUCATION: Instruct the client to report evidence of bleeding during medication therapy.

INTERPROFESSIONAL CARE

- Pain management services can be consulted if pain persists or is uncontrolled.
- Cardiac rehabilitation care can be consulted if the client has prolonged weakness and needs assistance with increasing level of activity.
- Nutritional services can be consulted for diet modification to promote food choices low in sodium and saturated fat.

THERAPEUTIC PROCEDURES

- Percutaneous transluminal coronary angioplasty (PTCA)
- Bypass graft (also known as CABG)

CLIENT EDUCATION

- Cardiac rehabilitation should be consulted for a specific exercise program related to the heart.
- Nutritional services, such as a dietitian, can be consulted for diet modification or weight management.
- Instruct the client to monitor and report signs of infection, such as fever, incisional drainage, and redness.
- Teach the client to avoid straining, strenuous exercise, or emotional stress when possible.
- Regarding response to chest pain: follow instructions on use of sublingual nitroglycerin.
- If client is a smoker, encourage smoking cessation.
- Encourage the client to remain active and to exercise regularly.

COMPLICATIONS

Acute MI

A complication of angina not relieved by rest or nitroglycerin

NURSING ACTIONS
- Administer oxygen.
- Notify the provider immediately.

Heart failure/cardiogenic shock

Injury to the left ventricle can lead to decreased cardiac output and heart failure. Progressive heart failure can lead to cardiogenic shock.
- This is a serious complication of pump failure, commonly following an MI of 40% blockage.
- Manifestations include tachycardia; hypotension; inadequate urinary output; altered level of consciousness; respiratory distress (crackles and tachypnea); cool, clammy skin; decreased peripheral pulses; and chest pain.

NURSING ACTIONS
- Administer oxygen. Intubation and ventilation can be required.
- Administer IV morphine, diuretics, and/or nitroglycerin to decrease preload. Administer IV vasopressors and/or positive inotropes to increase cardiac output and maintain organ perfusion.
- Maintain continuous hemodynamic monitoring.

Ischemic mitral regurgitation

Evidenced by development of a new cardiac murmur.

NURSING ACTIONS
- Administer oxygen.
- Notify the provider immediately.

Ventricular aneurysms/rupture

Can be due to necrosis from MI. Can present as sudden chest pain, dysrhythmias, and severe hypotension

NURSING ACTIONS
- Administer oxygen.
- Notify the provider immediately.

Dysrhythmias

- An inferior wall MI can lead to an injury to the AV node, resulting in bradycardia and second-degree AV heart block.
- An anterior wall MI can lead to an injury to the ventricle, resulting in premature ventricular contractions, bundle branch block, or complete heart block.

NURSING ACTIONS
- Monitor ECG and vital signs.
- Administer oxygen.
- Administer antidysrhythmic medications.
- Prepare for cardiac pacemaker if needed.

Application Exercises

1. A nurse is admitting a client who has a suspected myocardial infarction (MI) and a history of angina. Which of the following findings will help the nurse distinguish angina from an MI?

   A. Angina can be relieved with rest and nitroglycerin.

   B. The pain of an MI resolves in less than 15 min.

   C. The type of activity that causes an MI can be identified.

   D. Angina can occur for longer than 30 min.

2. A nurse on a cardiac unit is reviewing the laboratory findings of a client who has a diagnosis of myocardial infarction (MI) and reports that his dyspnea began 2 weeks ago. Which of the following cardiac enzymes would confirm the MI occurred 14 days ago?

   A. CK-MB

   B. Troponin I

   C. Troponin T

   D. Myoglobin

3. A nurse is caring for a client who asks why her provider prescribed a daily aspirin. Which of the following is an appropriate response by the nurse?

   A. "Aspirin reduces the formation of blood clots that could cause a heart attack."

   B. "Aspirin relieves the pain due to myocardial ischemia."

   C. "Aspirin dissolves clots that are forming in your coronary arteries."

   D. "Aspirin relieves headaches that are caused by other medications."

4. A nurse is teaching a client who has angina about a new prescription for metoprolol. Which of the following statements by the client indicates understanding of the teaching?

   A. "I should place the tablet under my tongue."

   B. "I should have my clotting time checked weekly."

   C. "I will report any ringing in my ears."

   D. "I will call my doctor if my pulse rate is less than 60."

5. A nurse is presenting a community education program on recommended lifestyle changes to prevent angina and myocardial infarction. Which of the following changes should the nurse recommend be made first?

   A. Diet modification

   B. Relaxation exercises

   C. Smoking cessation

   D. Taking omega-3 capsules

Application Exercises Key

1. A. **CORRECT:** Angina can be relieved by rest and nitroglycerin.

    B. Pain associated with an MI usually lasts longer than 30 min and requires opioid analgesics for relief.

    C. There is no specific type of activity that causes an MI. It can occur following rest.

    D. The pain of angina usually occurs for 15 min or less.

    Ⓝ *NCLEX® Connection: Physiological Adaptation, Hemodynamics*

2. A. The creatinine kinase MB levels are no longer evident after 3 days.

    B. Troponin I levels are no longer evident after 7 to 10 days.

    C. **CORRECT:** The Troponin T level will still be evident 10 to 14 days following an MI.

    D. Myoglobin levels are no longer evident after 24 hr.

    Ⓝ *NCLEX® Connection: Reduction of Risk Potential, Laboratory Values*

3. A. **CORRECT:** Aspirin decreases platelet aggregation that can cause a myocardial infarction.

    B. One aspirin per day is not sufficient to alleviate ischemic pain.

    C. Aspirin does not dissolve clots.

    D. Other medications can cause headaches, but one aspirin per day is not administered as an analgesic.

    Ⓝ *NCLEX® Connection: Pharmacological and Parenteral Therapies, Medication Administration*

4. A. Lopressor is administered orally, not sublingually.

    B. Lopressor does not affect bleeding or clotting time. The client should have CBC and blood glucose checked periodically.

    C. Ringing in the ears is not an adverse effect of the medication. Dry mouth and mucous membranes can occur.

    D. **CORRECT:** The client is advised to notify the provider if bradycardia (pulse rate less than 60) occurs.

    Ⓝ *NCLEX® Connection: Pharmacological and Parenteral Therapies, Medication Administration*

5. A. The nurse should recommend changing the diet to decrease consumption of sodium and saturated fat; however, there is another change the clients should plan to make first.

    B. The nurse should recommend using relaxation exercise to cope with stress; however, there is another change the clients should plan to make first.

    C. **CORRECT:** According to the airway, breathing, and circulation (ABC) priority-setting framework, the first change the nurse should recommend the clients take is to stop smoking. Nicotine causes vasoconstriction, elevates blood pressure, and narrows coronary arteries.

    D. The nurse should recommend taking omega-3 capsules to increase consumption of good cholesterol; however, there is another change the clients should plan to make first.

    Ⓝ *NCLEX® Connection: Health Promotion and Maintenance, Health Promotion/Disease Prevention*

PRACTICE Active Learning Scenario

A nurse is teaching a client who has new diagnosis of angina about coronary syndrome. What information should the nurse include in the teaching? Use the ATI Active Learning Template: System Disorder to complete this item.

RISK FACTORS: Describe five.

CLIENT EDUCATION: Describe at least two teaching points the nurse can use to help the client decrease risk of having angina or an MI.

EXPECTED FINDINGS

- List five subjective findings.
- Describe four physical assessment findings.

PRACTICE Answer

Using the ATI Active Learning Template: System Disorder

RISK FACTORS

- Male gender or postmenopausal women
- Sedentary lifestyle
- Hypertension
- Substance use (tobacco, cocaine, methamphetamine, excessive alcohol)
- Hyperlipidemia
- Metabolic disorders (diabetes mellitus, hyperthyroidism)
- Stress (with ineffective coping skills)

CLIENT EDUCATION

- Teach the client to have routine cholesterol, blood pressure, and blood sugar screenings.
- Encourage the client to participate in regular physical activity for exercise and stress reduction.

EXPECTED FINDINGS

- Subjective findings: Feeling of impending doom; chest pain, pressure, or crushing radiating to the arm or jaw; nausea; dizziness; anxiety
- Physical assessment findings: Pale, cool, clammy skin; tachycardia; tachypnea; diaphoresis

Ⓝ *NCLEX® Connection: Physiological Adaptation, Alterations in Body Systems*

UNIT 4   NURSING CARE OF CLIENTS WHO HAVE
CARDIOVASCULAR DISORDERS
SECTION: CARDIAC DISORDERS

CHAPTER 32   *Heart Failure and Pulmonary Edema*

Heart failure occurs when the heart muscle is unable to pump effectively, resulting in inadequate cardiac output, myocardial hypertrophy, and pulmonary/systemic congestion. The heart is unable to maintain adequate circulation to meet tissue needs.

Heart failure is the result of an acute or chronic cardiopulmonary problem, such as systemic hypertension, myocardial infarction (MI), pulmonary hypertension, dysrhythmias, valvular heart disease, pericarditis, or cardiomyopathy. (32.1)

Pulmonary edema is a severe, life-threatening accumulation of fluid in the alveoli and interstitial spaces of the lung that can result from severe heart failure.

Heart failure

New York Heart Association's functional classification scale

The severity of heart failure is graded on the New York Heart Association's (NYHA) functional classification scale indicating the level of activity it takes to make the client symptomatic (chest pain or shortness of breath).

CLASS I: Client exhibits no symptoms with activity.

CLASS II: Client has symptoms with ordinary exertion.

CLASS III: Client displays symptoms with minimal exertion.

CLASS IV: Client has symptoms at rest.

American College of Cardiology and American Heart Association staging heart failure

American College of Cardiology and American Heart Association developed an evidence-based guidelines for staging and managing heart failure in comparison with the NYHA system.

A: High risk for developing heart failure

B: Cardiac structural abnormalities or remodeling but no heart failure symptoms

C: Current or prior symptoms of heart failure

D: Refractory end-stage heart failure

Low-output heart failure

Low-output heart failure can initially occur on either the left or right side of the heart.
- Left-sided heart (ventricular) failure results in inadequate left ventricle (cardiac) output and consequently in inadequate tissue perfusion.
  ○ Systolic heart (ventricular) failure (ejection fraction below 40%, pulmonary and systemic congestion)
  ○ Diastolic heart (ventricular) failure (inadequate relaxation or "stiffening" prevents ventricular filling)
- Right-sided heart (ventricular) failure results in inadequate right ventricle output and systemic venous congestion (peripheral edema).

High-output heart failure

An uncommon form of heart failure is high-output failure, in which cardiac output is normal or above normal.

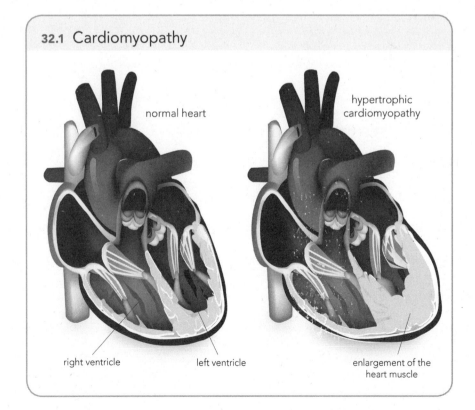

32.1 Cardiomyopathy

normal heart

hypertrophic cardiomyopathy

right ventricle   left ventricle   enlargement of the heart muscle

HEALTH PROMOTION AND DISEASE PREVENTION

- Maintain an exercise routine to remain physically active, and consult with the provider before starting any exercise regimen.
- Consume a diet low in sodium, along with fluid restrictions, and consult with the provider regarding diet specifications.
- Refrain from smoking.
- Follow medication regimen, and follow up with the provider as needed.

ASSESSMENT

RISK FACTORS

- Systolic blood pressure is elevated in older adults, putting them at risk for coronary artery disease and heart failure. Ⓖ
- Some medications can increase the risk of heart failure or worsen manifestations in older adult clients.

Left-sided heart (ventricular) failure

- Hypertension
- Coronary artery disease, angina, MI
- Valvular disease (mitral and aortic)

Right-sided heart (ventricular) failure

- Left-sided heart (ventricular) failure
- Right ventricular MI
- Pulmonary problems (COPD, pulmonary fibrosis)

High-output heart failure

- Increased metabolic needs
- Septicemia (fever)
- Anemia
- Hyperthyroidism

Cardiomyopathy

- Coronary artery disease
- Infection or inflammation of the heart muscle
- Various cancer treatments
- Prolonged alcohol use
- Heredity

EXPECTED FINDINGS

The presence of other chronic illnesses (lung disease, kidney failure) can mask the presence of heart failure in older adult clients. Ⓖ

Left-sided failure

- Dyspnea, orthopnea (shortness of breath while lying down), nocturnal dyspnea
- Fatigue
- Displaced apical pulse (hypertrophy)
- S_3 heart sound (gallop)
- Pulmonary congestion (dyspnea, cough, bibasilar crackles)
- Frothy sputum (can be blood-tinged)
- Altered mental status
- Manifestations of organ failure, such as oliguria (decrease in urine output)

Right-sided failure

- Jugular vein distention
- Ascending dependent edema (legs, ankles, sacrum)
- Abdominal distention, ascites
- Fatigue, weakness
- Nausea and anorexia
- Polyuria at rest (nocturnal)
- Liver enlargement (hepatomegaly) and tenderness
- Weight gain

Cardiomyopathy (leading to heart failure)

Blood circulation to the lungs is impaired when the cardiac pump is compromised. **(32.1)**

FOUR TYPES
- Dilated (most common)
- Hypertrophic
- Arrhythmogenic right ventricular
- Restrictive

MANIFESTATIONS
- Fatigue, weakness
- Heart failure (left with dilated type, right with restrictive type)
- Dysrhythmias (heart block)
- S_3 gallop
- Cardiomegaly (enlarged heart), more severe with dilated type
- Angina (hypertrophic type)

LABORATORY TESTS

Human B-type natriuretic peptides (hBNP)

In clients who have dyspnea, elevated hBNP confirms a diagnosis of heart failure rather than a problem originating in the respiratory system. hBNP levels direct the aggressiveness of treatment interventions.
- Less than 100 pg/mL indicates no heart failure.
- 100 to 300 pg/mL suggests heart failure is present.
- Greater than 300 pg/mL indicates mild heart failure.
- Greater than 600 pg/mL indicates moderate heart failure.
- Greater than 900 pg/mL indicates severe heart failure.

DIAGNOSTIC PROCEDURES

Hemodynamic monitoring

- Heart failure generally results in increased central venous pressure (CVP), increased pulmonary wedge pressure (PAWP), increased pulmonary artery pressure (PAP), and decreased cardiac output (CO). See **CHAPTER 30: INVASIVE CARDIOVASCULAR PROCEDURES** for detailed information related to hemodynamic monitoring.
- Mixed venous oxygen saturation (SvO_2) is directly related to cardiac output. A drop in SvO_2 indicates worsening cardiac function.

Ultrasound

Two-dimensional or three-dimensional ultrasound (also called cardiac ultrasound or echocardiogram) is used to measure the systolic and diastolic functioning of the heart.

Left ventricular ejection fraction: The volume of blood pumped from the left ventricle into the arteries upon each beat. Expected reference range is 55% to 70%.

Right ventricular ejection fraction: The volume of blood pumped from the right ventricle to the lungs upon each beat. Expected reference range is 45% to 60%.

Transesophageal echocardiography (TEE)

Uses a transducer placed in the esophagus behind the heart to obtain a detailed view of cardiac structures. The nurse prepares the client for a TEE in the same manner as for an upper endoscopy.

Chest x-ray

A chest x-ray can reveal cardiomegaly and pleural effusions.

ECG, cardiac enzymes, electrolytes, and ABGs

Electrocardiogram (ECG), cardiac enzymes, electrolytes, and ABGs are used to assess factors contributing to heart failure and/or the impact of heart failure.

PATIENT-CENTERED CARE

NURSING CARE

- Monitor daily weight and I&O.
- Assess for shortness of breath and dyspnea on exertion.
- Administer oxygen as prescribed.
- Monitor vital signs and hemodynamic pressures.
- Position the client to maximize ventilation (high-Fowler's).
- Check ABGs, electrolytes (especially potassium if on diuretics), SaO_2, and chest x-ray findings.
- Assess for signs of medication toxicity (digoxin toxicity).
- Encourage bed rest until the client is stable.
- Encourage energy conservation by assisting with care and ADLs.
- Maintain dietary restrictions as prescribed (restricted fluid intake, restricted sodium intake).
- Provide emotional support to the client and family.

MEDICATIONS

Herbal medications can stimulate the cardiovascular system. Obtain a list of herbal supplements the client takes, and advise the client of potential contraindications. Q**EBP**

Diuretics

Diuretics are used to decrease preload.

Loop diuretics, such as furosemide and bumetanide

Thiazide diuretics, such as hydrochlorothiazide

Potassium-sparing diuretics, such as spironolactone

NURSING CONSIDERATIONS
- Administer furosemide IV no faster than 20 mg/min.
- Loop and thiazide diuretics can cause hypokalemia, and potassium supplementation can be required.

CLIENT EDUCATION: Teach clients taking loop or thiazide diuretics to ingest foods and drinks that are high in potassium to counter the effects of hypokalemia. Q**s**

Afterload-reducing agents

Afterload-reducing agents help the heart pump more easily by altering the resistance to contraction. These are contraindicated for clients who have renal deficiency.

Angiotensin-converting enzyme (ACE) inhibitors, such as enalapril and captopril

Angiotensin receptor II blockers, such as losartan

Calcium channel blockers, such as diltiazem and nifedipine

Phosphodiesterase-3 inhibitors, such as milrinone

NURSING CONSIDERATIONS
- Monitor clients taking ACE inhibitors for hypotension following the initial dose.
- ACE inhibitors can cause angioedema (swelling of the tongue and throat), decreased sense of taste, or skin rash.
- Monitor for increased levels of potassium.

CLIENT EDUCATION: ACE INHIBITORS
- Inform the client that this medication can cause a dry cough.
- Notify the provider if the client observes a rash or has a decreased sense of taste.
- Notify the provider if swelling of the face or extremities occurs.
- Remind the client that blood pressure needs to be monitored for 2 hr after the initial dose to detect hypotension.

Inotropic agents

Inotropic agents, such as digoxin, dopamine, dobutamine, and milrinone, are used to increase contractility and thereby improve cardiac output.

NURSING CONSIDERATIONS
- For a client taking digoxin, take the apical heart rate for 1 min. Hold the medication if apical pulse is less than 60/min, and notify the provider.
- Observe the client for nausea and vomiting.
- Dopamine, dobutamine, and milrinone are administered via IV. The ECG, blood pressure, and urine output must be closely monitored.

CLIENT EDUCATION
Teach clients who are self-administering digoxin to:
- Count pulse for 1 min before taking the medication. If the pulse rate is irregular or the pulse rate is outside of the limitations set by the provider (usually less than 60/min or greater than 100/min), instruct the client to hold the dose and contact the provider. Qs
- Take the digoxin dose at the same time each day.
- Do not take digoxin at the same time as antacids. Separate the two medications by at least 2 hr.
- Report signs of toxicity, including fatigue, muscle weakness, confusion, and loss of appetite.
- Regularly have digoxin and potassium levels checked.

Beta-adrenergic blockers (beta-blockers)

Medications such as carvedilol and metoprolol can be used to improve the condition of the client who has sustained increased levels of sympathetic stimulation and catecholamines. This includes clients who have chronic heart failure.

NURSING CONSIDERATIONS
- Monitor blood pressure, pulse, activity tolerance, and orthopnea.
- Check orthostatic blood pressure readings.

CLIENT EDUCATION
- Instruct the client to weigh daily.
- Advise the client to regularly check blood pressure.
- Tell the client to follow the provider's instructions for increasing medication dosage.

Vasodilators

Nitroglycerin and isosorbide mononitrate prevent coronary artery vasospasm and reduce preload and afterload, decreasing myocardial oxygen demand.

NURSING CONSIDERATIONS
- Vasodilators are given to treat angina and help control blood pressure.
- Use cautiously with other antihypertensive mediations.
- Vasodilators can cause orthostatic hypotension.

CLIENT EDUCATION
- Remind the client that a headache is a common side effect of this medication.
- Encourage the client to sit and lie down slowly.

Human B-type natriuretic peptides

hBNPs, such as nesiritide, are used to treat acute heart failure by causing natriuresis (loss of sodium and vasodilation). They are administered IV.

NURSING CONSIDERATIONS
- hBNPs can cause hypotension, as well as a number of cardiac effects, including ventricular tachycardia and bradycardia.
- BNP levels will increase while on this medication.
- Monitor ECG, blood pressure, and other parameters.

CLIENT EDUCATION
- The client can be asymptomatic with a low blood pressure.
- Remind the client to sit and lie down slowly.

Anticoagulants

Anticoagulants, such as warfarin, can be prescribed if the client has a history of thrombus formation.

NURSING CONSIDERATIONS
- Assess for contraindications: active bleeding, peptic ulcer disease, history of cerebrovascular accident, and recent trauma.
- Monitor bleeding times: PT, aPTT, INR, and CBC.

CLIENT EDUCATION
- Remind the client of the risk for bruising and bleeding while on this medication.
- Instruct the client to have blood monitored routinely to check bleeding times.

INTERPROFESSIONAL CARE

Cardiology and pulmonary services should be consulted to manage heart failure.

Respiratory services should be consulted for inhalers, breathing treatments, and suctioning for airway management.

Cardiac rehabilitation services can be consulted if the client has prolonged weakness and needs assistance with increasing level of activity.

Nutritional services can be consulted for diet modification to promote low-sodium, and low-saturated fat food choices.

THERAPEUTIC PROCEDURES

Ventricular assist device (VAD)

A VAD is a mechanical pump that assists a heart that is too weak to pump blood through the body. It is used in clients who are eligible for heart transplants or who have severe end-stage heart failure and are not candidates for heart transplants. Heart transplantation is the treatment of choice for clients who have severe dilated cardiomyopathy.

NURSING ACTIONS
- Prepare the client for the procedure (NPO status and informed consent).
- Monitor postoperatively: vital signs, SaO$_2$, incision drainage, and pain management.

Heart transplantation

- Heart transplantation is a possible option for clients who have end-stage heart failure. Immunosuppressant therapy is required post-transplantation to prevent rejection.
- Eligibility for transplantation depends on several factors, including life expectancy, age, psychosocial status, and absence of drug and alcohol use disorders.

NURSING ACTIONS
- Prepare the client for the procedure (NPO status and informed consent). Laboratory reports and results of diagnostic testing should be available as prescribed.
- Monitor postoperatively: vital signs, SaO₂, incision drainage, and pain management.
- Monitor for complications. Organ transplant recipients are at risk for infection, thrombosis, and rejection. See **CHAPTER 58: KIDNEY TRANSPLANT** for details related to these complications.

CLIENT EDUCATION: Instruct the client to:
- Take medications as prescribed.
- Take diuretics in the early morning and early afternoon.
- Maintain fluid and sodium restriction: a dietary consult can be useful.
- Increase dietary intake of potassium (cantaloupe or bananas) if the client is taking potassium-losing diuretics, such as loop and thiazide diuretics.
- Check weight daily at the same time, and notify the provider for a weight gain of 2 lb in 24 hr or 5 lb in 1 week.
- Schedule regular follow-up visits with the provider.
- Get vaccinations (pneumococcal and yearly influenza vaccines).

COMPLICATIONS

Acute pulmonary edema

Acute pulmonary edema is a life-threatening medical emergency.

EXPECTED FINDINGS: anxiety, tachycardia, acute respiratory distress, dyspnea at rest, change in level of consciousness, and an ascending fluid level within the lungs (crackles, cough productive of frothy, blood-tinged sputum).

NURSING ACTIONS
- Administer prescribed medications to improve cardiac output.
- Teach the client about measures to improve tolerance to activity, such as alternating periods of activity with periods of rest.
- Prompt response to this emergency includes the following.
  ○ Positioning the client in high-Fowler's position.
  ○ Administration of oxygen, positive airway pressure, and/or intubation and mechanical ventilation.
  ○ IV morphine (to decrease anxiety, respiratory distress, and decrease venous return).
  ○ IV administration of rapid-acting loop diuretics, such as furosemide .
  ○ Effective intervention should result in diuresis (carefully monitor output), reduction in respiratory distress, improved lung sounds, and adequate oxygenation.

Cardiogenic shock

This is a serious complication of pump failure that occurs commonly following an MI and injury to greater than 40% of the left ventricle.

EXPECTED FINDINGS: include tachycardia, hypotension, inadequate urinary output, altered level of consciousness, respiratory distress (crackles, tachypnea), cool, clammy skin, decreased peripheral pulses, and chest pain.

NURSING ACTIONS
- Monitor breath sounds. Assess for crackles or wheezing.
- Monitor heart sounds.
- Administration of oxygen, intubation, and ventilation can be required.
- Administer IV morphine, diuretics, and/or nitroglycerin to decrease preload. Administer IV vasopressors and/or positive inotropes to increase cardiac output and maintain organ perfusion.
- Provide continuous hemodynamic monitoring.

Pericardial tamponade

Cardiac tamponade can result from fluid accumulation in the pericardial sac.

EXPECTED FINDINGS: include hypotension, jugular venous distention, muffled heart sounds, and paradoxical pulse (variance of 10 mm Hg or more in systolic blood pressure between expiration and inspiration).

DIAGNOSTIC PROCEDURES: Hemodynamic monitoring will reveal intracardiac and pulmonary artery pressures similar and elevated (plateau pressures).

NURSING ACTIONS
- Notify the provider immediately.
- Administer IV fluids to combat hypotension as prescribed while monitoring for fluid overload.
- Obtain a chest x-ray or echocardiogram to confirm diagnosis.
- Prepare the client for pericardiocentesis (informed consent, gather materials, administer medications as appropriate).
- Monitor hemodynamic pressures as they normalize.
- Monitor heart rhythm; changes indicate improper positioning of the needle.
- Monitor for reoccurrence of findings after the procedure.

Pulmonary edema

Cardiogenic factors are the most common cause of pulmonary edema. It is a complication of various heart and lung diseases and usually occurs from increased pulmonary vascular pressure secondary to severe cardiac dysfunction.

Noncardiac pulmonary edema can occur due to barbiturate or opiate overdose, inhalation of irritating gases, rapid administration of IV fluids, and after a pneumonectomy evacuation of pleural effusion.

Neurogenic pulmonary edema develops following a head injury.

OLDER ADULTS: Increased risk for pulmonary edema occurs related to decreased cardiac output and heart failure. ©

- Increased risk for fluid and electrolyte imbalances occurs when the older adult client receives treatment with diuretics.
- For older adults, IV infusions must be administered at a slower rate to prevent circulatory overload.

HEALTH PROMOTION AND DISEASE PREVENTION

- Maintain an exercise routine to remain physically active, and consult with the provider before starting any exercise regimen.
- Consume a diet low in sodium along with fluid restrictions, and consult with the provider regarding diet specifications.
- Refrain from smoking.
- Follow medication regimen, and follow up with the provider as needed.

ASSESSMENT

RISK FACTORS

- Acute MI Q**EBP**
- Fluid volume overload
- Hypertension
- Valvular heart disease
- Postpneumonectomy
- Postevacuation of pleural effusion
- Acute respiratory failure
- Left-sided heart failure
- High altitude exposure or deep-sea diving
- Trauma
- Sepsis
- Drug overdose

EXPECTED FINDINGS

- Anxiety
- Inability to sleep
- Persistent cough with pink, frothy sputum (cardinal sign)
- Tachypnea, dyspnea, and orthopnea
- Hypoxemia (SaO_2 expected reference range greater than 95%)
- Cyanosis (later stage)
- Crackles
- Tachycardia
- Reduced urine output
- Confusion, stupor
- S_3 heart sound (gallop)
- Increased pulmonary artery occlusion pressure

PATIENT-CENTERED CARE

NURSING CARE

- Monitor vital signs every 15 min until stable.
- Monitor intake and output.
- Monitor hemodynamic status (pulmonary wedge pressures, cardiac output).
- Check ABGs, electrolytes (especially potassium if on diuretics), SaO_2, and chest x-ray findings.
- Maintain a patent airway. Suction as needed.
- Position the client in high-Fowler's position with feet and legs dependent or sitting on the side of the bed to decrease preload.
- Administer high-flow oxygen using a face mask or nonrebreather mask. Bilevel positive airway pressure or intubation/ventilation can become necessary. Be prepared to intervene quickly.
- Restrict fluid intake (slow or discontinue infusing IV fluids).
- Monitor hourly urine output. Watch for intake greater than output or hourly urine less than 30 mL/hr.

MEDICATIONS

Rapid-acting diuretics, such as furosemide and bumetanide, promote fluid excretion.

Morphine decreases sympathetic nervous system response and anxiety and promotes mild vasodilation.

Vasodilators (nitroglycerin, sodium nitroprusside) decrease preload and afterload.

Inotropic agents, such as digoxin and dobutamine, improve cardiac output.

Antihypertensives, such as ACE inhibitors and beta-blockers, decrease afterload

CLIENT EDUCATION

- Provide emotional support for the client and family.
- Instruct the client on effective breathing techniques.
- Instruct the client on medications.
- Stress the importance of continuing to take medications even if the client is feeling better.
- Teach common adverse effects of medications, and reasons to contact the provider.
- Instruct the client on a low-sodium diet and fluid restriction.
- The client should measure weight daily at the same time. Notify the provider of a gain of more than 2 lb in 1 day or 5 lb in 1 week.
- Instruct the client to report swelling of feet or ankles or any shortness of breath or angina.

Application Exercises

1. A nurse is caring for a client who has heart failure and reports increased shortness of breath. The nurse increases the client's oxygen per protocol. Which of the following actions should the nurse take first?

   A. Obtain the client's weight.

   B. Assist the client into high-Fowler's position.

   C. Auscultate lungs sounds.

   D. Check oxygen saturation with pulse oximeter.

2. A nurse is teaching a client who has heart failure about the need to limit sodium in the diet to 2,000 mg daily. Which of the following foods should the nurse recommend for the client? ? (Select all that apply.)

   A. 1 slice cheddar cheese

   B. 1 medium beef hot dog

   C. 3 oz Atlantic salmon

   D. 3 oz roasted chicken breast

   E. 2 oz lean baked ham

3. A nurse is completing the admission assessment of a client who has suspected pulmonary edema. Which of the following manifestation are expected findings? (Select all that apply.)

   A. Tachypnea

   B. Persistent cough

   C. Increased urinary output

   D. Thick, yellow sputum

   E. Orthopnea

4. A nurse is completing discharge teaching with a client who has heart failure and is encouraged to increase potassium in his diet. Which of the following food selections should the nurse include as having the highest source of potassium?

   A. 1 medium apple

   B. 1 medium baked potato

   C. 1 slice toast with 1 tbsp peanut butter

   D. 1 large scrambled egg

5. A nurse is providing discharge teaching for a client who has heart failure and is on a fluid restriction of 2,000 mL/day. The client asks the nurse how to determine the appropriate amount of fluids he is allowed. Which of the following statements is an appropriate response by the nurse?

   A. "Pour the amount of fluid you drink into an empty 2-liter bottle to keep track of how much you drink."

   B. "Each glass contains 8 ounces. There are 30 milliliters per ounce, so you can have a total of 8 glasses or cups of fluid each day."

   C. "This is the same as 2 quarts, or about the same as two pots of coffee."

   D. "Take sips of water or ice chips so you will not take in too much fluid."

PRACTICE Active Learning Scenario

A nurse in a cardiac rehabilitation program is teaching a class on heart failure to a group of clients. What should the nurse include in this presentation? Use the ATI Active Learning Template: System Disorder to complete this item.

ALTERATION IN HEALTH (DIAGNOSIS): Describe the difference between left- and right-sided heart failure.

LABORATORY TESTS: Describe one and its importance.

DIAGNOSTIC PROCEDURES: Describe two.

MEDICATIONS: Describe two groups of medications and an example of one medication for each group.

Application Exercises Key

1. A. Obtaining the client's weight is an appropriate action. However, another action is the priority

    B. **CORRECT:** Using the airway, breathing, and circulation (ABC) priority approach to client care, the first action the nurse should take is to assist the client into high-Fowler's position. This will decrease venous return to the heart (preload) and help relieve lung congestion.

    C. Auscultating lung sounds is an appropriate action. However, another action is the priority.

    D. Checking oxygen saturation is an appropriate action. However, another action is the priority.

    Ⓝ *NCLEX® Connection: Physiological Adaptation, Medical Emergencies*

2. A. **CORRECT:** One slice cheddar cheese contains 180 mg sodium.

    B. A medium beef hot dog contains 557 mg sodium. Foods should be less than 300 mg per serving for a 2,000 mg sodium-restricted diet.

    C. **CORRECT:** Three ounces Atlantic salmon contains 37 mg sodium.

    D. **CORRECT:** Three ounces roasted chicken breast contains 62 mg sodium.

    E. Two ounces lean baked ham contains 782 mg sodium. Foods should be less than 300 mg per serving for a 2,000 mg sodium-restricted diet.

    Ⓝ *NCLEX® Connection: Basic Care and Comfort, Nutrition and Oral Hydration*

3. A. **CORRECT:** Tachypnea is an expected finding in a client who has pulmonary edema.

    B. **CORRECT:** A persistent cough with pink, frothy sputum is an expected finding in a client who has pulmonary edema.

    C. Decreased urinary output is an expected finding in a client who has pulmonary edema.

    D. Pink, frothy sputum is an expected finding in a client who has pulmonary edema.

    E. **CORRECT:** Orthopnea is an expected finding in a client who has pulmonary edema.

    Ⓝ *NCLEX® Connection: Physiological Adaptation, Pathophysiology*

4. A. One medium apple contains 195 mg potassium. The nurse should recommend a different food because another choice contains more potassium.

    B. **CORRECT:** A medium baked potato is the best food source of potassium because it contains 926 mg potassium per serving.

    C. One slice toast with 1 tbsp peanut butter contains 148 mg potassium per serving. Another choice contains more potassium.

    D. One large egg scrambled contains 81 mg potassium per serving. Another choice that contains more potassium.

    Ⓝ *NCLEX® Connection: Basic Care and Comfort, Nutrition and Oral Hydration*

5. A. **CORRECT:** Pouring the amount of fluid consumed into an empty 2 L bottle provides a visual guide for the client as to the amount consumed and how to plan daily intake.

    B. Glasses and cups vary in size and can contain more than 8 oz.

    C. Offering a vague frame of reference does not assist with accurate fluid measurement.

    D. Suggesting that the client take sips of water or ice chips does not assist with accurate fluid measurement.

    Ⓝ *NCLEX® Connection: Basic Care and Comfort, Nutrition and Oral Hydration*

PRACTICE Answer

Using the ATI Active Learning Template: System Disorder

ALTERATION IN HEALTH (DIAGNOSIS): Left-sided heart failure results in inadequate output from the left ventricle, leading to poor tissue perfusion. Systolic failure includes an ejection fraction below 40% with pulmonary and systemic congestion. Diastolic failure includes stiffening or inadequate relaxation of the ventricle. Right-sided heart failure results in inadequate output from the right ventricle, leading to systemic venous congestion and peripheral edema.

LABORATORY TESTS: Human B-type natriuretic peptides (hBNP) confirms a diagnosis of heart failure, and findings direct the aggressiveness of the treatment.

DIAGNOSTIC PROCEDURES
- Hemodynamic monitoring
- Ultrasound
- Chest x-ray
- Electrocardiogram

MEDICATIONS
- Diuretics: furosemide, bumetanide, hydrochlorothiazide, spironolactone
- Afterload-reducing agents: enalapril, captopril, losartan, diltiazem, nifedipine, milrinone

Ⓝ *NCLEX® Connection: Physiological Adaptation, Alterations in Body Systems*

UNIT 4 NURSING CARE OF CLIENTS WHO HAVE
CARDIOVASCULAR DISORDERS
SECTION: CARDIAC DISORDERS

CHAPTER 33 *Valvular Heart Disease*

Valvular heart disease describes an abnormality or dysfunction of any of the heart's four valves: the mitral and aortic valves (left side), the tricuspid (rare, might occur as a result of endocarditis or IV drug use), and pulmonic valves (right side).

It affects the efficiency of the heart as a pump and reduces stroke volume. Over time, there might be remodeling of the heart itself (hypertrophy) and heart failure.

With age, fibrotic thickening occurs in the mitral and aortic valves. The aorta is stiffer in older adult clients, increasing systolic blood pressure and stress on the mitral valve. (33.1) ⓒ

HEALTH PROMOTION AND DISEASE PREVENTION

- Prevent and treat bacterial infections.
- Encourage clients to consume a diet low in sodium and to follow fluid restrictions prescribed by the provider to prevent heart failure.
- Control chronic illnesses (diabetes mellitus, hypertension, hypercholesterolemia).
- Encourage increased activity and exercise to boost high-density lipoprotein (HDL) levels.

ASSESSMENT

- Valvular heart disease is classified as:
  - **Stenosis:** Narrowed opening that impedes blood moving forward.
  - **Insufficiency/Improper closure:** Some blood flows backward (regurgitation).
- Valvular heart disease can have congenital or acquired causes.
  - **Congenital** valvular heart disease can affect all four valves and cause either stenosis or insufficiency.
  - **Acquired** valvular heart disease is classified as one of three types:
    - **Degenerative disease:** Due to damage over time from mechanical stress, atherosclerosis, and hypertension. Most common in developed countries.
    - **Rheumatic disease:** Gradual fibrotic changes, calcification of valve cusps. Most common in developing countries.
    - **Infective endocarditis:** Infectious organisms destroy the valve. Streptococcal infections are a common cause.

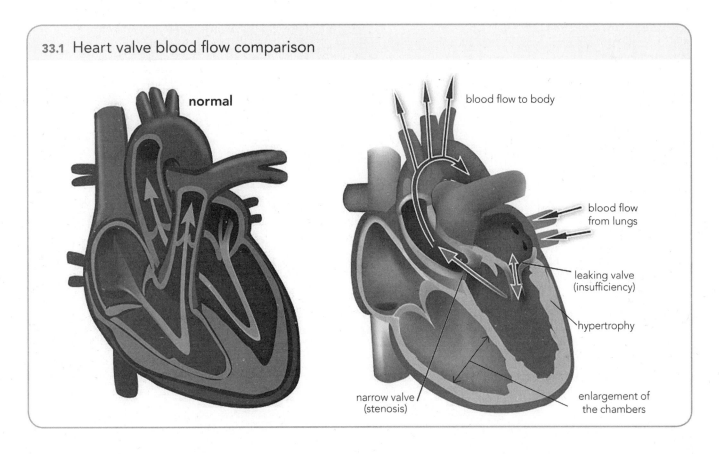

33.1 Heart valve blood flow comparison

normal

blood flow to body

blood flow from lungs

leaking valve (insufficiency)

hypertrophy

narrow valve (stenosis)

enlargement of the chambers

RISK FACTORS

- Hypertension
- Rheumatic fever (mitral stenosis and insufficiency)
- Infective endocarditis
- Congenital malformations
- Marfan syndrome (connective tissue disorder that affects the heart and other areas of the body)
- In older adult clients, the predominant causes of valvular heart disease are degenerative calcification and atherosclerosis, papillary muscle dysfunction, and infective endocarditis. ©

EXPECTED FINDINGS

- Clients who have valvular heart disease are often asymptomatic until late in the progression of the disease.
- A murmur is heard with turbulent blood flow. The location of the murmur and timing (diastolic versus systolic) help determine the valve involved. Murmurs are graded on a scale of I (very faint) to VI (extremely loud).
- Left-sided valve damage causes increased pulmonary artery pressure, left ventricular hypertrophy, and decreased cardiac output, resulting in orthopnea, paroxysmal nocturnal dyspnea (PND), and fatigue. **(33.2)**

DIAGNOSTIC PROCEDURES

Chest x-ray shows chamber enlargement (with stenosis and insufficiencies) and pulmonary congestion (with aortic stenosis).

12-lead electrocardiogram (ECG) shows chamber hypertrophy.

Echocardiogram shows chamber size, hypertrophy, specific valve dysfunction, ejection function, and amount of regurgitant flow.

Transesophageal echocardiography (TEE)

Exercise tolerance testing/stress echocardiography is used to assess the impact of the valve problem on cardiac functioning during stress.

Radionuclide studies determine ejection fraction during activity and rest.

Angiography is used to evaluate the coronary arteries and the degree of atherosclerosis. Cardiac catheterization might be used as a diagnostic tool in valvular disease.

PATIENT-CENTERED CARE

NURSING CARE

- Monitor current weight and note recent changes.
- Assess heart rhythm (can be irregular or bradycardic, assess for murmur).
- Administer oxygen and medications as prescribed.
- Assess hemodynamic monitoring. Maintain fluid and sodium restrictions.
- Assist the client to conserve energy.

MEDICATIONS

Diuretics

Diuretics are used to treat heart failure by removing excessive extracellular fluid.
- Loop diuretics, such as furosemide
- Thiazide diuretics, such as hydrochlorothiazide
- Potassium-sparing diuretics, such as spironolactone

NURSING CONSIDERATIONS
- Administer furosemide IV slow over 1 to 2 minutes.
- Loop and thiazide diuretics can cause hypokalemia, and a potassium supplement might be required.

CLIENT EDUCATION: Teach clients who are taking loop or thiazide diuretics to ingest foods (dried fruits, nuts, spinach, citrus fruits, bananas and potatoes) and drinks that are high in potassium to counter hypokalemia effect.

33.2 Left-sided valve damage

Mitral stenosis	Mitral insufficiency	Aortic stenosis	Aortic insufficiency
Apical diastolic murmur	Systolic murmur at the apex	Systolic murmur	Diastolic murmur
Dyspnea on exertion	S_3 sounds	Dyspnea on exertion	Sinus tachycardia
Orthopnea	Fatigue and weakness	S_4 sounds	Exertional dyspnea
Atrial fibrillation	Atrial fibrillation	Angina	Orthopnea
Palpitations	Dyspnea on exertion	Syncope	Palpitations
Fatigue	Orthopnea	Fatigue	Fatigue
Jugular venous distention	Atypical chest pain	Orthopnea	Nocturnal angina with diaphoresis
Pitting edema	Palpitations	PND	Widened pulse pressure
Hemoptysis	Jugular venous distention	Narrowed pulse pressure	Bounding arterial pulse on palpation (Corrigan's pulse)
Dry cough	Pitting edema		Elevated systolic and diminished diastolic pressures
Repeated respiratory infections	Crackles in lungs		PND
PND	Possible diminished lung sounds		
Hepatomegaly	PND		
	Hepatomegaly		

Afterload-reducing agents

Afterload-reducing agents help the heart pump more easily by altering the resistance to contraction.
- Angiotensin-converting enzyme (ACE) inhibitors (enalapril , captopril, lisinopril)
- Angiotensin-receptor blockers (losartan, valsartan)
- Beta-blockers, metoprolol, carvedilol
- Calcium-channel blockers (felodipine, nifedipine, amlodipine)
- Vasodilators, such as hydralazine

NURSING CONSIDERATIONS: Monitor clients taking ACE inhibitors for initial dose hypotension.

Inotropic agents

Inotropic agents, such as digoxin, are used to increase contractility and thereby improve cardiac output.

CLIENT EDUCATION
Teach clients who are self-administering digoxin to:
- Count pulse for 1 minute before taking the medication. If the pulse rate is irregular or the pulse rate is outside of the limitations set by the provider (usually less than 60/min or greater than 100/min), the client should hold the dose and contact the provider.
- Take the dose of digoxin at the same time every day.
- Do not take digoxin at the same time as antacids. Separate the two medications by at least 2 hr
- Report signs of toxicity, including fatigue, muscle weakness, confusion, visual changes, and loss of appetite.

Anticoagulants

Anticoagulation therapy is used for clients who have a mechanical valve replacement, atrial fibrillation, or severe left ventricle dysfunction.

THERAPEUTIC PROCEDURES

NURSING ACTIONS: Postsurgery care is similar to coronary artery bypass surgery (care for sternal incision, activity limited for 6 weeks, report fever).

Percutaneous balloon valvuloplasty

This procedure can open aortic or mitral valves affected by stenosis. A catheter is inserted through the femoral artery and advanced to the heart. A balloon is inflated at the stenotic lesion to open the fused commissures and improve leaflet mobility.

Valve replacement

This procedure replaces damaged heart valves with mechanical, xenografts (from other species), allografts (from cadavers), or autografts (formed from the client's pulmonic valve and a portion of the pulmonary artery). It is often done with an open-heart approach, although minimally invasive surgery is also performed in some instances.
- Mechanical valves require lifelong anticoagulant therapy.
- Tissue valves need to be replaced every 7 to 10 years.

Miscellaneous surgical management

- Other surgeries used in the treatment of valvular disorders include chordae tendineae reconstruction, commissurotomy (relieve stenosis on leaflets), annuloplasty ring insertion (correct dilatation of valve annulus by narrowing the opening), and leaflet repair.
- Medical management is appropriate for many older adult clients; surgery is indicated when manifestations interfere with daily activities. The goal of surgery can be to improve the quality of life rather than to prolong life. ©

INTERPROFESSIONAL CARE

- Respiratory services should be consulted for inhalers, breathing treatments, and suctioning for airway management.
- Cardiology can be consulted for cardiac management.
- Nutritional services can be contacted for weight loss or gain related to medications or diagnosis.
- Rehabilitative care might need to be consulted if the client has prolonged weakness and needs assistance with increasing level of activity.

CLIENT EDUCATION

- Stress the importance of prophylactic antibiotic use before any invasive dental or respiratory procedure. Qs
- Weigh daily and notify the provider of 3 lb (1.4 kg) gain in 1 day or 5 lb (2.3 kg) gain in 1 week.
- Coordinate activities with planned rest periods.
- Encourage the client to follow the prescribed exercise program.
- Encourage adherence to dietary restrictions, including avoidance of caffeine and alcohol; consider nutritional consultation.
- Teach the client energy conservation.
- Open wounds need to be cleaned carefully and antibiotic ointment should be used.
- Fever should be reported immediately to the health care provider.
- Petechial rash or shortness of breath should be reported to the health care provider.
- Read labels of over-the-counter medication to avoid those which include alcohol, ephedrine, or epinephrine (might cause dysrhythmias).
- Teach symptoms of heart failure; report to provider immediately.

COMPLICATIONS

Heart failure

Heart failure is the inability of the heart to maintain adequate circulation to meet tissue needs for oxygen and nutrients. Ineffective valves result in heart failure.

NURSING ACTIONS: Monitoring the client's heart failure class (I to IV) is often the gauge for surgical intervention for valvular problems.

Application Exercises

1. A nurse is completing discharge teaching with a client who had a surgical placement of a mechanical heart valve. Which of the following statements by the client indicates understanding of the teaching?

   A. "I will be glad to get back to my exercise routine right away."

   B. "I will have my prothrombin time checked on a regular basis."

   C. "I will talk to my dentist about no longer needing antibiotics before dental exams."

   D. "I will continue to limit my intake of foods containing potassium."

2. A nurse is completing the admission physical assessment of client who has a history of mitral valve insufficiency. Which of the following findings should the nurse expect?

   A. S4 heart sound

   B. Petechiae

   C. Crackles in lung bases

   D. Splenomegaly

3. A nurse is reviewing the health record of a client who is being evaluated for possible valvular heart disease. The nurse should recognize which of the following data as risk factors for this condition? (Select all that apply.)

   A. Surgical repair of an atrial septal defect at age 2

   B. Measles infection during childhood

   C. Hypertension for 5 years

   D. Weight gain of 10 lb in past year

   E. Diastolic murmur present

4. A nurse is caring for a 72-year-old client who is to undergo a percutaneous balloon valvuloplasty. The client's daughter asks the nurse to explain the expected outcome of this procedure. Which of the following responses should the nurse give?

   A. "This will improve blood flow in your mother's coronary arteries."

   B. "This will permit your mother to resume her activities of daily living."

   C. "This will prolong your mother's life."

   D. "This will reverse the effects to the damaged area."

5. A nurse educator is reviewing expected findings in a client who has right-sided valvular heart disease with a group of nurses. Which of the following findings should the nurse include in the discussion? (Select all that apply.)

   A. Dyspnea

   B. Client report of fatigue

   C. Bradycardia

   D. Pleural friction rub

   E. Peripheral edema

PRACTICE Active Learning Scenario

A nurse educator is preparing a poster on valvular heart disease to be displayed at a health fair. What content should be included on the poster? Use the ATI Active Learning Template: System Disorder to complete this item.

ALTERATION IN HEALTH (DIAGNOSIS)
- Describe the difference between valve stenosis and insufficiency.
- Describe the difference between acquired and congenital valvular heart disease.

CLIENT EDUCATION: Describe two actions to prevent valvular disease.

Application Exercises Key

1. A. The client will be on activity limitation for 6 weeks following surgery for a heart valve replacement.

   B. **CORRECT:** Anticoagulant therapy with warfarin (Coumadin) is necessary for the client following placement of a mechanical heart valve; the client's prothrombin time will be checked on a regular basis.

   C. Antibiotic therapy is recommended prior to dental work following placement of a heart valve.

   D. Dietary recommendations include limiting foods containing sodium.

   Ⓝ *NCLEX® Connection: Physiological Adaptation, Alterations in Body Systems*

2. A. An S_3 heart sound is an expected finding in a client who has mitral valve insufficiency. An S4 heart sound is an expected finding for a client who has aortic stenosis.

   B. Petechiae is an expected finding in a client who has infective endocarditis.

   C. **CORRECT:** Crackles in the lung bases is an expected finding in a client who has pulmonary congestion due to mitral valve insufficiency.

   D. Hepatomegaly, not splenomegaly, is an expected finding in a client who has left-sided heart valve damage.

   Ⓝ *NCLEX® Connection: Physiological Adaptation, Pathophysiology*

3. A. **CORRECT:** A history of congenital malformations is a risk factor for valvular heart disease.

   B. Having a streptococcal infection or rheumatic fever during childhood is a risk factor for valvular heart disease.

   C. **CORRECT:** Hypertension places a client at risk for valvular heart disease.

   D. A sudden weight gain of 10 lb could indicate fluid collection related to left-sided valvular heart disease.

   E. **CORRECT:** A murmur indicates turbulent blood flow, which is often due to valvular heart disease.

   Ⓝ *NCLEX® Connection: Health Promotion and Maintenance, Health Promotion/Disease Prevention*

4. A. A valvuloplasty improves blood flow through a heart valve by opening the fused commissures and allowing valve leaflets greater mobility. It does not improve blood flow in the coronary arteries.

   B. **CORRECT:** Surgery is indicated for older adult clients when manifestations interfere with activities of daily living.

   C. Surgical interventions can improve the client's quality of life, but they will not necessarily prolong life.

   D. A valvuloplasty improves blood flow through a heart valve by opening the fused commissures and allowing valve leaflets greater mobility. It does not reverse the damage that has already occurred to the valve.

   Ⓝ *NCLEX® Connection: Reduction of Risk Potential, Therapeutic Procedures*

5. A. **CORRECT:** Dyspnea is a manifestation of right-sided valvular heart disease.

   B. **CORRECT:** A client's report of fatigue is a manifestation of right-sided valvular heart disease.

   C. A normal or rapid pulse and an irregularly irregular rhythm are manifestations of right-sided valvular heart disease.

   D. A pleural friction rub is a manifestation of pleurisy or pneumonia.

   E. **CORRECT:** Peripheral edema is a manifestation of right-sided valvular heart disease.

   Ⓝ *NCLEX® Connection: Physiological Adaptation, Pathophysiology*

PRACTICE Answer

Using ATI Active Learning Template: System Disorder

ALTERATION IN HEALTH (DIAGNOSIS)

- Stenosis is the narrowed opening of a heart valve, which prevents blood from moving forward. Insufficiency is the improper closure of a valve resulting in blood flowing backward (regurgitation) through the valve.
- Congenital valvular heart disease can affect all four valves and can cause either stenosis or insufficiency. Acquired valvular heart disease occurs due to degenerative changes from mechanical stress over time; rheumatic disease, which causes calcifications, and fibrotic changes, often to the mitral valve; and infective endocarditis, in which infectious organisms destroy the valve.

Ⓝ *NCLEX® Connection: Physiological Adaptation, Pathophysiology*

CLIENT EDUCATION

- Prevent and manage hypertension.
- Early detection and prevention of rheumatic fever.
- Consume a low-sodium diet.

UNIT 4 NURSING CARE OF CLIENTS WHO HAVE
CARDIOVASCULAR DISORDERS
SECTION: CARDIAC DISORDERS

CHAPTER 34 *Inflammatory Disorders*

Inflammation related to the heart is an extended inflammatory response that often leads to the destruction of healthy tissue. This primarily includes the layers of the heart.

Inflammatory disorders related to the cardiovascular system that nurses should be familiar with include pericarditis, myocarditis, rheumatic endocarditis, and infective endocarditis.

HEALTH PROMOTION AND DISEASE PREVENTION

- Early treatment of streptococcal infections can prevent rheumatic fever.
- Prophylactic treatments (including antibiotics for clients who have cardiac defects) can prevent infective endocarditis.
- Influenza and pneumonia immunizations are important for all clients (especially older adults) in order to decrease the incidence of myocarditis. Ⓒ

ASSESSMENT

RISK FACTORS

- Congenital heart defect/cardiac anomalies
- Intravenous substance use
- Heart valve replacement
- Immunosuppression
- Rheumatic fever and other infections
- School-age children who have long duration of streptococcus infection
- Malnutrition
- Overcrowding
- Lower socioeconomic status

EXPECTED FINDINGS

Pericarditis: Inflammation of the pericardium
- Commonly follows a respiratory infection.
- Can be due to a myocardial infarction.
- Findings include chest pressure/pain aggravated by breathing (mainly inspiration), coughing, and swallowing; pericardial friction rub auscultated at left lower sternal border; shortness of breath; and relief of pain when sitting and leaning forward.

Myocarditis: Inflammation of the myocardium
- Can be due to a viral, fungal, or bacterial infection, or a systemic inflammatory disease (Crohn's disease).
- Findings include tachycardia, murmur, friction rub auscultated in the lungs, cardiomegaly, chest pain, and dysrhythmias.

Rheumatic endocarditis: An infection of the endocardium due to a complication of rheumatic fever.
- Preceded by group A beta-hemolytic streptococcal pharyngitis.
- Produces lesions in the heart.
- Findings include fever, chest pain, joint pain, tachycardia, shortness of breath, rash on trunk and extremities, friction rub, murmur, and muscle spasms.

Infective endocarditis: Infection of the endocardium due to staphylococci, streptococci, fungi or other infectious organisms
- Most common in clients who have structural cardiac malformations, cardiac devices (pacemaker), prosthetic heart valves, or IV substance use disorder.
- Invasive procedures, such as dental procedures, body piercing, and tattooing, can cause bacteremia, which can lead to infective endocarditis in at-risk clients.
- Findings include fever, flu-like manifestations, murmur, petechiae (on the trunk and mucous membranes), positive blood cultures, and splinter hemorrhages (red streaks under the nail beds).

LABORATORY TESTS Q EBP

- Blood cultures to detect a bacterial infection.
- An elevated WBC count can be indicative of a bacterial infection.
- Cardiac enzymes can be elevated with pericarditis.
- Elevated ESR and CRP indicate inflammation in the body.
- Throat cultures to detect a streptococcal infection, which can lead to rheumatic fever.

DIAGNOSTIC PROCEDURES

Electrocardiography (ECG)

Can detect a heart block, which is associated with rheumatic fever or demonstrate ST segment elevation in almost all leads in the case of pericarditis.

Echocardiography

Can reveal inflamed heart layers or pericardial effusion.

PATIENT-CENTERED CARE

NURSING CARE

- Auscultate heart sounds. (Listen for murmur or friction rub.)
- Review ABGs, SaO₂, and chest x-ray results.
- Administer oxygen as prescribed.
- Monitor vital signs. (Watch for fever.)
- Monitor ECG, and notify the provider of changes.
- Monitor for cardiac tamponade and heart failure.
- Obtain throat cultures to identify bacteria to be treated by antibiotic therapy.
- Administer antibiotics as prescribed.
- Administer antipyretics as prescribed.
- Assess onset, quality, duration, and severity of pain.
- Administer pain medication as prescribed.
- Encourage bed rest.
- Provide emotional support to the client and family, and encourage verbalization of feelings regarding the illness.

MEDICATIONS

Penicillin

Antibiotic given to treat infection

NURSING CONSIDERATIONS
- Monitor for skin rash and hives.
- Monitor electrolyte and kidney levels.

CLIENT EDUCATION
- Instruct clients to report skin rash or hives.
- Inform clients that the medication can cause gastrointestinal (GI) distress.

Ibuprofen

NSAID (nonsteroidal anti-inflammatory drug) given to treat fever and inflammation

NURSING CONSIDERATIONS
- Do not use with clients who have peptic ulcer disease.
- Watch for indications of GI distress.
- Monitor platelets, and liver and kidney function levels.

CLIENT EDUCATION
- Instruct clients to take the medication with food.
- Inform clients that the medication can cause GI distress.
- Instruct clients to avoid alcohol consumption while taking the medication.

Prednisone

Glucocorticosteroid given to treat inflammation

NURSING CONSIDERATIONS
- Use in low doses.
- Monitor blood pressure.
- Monitor electrolytes and blood sugar levels.
- Clients can have impaired would healing when taking this medication.

CLIENT EDUCATION
- Instruct clients to take the medication with food.
- Instruct clients to avoid stopping the medication abruptly.
- Instruct clients to report unexpected weight gain.

Amphotericin B

Antifungal given to treat fungal infection

NURSING CONSIDERATIONS: Monitor liver and kidney function levels.

CLIENT EDUCATION: Inform clients that the medication can cause GI distress.

INTERPROFESSIONAL CARE

- Cardiology services are consulted to manage cardiac dysfunction.
- Infectious disease services can be consulted to manage infection.
- Physical therapy can be consulted to increase the client's level of activity once prescribed.

THERAPEUTIC PROCEDURES

Pericarditis

Pericardiocentesis is the insertion of a needle into the pericardium to aspirate pericardial fluid. This can be done in the emergency department or a procedure room.

NURSING ACTIONS
- Pericardial fluid can be sent to the laboratory for culture and sensitivity.
- Monitor for reoccurrence of cardiac tamponade.

Infective endocarditis

Valve debridement, draining of abscess, and repairing congenital shunts are procedures involved with infective endocarditis.

NURSING ACTIONS: Monitor for indications of bleeding, infection, and alteration in cardiac output.

CLIENT EDUCATION

- Encourage the client to take rest periods as needed.
- Encourage the client to wash hands to prevent infection.
- Encourage the client to avoid crowded areas to reduce the risk of infection.
- Educate the client about the importance of good oral hygiene and the prevention of infection.
- Educate the client about the importance of taking medications as prescribed.
- Ask the client to demonstrate the administration of intravenous antibiotics and management before discharge.
- Encourage the client to participate in cessation of tobacco use if applicable.
- Educate the client and family about the illness, and encourage them to express their feelings.
- Advise all providers, including dentists, of history of endocarditis so that antibiotic prophylaxis is prescribed if needed. Qs

CARE AFTER DISCHARGE

- Home health services can be indicated if the client had surgery. Qᴛᴄ
- Intravenous antibiotic therapy can be given by the home health service.
- Pharmaceutical services can be indicated for IV supplies and medications.
- Rehabilitation services can be indicated to help the client increase the level of activity.

COMPLICATIONS

Cardiac tamponade

Cardiac tamponade can result from fluid accumulation in the pericardial sac.

- Manifestations include dyspnea, dizziness, report of "tightness" in the chest, increasing restlessness, pulsus paradoxus (a decrease of 10 mm Hg or more in systolic blood pressure during inspiration), tachycardia, muffled heart sounds, and jugular venous distention.
- Hemodynamic monitoring reveals intracardiac and pulmonary artery pressures similar and elevated (plateau pressures).

NURSING ACTIONS

- Notify the provider immediately.
- Administer IV fluids to combat hypotension as prescribed.
- Obtain a chest x-ray or echocardiogram to confirm the diagnosis.
- Prepare the client for pericardiocentesis (informed consent, gather materials, administer medications as prescribed).
  - Monitor hemodynamic pressures as they normalize.
  - Monitor heart rhythm as changes indicate improper positioning of the needle.
  - Monitor for reoccurrence of manifestations after the procedure.

PRACTICE Active Learning Scenario

A nurse is reviewing discharge teaching with a client who has myocarditis. What should the nurse include in the teaching? Use the ATI Active Learning Template: System Disorder to complete this item.

CLIENT EDUCATION
- Identify at least two referral facilities and the services they can provide.
- Describe at least four actions the client should take when at home.

Application Exercises

1. A nurse is caring for a client who has pericarditis. Which of the following findings should the nurse expect?

   A. Petechiae

   B. Murmur

   C. Rash

   D. Friction rub

2. A nurse is caring for four clients. Which of the following clients should the nurse identify as being at risk of acquiring rheumatic endocarditis?

   A. Older adult who has chronic obstructive pulmonary disease

   B. Child who has streptococcal pharyngitis

   C. Middle-age adult who has lupus erythematosus

   D. Young adult who recently received a body tattoo

3. A nurse in a clinic is caring for a client who has been on long-term NSAID therapy to treat myocarditis. Which of the following laboratory findings should the nurse report to the provider?

   A. Platelets 100,000/mm³

   B. Serum glucose 110 mg/dL

   C. Serum creatinine 0.7 mg/dL

   D. Amino alanine transferase (ALT) 30 IU/L

4. A nurse is assessing a client who has splinter hemorrhages in her nail beds and reports a fever. The nurse should identify these findings as manifestations of which of the following disorders?

   A. Infective endocarditis

   B. Pericarditis

   C. Myocarditis

   D. Rheumatic endocarditis

5. A nurse is admitting a client who has suspected rheumatic endocarditis. The nurse should anticipate a prescription from the provider for which of the following laboratory tests to assist in confirmation of this diagnosis?

   A. Arterial blood gases

   B. Serum albumin

   C. Liver enzymes

   D. Throat culture

Application Exercises Key

1. A. Petechiae are an expected finding in a client who has endocarditis.

    B. A murmur is an expected finding in a client who has myocarditis and endocarditis.

    C. Rash is an expected finding in a client who has rheumatic endocarditis.

    D. **CORRECT:** A friction rub can be heard during auscultation of a client who has pericarditis.

    Ⓝ *NCLEX® Connection: Physiological Adaptation, Pathophysiology*

2. A. An older adult who has chronic obstructive pulmonary disease is not at risk for rheumatic endocarditis unless he develops rheumatic fever.

    B. **CORRECT:** A child who has streptococcal pharyngitis is at risk for developing rheumatic fever which could result in rheumatic endocarditis.

    C. A middle-age adult who has lupus erythematosus is not at risk for rheumatic endocarditis unless he develops rheumatic fever.

    D. A young adult who receives a body tattoo is at increased risk for infective endocarditis but is not at risk for rheumatic endocarditis unless he develops rheumatic fever.

    Ⓝ *NCLEX® Connection: Health Promotion and Maintenance, Health Promotion/Disease Prevention*

3. A. **CORRECT:** Long-term NSAID therapy can lower platelets. This finding is outside the expected reference range and should be reported to the provider.

    B. Serum glucose is not affected by long-term NSAID therapy. This finding is within the expected reference range.

    C. Kidney function, which is monitored by serum creatinine level, is affected by long-term NSAID therapy. This finding is within the expected reference range.

    D. Liver function, which is monitored by the ALT level, is affected by long-term NSAID therapy. This finding is within the expected reference range.

    Ⓝ *NCLEX® Connection: Reduction of Risk Potential, Laboratory Values*

4. A. **CORRECT:** Splinter hemorrhages in nail beds and a report of fever are findings associated with infective endocarditis.

    B. A client who has pericarditis would report chest pain.

    C. A client who has myocarditis would report a rapid heart rate.

    D. A client who has rheumatic endocarditis would report joint pain.

    Ⓝ *NCLEX® Connection: Physiological Adaptation, Illness Management*

5. A. Arterial blood gases are used to monitor the respiratory status of a client who has suspected rheumatic endocarditis, but they do not confirm the diagnosis.

    B. Serum albumin monitors the nutrition status of a client who has a suspected inflammatory disorder, but it does not confirm the diagnosis.

    C. Liver enzymes monitor a client's response to antibiotic therapy, which is used to treat rheumatic endocarditis, but they do not confirm the diagnosis.

    D. **CORRECT:** A throat culture can reveal the presence of streptococcus, which is the leading cause of rheumatic endocarditis.

    Ⓝ *NCLEX® Connection: Reduction of Risk Potential, Laboratory Values*

PRACTICE Answer

Using the ATI Active Learning Template: System Disorder

CLIENT EDUCATION

Referral facilities

- Home health: postoperative care, home administration of intravenous antibiotic therapy
- Pharmaceutical services: intravenous antibiotic therapy, provision of supplies and medications
- Rehabilitation services: assistance with monitoring and increasing activity level

Client discharge activities

- Rest as needed.
- Wash hands to prevent infection.
- Avoid crowded areas to reduce the risk of infection.
- Maintain good oral hygiene to prevent infection.
- Take medications as prescribed.
- Administer and manage IV antibiotics.
- Participate in a tobacco use cessation program.

Ⓝ *NCLEX® Connection: Physiological Adaptation, Pathophysiology*

UNIT 4 NURSING CARE OF CLIENTS WHO HAVE
CARDIOVASCULAR DISORDERS
SECTION: VASCULAR DISORDERS

CHAPTER 35 *Peripheral Vascular Diseases*

Peripheral vascular diseases include peripheral arterial disease (PAD) and peripheral venous disorders, both of which interfere with normal blood flow. PAD affects arteries (blood vessels that carry blood away from the heart), and peripheral venous disease affects veins (blood vessels that carry blood toward the heart).

Peripheral arterial disease

- PAD results from atherosclerosis that usually occurs in the arteries of the lower extremities and is characterized by inadequate flow of blood.
- Atherosclerosis is caused by a gradual thickening of the intima and media of the arteries, ultimately resulting in the progressive narrowing of the vessel lumen. Plaques can form on the walls of the arteries, making them rough and fragile.
- Progressive stiffening of the arteries and narrowing of the lumen decreases the blood supply to affected tissues and increases resistance to blood flow.
- Atherosclerosis is actually a type of arteriosclerosis, which means "hardening of the arteries" and alludes to the loss of elasticity of arteries over time due to thickening of their walls.
- PAD is classified as inflow (distal aorta and iliac arteries) or outflow (femoral, popliteal, and tibial arteries) and can range from mild to severe. Tissue damage occurs below the arterial obstruction.
- Buerger's disease, subclavian steal syndrome, thoracic outlet syndrome, Raynaud's disease, and popliteal entrapment are examples of PAD.

ASSESSMENT

RISK FACTORS

- Hypertension
- Hyperlipidemia
- Diabetes mellitus
- Cigarette smoking
- Obesity
- Sedentary lifestyle
- Familial predisposition
- Female gender
- Age: Older adult clients Ⓖ

EXPECTED FINDINGS

- Burning, cramping, and pain in the legs during exercise (intermittent claudication)
- Numbness or burning pain primarily in the feet when in bed
- Pain that is relieved by placing legs at rest in a dependent position

PHYSICAL ASSESSMENT FINDINGS

- Bruit over femoral and aortic arteries
- Decreased capillary refill of toes (greater than 3 seconds)
- Decreased or nonpalpable pulses
- Loss of hair on lower calf, ankle, and foot
- Dry, scaly, mottled skin
- Thick toenails
- Cold and cyanotic extremity
- Pallor of extremity with elevation
- Dependent rubor (redness) of the extremity
- Muscle atrophy
- Ulcers and possible gangrene of toes

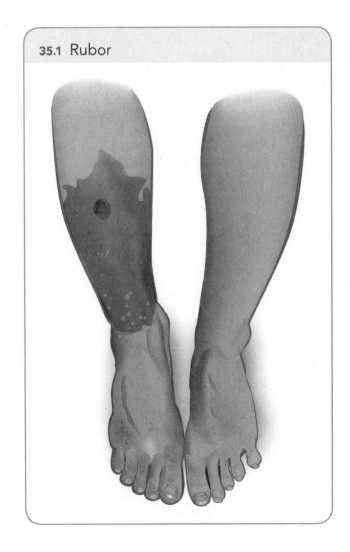

35.1 Rubor

DIAGNOSTIC PROCEDURES

Arteriography

- Arteriography of the lower extremities involves arterial injection of contrast medium to visualize areas of decreased arterial flow on an x-ray. Q🅴🅱🅿
- It is usually done only to determine isolated areas of occlusion that can be treated during the procedure with percutaneous transluminal angioplasty and possible stent placement.

NURSING ACTIONS
- Observe for bleeding and hemorrhage.
- Palpate pedal pulses to identify possible occlusions.

Exercise tolerance testing

A stress test is done with or without the use of a treadmill (medications such as dipyridamole and adenosine may be given to mimic the effects of exercise in clients who cannot tolerate a treadmill) with measurement of pulse volumes and blood pressures prior to and following the onset of manifestations or 5 min of exercise. Delays in return to normal pressures and pulse waveforms indicate arterial disease. It is used to evaluate claudication during exercise.

Plethysmography

- Plethysmography is used to determine the variations of blood passing through an artery, thus identifying abnormal arterial flow in the affected limb.
- Blood pressure cuffs are attached to the client's upper extremities, a lower extremity, and the plethysmograph machine. Variations in peripheral pulses between the upper and lower extremity are recorded.
- A decrease in pulse pressure of the lower extremity indicates a possible blockage in the leg.

Segmental systolic blood pressure measurements

- A Doppler probe is used to take various blood pressure measurements (thigh, calf, ankle, brachial) for comparison. In the absence of PAD, pressures in the lower extremities are higher than those of the upper extremities.
- With arterial disease, the pressures in the thigh, calf, and ankle are lower.

Magnetic resonance angiography

A contrast medium, such as gadolinium, is injected to help visualize blood flow through peripheral arteries.

Ankle-brachial index (ABI)

The ankle pressure is compared to the brachial pressure. The expected finding for ABI is 0.9 to 1.3. ABI less than 0.9 in either leg is diagnostic for PAD.

Doppler-derived maximal systolic acceleration

A technique that is especially helpful for evaluating PAD in clients who have diabetes mellitus.

PATIENT-CENTERED CARE

NURSING CARE

- Encourage the client to exercise to build up collateral circulation.
  - Initiate exercise gradually and increase slowly.
  - Instruct the client to walk until the point of pain, stop and rest, and then walk a little farther.
- Promote vasodilation and avoid vasoconstriction.
  - Provide a warm environment for the client.
  - Have the client wear insulated socks.
  - Tell the client to never apply direct heat, such as a heating pad, to the affected extremity because sensitivity is decreased, and this can cause a burn.
  - Instruct the client to avoid exposure to cold (causes vasoconstriction and decreased arterial flow).
  - Instruct the client to avoid stress, caffeine, and nicotine, which also cause vasoconstriction.
    - Vasoconstriction is avoided when the client completely abstains from smoking or chewing tobacco. Q🅴🅱🅿
    - Vasoconstriction of vessels lasts up to 1 hr after smoking or chewing tobacco.

POSITIONING
- Instruct the client to avoid crossing the legs.
- Tell the client to refrain from wearing restrictive garments.
- Tell the client to elevate the legs to reduce swelling, but not to elevate them above the level of the heart because extreme elevation slows arterial blood flow to the feet.

MEDICATIONS

Antiplatelet medications

Aspirin, clopidogrel, pentoxifylline
Antiplatelet medications reduce blood viscosity by decreasing blood fibrinogen levels, enhancing erythrocyte flexibility, and increasing blood flow in the extremities. Medications such as aspirin and clopidogrel may be prescribed. Pentoxifylline, sometimes referred to as a hemorheologic medication, was one of the first to be used and is still used, but less commonly than other medications. It may be given to specifically treat intermittent claudication in clients who have PAD.

CLIENT EDUCATION
- Inform the client that the medication's effects might not be apparent for several weeks.
- Advise the client to monitor for evidence of bleeding, such as abdominal pain, coffee-ground emesis, or black, tarry stools.

Statins

Simvastatin, atorvastatin: Can relieve manifestations associated with PAD (intermittent claudication).

THERAPEUTIC PROCEDURES

Percutaneous transluminal angioplasty and laser-assisted angioplasty

- Percutaneous transluminal angioplasty is an invasive intra-arterial procedure using a balloon and stent to open and help maintain the patency of the vessel.
- Laser-assisted angioplasty is an invasive procedure in which a laser probe is advanced through a cannula to the site of stenosis.
  - The laser is used to vaporize atherosclerotic plaque and open the artery.

NURSING CONSIDERATIONS

- The priority action is to observe for bleeding at the puncture site. Qs
- Monitor vital signs, peripheral pulses, and capillary refill.
- Keep the client on bed rest with his limb straight for 2 to 6 hr before ambulation.
- Anticoagulant therapy is used during the procedure, followed by antiplatelet therapy for 1 to 3 months.

Mechanical rotational abrasive atherectomy

Uses a rotational device to scrape plaque from the inside of the client's peripheral artery. The device is designed to cause minimal damage to the surface of the artery.

NURSING CONSIDERATIONS

- The priority action is to observe for bleeding at the puncture site. Qs
- Monitor vital signs, peripheral pulses, and capillary refill.
- Keep the client on bed rest with his limb straight for 2 to 6 hr before ambulation.
- Anticoagulant therapy is used during the procedure, followed by antiplatelet therapy for 1 to 3 months.

Arterial revascularization surgery

Used with clients who have severe claudication and/or limb pain at rest, or with clients who are at risk for losing a limb due to poor arterial circulation.

- Bypass grafts are used to reroute the circulation around the arterial occlusion.
- Grafts can be harvested from the client (autologous) or made from synthetic materials.

NURSING ACTIONS

- The priority action is to maintain adequate circulation in the repaired artery. The location of the pedal or dorsalis pulse should be marked, and its pulsatile strength compared with the contralateral leg on a scheduled basis using a Doppler. Qs
- Color, temperature, sensation, and capillary refill should be compared with the contralateral extremity on a scheduled basis.
- Assess for warmth, redness, and possibly edema of the affected limb as a result of increased blood flow.
- Monitor for pain. Pain can be severe due to the reestablishment of blood flow to the extremity.
- Monitor blood pressure. Hypotension can result in an increased risk of clotting or graft collapse, while hypertension increases the risk for bleeding from sutures.
- Instruct the client to limit bending of the hip and knee to decrease the risk of clot formation.

CLIENT EDUCATION

- Instruct the client to avoid crossing or raising legs above the level of the heart.
- Instruct the client to wear loose clothing.
- Instruct the client on wound care if revascularization surgery was done.
- Discourage smoking and cold temperatures.
- Instruct the client about foot care (keep feet clean and dry, wear good-fitting shoes, never go barefoot, cut toenails straight across or have the podiatrist cut nails).

COMPLICATIONS

Graft occlusion

Graft occlusion is a serious complication of arterial revascularization and often occurs within the first 24 hr following surgery.

NURSING ACTIONS

- Promptly notify the surgeon of manifestations of occlusion, such as absent or reduced pedal pulses, increased pain, or change in extremity color or temperature. Qs
- Be prepared to assist with treatment, which can include an emergency thrombectomy (removal of a clot), local intra-arterial thrombolytic therapy with an agent such as tissue plasminogen activator, infusion of a platelet inhibitor, or a combination of these. With these treatments, assess for indications of bleeding.

Wound or graft infection

An infection of the surgical wound or graft is a potentially life-threatening complication.

NURSING ACTIONS

- Use sterile technique when changing the surgical dressing or providing wound care.
- Indications of infection include localized induration, warmth, tenderness, erythema, edema, purulent drainage, and an elevated WBC. Promptly report findings to the provider.

Compartment syndrome

Compartment syndrome is considered a medical emergency. Tissue pressure within a confined body space can restrict blood flow, and the resulting ischemia can lead to irreversible tissue damage.

NURSING ACTIONS

- Manifestations of compartment syndrome include tingling, numbness, worsening pain, edema, pain on passive movement, and unequal pulses. Immediately report findings to the provider.
- Loosen dressings.
- Prepare to assist with fasciotomy (surgical opening into the tissues), which can be necessary to prevent further injury and to save the limb.

Peripheral venous disorders

Peripheral venous disorders are problems with the veins that interfere with adequate return of blood flow from the extremities.

- There are superficial and deep veins in the lower extremities that have valves that prevent backflow of blood as it returns to the heart. The action of the skeletal muscles of the lower extremities during walking and other activities also promotes venous return.
- Three peripheral venous disorders that nurses should be familiar with are venous thromboembolism (VTE), venous insufficiency, and varicose veins.

VTE is a blood clot believed to form as a result of venous stasis, endothelial injury, or hypercoagulability. Thrombus formation can lead to a pulmonary embolism, which is a life-threatening complication. Thrombophlebitis refers to a thrombus that is associated with inflammation. **(35.3, 35.4)**

Venous insufficiency occurs secondary to incompetent valves in the deeper veins of the lower extremities, which allows pooling of blood and dilation of the veins. The veins' inability to carry fluid and wastes from the lower extremities precipitates the development of swelling, venous stasis ulcers, and in advanced cases, cellulitis.

Varicose veins are enlarged, twisted and superficial veins that can occur in any part of the body; however, they are commonly observed in the lower extremities and in the esophagus. **(35.5)**

35.2 Compartment syndrome

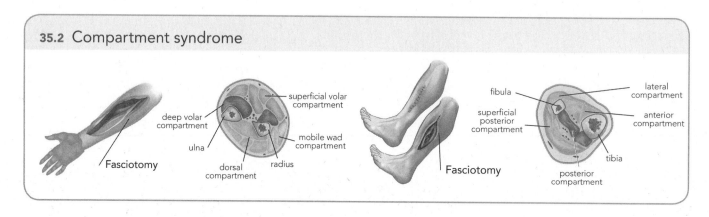

35.3 Deep-vein thrombosis

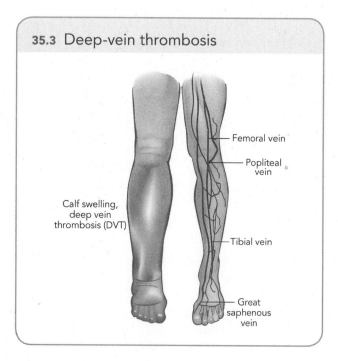

35.4 Thrombophlebitis

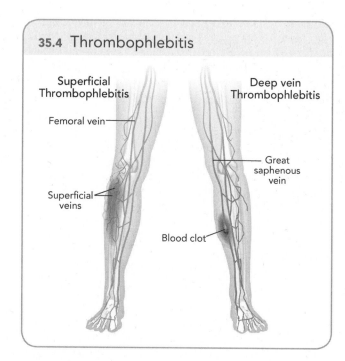

ASSESSMENT

RISK FACTORS

Venous thromboembolism: Associated with Virchow's triad (hypercoagulability, impaired blood flow, damage to blood vessels)
- Hip surgery, total-knee replacement, open prostate surgery
- Heart failure
- Immobility
- Pregnancy
- Oral contraceptives
- Active cancer

Venous Insufficiency
- Sitting or standing in one position for a long period of time
- Obesity
- Pregnancy
- Thrombophlebitis

Varicose veins
- Female gender
- Age older than 30 years and an occupation requiring prolonged standing
- Pregnancy
- Obesity
- Systemic diseases (heart disease)
- Family history

EXPECTED FINDINGS

Limb pain: Aching pain and feeling of fullness or heaviness in the legs after standing

PHYSICAL ASSESSMENT FINDINGS
- **Deep vein thrombosis (DVT) and thrombophlebitis**
  - Client can be asymptomatic.
  - Calf or groin pain, tenderness, and a sudden onset of edema of the extremity. ⓠEBP
  - Warmth, edema, and induration and hardness over the involved blood vessel.
  - Changes in circumferences of right and left calf and thigh over time; localized edema over the affected area.

  ! Shortness of breath and chest pain can indicate that the embolus has moved to the lungs (pulmonary embolism).

- **Venous insufficiency**
  - Stasis dermatitis is a brown discoloration along the ankles that extends up the calf relative to the level of insufficiency.
  - Edema
  - Stasis ulcers (typically found around ankles)
- **Varicose veins**
  - Distended, superficial veins that are visible just below the skin and are tortuous in nature
  - Clients often report muscle cramping and aches, pain after sitting, and pruritus.

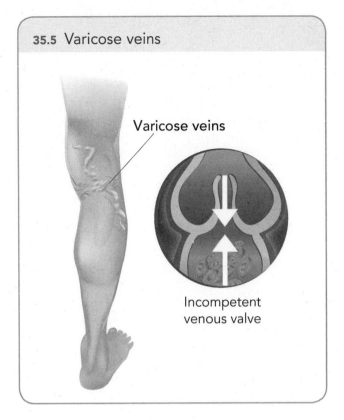

35.5 Varicose veins

Varicose veins

Incompetent venous valve

LABORATORY TESTS

D-dimer test measures fibrin degradation products present in the blood produced from fibrinolysis. A positive test indicates that thrombus formation has possibly occurred.

DIAGNOSTIC PROCEDURES

DVT and thrombophlebitis

- Venous duplex ultrasonography uses high-frequency sound waves to provide a real-time picture of the blood flow through a blood vessel.
- Doppler flow study produces an audible sound when venous circulation is normal and little or no sound when veins are thrombosed.
- Impedance plethysmography can be used to determine the variations of blood passing through a vein, thus identifying abnormal venous flow in the affected limb.
- If the above tests are negative for a DVT, but one is still suspected, a venogram, which uses contrast material, or magnetic resonance imaging might be needed for accurate diagnosis.

Varicose veins: Trendelenburg test

NURSING ACTIONS
- Place the client in a supine position with legs elevated.
- When the client sits up, the veins will fill from the proximal end if varicosities are present (veins normally fill from the distal end).

PATIENT-CENTERED CARE

NURSING CARE

DVT and thrombophlebitis

- Encourage the client to rest.
  - Facilitate bed rest and elevation of the extremity above the level of the heart as prescribed. (Avoid using a knee gatch or pillow under knees.)
- Administer intermittent or continuous warm moist compresses as prescribed.
- Do not massage the affected limb. Qs
- Provide thigh-high compression or antiembolism stockings.
- Prepare the client for an inferior vena cava interruption surgery (a filter traps emboli and prevents them from reaching the heart) as indicated.

Venous insufficiency

- Elevate legs for at least 20 min, four to five times a day.
- Elevate the legs above the heart when in bed.
- Instruct clients to avoid crossing legs and wearing constrictive clothing or stockings.
- Instruct clients to wear elastic compression stockings and apply them after the legs have been elevated and when swelling is at a minimum. QEBP

MEDICATIONS

DVT and thrombophlebitis: anticoagulants

Unfractionated heparin
- Given IV to prevent formation of other clots and to prevent enlargement of the existing clot.
- It has significant adverse effects and must be given in the facility. Prior to discharge, the client will be converted to oral anticoagulation therapy with warfarin.
- NURSING ACTIONS
  - Monitor aPTT to allow for adjustments of heparin dosage.
  - Monitor platelet counts for heparin-induced thrombocytopenia. Qs
  - Ensure that protamine sulfate, the antidote for heparin, is available if needed for excessive bleeding.
  - Monitor for hazards and adverse effects associated with anticoagulant therapy.

Low-molecular weight heparin
- Given subcutaneously and is based on a client's weight.
- Enoxaparin is used for the prevention and treatment of DVT. It is usually given in the facility, but the twice-daily injections can be given in the home setting.
- NURSING ACTIONS
  - Instruct the client to observe for evidence of bleeding.
  - Instruct the client on bleeding precautions that should be taken (use electric instead of bladed razor and brush teeth with a soft toothbrush). Qs

Warfarin
- Inhibits synthesis of the four vitamin K–dependent clotting factors.
- The therapeutic effect takes 3 to 4 days to develop, so administration of the medication is begun while the client is still on heparin.
- NURSING ACTIONS
  - Monitor for bleeding.
  - Monitor PT and INR.
  - Ensure that vitamin K (the antidote for warfarin) is available in case of excessive bleeding.
  - Instruct the client about food sources of vitamin K (green leafy vegetables) and to avoid fluctuations in the amount and frequency of consumption.
  - Instruct the client about observing for evidence of bleeding.
  - Instruct the client on bleeding precautions that should be taken (use electric instead of bladed razor, and brush teeth with soft toothbrush).

DVT and thrombophlebitis: thrombolytic therapy

Thrombolytic therapy dissolves clots that have already developed. Therapy must be started within 5 days after the development of the clot for the therapy to be effective. Tissue plasminogen activator, a thrombolytic agent, and platelet inhibitors (such as abciximab and eptifibatide) can be effective in dissolving a clot or preventing new clots during the first 24 hr. Administering the medication in a manner that provides direct contact with the thrombus can be more effective and lessen the chance of bleeding.

NURSING ACTIONS
- Monitor for bleeding (e.g., intracerebral bleeding).
- Instruct the client about bleeding precautions that should be taken. (Use electric instead of bladed razor and brush teeth with a soft toothbrush.)

THERAPEUTIC PROCEDURES

DVT

An **inferior vena cava filter** can be inserted when a client is unresponsive to medical therapy or when anticoagulation is contraindicated. It is inserted via the femoral vein and passed into the inferior vena cava where it traps emboli before they progress to the lungs.

Varicose veins

Sclerotherapy
- A sclerosing irritating chemical solution is injected into the varicose vein to produce localized inflammation, which will close the lumen of the vessel over time.
- For larger vessels, an incision and drainage of the trapped blood in a sclerosed vein might need to be performed 2 to 3 weeks after the injection.
- Pressure dressings are applied for approximately 1 week after each procedure to keep the vessel free of blood.
- CLIENT EDUCATION
  - Instruct the client to wear elastic stockings for the prescribed time.
  - Mild analgesics, such as acetaminophen, can be taken for discomfort.

Vein stripping

- Vein stripping is the removal of large varicose veins that cannot be treated with less-invasive procedures.
- PREOPERATIVE NURSING ACTIONS
  - Assist the provider with vein marking.
  - Evaluate pulses as a baseline for postoperative comparison.
- POSTOPERATIVE NURSING ACTIONS
  - Maintain elastic bandages on the legs.
  - Monitor groin and leg for bleeding through the elastic bandages.
  - Monitor extremity for edema, warmth, color, and pulses.
  - Elevate legs above the level of the heart.
  - Encourage the client to engage in range-of-motion exercises of the legs.
- CLIENT EDUCATION
  - Emphasize the importance of wearing elastic stockings after bandage removal.
  - Instruct the client to elevate the legs when sitting, and avoid dangling them over the side of the bed.

Endovenous laser treatment: This type of treatment uses a laser fiber that is inserted into the vessel proximal to the area to be treated and then threaded to the involved area, where heat from the laser is used to close the dilated vein.

Application of radio frequency energy: This type of treatment uses a small catheter with a radio frequency electrode, instead of a laser, that is inserted into the vessel proximal to the area to be treated that scars and closes a dilated vein.

INTERPROFESSIONAL CARE

Venous insufficiency

- Care of venous stasis ulcers requires long-term management.
- Consultation with a dietitian and wound care specialist facilitate the healing process. Q_{TC}

COMPLICATIONS

Ulcer formation

- Venous stasis ulcers often form over the medial malleolus. Venous ulcers are chronic, hard to heal, and often recur. They can lead to amputation or death. **(34.6)**
- Clients who have neuropathy might not feel as much discomfort from the ulcer as its appearance can warrant.

NURSING ACTIONS

- Administer and assist with treatments to improve circulation (wound vacuum, hyperbaric chamber).
- Assess and treat pain as prescribed.
- Apply oxygen-permeable polyethylene films to superficial ulcers.
- Apply occlusive hydrocolloid dressings on deeper ulcers to promote granulation tissue and reepithelialization. Q_{EBP}
- Leave a dressing on for 3 to 7 days.
- If a wound needs chemical debridement, apply prescribed topical enzymatic agents to debride the ulcer, eliminate necrotic tissue, and promote healing.
- Administer systemic antibiotics as prescribed.

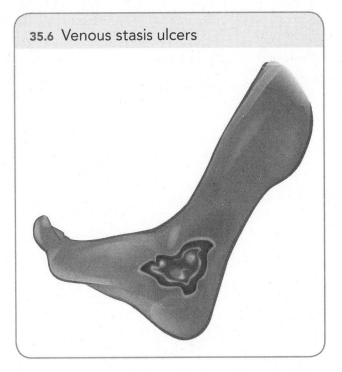

35.6 Venous stasis ulcers

CLIENT EDUCATION

- Recommend a diet high in zinc, protein, iron, and vitamins A and C.
- Instruct clients on the use of compression stockings.
- Prepare for oxygen therapy and blood gas analysis while continuing to monitor and assess the client for other manifestations.
- Prepare to administer prescribed anticoagulation.

Pulmonary embolism

A pulmonary embolism occurs when a thrombus is dislodged, becomes an embolus, and lodges in a pulmonary vessel. This can lead to obstruction of pulmonary blood flow, decreased systemic oxygenation, pulmonary tissue hypoxia, and possible death.

NURSING ACTIONS

- Manifestations include sudden onset dyspnea, pleuritic chest pain, restlessness, apprehension, feelings of impending doom, cough, and hemoptysis.
- Findings include tachypnea, crackles, pleural friction rub, tachycardia, S_3 or S_4 heart sounds, diaphoresis, low-grade fever, petechiae over chest and axillae, and decreased arterial oxygen saturation.
- Notify the provider immediately. Reassure the client. Assist the client to a position of comfort with the head of the bed elevated. Q_S
- Prepare for oxygen therapy and blood gas analysis while continuing to monitor and assess the client for other manifestations.
- Prepare to administer prescribed anticoagulation.

Application Exercises

1. A nurse is caring for a client who has chronic venous insufficiency and a prescription for thigh-high compression stockings. Which of the following actions should the nurse take?

   A. Elevate the legs for 10 min, two to three times daily while wearing stockings.

   B. Apply the stockings in the morning upon awakening and before getting out of bed.

   C. Roll the stockings down to the knees to relieve discomfort on the legs.

   D. Remove the stockings while out of bed for 1 hr, four times a day, to allow the legs to rest.

2. A nurse is assessing a client who has chronic peripheral arterial disease (PAD). Which of the following findings should the nurse expect?

   A. Edema around the ankles and feet

   B. Ulceration around the medial malleoli

   C. Scaling eczema of the lower legs with stasis dermatitis

   D. Pallor on elevation of the limbs, and rubor when the limbs are dependent

3. A nurse is teaching a client who has a new diagnosis of severe peripheral arterial disease. Which of the following instructions should the nurse include?

   A. Wear tightly fitted insulated socks with shoes when going outside.

   B. Elevate both legs above the heart when resting.

   C. Apply a heating pad to both legs for comfort.

   D. Place both legs in dependent position while sleeping.

4. A nurse is teaching a client who has a new prescription for clopidogrel. Which of the following instructions should the nurse include in the teaching? (Select all that apply.)

   A. Avoid the consuming grapefruit while taking this medication.

   B. Monitor for the presence of black, tarry stools.

   C. Take this medication when you have pain.

   D. Schedule a weekly PT test.

   E. Limit food sources containing vitamin K while taking this medication.

5. A nurse is caring for a client who has a deep-vein thrombosis (DVT) and has been taking unfractionated heparin for 1 week. Two days ago, the provider also prescribed warfarin. The client asks the nurse about receiving both heparin and warfarin at the same time. Which of the following statements should the nurse give?

   A. "I will remind your provider that you are already receiving heparin."

   B. "Your laboratory findings indicated that two anticoagulants were needed."

   C. "It takes 3 to 4 days before the therapeutic effects of warfarin are achieved, and then the heparin can be discontinued."

   D. "Only one of these medications is being given to treat your deep-vein thrombosis."

PRACTICE Active Learning Scenario

A nurse is developing a poster presentation on peripheral arterial disease (PAD) for a community health fair. What content should the nurse include on the poster? Use the ATI Active Learning Template: System Disorder to complete this item.

ALTERATION IN HEALTH (DIAGNOSIS)

RISK FACTORS: Describe at least six.

EXPECTED FINDINGS: Describe at least six findings.

CLIENT EDUCATION: Describe at least two actions by the client related to proper positioning and two actions related to promoting vasodilation.

Application Exercises Key

1. A. The client who has venous insufficiency should sit with legs elevated for at least 20 min, four to five times daily.

B. **CORRECT:** Applying stockings in the morning upon awakening and before getting out of bed reduces venous stasis and assists in the venous return of blood to the heart. Legs are less edematous at this time.

C. Rolling stockings down can restrict circulation and cause edema.

D. Stockings should remain in place throughout the day and are removed before going to bed to provide continuous venous support. If the stockings are removed, such as for a bath or shower, then the legs should be elevated before the stockings are reapplied.

(N) *NCLEX® Connection: Reduction of Risk Potential, Potential for Complications of Diagnostic Tests/Treatments/Procedures*

2. A. Edema around the ankles and feet is an expected finding in a client who has venous stasis.

B. Ulceration around the medial malleoli is an expected finding in a client who has venous stasis.

C. Scaling eczema of the lower legs with stasis dermatitis is an expected finding in a client who has venous stasis.

D. **CORRECT:** In a client who has chronic PAD, pallor is seen in the extremities when the limbs are elevated, and rubor occurs when they are lowered.

(N) *NCLEX® Connection: Physiological Adaptation, Pathophysiology*

3. A. While insulated socks can promote warmth, they should be loose fitting to promote circulation.

B. The client should avoid elevating the legs above the heart while resting. This can cause a restriction in arterial blood flow to the feet.

C. The client should not apply a heating pad to his legs due to the loss in sensation as a result of the disease. Applying direct heat to the legs can burn the client.

D. **CORRECT:** The nurse should instruct the client to place his legs in a dependent position, such as hanging off the edge of the bed while sleeping. This can alleviate swelling and discomfort of the legs.

(N) *NCLEX® Connection: Physiological Adaptation, Illness Management*

4. A. **CORRECT:** The nurse should instruct the client to avoid consuming grapefruit while taking clopidogrel. Grapefruit interferes with absorption of clopidogrel and can cause severe complications.

B. **CORRECT:** The nurse should instruct the client to monitor for evidence of GI bleeding, such as abdominal pain, coffee-ground emesis, or black, tarry stools. If this occurs, the client should report this to the provider.

C. The client should take clopidogrel routinely as prescribed because it can take several weeks to be effective.

D. PT and INR levels are monitored regularly in a client taking warfarin.

E. A client who is taking warfarin should be advised about food sources containing vitamin K.

(N) *NCLEX® Connection: Pharmacological and Parenteral Therapies, Adverse Effects/Contraindications/Side Effects/Interactions*

5. A. Warfarin is prescribed for 3 to 4 days before discontinuing IV heparin.

B. IV heparin is monitored to achieve adequate therapeutic levels in treating a DVT.

C. **CORRECT:** Warfarin depresses synthesis of clotting factors but does not have an effect on clotting factors that are present. It takes 3 to 4 days for the clotting factors that are present to decay and for the therapeutic effects of warfarin to occur.

D. Heparin and warfarin are both effective in treating DVT.

(N) *NCLEX® Connection: Pharmacological and Parenteral Therapies, Medication Administration*

PRACTICE Answer

Using the ATI Active Learning Template: System Disorder

ALTERATION IN HEALTH (DIAGNOSIS): PAD is inadequate blood flow of the lower extremities due to atherosclerosis. The intima and media of the arteries become thickened, and plaque can form on the walls of the arteries, making them rough and fragile. The arteries progressively stiffen and the lumen narrows, decreasing blood supply to tissues and increasing resistance to blood flow. It is classified as either an inflow or outflow type of PAD.

RISK FACTORS
• Hypertension
• Hyperlipidemia
• Diabetes mellitus
• Cigarette smoking
• Obesity
• Sedentary lifestyle
• Familial predisposition
• Age: older adults clients
• Female gender

EXPECTED FINDINGS
• Bruits over femoral and aortic arteries
• Decreased capillary refill of toes (greater than 3 seconds)
• Decreased or nonpalpable pulses
• Loss of hair on the lower extremities
• Dry, scaly, mottled skin
• Thick toenails
• Cold, cyanotic extremity
• Pallor of extremity with elevation
• Dependent rubor
• Muscle atrophy
• Ulcers and possible gangrene of toes

CLIENT EDUCATION
• Teach actions related to positioning.
  ○ Tell the client to avoid crossing the legs.
  ○ Remind the client to avoid wearing restrictive garments.
  ○ Teach the client to keep legs elevated to reduce swelling, but not above the level of the heart.
• Teach actions to promote vasodilation.
  ○ Instruct clients to maintain a warm environment.
  ○ Tell clients to wear insulated socks.
  ○ Remind clients to avoid applying direct heat to the extremity.
  ○ Teach clients to avoid exposure to cold.
  ○ Instruct clients to avoid stress, caffeine, and nicotine.

(N) *NCLEX® Connection: Physiological Adaptation, Illness Management*

CHAPTER 36 *Hypertension*

For an adult client, hypertension occurs when systolic blood pressure is at or greater than 140 mm Hg or diastolic blood pressure is at or greater than 90 mm Hg for two or more assessments of blood pressure. For clients older than 60 years, blood pressure should be less than 150/90.

Essential hypertension, also called primary hypertension, accounts for most cases of hypertension. There is no known cause. Secondary hypertension can be caused by disease states, such as kidney disease, or as an adverse effect of some medications. Treatment for secondary hypertension occurs by removing the cause (adrenal tumor, medication).

Clients who have a systolic blood pressure of 120 to 139 mm Hg or a diastolic blood pressure of 80 to 89 mm Hg are considered to have prehypertension. Lifestyle changes are necessary for these clients to help prevent cardiovascular disease.

Prolonged, untreated, or poorly controlled hypertension can cause peripheral vascular disease that primarily affects the heart, brain, eyes, and kidneys. The risk of developing complications increases as blood pressure increases.

Hypertrophy of the left ventricle can develop as the heart pumps against resistance caused by the hypertension.

HEALTH PROMOTION AND DISEASE PREVENTION

- Maintain body mass index of less than 30.
- Clients who have diabetes mellitus should keep blood glucose within a recommended reference range.
- Limit caffeine and alcohol intake.
- Use stress-management techniques during times of stress.
- Stop smoking. Nicotine patches or engaging in a smoking cessation class are potential strategies.
- Engage in exercise that provides aerobic benefits at least 3 times a week.
- Limit sodium and fat intake.

ASSESSMENT

Four bodily mechanisms regulate blood pressure.

Arterial baroreceptors
- Baroreceptors are located in the carotid sinus, aorta, and left ventricle.
- They control blood pressure by altering the heart rate. They also cause vasoconstriction or vasodilation.

Regulation of body-fluid volume: Properly functioning kidneys retain fluid when a client is hypotensive and excrete fluid when a client is hypertensive.

Renin-angiotensin-aldosterone system: Renin is converted into angiotensin II, which causes vasoconstriction and controls aldosterone release, causing the kidneys to reabsorb sodium and inhibit fluid loss.

Vascular autoregulation: This maintains consistent levels of tissue perfusion.

RISK FACTORS

Essential hypertension
- Positive family history
- Excessive sodium intake
- Physical inactivity
- Obesity
- High alcohol consumption
- African American
- Smoking
- Hyperlipidemia
- Stress
- Age greater than 60 or postmenopausal

Secondary hypertension
- Kidney disease
- Cushing's disease (excessive glucocorticoid secretion)
- Primary aldosteronism (causes hypertension and hypokalemia)
- Pheochromocytoma (excessive catecholamine release)
- Brain tumors, encephalitis
- Medications such as estrogen, steroids, and sympathomimetics
- Pregnancy

EXPECTED FINDINGS

- Clients who have hypertension can experience few or no manifestations. Monitor for the following.
  - Headaches, particularly in the morning
  - Facial flushing
  - Dizziness
  - Fainting
  - Retinal changes, visual disturbances
  - Nocturia

PHYSICAL ASSESSMENT FINDINGS

- When a blood pressure reading is elevated, take it in both arms and with the client sitting and standing.
- There are **levels of hypertension**, as defined by the Joint National Committee on Prevention, Detection, Evaluation, and Treatment of High Blood Pressure.
  - **Prehypertension:** systolic 120 to 139 mm Hg; diastolic 80 to 89 mm Hg
  - **Stage I hypertension:** systolic 140 to 159 mm Hg; diastolic 90 to 99 mm Hg
  - **Stage II hypertension:** systolic greater than or equal to 160 mm Hg; diastolic greater than or equal to 100 mm Hg

LABORATORY TESTS

No laboratory tests exist to diagnose hypertension. However, several laboratory tests can identify the causes of secondary hypertension and target organ damage.
- **BUN, creatinine** elevation is indicative of kidney disease.
- **Elevated serum corticoids** detect Cushing's disease.
- **Blood glucose and cholesterol studies** can identify contributing factors related to blood vessel changes.

DIAGNOSTIC PROCEDURES

ECG evaluates cardiac function. Tall R-waves are often seen with left-ventricular hypertrophy.

Chest x-ray can show cardiomegaly.

PATIENT-CENTERED CARE

NURSING CARE

Discuss with the client factors that increase the risk of hypertension and how the client can manage them.

MEDICATIONS

Medications are added to treat hypertension that is not responsive to lifestyle changes alone. Diuretics are often first-line medications. However, clients can require a combination of medications to control hypertension.

CLIENT EDUCATION: Instruct clients who are taking antihypertensives to change positions slowly, and to be careful when getting out of bed, driving, and climbing stairs until the medication's effects are fully known. Qs

Diuretics

- **Thiazide diuretics**, such as hydrochlorothiazide, inhibit water and sodium reabsorption, and increase potassium excretion.
- Other diuretics can treat hypertension that is not responsive to thiazide diuretics.
  - **Loop diuretics**, such as furosemide, decrease sodium reabsorption and increase potassium excretion. **Potassium-sparing diuretics**, such as spironolactone, affect the distal tubule and prevent reabsorption of sodium in exchange for potassium.

NURSING CONSIDERATIONS: Monitor potassium levels and watch for muscle weakness, irregular pulse, and dehydration. Thiazide and loop diuretics can cause hypokalemia, and potassium-sparing diuretics can cause hyperkalemia.

CLIENT EDUCATION
- Encourage the client to keep all appointments with the provider to monitor efficacy of pharmacological treatment and possible electrolyte imbalance (hyponatremia, hyperkalemia).
- If the client is taking a potassium-depleting diuretic, encourage consumption of potassium-rich foods, such as bananas.

Calcium-channel blockers

Verapamil, amlodipine, and diltiazem alter the movement of calcium ions through the cell membrane, causing vasodilation and lowering blood pressure.

NURSING CONSIDERATIONS
- Monitor blood pressure and pulse, and change the client's position slowly. Hypotension is a common adverse effect.
- Use calcium-channel blockers cautiously with clients who have heart failure.

CLIENT EDUCATION
- Constipation can occur with verapamil, so encourage intake of foods that are high in fiber.
- A decrease or increase in heart rate and atrioventricular (AV) block can occur. Teach the client how to take her pulse and to call the provider if it is irregular or lower than the established rate.
- Instruct the client to avoid grapefruit juice, which potentiates the medication's effects, increases hypotensive effects, and increases the risk of medication toxicity.

ANGIOTENSIN-CONVERTING ENZYME (ACE) INHIBITORS

ACE inhibitors, such as lisinopril and enalapril, prevent the conversion of angiotensin I to angiotensin II, which prevents vasoconstriction.

NURSING CONSIDERATIONS
- Monitor blood pressure and pulse. Hypotension is a common adverse effect.
- Monitor for evidence of heart failure, such as edema. ACE inhibitors can cause heart and kidney complications.

CLIENT EDUCATION
- Teach the client to report a cough, which is an adverse effect of ACE inhibitors. The client should notify the provider of this adverse effect, as the medication can be discontinued due to its persistent nature and occasional relationship to angioedema (swelling of the tissues in the throat that can progress to a life-threatening obstruction). Qs
- Teach the client to reports manifestations of heart failure (edema).

Angiotensin-II receptor antagonists

Also called angiotensin-receptor blockers (ARBs), these medications, such as valsartan and losartan, are a good option for clients taking ACE inhibitors who report cough or have hyperkalemia. ARBs do not require a dosage adjustment for older adult clients.

NURSING CONSIDERATIONS: Monitor for manifestations of angioedema or heart failure. Angioedema is a serious, but uncommon adverse effect, and heart failure can result from taking this medication.

CLIENT EDUCATION
- Teach the client to change positions slowly.
- Teach the client to report findings of angioedema (swollen lips or face) or heart failure (edema).
- Reinforce to client to avoid foods that are high in potassium and to have serum potassium levels monitored because ARBS can cause hyperkalemia.

Aldosterone-receptor antagonists

Aldosterone-receptor antagonists, such as eplerenone, block aldosterone action. The blocking effect of eplerenone on aldosterone receptors promotes the retention of potassium and excretion of sodium and water.

NURSING CONSIDERATIONS
- Monitor kidney function, triglycerides, sodium, and potassium levels. The risk of adverse effects increases with deteriorating kidney function. Hypertriglyceridemia, hyponatremia, and hyperkalemia can occur as the dose increases.
- Monitor potassium levels every 2 weeks for the first few months and every 2 months thereafter. The client should avoid taking potassium supplements or potassium-sparing diuretics.

CLIENT EDUCATION
- Teach the client about potential food, medication, and herbal interactions. Grapefruit juice and St. John's wort can increase adverse effects.
- Instruct the client not to take salt substitutes with potassium or other foods that are rich in potassium.

Beta blockers

Beta blockers, such as metoprolol and atenolol, are for clients who have unstable angina or MI. They decrease cardiac output and block the release of renin, subsequently decreasing vasoconstriction of the peripheral vasculature.

NURSING CONSIDERATIONS
- Monitor blood pressure and pulse.
- These medications can mask hypoglycemia in clients who have diabetes mellitus.

CLIENT EDUCATION
- Teach the client that these medications can cause fatigue, weakness, depression, and sexual dysfunction.
- Advise the client not to suddenly stop taking the medication without consulting with the provider. Stopping suddenly can cause rebound hypertension.
- Teach the client manifestations of hypoglycemia that do not include tachycardia, which beta blockers suppress.

Central-alpha₂ agonists

Central-alpha$_2$ agonists, such as clonidine, reduce peripheral vascular resistance and decrease blood pressure by inhibiting the reuptake of norepinephrine.

NURSING CONSIDERATIONS
- Monitor blood pressure and pulse.
- This medication is not for first-line management of hypertension.

CLIENT EDUCATION: Teach the client that adverse effects include sedation, orthostatic hypotension, and impotence.

Alpha-adrenergic Antagonists

Alpha-adrenergic antagonists, such as prazosin, reduce blood pressure by causing vasodilation.

NURSING CONSIDERATIONS
- Start treatment with a low dose of the medication, usually given at night.
- Monitor blood pressure for 2 hr after initiation of treatment.

CLIENT EDUCATION: Advise the client to rise slowly to prevent postural hypotension. Tell the client to use caution when driving until the effects of the medication are known. Qs

CLIENT EDUCATION

- Instruct client to report manifestations of electrolyte imbalance (hyperkalemia, hypokalemia, hyponatremia).
- Express to the client and family the importance of adhering to the medication regimen, even if the client does not have any manifestations of hypertension.
- Provide verbal and written education to the client regarding medications and their adverse effects.
- Ensure that the client has the resources necessary to pay for and obtain prescribed antihypertensive medication.
- Encourage the client to schedule regular provider appointments to monitor hypertension and cardiovascular status.
- Teach the client or a significant other how to monitor blood pressure at home.
- Encourage the client to report findings and adverse effects, as they can be indicative of additional problems. Medications can often be changed to alleviate adverse effects.
- Older adult clients are more likely to experience medication interactions and orthostatic hypotension. Ⓖ
- Treatment involves the client making lifestyle changes.

Nutrition
- Monitor for hyperkalemia with salt substitute use.
- Consume less than 2.3 g/day of sodium.
- Consume a diet low in fat, saturated fat, and cholesterol.
- Limit alcohol intake to 2 servings per day for men and 1 serving per day for women. A serving of alcohol is equivalent to 1.5 oz liquor, 5 oz wine, or 12 oz beer.
- Dietary approaches to stop hypertension (DASH) are effective in the prevention and treatment of hypertension. QEBP
- The DASH diet is high in fruits, vegetables, and low-fat dairy foods.
- Avoid foods high in sodium and fat (trans and saturated fat).
- Consume foods rich in calcium, and magnesium.
- Clients not taking a potassium–sparing medication should increase potassium consumption.

Weight reduction and maintenance
- Begin slowly and gradually advance the program with the guidance of the provider and physical therapist.
- Exercise at least three times a week in a manner that provides aerobic benefits.

Smoking cessation: Explore smoking cessation options such as nicotine replacement therapy, medications such as bupropion or varenicline, and support groups. QPCC

Stress reduction: Encourage the client to try yoga, massage, hypnosis, or other forms of relaxation.

COMPLICATIONS

Hypertensive crisis

Hypertensive crisis often occurs when clients do not follow the medication therapy regimen.

NURSING ACTIONS
- Recognize manifestations.
  - Severe headache
  - Extremely high blood pressure (generally, systolic blood pressure greater than 240 mm Hg, diastolic greater than 120 mm Hg)
  - Blurred vision, dizziness, and disorientation
  - Epistaxis
- Administer IV antihypertensive therapies, such as nitroprusside, nicardipine, and labetalol.
- Before, during, and after administration of an IV antihypertensive, monitor blood pressure every 5 to 15 min.
- Assess neurological status, such as pupils, level of consciousness, and muscle strength, to monitor for cerebrovascular change.
- Monitor the ECG to assess cardiac status.

Application Exercises

1. A nurse is screening a male client for hypertension. The nurse should identify that which of the following actions by the client increase his risk for hypertension? (Select all that apply.)

   A. Drinking 8 oz nonfat milk daily

   B. Eating popcorn at the movie theater

   C. Walking 1 mile daily at 12 min/mile pace

   D. Consuming 36 oz beer daily

   E. Getting a massage once a week

2. A nurse in an urgent care clinic is obtaining a history from a client who has type 2 diabetes mellitus and a recent diagnosis of hypertension. This is the second time in 2 weeks that the client experienced hypoglycemia. Which of the following client data should the nurse report to the provider?

   A. Takes psyllium daily as a fiber laxative

   B. Drinks skim milk daily as a bedtime snack

   C. Takes metoprolol daily after meals

   D. Drinks grapefruit juice daily with breakfast

3. A nurse is caring for a client who is admitted to the emergency department with a blood pressure of 266/147 mm Hg. The client reports a headache and double vision. The client states that she ran out of her diltiazem 3 days ago, and is unable to purchase more. Which of the following actions should the nurse take first?

   A. Administer acetaminophen for headache.

   B. Provide teaching regarding the importance of not abruptly stopping an antihypertensive.

   C. Obtain IV access and prepare to administer an IV antihypertensive.

   D. Call social services for a referral for financial assistance in obtaining prescribed medication.

4. A nurse is providing teaching for a client who has a new diagnosis of hypertension and a new prescription for spironolactone 25 mg/day. Which of the following statements by the client indicates an understanding of the teaching?

   A. "I should eat a lot of fruits and vegetables, especially bananas and potatoes."

   B. "I will report any changes in heart rate to my provider."

   C. "I should replace the salt shaker on my table with a salt substitute."

   D. "I will decrease the dose of this medication when I no longer have headaches and facial redness."

5. A nurse is providing discharge teaching for a client who has a prescription for furosemide 40 mg PO daily. The nurse should instruct the client to take this medication at which of the following times of day?

   A. Morning

   B. Immediately after lunch

   C. Immediately before dinner

   D. Bedtime

PRACTICE Active Learning Scenario

A nurse is preparing a community education presentation on hypertension. What information should the nurse include in the presentation? Use the ATI Active Learning Template: System Disorder to complete this item.

ALTERATION IN HEALTH (DIAGNOSIS): Describe hypertension to include essential, secondary, and prehypertension.

RISK FACTORS: Describe at least four risk factors each for essential and secondary hypertension.

EXPECTED FINDINGS
- Describe at least three expected subjective data findings for hypertension.
- Describe the objective data stages of hypertension.

1. A. Consuming low-fat beverages and foods lowers the risk for developing hypertension.

   B. **CORRECT:** Popcorn at a movie theater contains a large quantity of sodium and fat, which increases the risk for hypertension.

   C. Engaging in regular exercise, such as walking, lowers the risk of developing hypertension.

   D. **CORRECT:** Consuming more than 24 oz beer per day for a male client increases the risk for hypertension.

   E. Stress management activities, such as a massage, lower the risk of hypertension.

   Ⓝ *NCLEX® Connection: Health Promotion and Maintenance, Health Promotion/Disease Prevention*

2. A. Adverse effects of psyllium do not include hypoglycemia.

   B. Skim milk increases blood glucose levels and lowers cholesterol.

   C. **CORRECT:** Metoprolol can mask the effects of hypoglycemia in clients who have diabetes mellitus.

   D. Grapefruit juice increases blood glucose levels.

   Ⓝ *NCLEX® Connection: Pharmacological and Parenteral Therapies, Adverse Effects/Contraindications/Side Effects/Interactions*

3. A. Administering acetaminophen will treat the client's pain, but there is another action that the nurse should take first.

   B. Providing teaching regarding medication administration can help promote future compliance with taking medication, but there is another action that the nurse should take first.

   C. **CORRECT:** The greatest risk to the client is injury due to a blood pressure of 266/147 mm Hg, which can be life-threatening and should be lowered as soon as possible. Obtaining IV access will permit administration of an IV hypertensive, which will act more rapidly than by the oral route.

   D. Calling social services will help connect the client with financial resources, but there is another action that the nurse should take first.

   Ⓝ *NCLEX® Connection: Pharmacological and Parenteral Therapies, Medication Administration*

4. A. The nurse should teach the client that potatoes and bananas are high in potassium, and can lead to hyperkalemia when taken with a potassium-sparing diuretic such as spironolactone.

   B. **CORRECT:** The nurse should teach the client to monitor her heart rate and report any changes to her provider.

   C. The nurse should teach the client that salt substitutes are commonly high in potassium and can lead to hyperkalemia when taken with a potassium-sparing diuretic such as spironolactone.

   D. The nurse should teach the client to continue taking her medication as prescribed even if she does not have any manifestations of hypertension.

   Ⓝ *NCLEX® Connection: Pharmacological and Parenteral Therapies, Medication Administration*

5. A. **CORRECT:** The client should take furosemide, a diuretic, in the morning so that the peak action and duration of the medication occurs during waking hours.

   B. Taking furosemide at this time increases the likelihood of interruption of the client's sleep due to the need to urinate.

   C. Taking furosemide at this time increases the likelihood of interruption of the client's sleep due to the need to urinate.

   D. Taking furosemide at this time increases the likelihood of interruption of the client's sleep due to the need to urinate.

   Ⓝ *NCLEX® Connection: Pharmacological and Parenteral Therapies, Medication Administration*

PRACTICE Answer

Using the ATI Active Learning Template: System Disorder

ALTERATION IN HEALTH (DIAGNOSIS)

- Hypertension is when systolic blood pressure is at or above 140 mm Hg or diastolic blood pressure is at or greater than 90 mm Hg for an adult client or greater than 150/90 mm Hg for a client older than 60.
- Essential (primary) hypertension has no known cause.
- Secondary hypertension is caused by diseases such as kidney disorders, or as an adverse effect of a medication. Treatment occurs by removing the cause.
- Prehypertension is when a client has a systolic blood pressure of 120 to 139 mm Hg or a diastolic blood pressure of 80 to 89 Hg.

RISK FACTORS

- Primary hypertension: Positive family history, excessive sodium intake, physical inactivity, obesity, high alcohol consumption, African-American, nicotine use, hyperlipidemia, stress, age greater than 60, postmenopausal
- Secondary hypertension: Kidney disease, Cushing's disease, primary aldosteronism (caused by hypertension and hypokalemia), pheochromocytoma (excessive catecholamine release), brain tumors, encephalitis, and medications such as estrogen, steroids, and sympathomimetics

EXPECTED FINDINGS

Subjective data: Few or no manifestations

- Can include headaches, particularly in the morning
- Dizziness, fainting, retinal changes, visual disturbances, nocturia, facial flushing

Objective data stages: Obtain blood pressure readings in both arms with the client sitting and standing:

- Prehypertension: systolic 120 to 139 mm Hg, diastolic 80 to 89 mm Hg
- Stage I: systolic 140 to 159 mm Hg, diastolic 90 to 99 mm Hg
- Stage II: systolic greater than or equal to 160 mm Hg, diastolic greater than or equal to 100 mm Hg

Ⓝ *NCLEX® Connection: Physiological Adaptation, Illness Management*

CHAPTER 37 *Hemodynamic Shock*

Shock is a state of inadequate tissue perfusion that impairs cellular function and can lead to organ failure. Any condition that compromises oxygen delivery to organs and tissues can lead to shock. Shock is a rapidly progressing, life-threatening process. Early detection with rapid response is necessary to improve client outcome.

Older adult clients can have reduced compensatory mechanisms and rapidly progress through the stages of shock. Catecholamine secretions might not improve cardiac contractility or cause vasoconstriction as in younger adults due to decreased baroreceptor response. Decreased ability to compensate can cause sustained low cardiac output and blood pressure. ©

The type and stage of shock guide treatment.

TYPES OF SHOCK

The type of shock is identified by its underlying cause.

Cardiogenic: Failure of the heart to pump effectively due to a cardiac factor.

Hypovolemic: A decrease in intravascular volume of at least 15% to 30%.

Obstructive: Impairment of the heart to pump effectively as a result of a noncardiac factor.

Distributive: Widespread vasodilation and increased capillary permeability. This includes neurogenic, septic, and anaphylactic shock.

STAGES

All types of shock progress through the same stages and produce similar effects on body systems.

Initial: No visible changes in client parameters; only changes on the cellular level.

Compensatory (non-progressive): Measures to increase cardiac output to restore tissue perfusion and oxygenation.

Progressive: Compensatory mechanisms begin to fail.

Refractory: Irreversible shock and total body failure.

HEALTH PROMOTION AND DISEASE PREVENTION

Cardiogenic shock

Educate the client about ways to reduce the risk of a myocardial infarction (MI), such as exercise, diet, stress reduction, and smoking cessation.

Hypovolemic shock

- Advise the client to drink plenty of fluids when exercising or when in hot weather.
- Advise the client to obtain early medical attention with illness or trauma and with any evidence of dehydration or bleeding.
- Educate the client about the manifestations of dehydration, including thirst, decreased urine output, and dizziness.

Obstructive/neurogenic/hypovolemic shock

Educate the client about wearing seat belts and helmets, and the use of caution with dangerous equipment, machinery, or activities.

Septic shock

- Advise the client to obtain early medical attention with evidence of an infection, such as localized redness, swelling, drainage, fever, or urinary frequency and burning.
- Advise the client to complete the entire course of antibiotics as directed.

Anaphylactic shock

- Advise the client to wear a medical identification wristband, avoid allergens, and to have an epinephrine pen available at all times. Qs
- Teach the client and family how to use the epinephrine pen and to be alert to early manifestations of an allergic reaction.

ASSESSMENT

RISK FACTORS

Cardiogenic shock

- Cardiac pump failure due to a direct cardiac cause, such as MI, heart failure, cardiomyopathy, dysrhythmias, and valvular rupture or stenosis.
- Older adult clients are at increased risk for MI and cardiomyopathy.

Hypovolemic shock

- Excessive fluid loss from diuresis, vomiting, or diarrhea; or blood loss secondary to surgery, trauma, gynecologic/obstetric causes, burns, and diabetic ketoacidosis.
- Older adult clients are more prone to dehydration due to decreased fluid and protein intake and the use of medications, such as diuretics. Minimal amounts of fluid loss (vomiting, diarrhea) can cause the older adult client to become dehydrated. ©

Obstructive shock

Cardiac pump failure due to an indirect cardiac factor, such as blockage of great vessels, pulmonary artery stenosis, pulmonary embolism, cardiac tamponade, tension pneumothorax, and aortic dissection.

Distributive shock

Divided into three types:

Neurogenic: Loss of sympathetic tone causing massive vasodilation. Head trauma, spinal cord injury, and epidural anesthesia are among the causes.

Septic: Endotoxins and other mediators causing massive vasodilation. Most common cause is gram-negative bacteria.

> Urosepsis is more frequent in older adult clients due to increased use of catheters in long-term care facilities and late detection of urinary tract infection (decreased sensation of burning, urgency). ⑥

Anaphylactic: Allergen exposure results in an antigen–antibody reaction causing massive vasodilation. Common causes include antibiotics, foods (e.g., peanuts), latex, and bee stings.

EXPECTED FINDINGS

Manifestations can include chest pain, lethargy, somnolence, restlessness, anxiousness, dyspnea, diaphoresis, thirst, muscle weakness, nausea, and constipation.

PHYSICAL ASSESSMENT FINDINGS Q̲EBP
- Hypoxia, tachypnea progressing to greater than 40/min, hypocarbia
- Skin can be pale, mottled or dusky in color, cool, diaphoretic, warm, flushed with fever (distributive shock), and exhibit a rash (anaphylactic and septic shock).
- Angioedema (anaphylactic shock)
- Wheezing
- Decreased blood pressure with narrowed pulse pressure.
- Postural hypotension.
- Tachycardia
- Pulse that is weak, thready, or bounding (distributive shock)
- Decreased cardiac output
- Central venous pressure decreased (hypovolemic shock)
- Central venous pressure increased with increased systemic vascular resistance (cardiogenic shock)
- Decreased urine output
- Seizures

LABORATORY TESTS

ABGs: Decreased tissue oxygenation (decreased pH, decreased PaO_2, increased $PaCO_2$)

Serum lactic acid: Increases due to anaerobic metabolism

Serum glucose and electrolytes: Serum glucose can increase during shock.

Cardiogenic shock

Cardiac enzymes: Creatine phosphokinase, troponin

Hypovolemic shock

Hgb and Hct: Decreased with hemorrhage, increased with dehydration

Septic shock

Cultures: Blood, urine, wound

Coagulation tests: PT, INR, aPTT

DIAGNOSTIC PROCEDURES

Hemodynamic monitoring

Arterial line insertion: Needed for continuous blood pressure monitoring and blood specimens for ABGs and other tests

Pulmonary artery catheter insertion: A pulmonary artery catheter is inserted to measure central venous pressure, pulmonary artery pressures, and cardiac output. Continuous hemodynamic monitoring is important to manage fluids and dosage of inotropic medications.

NURSING ACTIONS
- Monitor ECG during catheter insertion.
- Have resuscitation medications and equipment ready.
- Monitor hemodynamic waveforms and readings.
- Confirm catheter placement using a chest x-ray. Q̲s

CLIENT EDUCATION: Explain all procedures to the client. The client can be anxious and scared.

Cardiogenic and obstructive shock

ECG: Assess for ECG changes associated with MI and dysrhythmias. Q̲EBP

Echocardiogram: Used for cardiomegaly, cardiomyopathy, evaluation of cardiac contractility and function, ejection fraction, and valve function

Computerized tomography (CT): Used for cardiomegaly, cardiac tamponade, pulmonary emboli, cardiomyopathy, aortic dissection or aneurysm, and pericardial effusion

Cardiac catheterization: Used to identify coronary artery blockage

Chest x-ray: Used to diagnose cardiomegaly and pneumothorax, and to evaluate lungs

Hypovolemic shock: miscellaneous diagnostic procedures

Investigate possible sources of bleeding.
- Blood in nasogastric drainage or stools
- Esophagogastroduodenoscopy
- CT scan of abdomen

NURSING ACTIONS
- Continuously monitor airway and vital signs.
- Provide hemodynamic support by administration of fluids and medications because a client who has suspected shock can be hemodynamically unstable.
- Have resuscitation equipment available when transporting the client to and from procedures.

CLIENT EDUCATION: Explain all procedures to the client.

PATIENT-CENTERED CARE

NURSING CARE

- Monitor the following.
  - Oxygenation status (priority)
  - Vital signs
  - Cardiac rhythm with continuous cardiac monitoring
  - Urine output: hourly, report if less than 20 mL/hr
  - Level of consciousness
  - Skin color, temperature, moisture, capillary refill, turgor
- Explain procedures and findings to the client and family while providing reassurance.
- Place the client on high-flow oxygen, such as a 100% nonrebreather face mask. If the client has COPD, insert a 2 L/min nasal cannula and increase the oxygen flow as needed.
- Be prepared to intubate the client. Have emergency resuscitation equipment ready. Qs
- Maintain patent IV access.
- For hypotension, place the client flat with his legs elevated to increase venous return.
- If change in status occurs, notify the rapid response team and provider of the findings.
- Prepare for and maintain client care during transfer to the intensive care unit, surgery, other specialty unit, or diagnostic area.
- Prepare for and perform hemodynamic monitoring.
  - Monitor central venous pressure, pulmonary artery pressures, cardiac output, and pulse pressure.
  - Titrate continuous IV drips to maintain hemodynamic parameters as prescribed.

MEDICATIONS

Inotropic agents

Milrinone lactate, dobutamine

ACTIONS: Strengthens cardiac contraction and increases cardiac output

NURSING CONSIDERATIONS
- Administer by continuous IV infusion with constant hemodynamic monitoring.
- Can titrate agent to maintain prescribed hemodynamic parameters.
- Agent can cause vasodilation in some clients.
- Agents are often administered in combination with a vasopressor.

Vasopressors

Dopamine hydrochloride, norepinephrine

ACTIONS
- Strengthens cardiac contraction and increases cardiac output
- Increases kidney perfusion at low doses
- Decreases kidney perfusion at high doses

NURSING CONSIDERATIONS
- Administer by continuous IV infusion with constant hemodynamic monitoring.
- Can titrate vasopressor to maintain prescribed hemodynamic parameters.
- Monitor urine output.
- Administer through a central line to prevent extravasation. Rapid onset occurs in 5 min, and short duration occurs in 10 min. QEBP

Pituitary hormone: Vasopressin

ACTIONS: Causes vasoconstriction, increases systemic vascular resistance, increases blood pressure

NURSING CONSIDERATIONS
- Administer by continuous IV infusion with constant hemodynamic monitoring.
- Can titrate to maintain prescribed hemodynamic parameters.
- Monitor urine output.
- Administer through a central line to prevent extravasation. Rapid onset occurs in 5 min, and short duration occurs in 10 min.

Sympathomimetics: Epinephrine

ACTIONS
- Rapid-acting bronchodilator
- Increases heart rate and cardiac output

NURSING CONSIDERATIONS
- Monitor blood pressure, pulse, and cardiac output.
- Epinephrine can cause sloughing if it infiltrates tissue.

Opioid analgesics: Morphine sulfate

ACTIONS: Pain management

NURSING CONSIDERATIONS
- Monitor respirations of clients who are nonventilated.
- Monitor blood pressure, heart rate, and SaO_2.
- Monitor ABGs.
- Use opioid analgesics cautiously in conjunction with hypnotic sedatives.
- Assess and document the client's pain level and response to medication.
- Use cautiously due to risk of increased vasodilation and hypotension.
- Have naloxone and resuscitation equipment available for severe respiratory depression in a client who is nonventilated. Qs

Proton-pump inhibitors: Pantoprazole

ACTIONS: Protects against stress ulcer development

NURSING CONSIDERATIONS: Do not mix with other medications.

Anticoagulants

Low-molecular weight heparin, enoxaparin sodium

ACTIONS: Deep-vein thrombosis prophylaxis

NURSING CONSIDERATIONS
- Administer subcutaneously, usually in abdomen.
- Do not rub injection site.

Isotonic crystalloids or colloids (including blood products)

0.9% sodium chloride or lactated Ringer's

ACTIONS: Hypovolemic shock: volume replacement

NURSING CONSIDERATIONS: Use vasopressors only if blood pressure remains low after volume is replaced.

> **!** During hypovolemic shock, replace volume first.

Antihistamines: Diphenhydramine

ACTIONS
- Used to treat anaphylactic shock
- Blocks histamine at receptor sites

NURSING CONSIDERATIONS: Can cause drowsiness, hypotension, and tachycardia.

Vasodilator: Sodium nitroprusside

ACTIONS
- Used to treat cardiogenic shock
- Reduces afterload and preload
- Causes vasodilation
- Decreases cardiac output and afterload

NURSING CONSIDERATIONS
- Assess blood pressure every 15 min.
- Administer with caution because it is a potent vasodilator.
- Protect the solution from light.

Corticosteroids: Hydrocortisone, methylprednisolone

ACTIONS: Reduces WBC migration and decreases inflammation

NURSING CONSIDERATIONS
- Hydrocortisone can cause hypertension.
- Discontinue medication gradually.
- Administer hydrocortisone with an antiulcer medication to prevent peptic ulcer formation.
- Monitor weight and blood pressure.
- Monitor glucose and electrolytes.

Antibiotics sensitive to cultured organism(s)

Because septic shock is most commonly caused by gram-negative bacteria, the Joint Commission's National Patient Safety Goals recommends the administration of IV antibiotics that are effective against gram-negative bacteria within 1 hr of a septic shock diagnosis. Qs

Vancomycin
Antibiotics sensitive to the cultured organism, such as vancomycin, can then be prescribed once the causative organism is identified.

ACTIONS
- Used to treat septic shock.
- Inhibits cell growth or reproduction of causative organism.

NURSING CONSIDERATIONS
- Monitor for hypersensitivity reaction.
- Administer IV vancomycin slowly.
- Culture infected area prior to administration of the first dose of vancomycin.
- Monitor the IV site for infiltration.
- Do not administer vancomycin with other medications.
- Monitor coagulopathy and kidney function.

THERAPEUTIC PROCEDURES

Intubation and mechanical ventilation

An artificial airway is inserted, and the client's respirations are controlled by mechanical ventilation.

PREINTUBATION NURSING ACTIONS
- Monitor ECG, SaO_2, breath sounds, and color.
- Sedate the client as needed.
- Preoxygenate with 100% oxygen.
- Assist with ventilation using a manual resuscitation bag and a face mask.
- Have suction equipment, manual emergency resuscitation, and a face mask readily available.
- Suction secretions as needed.

POSTINTUBATION NURSING ACTIONS
- Assess bilateral breath sounds, symmetrical chest movement, and a chest x-ray to confirm placement of the endotracheal tube.
- Secure the endotracheal tube per facility guidelines.
- Assess the balloon cuff for air leak periodically.

Positive end expiratory pressure (PEEP)
- Positive pressure is applied at the end of expiration to keep the alveoli expanded to promote gas exchange.
- PEEP is added to the ventilator setting to increase oxygenation and improve lung expansion.

CLIENT EDUCATION
- Explain all procedures to the client.
- Provide reassurance to the client and family. Experiencing shock, as well as the treatments involved, can be frightening.
- Explain to the client and family that the client will be unable to talk with the endotracheal tube in place. Qpcc

Needle decompression and chest tube insertion

This procedure is used to relieve pressure from a tension pneumothorax that can be causing obstructive shock.

NURSING ACTIONS
- Monitor ECG, SaO_2, breath sounds, and color.
- Sedate as needed.
- Set up a water seal chest-drainage system and attach it to suction.
- Apply a dressing.
- Assess the chest tube for air leaks.
- Monitor and document the drainage.
- Obtain a chest x-ray postprocedure.

CLIENT EDUCATION

- Explain that needle decompression provides temporary relief while chest tube insertion allows for lung reinflation.
- Provide reassurance to the client and family. Experiencing shock, as well as the treatments involved, can be frightening. Qpcc

Pericardiocentesis

Pericardial fluid that is causing cardiac tamponade and obstructive shock is drained.

NURSING ACTIONS

- Monitor ECG, SaO_2, breath sounds, and color.
- Sedate as needed.
- Obtain a postprocedure chest x-ray.

CLIENT EDUCATION

- Explain that additional procedures are often necessary to resolve acute tamponade (pericardial window, pericardiectomy).
- Provide reassurance to the client and family. Experiencing shock, as well as the treatments involved, can be frightening.

Surgical interventions

Surgery might be needed to correct the cause of shock, such as a hemorrhaging ulcer, wound, artery or vein.

PREPROCEDURE NURSING ACTIONS

- Manage the airway and provide supplemental oxygen and intubation if needed.
- Provide hemodynamic support with fluids and medications to stabilize the client prior to surgical intervention, if possible.

POSTPROCEDURE NURSING ACTIONS

- Continue to monitor blood pressure, ECG, pulmonary artery pressures, cardiac output, central venous pressure, and urine output.
- Titrate and administer medications as prescribed.
- Assess the surgical site for bleeding.
- Monitor airway, breath sounds, and ABGs.
- Monitor CBC.

CLIENT EDUCATION

- Explain all procedures to the client.
- Provide reassurance, and calm the client and family. Experiencing shock, as well as the treatments involved, can be frightening.

INTERPROFESSIONAL CARE

Respiratory therapy: The respiratory therapist typically manages the ventilator, adjusts the settings, and provides chest physical therapy to improve ventilation and chest expansion. The respiratory therapist can also suction the endotracheal tube and administer inhalation medications, such as bronchodilators.

COMPLICATIONS

Multiple organ dysfunction syndrome (MODS)

MODS can develop from severe hypotension and reperfusion of ischemic cells, causing further tissue injury. Inadequate tissue perfusion can cause organ failure in the lungs (adult respiratory distress syndrome), kidneys, heart (decreased coronary artery perfusion, decreased cardiac contractility), and the gastrointestinal tract (necrosis).

NURSING ACTIONS

- Assess organ function, and provide support measures that can increase tissue perfusion and improve organ function (ventilatory support, inotropic medications).
- Implement measures to compensate for dysfunction (administration of clotting factors, dialysis).

Disseminated intravascular coagulation (DIC)

DIC is a complication of septic shock. Thousands of small clots form within organ capillaries (liver, kidney, heart, brain), creating hypoxia and anaerobic metabolism. As a result of massive, multiple clot formation, platelets and other clotting factors such as fibrinogen are depleted and the client is at increased risk for hemorrhage. The client can develop diffuse petechiae and ecchymoses, and blood can leak from membranes and puncture sites.

NURSING ACTIONS

- Assess client preference related to transfusion of blood products. Some clients may not accept this treatment for various reasons (religion, fear of contamination). Qpcc
- Administer platelets, clotting factors, and other blood products as prescribed.
- Monitor hemodynamic levels.
- Monitor results of laboratory tests (PT, PTT, serum fibrinogen, fibrin degradation products).
- Assess for further indications of bleeding.
- Apply pressure to leaking IV/central line/arterial line sites.

CLIENT EDUCATION: Explain procedures and care to the client and family.

Application Exercises

1. A nurse is caring for a client who has a prescription for an afterload-reducing medication. The nurse should identify that this medication is administered for which of the following types of shock?

   A. Cardiogenic

   B. Obstructive

   C. Hypovolemic

   D. Distributive

2. A nurse is planning care for a client who has septic shock. Which of the following actions is the priority for the nurse to take?

   A. Maintain adequate fluid volume with IV infusions.

   B. Administer antibiotic therapy.

   C. Monitor hemodynamic status.

   D. Administer vasopressor medication.

3. A nurse in the emergency department is caring for a client who had an allergic reaction related to a bee sting. The client is experiencing wheezing and swelling of the tongue. Which of the following medications should the nurse anticipate administering first?

   A. Methylprednisolone IV bolus

   B. Diphenhydramine subcutaneously

   C. Epinephrine IV

   D. Albuterol inhaler

4. A nurse in the emergency department is completing an assessment on a client who is in shock. Which of the following findings should the nurse expect? (Select all that apply.)

   A. Heart rate 60/min

   B. Seizure activity

   C. Respiratory rate 42/min

   D. Increased urine output

   E. Weak, thready pulse

5. A nurse in a cardiac unit is assisting with the admission of a client who is to undergo hemodynamic monitoring. Which of the following actions should the nurse anticipate performing?

   A. Administer large volumes of IV fluids.

   B. Assist with insertion of pulmonary artery catheter.

   C. Position the client laterally to calculate the phlebostatic axis.

   D. Gather supplies for insertion of a peripheral IV catheter.

PRACTICE Active Learning Scenario

A nurse educator is reviewing care of a client who is in shock with a group of newly hired nurse. What should the nurse educator include in this discussion? Use the ATI Active Learning Template: System Disorder to complete this item.

RISK FACTORS: List each type of shock and at least one risk factor for each.

EXPECTED FINDINGS: Describe expected findings related to blood pressure, pulse, respirations, and urine output.

Application Exercises Key

1. A. **CORRECT:** The nurse should identify that a prescription to reduce afterload will allow the heart to pump more effectively, which is needed for the client who has cardiogenic shock.

   B. In obstructive shock, the high afterload is due to obstruction of blood flow. Afterload-reducing agents will not remove the obstruction.

   C. Fluid replacement and reduction of further fluid loss are the focus of management of hypovolemic shock.

   D. Afterload-reducing medication is not administered to a client who has distributive shock because the client already has decreased afterload.

   Ⓝ *NCLEX® Connection: Pharmacological and Parenteral Therapies, Expected Actions/Outcomes*

2. A. The nurse should maintain the client's fluid volume by administration of IV fluids. However, another action is the priority.

   B. **CORRECT:** The greatest risk to the client is injury from elimination endotoxins and mediators from bacteria, which will reduce the vasodilation from occurring. The priority intervention for the nurse is to administer antibiotics.

   C. The nurse should monitor hemodynamic status to monitor the blood pressure inside the veins, arteries and heart. However, another action is the priority.

   D. The nurse should administer vasopressor medication to increase the contractility of the heart muscle and to cause vasoconstriction. However, another action is the priority.

   Ⓝ *NCLEX® Connection: Physiological Adaptation, Medical Emergencies*

3. A. The nurse should administer methylprednisolone to treat the inflammatory response to the bee sting. However, the nurse should administer another medication first.

   B. The nurse should administer diphenhydramine to treat the client's itching related to the bee sting. However, the nurse should administer another medication first.

   C. **CORRECT:** When using the airway, breathing, circulation approach to client care, the nurse should place the priority on administering epinephrine to the client. This is a rapid-acting medication that promotes effective oxygenation and is used to treat anaphylactic shock.

   D. The nurse should administer albuterol to assist with the client's breathing. However, the nurse should administer another medication first.

   Ⓝ *NCLEX® Connection: Pharmacological and Parenteral Therapies, Medication Administration*

4. A. Tachycardia is an expected finding in a client who is in shock.

   B. **CORRECT:** Seizure activity can be present in a client who is in shock.

   C. **CORRECT:** Tachypnea is an expected finding in a client who is in shock.

   D. Decreased urine output is in expected finding in a client who is in shock.

   E. **CORRECT:** A weak, thready pulse is an expected finding in a client who is in shock.

   Ⓝ *NCLEX® Connection: Physiological Adaptation, Medical Emergencies*

5. A. Patency of the catheter is maintained with a slow continuous infusion of 0.9% sodium chloride. The catheter is used for blood sampling and pressure monitoring, not fluid administration.

   B. **CORRECT:** A pulmonary artery catheter and pressure-monitoring system are inserted for hemodynamic monitoring.

   C. Calculation of the phlebostatic axis is performed with the client in a supine position.

   D. An arterial line is needed to obtain blood samples for ABGs and other blood tests as part of hemodynamic monitoring.

   Ⓝ *NCLEX® Connection: Physiological Adaptation, Hemodynamics*

PRACTICE Answer

Using the ATI Active Learning Template: System Disorder

RISK FACTORS

- Cardiogenic: Pump failure due to myocardial infarction, heart failure, cardiomyopathy, dysrhythmia, and valvular rupture or stenosis
- Hypovolemic: Excessive fluid loss from diuresis, vomiting, diarrhea, blood loss
- Obstructive: Blockage of great vessels, pulmonary artery stenosis, pulmonary embolism, cardiac tamponade, tension pneumothorax, and aortic dissection
- Septic: Endotoxins (gram-negative bacteria) and mediators causing massive vasodilation
- Neurogenic: Loss of sympathetic tone causing massive vasodilation due to trauma, spinal shock, epidural anesthesia
- Anaphylactic: Antigen-antibody reaction causing massive vasodilation due to allergens (inhaled, swallowed, contacted, or introduced IV)

Ⓝ *NCLEX® Connection: Physiological Adaptation, Medical Emergencies*

EXPECTED FINDINGS

- Blood pressure: Decreased blood pressure with narrowed pulse pressure, postural hypotension.
- Pulse: Tachycardia, can be weak or thready, bounding with distributive shock
- Respirations: Tachypnea progressing to greater than 40/min, hypocarbia, hypoxia
- Urine output: Decreased

UNIT 4   NURSING CARE OF CLIENTS WHO HAVE
CARDIOVASCULAR DISORDERS
SECTION: VASCULAR DISORDERS

CHAPTER 38 *Aneurysms*

A weakness in a section of a dilated artery that causes a widening or ballooning in the wall of the blood vessel is called an aneurysm. Aneurysms can occur in two forms. They can be saccular (only affecting one side of the artery), or fusiform (involving the complete circumference of the artery).

Aortic dissection (also known as a dissecting aneurysm) can occur when blood accumulates within the artery wall (hematoma) following a tear in the lining of the artery (usually due to hypertension). This is a life-threatening condition.

HEALTH PROMOTION AND DISEASE PREVENTION

- Promote smoking cessation.
- Maintain appropriate weight for height and body frame.
- Encourage a healthy diet and physical activity.
- Control blood pressure with regular monitoring and medication if needed.

ASSESSMENT

RISK FACTORS

- Male gender
- Atherosclerosis (most common cause)
- Uncontrolled hypertension
- Tobacco use
- Hyperlipidemia
- Family history
- Blunt force trauma
- History of syphilis
- With age, arterial stiffening caused by loss of elastin in arterial walls, thickening of intima of arteries, and progressive fibrosis of media occurs. Older adult clients are more prone to aneurysms and have a higher mortality rate from aneurysms than younger individuals. Ⓖ

EXPECTED FINDINGS

Initially, clients are often asymptomatic.

Abdominal aortic aneurysm (AAA)

Most common, related to atherosclerosis
- Constant gnawing feeling in abdomen
- Flank or back pain
- Pulsating abdominal mass (do not palpate; can cause rupture Ⓠs)
- Bruit over the area of the aneurysm
- Elevated blood pressure (unless in cardiac tamponade or rupture of aneurysm)

Thoracic aortic aneurysm

- Severe back pain (most common)
- Hoarseness, cough, shortness of breath, and difficulty swallowing
- Decrease in urinary output (secondary to hypovolemic shock)

Aortic dissections

Often associated with Marfan syndrome
- Sudden onset of "tearing," "ripping," and "stabbing" abdominal or back pain
- Hypovolemic shock
  - Diaphoresis, nausea, vomiting, faintness, apprehension
  - Decreased or absent peripheral pulses
  - Neurological deficits
  - Hypotension and tachycardia (initial)
  - Oliguria

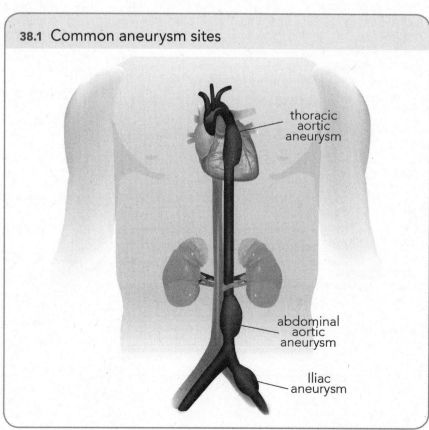

38.1 Common aneurysm sites

thoracic aortic aneurysm

abdominal aortic aneurysm

Iliac aneurysm

DIAGNOSTIC PROCEDURES

X-ray: Can be used to detect the presence of an aneurysm.

Computed tomography (CT) and ultrasonography: Used to assess the size and location of aneurysms. Often repeated at periodic intervals to monitor the progression of an aneurysm.

Transesophageal echocardiography (TEE): Useful in diagnosing thoracic aneurysms and aortic dissections.

PATIENT-CENTERED CARE

NURSING CARE

- Take vital signs every 15 min until stable, then every hour. Monitor for an increase in blood pressure.
- Assess the onset, quality, duration, and severity of pain.
- Assess temperature, circulation, and range of motion of extremities.
- Continuously monitor cardiac rhythm.
- Monitor hemodynamic findings.
- Monitor ABGs, SaO$_2$, electrolytes, and CBC findings.
- Monitor hourly urine output. Greater than 30 mL/hr indicates adequate kidney perfusion.
- Administer oxygen as prescribed.
- Obtain and maintain IV access.
- Administer medications as prescribed.

> ! All aneurysms can be life-threatening and require medical attention.

MEDICATIONS

- The priority intervention is to reduce systolic blood pressure to between 100 and 120 mm Hg during an emergency. Long-term goal includes maintaining systolic blood pressure at or less than 130 to 140 mm Hg. **Qs**
- Administer antihypertensive agents as prescribed. Often, more than one is prescribed (beta blockers and calcium blockers).

THERAPEUTIC PROCEDURES

Abdominal aortic aneurysm resection

Excision of the aneurysm and the placement of a synthetic graft (elective or emergency)
- Elective surgery is used to manage AAA of 5.5 cm diameter or greater (2% to 5% mortality rate).
- Emergency surgery is indicated for a rupturing aneurysm.
- Risks include significant blood loss and the consequences of reduced cardiac output and tissue ischemia (myocardial infarction, acute kidney injury, respiratory distress, and paralytic ileus).

NURSING ACTIONS
- Priority interventions include monitoring the arterial pressure, heart rhythm, and hemodynamic findings, as well as monitoring for evidence of graft occlusion or rupture postoperatively.
- Monitor vital signs and circulation (pulses distal to graft) every 15 min.
- Maintain the head of the bed below 45° to prevent flexion of the graft. **Q EBP**
- Report evidence of graft occlusion or rupture immediately (changes in pulses, coolness of extremity below graft, white or blue extremities or flanks, severe pain, abdominal distention, decreased urine output). **Qs**
- Monitor and maintain blood pressure within the prescribed parameters. Prolonged hypotension can cause thrombi to form within the graft; severe hypertension can cause leakage or rupture at the arterial anastomosis suture line.
- Maintain a warm environment to prevent temperature-induced vasoconstriction.
- Administer IV fluids at prescribed rates to ensure adequate hydration and kidney perfusion.
- Monitor for altered kidney perfusion and acute kidney injury caused by clamping aorta during surgery (urine output less than 30 mL/hr, weight gain, elevated BUN or serum creatinine).
- Auscultate lung sounds. Encourage coughing and deep breathing every 2 hr. Encourage splinting with coughing.
- Assess onset, quality, duration, and severity of pain. Administer pain medication as prescribed.
- Monitor bowel sounds, and observe for abdominal distention. Maintain nasogastric suction as prescribed.
- Prevent thromboembolism. Maintain sequential compression devices. Encourage early ambulation. Administer antiplatelet or anticoagulant medications.
- Monitor for infection.
- Administer antibiotics as prescribed to maintain adequate blood levels of the medication.

Percutaneous aneurysm repair

Insertion of endothelial stent grafts for aneurysm repair avoids abdominal incision and shortens the postoperative period (can be used to repair thoracic and abdominal aortic aneurysms).

NURSING ACTIONS: Nursing care after the procedure is similar to care following an arteriogram or cardiac catheterization (monitor pedal pulse). Refer to **CHAPTER 30: INVASIVE CARDIOVASCULAR PROCEDURES**.

Thoracic aortic aneurysm repair

Procedure similar to thoracic surgery, such as open heart. The course of action depends on the location of the aneurysm. Cardiopulmonary bypass is commonly used for this procedure.

NURSING ACTIONS

- Nursing care after the procedure is similar to care following coronary artery bypass graft surgery. (Monitor respiratory status. Respiratory distress is common after this type of procedure.)
- Cardiac rehabilitation services are often consulted for prolonged weakness and assistance in increasing the client's level of activity.
- Nutritional services can be consulted for food choices that are low in fat and cholesterol.

CLIENT EDUCATION

- Monitor and maintain blood pressure. Emphasize importance of staying within parameters set by the provider. Taking medications as prescribed prevents complications (rupture). Qs
- Promote follow-up on scheduled CT scans to monitor aneurysm size (nonsurgical client). Collaborate with case management services to assist with transportation needs.
- Promote smoking cessation if the client smokes. Qpcc
- Prevent infection (good hand hygiene, wound care management). Report evidence of infection following surgical intervention (wound redness, edema, drainage; elevated temperature).
- Encourage proper diet (low-fat, high-protein, vitamins A and C, zinc to promote wound healing).
- Review manifestations of aneurysm rupture (abdominal fullness or pain, chest or back pain, shortness of breath, cough, difficulty swallowing, hoarseness). Instruct the client to report these immediately.
- Avoid strenuous activity, and restrict heavy lifting to less than 15 lb (surgical client).

INTERPROFESSIONAL CARE

- Cardiology services can assist in managing and treating hypertension.
- Radiology should be consulted for diagnostic studies to diagnose and monitor an aneurysm.
- Vascular services may be consulted for surgical intervention.

COMPLICATIONS

Rupture

- Aneurysm rupture is a life-threatening emergency, often resulting in massive hemorrhage, shock, and death.
- Treatment requires simultaneous resuscitation and immediate surgical repair.
- Older adult clients who have an aneurysm greater than 6 cm (2.4 in) along with hypertension are at greater risk death due to spontaneous rupture than of dying during surgical repair. Ⓖ

Thrombus formation

- A thrombus can form inside the aneurysm. Emboli can be dislodged, blocking arteries distal to the aneurysm, which causes ischemia and shuts down other body systems.
- Assess circulation distal to aneurysm, including pulses and color and temperature of the lower extremities. Monitor urine output.

Application Exercises

1. A nurse in the emergency department is admitting a client who has a possible dissecting abdominal aortic aneurysm. Which of the following actions is the priority for the nurse to take?

   A. Administer pain medication as prescribed.

   B. Provide a warm environment.

   C. Administer IV fluids as prescribed.

   D. Initiate a 12-lead ECG.

2. A nurse is reviewing manifestations of a thoracic aortic aneurysm with a newly hired nurse. Which of the following findings should the nurse include in the discussion? (Select all that apply.)

   A. Cough

   B. Shortness of breath

   C. Upper chest pain

   D. Diaphoresis

   E. Altered swallowing

3. A nurse is planning postoperative care for a client following a surgical placement of a synthetic graft to repair an aneurysm. Which of the following interventions should the nurse include in the plan of care? (Select all that apply.)

   A. Assess pedal pulses.

   B. Monitor for an increase in pain below the graft site.

   C. Maintain the client in high-Fowler's position.

   D. Administer prescribed antiplatelet agents.

   E. Report hourly urine output of 60 mL.

4. A nurse is teaching a client who has a new diagnosis of an aneurysm. The client asks the nurse to explain what causes an aneurysm to rupture. Which of the following statements should the nurse give?

   A. "This happens when the wall of an artery becomes thin and flexible."

   B. "This happens when there is turbulence in blood flow in the artery."

   C. "It is due to abdominal enlargement."

   D. "It is due to hypertension."

5. A nurse is admitting a client who has a suspected occlusion of a graft of the abdominal aorta. Which of the following manifestations should the nurse expect?

   A. Increase in urine output

   B. Bounding pedal pulse

   C. Increase in abdominal girth

   D. Redness of the lower extremities

Application Exercises Key

1. A. The nurse should administer pain medication to alleviate the client's pain and discomfort related to the aneurysm. However, another action is the priority.

   B. The nurse should provide a warm environment due to impaired blood flow and decreasing blood pressure related to the aneurysm. However, another action is the priority.

   C. **CORRECT:** When using the airway, breathing, circulation approach to client care, the nurse should determine that the priority is on administering IV fluids to the client. The client is at risk of inadequate circulatory volume due to profuse sweating related to the pain and feeling of fullness related to the aneurysm.

   D. The nurse should initiate a 12-lead ECG to determine the cardiac rhythm related to the aneurysm. However, another action is the priority.

   Ⓝ *NCLEX® Connection: Physiological Adaptation, Medical Emergencies*

2. A. **CORRECT:** Cough is a manifestation of a thoracic aortic aneurysm.

   B. **CORRECT:** Shortness of breath is a manifestation of a thoracic aortic aneurysm.

   C. Report of severe back pain is a finding of thoracic aortic aneurysm.

   D. Diaphoresis is a finding of dissecting aortic aneurysm.

   E. **CORRECT:** Difficulty swallowing is a manifestation of a thoracic aortic aneurysm.

   Ⓝ *NCLEX® Connection: Physiological Adaptation, Pathophysiology*

3. A. **CORRECT:** The nurse should assess the pulses distal to the graft site to detect possible occlusion of the graft.

   B. **CORRECT:** The nurse should monitor for an increase pain below the graft site. This can be an indication of graft occlusion or rupture.

   C. The head of the bed should be maintained at less than 45° to prevent flexion of the graft.

   D. **CORRECT:** The nurse should administer antiplatelet agents and anticoagulants as prescribed to prevent thrombus formation.

   E. Urine output of 60 mL/hr is an expected finding.

   Ⓝ *NCLEX® Connection: Reduction of Risk Potential, Therapeutic Procedures*

4. A. An aneurysm ruptures as a result of thickening in the intima of the artery and a lack of elasticity in the vessel wall, which is typically under pressure due to hypertension.

   B. A bruit is objective data that indicates the presence of an aneurysm, not the cause of rupture.

   C. Abdominal distention can occur when an aneurysm ruptures, but it is not the cause of the rupture.

   D. **CORRECT:** The nurse should explain to the client that aneurysm ruptures as a result of hypertension increasing pressure within the arterial walls.

   Ⓝ *NCLEX® Connection: Physiological Adaptation, Pathophysiology*

5. A. Decreased urine output is an expected finding with occlusion of a graft of the aorta.

   B. Decreased or absent pedal pulse is an expected finding with occlusion of a graft of the aorta.

   C. **CORRECT:** Abdominal distention is an expected finding with occlusion of a graft of the aorta.

   D. Pallor or cyanosis of the extremities is an expected finding with occlusion of a graft of the aorta.

   Ⓝ *NCLEX® Connection: Physiological Adaptation, Pathophysiology*

PRACTICE Active Learning Scenario

A nurse manager is presenting an in-service to a group of nurses about care of the client who has an aneurysm. What information should the nurse manager include in the in-service? Use the ATI Active Learning Template: System Disorder to complete this item.

RISK FACTORS: Describe three.

DIAGNOSTIC PROCEDURES: Describe two.

NURSING CARE: Describe at least four nursing actions.

PRACTICE Answer

Using the ATI Active Learning Template: System Disorder

RISK FACTORS
- Male gender
- Atherosclerosis
- Uncontrolled hypertension
- Tobacco use
- Hyperlipidemia
- Family history
- Blunt force trauma
- History of syphilis
- Age-related changes to the artery (loss of elastin, thickening of the intima, progressive fibrosis)

DIAGNOSTIC PROCEDURES
- X-rays
- CT scans
- Ultrasonography
- Transesophageal echocardiography

NURSING CARE
- Take vital signs every 15 min until stable. Then monitor for increased blood pressure hourly.
- Assess pain (onset, quality, duration, severity).
- Assess temperature, circulation, and range of motion of extremities.
- Monitor cardiac rhythm continuously.
- Monitor hemodynamic findings.
- Monitor ABGs, SaO_2, electrolytes, and CBC laboratory findings.
- Monitor hourly urine output.
- Administer oxygen as prescribed.
- Obtain and maintain IV access.
- Administer medications as prescribed.

Ⓝ *NCLEX® Connection: Physiological Adaptation, Pathophysiology*

NCLEX® Connections

When reviewing the following chapters, keep in mind the relevant topics and tasks of the NCLEX outline, in particular:

Client Needs: Pharmacological and Parenteral Therapies

BLOOD AND BLOOD PRODUCTS
Identify the client according to facility/agency policy prior to administration of red blood cells/ blood products.

Check the client for appropriate venous access for red blood cell/blood product administration.

Administer blood products and evaluate client response.

Client Needs: Reduction of Risk Potential

LABORATORY VALUES
Identify laboratory values for ABGs, BUN, cholesterol, glucose, hematocrit, hemoglobin, glycosylated hemoglobin, platelets, potassium, sodium, WBC, creatinine, PT, PTT & APTT, INR.

Educate client about the purpose and procedure of prescribed laboratory tests.

Client Needs: Physiological Adaptation

ALTERATIONS IN BODY SYSTEMS: Apply knowledge of nursing procedures, pathophysiology and psychomotor skills when caring for a client with an alteration in body systems.

FLUID AND ELECTROLYTE IMBALANCES: Manage the care of the client with a fluid and electrolyte imbalance.

HEMODYNAMICS: Intervene to improve the client's cardiovascular status.

UNIT 5 NURSING CARE OF CLIENTS WHO
HAVE HEMATOLOGIC DISORDERS
SECTION: DIAGNOSTIC AND THERAPEUTIC PROCEDURES

CHAPTER 39 *Hematologic Diagnostic Procedures*

Hematologic assessment and diagnostic procedures evaluate blood function by testing indicators such as erythrocytes (RBCs), leukocytes (WBCs), platelets, and coagulation times. By testing the blood, diagnosis of a disease and efficacy of treatment can be determined.

Bone marrow is responsible for the production of many blood cells including RBCs, WBCs, and platelets. A bone marrow biopsy provides diagnostic information about how the bone marrow is functioning.

39.1 Expected reference ranges for blood diagnostic procedures

	EXPECTED REFERENCE RANGE	INTERPRETATION OF FINDINGS
RBC	Females: 4.2 to 5.4 million/uL Males: 4.7 to 6.1 million/uL	Elevated level: erythrocytosis, polycythemia vera, severe dehydration Decreased level: anemia, hemorrhage, kidney disease
WBC	5,000 to 10,000/mm³	Elevated level: infection, inflammation. Decreased level: immunosuppression, autoimmune disease
MCV	80 to 95 fL	Elevated level: macrocytic (large) RBCs, megaloblastic anemia. Decreased level microcytic (small) RBCs, iron deficiency anemia.
MCH	27 to 31 pg/cell	Elevated/decreased level: same as above for MCV
TIBC	250 to 460 mcg/dL	Elevated level: iron deficiency anemia, polycythemia vera Decreased level: malnutrition, cirrhosis, pernicious anemia
IRON	Females: 60 to 160 mcg/dL Males: 80 to 180 mcg/dL	Elevated level: hemochromatosis, iron excess, liver disorder, or lead toxicity. Decreased level: iron deficiency anemia, chronic blood loss, inadequate dietary intake of iron.
PLATELETS	150,000 to 400,000 mm³	Increased level: malignancy, polycythemia vera, rheumatoid arthritis. Decreased level: enlarged spleen, hemorrhage, leukemia
HGB	Females: 12 to 16 g/dL Males: 14 to 18 g/dL Elderly: levels slightly decreased	Elevated level: erythrocytosis, COPD, severe dehydration Decreased level: anemia, hemorrhage, kidney disease
HCT	Females: 37 to 47% Males: 42 to 52% Elderly: levels slightly decreased	Elevated /decreased level: same as above for Hgb
APTT	30 to 40 seconds (1.5 to 2.5 times the control value if receiving heparin therapy)	Increased time: vitamin K deficiency, disseminated intravascular coagulation (DIC), liver disease, heparin administration Decreased time: extensive cancer
PT	11 to 12.5 seconds, 85 to 100%, or 1:1.1 client-control ratio	Increased time: of clotting factors II, V, VII, or X, liver disease, warfarin therapy, disseminated intravascular coagulation Decreased time: vitamin K excess, pulmonary embolus, thrombophlebitis
INR	0.8 to 1.1 (desired goal of 2 to 3 on warfarin therapy)	Measures the mean of PT to provide a universally recognized value. Elevated level: warfarin therapy Decreased level: cancer disorders
D-DIMER	Less than 0.4 mcg/mL	Positive result: disseminated intravascular coagulation, malignancy Negative result: can rule out pulmonary embolus or deep vein thrombosis
FIBRINOGEN LEVELS	200 to 400 mg/dL	Elevated level: acute inflammation, acute infection, heart disease Decreased levels: liver disease, advanced cancer, malnutrition
FIBRIN DEGRADATION PRODUCTS	Less than 10 mcg/mL	Elevated level: disseminated intravascular coagulation, massive trauma resulting in fibrinolysis Decreased level: anticoagulation therapy

Blood collection/testing

- Blood diagnostic procedures that nurses should be knowledgeable about include the following. **(39.1)**
  - Serum RBC count
  - Serum WBC count
  - Mean corpuscular volume (MCV)
  - Mean corpuscular Hgb (MCH)
  - Total iron-binding count (TIBC)
  - Iron
  - Platelets
  - Hemoglobin (Hgb)
  - Hematocrit (Hct)
  - Coagulation studies
    - Prothrombin time (PT)
    - Partial thromboplastin time (aPTT)
    - International normalized ratio (INR)
    - D-dimer
    - Fibrinogen levels
    - Fibrin degradation products
- CBC is a series of tests that includes RBC, WBC, MCV, MCH, Hgb, and Hct.

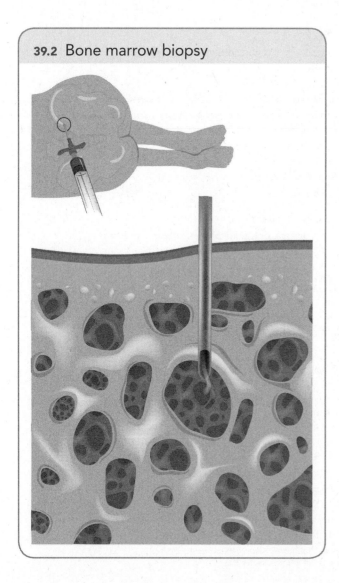

39.2 Bone marrow biopsy

CONSIDERATIONS

PREPROCEDURE

NURSING ACTIONS: Use standard precautions in collecting and handling blood for specimen collection.

INTRAPROCEDURE

NURSING ACTIONS

- Select the appropriate vial for the prescribed test.
- Collect a sufficient quantity of blood and fill to the indicated mark on the vial.
- Properly label the specimen. Deliver the specimen to the laboratory according to facility protocol for appropriate storage and analysis.
- For coagulation studies, draw blood at specific times and immediately send to the laboratory. Adjust the dose of anticoagulant therapy based on the results and prescription.

POSTPROCEDURE

NURSING ACTIONS

- Results of hematologic tests are usually available preliminarily within 24 to 48 hr, with final results in 72 hr.
- If results are out of the expected reference range, it is the nurse's responsibility to report the results to the provider for further intervention.

Bone marrow aspiration/biopsy

- A biopsy is the extraction of a very small amount of tissue, such as bone marrow, to definitively diagnose cell type and to confirm or rule out malignancy. A bone marrow tissue sample is removed by needle aspiration for cytological (histological) examination. **(39.2)**
- Biopsies are commonly performed with local anesthesia or conscious sedation in an ambulatory setting, intraoperatively, or during endoscopic procedures.

INDICATIONS

A bone marrow biopsy is commonly performed to diagnose causes of blood disorders, such as anemia or thrombocytopenia; to diagnose diseases of the bone marrow, such as leukemia, and infection; or to stage lymphoma or other forms of cancer.

CONSIDERATIONS

PREPROCEDURE

NURSING ACTIONS
- Ensure that the client has provided informed consent.
- Place the client in a prone or side-lying position to expose the iliac crest for the procedure.

CLIENT EDUCATION: Explain the procedure to the client. The biopsy site will be anesthetized with a local anesthetic, and the client might feel pressure and brief pain during the aspiration.

INTRAPROCEDURE

NURSING ACTIONS
- Inform the client that the test will last about 20 min.
- Administer a sedative if prescribed.
  - Older adult clients are at greater risk for complications associated with sedation for biopsy procedures due to chronic illnesses. Ⓒ
  - The nurse should take an older adult's kidney function into consideration when using analgesics for sedation.
- Cleanse the site with an antiseptic solution.
- Maintain sterility of equipment and supplies.
- Assist the provider with the procedure as needed.

POSTPROCEDURE

NURSING ACTIONS
- Apply pressure to the biopsy site to control bleeding.
- Place a sterile dressing over the biopsy site.
- Maintain the client on bed rest for 30 to 60 min.
- Monitor for evidence of infection (fever, increased WBCs, pain, and swelling at the site) and bleeding.
- Apply ice to the biopsy site to minimize bleeding and bruising.
- Postprocedure discomfort is usually relieved by mild analgesics.
- Avoid aspirin and other medications that affect clotting.

CLIENT EDUCATION
- Teach the client to report excessive bleeding and evidence of infection to the provider.
- Teach the client to check the biopsy site daily. Keep the dressing clean, dry, and intact.
- If sutures are in place, remind the client to return in 7 to 10 days to have them removed.

INTERPRETATION OF FINDINGS

After a procedure is completed, the tissue sample is sent to pathology for interpretation.

COMPLICATIONS

Infection

Infection can occur at the aspiration site.

NURSING ACTIONS: Monitor the site and keep the dressing clean and dry.

Bleeding

Bleeding can occur from the site.

NURSING ACTIONS: Report bleeding to the provider immediately.

PRACTICE Active Learning Scenario

A nurse is caring for a client who is having a bone marrow biopsy. What actions should the nurse take? Use the ATI Active Learning Template: Diagnostic Procedure to complete this item.

NURSING INTERVENTIONS (PRE, INTRA, POST): Describe two for each of the pre-, intra-, and postprocedure periods.

POTENTIAL COMPLICATIONS: Identify two.

CLIENT EDUCATION: Describe two discharge teaching points.

Application Exercises

1. A nurse in a clinic is caring for a client who has suspected anemia. Which of the following laboratory test results should the nurse expect?
   - A. Iron 90 mcg/dL
   - B. RBC 6.5 million/uL
   - C. WBC 4,800 mm³
   - D. Hgb 10 g/dL

2. A nurse is caring for a client who is receiving warfarin for anticoagulation therapy. Which of the following laboratory test results indicates to the nurse that the client needs an increase in the dosage?
   - A. aPTT 38 seconds
   - B. INR 1.1
   - C. PT 22 seconds
   - D. D-dimer negative

3. A nurse is providing teaching for a client who is scheduled for a bone marrow biopsy of the iliac crest. Which of the following statements made by the client indicates an understanding of the teaching?
   - A. "This test will be performed while I am lying flat on my back."
   - B. "I will need to stay in bed for about an hour after the test."
   - C. "This test will determine which antibiotic I should take for treatment."
   - D. "I will receive general anesthesia for the test."

Application Exercises Key

1. A. An iron level of 90 mcg/dL is within the expected reference range and is not an expected finding of anemia.

   B. RBC count of 6.5 million/uL is above the expected reference range. A decreased RBC count is an expected finding of anemia.

   C. WBC count of 4800 mm³ is below the expected reference range and is not an expected finding of anemia.

   D. **CORRECT:** Hgb of 10 g/dL is below the expected reference range and is an expected finding of anemia.

   Ⓝ *NCLEX® Connection: Reduction of Risk Potential, Laboratory Values*

2. A. aPTT is monitored for clients receiving heparin therapy. An aPTT of 38 seconds is within the expected reference range for clients not receiving heparin therapy.

   B. **CORRECT:** INR of 1.1 is within the expected reference range for a client who is not receiving warfarin. However, this value is subtherapeutic for anticoagulation therapy. The nurse should expect the client to receive an increased dosage of warfarin until the INR is 2 to 3.

   C. PT of 22 seconds is above the expected reference range for a client receiving warfarin therapy. This result indicates the client is at an increased risk for bleeding.

   D. A negative D-dimer test indicates the absence of a pulmonary embolus or deep vein thrombosis and is not used to determine the dosage needs for warfarin therapy.

   Ⓝ *NCLEX® Connection: Reduction of Risk Potential, Laboratory Values*

3. A. The nurse should inform the client that he will be placed in a prone or side-lying position during the test in order to expose the iliac crest.

   B. **CORRECT:** The nurse should inform the client of the need to stay on bed rest for 30 to 60 min following the test to reduce the risk for bleeding.

   C. The nurse should inform the client that a culture and sensitivity test determines the type of antibiotics needed to treat an infection.

   D. The nurse should inform the client that he will receive a sedative prior to the test and that a local anesthetic will be used at the site.

   Ⓝ *NCLEX® Connection: Reduction of Risk Potential, Diagnostic Tests*

PRACTICE Answer

Using the ATI Active Learning Template: Diagnostic Procedure

NURSING INTERVENTIONS (PRE, INTRA, POST)

Preprocedure
- Ensure that the client has signed the informed consent form.
- Position the client in a prone or side-lying position.
- Explain the procedure to the client. Inform the client that she might feel pressure and brief pain during the bone marrow aspiration.

Intraprocedure
- Administer sedative medication.
- Assist with the procedure.
- Inform the client that the procedure lasts about 20 min.
- Cleanse the site with an antiseptic solution.
- Maintain sterility of equipment and supplies.

Postprocedure
- Apply pressure to the biopsy site.
- Place a sterile dressing over the biopsy site.
- Monitor for evidence of infection and bleeding.
- Apply ice to the biopsy site.
- Administer mild analgesics. Avoid aspirin or medications that affect clotting.

POTENTIAL COMPLICATIONS
- Bleeding and infection
- Older adults at greater risk for complications associated with anesthesia

CLIENT EDUCATION
- Report excessive bleeding and evidence of infection to the provider.
- Check the biopsy site daily. Keep the dressing clean, dry and intact.
- If there are sutures, return in 7 to 10 days for removal.

Ⓝ *NCLEX® Connection: Reduction of Risk Potential, Diagnostic Tests*

CHAPTER 40 *Blood and Blood Product Transfusions*

Clients can receive transfusions of whole blood or components of whole blood for replacement due to blood loss or blood disease.

Blood components include packed RBCs, fresh frozen plasma, albumin, clotting factors, cryoprecipitate, and platelets.

TRANSFUSION TYPES

Standard donation: Transfusion from compatible donor blood.

Autologous transfusions: The client's blood is collected in anticipation of future transfusions (elective surgery). This blood is designated for and used only by the client. Clients can donate up to 6 weeks prior to the scheduled surgery. If the client's hemoglobin and hematocrit remain stable, donation can occur weekly to arrive at the desired amount of blood for the anticipated transfusion.

Intraoperative blood salvage: Blood loss during some surgeries (trauma-related, liver transplantation) is recycled through a device that filters blood into a transfusion bag for transfusion intraoperatively or postoperatively. Reinfusion must occur within 6 hr of salvaged blood collection.

INDICATIONS

POTENTIAL DIAGNOSES

Excessive blood loss: packed RBCs

Anemia (Hgb less than 6, or 6 to 10 g/dL, depending on findings): packed RBCs

Kidney failure: packed RBCs

Coagulation factor deficiencies such as hemophilia: fresh frozen plasma

Thrombocytopenia/platelet dysfunction (platelets less than 20,000 or less than 50,000 and actively bleeding): platelets

Hemophilia A: cryoprecipitate

Burns, hypoproteinemia: albumin

CONSIDERATIONS

PREPROCEDURE

- Incompatibility is a major concern when administering blood or blood products. Preventing incompatibility requires strict adherence to blood transfusion protocols.
- Blood is typed based on the presence of antigens.

40.1 Blood type compatibility

BLOOD TYPE	ANTIGEN	ANTIBODIES AGAINST	COMPATIBLE WITH
A	A	B	A, O
B	B	A	B, O
AB	AB	None	A, B, AB, O
O	None	A, B	O

- Another consideration is the Rh factor. Clients who are Rh-negative are born without the Rh antigen in their RBCs. As a result, they do not develop antibodies unless sensitization occurs. Once this occurs, any transfusion with Rh-positive blood will cause a reaction.

NURSING ACTIONS

- Explain the procedure to the client.
- Assess vital signs and the client's temperature prior to transfusion.
- Remain with the client during the initial 15 to 30 min of the transfusion. Most severe reactions occur within this time frame.
- Assess laboratory values (e.g., platelet count less than 20,000 and hemoglobin less than 6 g/dL).
- Verify the prescription for a specific blood product.
- Obtain consent for procedure if required.
- Obtain blood samples for compatibility determination, such as type and cross-match.
- Assess for a history of blood-transfusion reactions.
- Initiate large-bore IV access. An 18- or 20-gauge needle is standard for administering blood products.
- Obtain blood products from the blood bank. Inspect the blood for discoloration, excessive bubbles, or cloudiness.
- Prior to transfusion, two RNs (or an RN and a PN, depending on facility policy) must identify the correct blood product and client by looking at the hospital identification number (noted on the blood product) and the number identified on the client's identification band to make sure the numbers match.
- The nurse completing the blood product verification must be one of the nurses who administers the blood product.
- Prime the blood administration set with 0.9% sodium chloride only. Never add medications to blood products. Y-tubing with a filter is used to transfuse blood.
- Begin the transfusion, and use a blood warmer if indicated. Initiate the transfusion within 30 min of obtaining the blood product to reduce the risk of bacterial growth.
- OLDER ADULT CLIENTS Ⓖ
  - No larger than a 19-gauge needle is used.
  - Assess kidney function, fluid status, and circulation prior to blood product administration. Older adult clients are at an increased risk for fluid overload.
  - Use blood products that are less than 1 week old.

CLIENT EDUCATION: Explain the reason for the blood transfusion.

INTRAPROCEDURE

NURSING ACTIONS

- Remain with the client for the first 15 to 30 min of the infusion (reactions occur most often during the first 15 min) and monitor vital signs and rate of infusion per facility policy. Qs
- OLDER ADULT CLIENTS: Assess vital signs every 15 min throughout the transfusion because changes in pulse, blood pressure, and respiratory rate can indicate fluid overload, or can be the sole indicators of a transfusion reaction. Older adult clients who have cardiac or renal dysfunction are at an increased risk for heart failure and fluid-volume excess when receiving a blood transfusion. Administer the blood transfusion over 2 to 4 hr for older adult clients. Withhold administration of other IV fluids during blood product administration to prevent fluid overload. Ⓖ
- Notify the provider immediately if indications of a reaction occur.

POSTPROCEDURE

NURSING ACTIONS

- Obtain vital signs upon completion of the transfusion.
- Dispose of the blood-administration set according to facility policy.
- Complete paperwork, and file in the appropriate places.
- Document the client's response.

COMPLICATIONS

Acute hemolytic

ONSET: Immediate or can manifest during subsequent transfusions

FINDINGS

- Results from a transfusion of blood products that are incompatible with the client's blood type or Rh factor. Can occur following the transfusion of as few as 10 mL of a blood product.
- Can be mild or life-threatening, resulting in disseminated intravascular coagulation (DIC) or circulatory collapse.
- Findings include chills, fever, low-back pain, tachycardia, flushing, hypotension, chest tightening or pain, tachypnea, nausea, anxiety, hemoglobinuria, and an impending sense of doom.

NURSING ACTIONS

- Stop the transfusion.
- Remove the blood tubing from the IV access. Avoid infusing further blood products into the circulatory system.
- Initiate an infusion of 0.9% sodium chloride using new tubing.
- Monitor vital signs and fluid status.
- Send the blood bag and administration set to the lab for testing.

Febrile

ONSET: Commonly occurs within 2 hr of starting the transfusion

FINDINGS

- Results from the development of anti-WBC antibodies. Can be seen when the client has received multiple transfusions.
- Findings include chills, increase of 1° F (0.5° C) or greater from the pretransfusion temperature, flushing, hypotension, and tachycardia.

NURSING ACTIONS

- Use WBC filter for administration to prevent the reaction from occurring.
- Stop the transfusion and administer antipyretics.
- Initiate an infusion of 0.9% sodium chloride using new tubing.

Allergic

ONSET: During or up to 24 hr after transfusion

FINDINGS

- Results from a sensitivity reaction to a component of the transfused blood products.
- Findings are usually mild and include itching, urticaria, and flushing.
- The client can develop an anaphylactic transfusion reaction resulting in bronchospasm, laryngeal edema, and shock.

MILD REACTION NURSING ACTIONS

- Stop the transfusion.
- Initiate an infusion of 0.9% sodium chloride using new tubing.
- Administer an antihistamine, such as diphenhydramine.
- If the provider prescribes to restart the transfusion, do so slowly.

ANAPHYLACTIC REACTION NURSING ACTIONS

- Stop the transfusion.
- Administer epinephrine, oxygen, or CPR if indicated.
- Remove the blood tubing from the client's IV access.
- Initiate an infusion of 0.9% sodium chloride using new tubing.

Bacterial

ONSET: During or up to several hours after transfusion

FINDINGS

- Results from a transfusion of contaminated blood products.
- Findings include wheezing, dyspnea, chest tightness, cyanosis, hypotension, and shock.

NURSING ACTIONS

- Stop the transfusion.
- Administer antibiotics and an IV infusion of 0.9% sodium chloride using new tubing.
- Send a blood culture specimen to the lab for analysis.

Circulatory overload

ONSET: Can occur any time during the transfusion

FINDINGS
- Results from a transfusion rate that is too rapid for the client. Older adult clients or those who have a preexisting increased circulatory volume are at an increased risk.
- Findings include crackles, dyspnea, cough, anxiety, jugular vein distention, and tachycardia. Manifestations can progress to pulmonary edema.

NURSING ACTIONS
- Slow or stop the transfusion depending on the severity of manifestations.
- Position the client upright with feet lower than the level of the heart.
- Administer oxygen, diuretics, and morphine as prescribed.

PRACTICE Active Learning Scenario

A nurse is caring for a client who is receiving a blood transfusion. What nursing actions should the nurse anticipate if a transfusion reaction is suspected? Use the ATI Active Learning Template: Nursing Skill to complete this item.

INDICATIONS
- Describe the four types of reactions and the time of onset.
- Describe three medications that can be administered and for which reaction.

POTENTIAL COMPLICATIONS: Describe two nursing actions for each type of reaction.

Application Exercises

1. A nurse is preparing to administer packed RBCs to a client who has a Hgb of 8 g/dL. Which of the following actions should the nurse plan to take during the first 15 min of the transfusion?

   A. Obtain consent from the client for the transfusion.

   B. Assess for an acute hemolytic reaction.

   C. Explain the transfusion procedure to the client.

   D. Obtain blood culture specimens to send to the lab.

2. A nurse is caring for a client who is receiving a blood transfusion. Which of the following actions should the nurse expect if an allergic transfusion reaction is suspected? (Select all that apply.)

   A. Stop the transfusion.

   B. Monitor for hypertension.

   C. Maintain an IV infusion with 0.9% sodium chloride.

   D. Position the client in an upright position with the feet lower than the heart.

   E. Administer diphenhydramine.

3. A nurse is monitoring a client who began receiving a unit of packed RBCs 10 min ago. Which of the following findings should the nurse identify as an indication of a febrile transfusion reaction? (Select all that apply.)

   A. Temperature change from 37° C (98.6° F) pretransfusion to 37.2° C (99.0° F)

   B. Current blood pressure 178/90 mm Hg

   C. Heart rate change from 88/min pretransfusion to 120/min

   D. Client report of itching

   E. Client appears flushed

4. A nurse is providing preoperative teaching for a client who requests autologous donation in preparation for a scheduled orthopedic surgical procedure. Which of the following statements should the nurse include in the teaching?

   A. "You should make an appointment to donate blood 8 weeks prior to the surgery."

   B. "If you need an autologous transfusion, the blood your brother donates can be used."

   C. "You can donate blood each week if your hemoglobin is stable."

   D. "Any unused blood that is donated can be used for other clients."

5. A nurse preceptor is observing a newly licensed nurse on the unit who is preparing to administer a blood transfusion to an older adult client. Which of the following actions by the newly licensed nurse indicates an understanding of the procedure?

   A. Inserts an 18-gauge IV catheter in the client

   B. Verifies blood compatibility and expiration date of the blood with an assistive personnel (AP)

   C. Administers dextrose 5% in 0.9% sodium chloride IV with the transfusion

   D. Obtains vital signs every 15 min throughout the procedure.

Application Exercises Key

1. A. The nurse should obtain consent from the client for the transfusion prior to initiating the transfusion.

   B. **CORRECT:** The nurse should assess for an acute hemolytic reaction during the first 15 min of the transfusion. This form of a reaction can occur following the transfusion of as little as 10 mL of blood product.

   C. The nurse should explain the transfusion procedure to the client prior to initiating the transfusion.

   D. The nurse should obtain blood culture specimens from the client if a bacterial reaction is suspected.

   Ⓝ *NCLEX® Connection: Pharmacological and Parenteral Therapies, Blood and Blood Products*

2. A. **CORRECT:** The nurse should immediately stop the infusion if an allergic transfusion reaction is suspected.

   B. The nurse should monitor for hypotension if an allergic transfusion reaction is suspected due to the risk for shock.

   C. **CORRECT:** The nurse should administer 0.9% sodium chloride solution through new IV tubing if an allergic transfusion reaction is suspected.

   D. The nurse should position the client in an upright position with the feet lower than the level of the heart if a circulatory overload is suspected.

   E. **CORRECT:** The nurse should administer an antihistamine, such as diphenhydramine, if an allergic transfusion reaction is suspected.

   Ⓝ *NCLEX® Connection: Pharmacological and Parenteral Therapies, Blood and Blood Products*

3. A. A temperature increase of 1° F (0.5° C) is an indication of a febrile transfusion reaction.

   B. Hypotension is an indication of a febrile transfusion reaction.

   C. **CORRECT:** Tachycardia is an indication of a febrile transfusion reaction.

   D. The client's report of itching is an indication of an allergic transfusion reaction.

   E. **CORRECT:** A flushed appearance of the client can indicate a febrile transfusion reaction.

   Ⓝ *NCLEX® Connection: Pharmacological and Parenteral Therapies, Blood and Blood Products*

4. A. The client should donate blood for an autologous transfusion no sooner than 6 weeks prior to surgery.

   B. An autologous donation refers to the client's donation of blood for his own personal use.

   C. **CORRECT:** Beginning 6 weeks prior to surgery, the client can donate blood each week for autologous transfusion if his Hgb and Hct remain stable.

   D. An autologous donation is for use only by the client.

   Ⓝ *NCLEX® Connection: Reduction of Risk Potential, Therapeutic Procedures*

5. A. The nurse should use no larger than a 19-gauge needle in the older adult client.

   B. The nurse should verify the client's identity and blood compatibility, and expiration date of the blood with another nurse. This task is beyond the scope of practice for an assistive personnel.

   C. The nurse should administer blood products with 0.9% sodium chloride. IV solutions containing dextrose cannot be used.

   D. **CORRECT:** The nurse should check the older adult client's vital signs every 15 min throughout the transfusion to allow for early detection of fluid overload or other transfusion reaction.

   Ⓝ *NCLEX® Connection: Pharmacological and Parenteral Therapies, Blood and Blood Products*

PRACTICE Answer

Using the ATI Active Learning Template: Nursing Skill

INDICATIONS

Types of reactions and onset
- Acute hemolytic: immediate or during subsequent transfusions
- Febrile: within 2 hr of starting the transfusion
- Allergic: during or up to 24 hr after transfusion
- Bacterial: during or up to several hours after the transfusion
- Circulatory overload: any time during the transfusion

Medications
- Antipyretics (acetaminophen): febrile
- Antihistamines (diphenhydramine): mild allergic
- Antihistamines, corticosteroids, vasopressors, epinephrine: anaphylactic
- Antibiotics: bacterial
- Diuretics, morphine: circulatory overload

POTENTIAL COMPLICATIONS

Acute hemolytic
- Stop the transfusion.
- Remove the blood tubing.
- Initiate an infusion of 0.9% sodium chloride.
- Monitor vital signs and fluid status.
- Send the blood bag and administration set to the lab for testing.

Febrile
- Use a WBC filter to help prevent a febrile reaction.
- Stop the transfusion.
- Administer antipyretics.
- Initiate an infusion of 0.9% sodium chloride.

Mild allergic reaction
- Stop the transfusion.
- Initiate an infusion of 0.9% sodium chloride.
- Administer an antihistamine.
- If prescribed, restart the transfusion slowly to continue.

Anaphylactic reaction
- Stop the transfusion.
- Administer epinephrine and oxygen.
- Administer CPR if indicated.
- Remove the blood tubing from the client's IV access.
- Initiate an infusion of 0.9% sodium chloride.

Circulatory overload
- Slow or stop the transfusion depending on the severity.
- Position the client upright with feet lower than the level of the heart.
- Administer oxygen, diuretics, and morphine.

Bacterial
- Stop the transfusion.
- Administer antibiotics as prescribed.
- Initiate an infusion of 0.9% sodium chloride.
- Obtain blood samples for culture.

Ⓝ *NCLEX® Connection: Physiological Adaptation, Unexpected Response to Therapies*

CHAPTER 41 *Anemias*

Anemia is an abnormally low amount of circulating RBCs, Hgb concentration, or both. It is an indicator of an underlying disease or disorder. Anemia results in diminished oxygen-carrying capacity and delivery to tissues and organs. The goal of treatment is to restore and maintain adequate tissue oxygenation.

Iron-deficiency anemia due to inadequate intake is the most common cause of anemia in children, adolescents, and pregnant women. Iron-deficiency anemia due to blood loss (such as from a gastrointestinal ulcer) is the most common cause of anemia in women who are postmenopausal, as well as men. Women who are menstruating can develop anemia secondary to menorrhagia.

CAUSES OF ANEMIA

- Blood loss
- Inadequate RBC production (hypoproliferative)
- Increased RBC destruction (hemolytic)
- Deficiency of necessary components such as folic acid, iron, erythropoietin, and/or vitamin B_{12}

HEALTH PROMOTION AND DISEASE PREVENTION

- Women who are pregnant or menstruating should ensure that their diet contains adequate amounts of iron-rich foods. Otherwise, they should take an iron supplement.
- Individuals who are iron-deficient and have elevated cholesterol levels should integrate iron-rich foods that are not red or organ meats into their diets (iron-fortified cereal and breads, fish, poultry, and dried peas and beans).
- Clients should regularly consume foods high in folate (spinach, lentils, bananas) and folic acid fortified grains and juices.

ASSESSMENT

RISK FACTORS

Acute or chronic blood loss
- Trauma
- Menorrhagia
- Gastrointestinal bleed (ulcers, tumor)
- Intra or postsurgical blood loss or hemorrhage
- Chemical or radiation exposure

Increased hemolysis
- Defective Hgb (sickle-cell disease): RBCs become malformed during periods of hypoxia and obstruct capillaries in joints and organs
- Impaired glycolysis: glucose-6-phosphate-dehydrogenase (G6PD) deficiency anemia
- Immune disorder or destruction (transfusion reactions, autoimmune diseases)
- Mechanical trauma to RBCs (mechanical heart valve, cardiopulmonary bypass)

Inadequate dietary intake or malabsorption
- Iron deficiency
- Vitamin B_{12} deficiency: pernicious anemia due to deficiency of intrinsic factor produced by gastric mucosa, which is necessary for absorption of vitamin B_{12}
- Folic acid deficiency
- Pica, or a persistent eating of substances not normally considered food (nonnutritive substances), such as soil or chalk, for at least 1 month, can limit the amount of healthy food choices a client makes

Bone-marrow suppression
- Exposure to radiation or chemicals (such as insecticides or solvents)
- Aplastic anemia results in a decreased number of RBCs as well as decreased platelets and WBCs.

Age
- Older adult clients are at risk for nutrition-deficient anemias (iron, vitamin B_{12}, folate). Ⓖ
- Anemia can be misdiagnosed as depression or debilitation in older adult clients.
- Gastrointestinal bleeding is a common cause of anemia in older adult clients. Check stools for occult blood.

EXPECTED FINDINGS

- Possibly asymptomatic in mild cases
- Pallor
- Fatigue
- Irritability
- Numbness and tingling of extremities
- Dyspnea on exertion
- Sensitivity to cold
- Pain and hypoxia with sickle-cell crisis

PHYSICAL ASSESSMENT FINDINGS
- Shortness of breath/fatigue, especially upon exertion
- Tachycardia and palpitations
- Dizziness or syncope upon standing or with exertion
- Pallor with pale nail beds and mucous membranes
- Nail bed deformities (spoon-shaped nails)
- Smooth, sore, bright-red tongue (vitamin B_{12} deficiency)

LABORATORY TESTS

CBC count

- RBCs are the major carriers of hemoglobin in the blood.
- Hgb transports oxygen and carbon dioxide to and from the cells and can be used as an index of the oxygen-carrying capacity of the blood.
- Hct is the percentage of RBCs in relation to the total blood volume.

RBC indices

Used to determine the type and cause of most anemias

Mean corpuscular volume (MCV): Size of red blood cells
- Normocytic: Normal size
- Microcytic: Small cells
- Macrocytic: Large cells

Mean corpuscular Hgb (MCH): Determines the amount of Hgb per RBC
- Normochromic: Normal amount of Hgb per cell
- Hypochromic: Decreased Hgb per cell

Mean corpuscular Hgb concentration (MCHC): Indicates Hgb amount relative to the size of the cell

Iron studies

- Total iron-binding capacity (TIBC) reflects an indirect measurement of serum transferrin, a protein that binds with iron and transports it for storage.
- Serum ferritin is an indicator of total iron stores in the body.
- Serum iron measures the amount of iron in the blood. Low serum iron and elevated TIBC indicates iron-deficiency anemia.

Hgb electrophoresis

Separates normal Hgb from abnormal. It is used to detect thalassemia and sickle-cell disease.

Sickle-cell test

Evaluates the sickling of RBCs in the presence of decreased oxygen tension.

Schilling test

Measures vitamin B_{12} absorption with and without intrinsic factor. It is used to differentiate between malabsorption and pernicious anemia.

DIAGNOSTIC PROCEDURES

Bone-marrow aspiration/biopsy is used to diagnose aplastic anemia (failure of bone marrow to produce RBCs as well as platelets and WBCs).

PATIENT-CENTERED CARE

NURSING CARE

- Encourage increased dietary intake of the deficient nutrient (iron, vitamin B_{12}, folic acid).
- Monitor oxygen saturation to determine a need for oxygen therapy.
- Administer medications, as prescribed, at the proper time for optimal absorption, and using an appropriate technique.
- Teach the client and family about energy conservation in the client and the risk of the client experiencing dizziness upon standing.
- Teach the client about the time frame for resolution.

MEDICATIONS

Iron supplements

Ferrous sulfate, ferrous fumarate, ferrous gluconate
- Oral iron supplements are used to replenish serum iron and iron stores. Iron is an essential component of Hgb, and subsequently, oxygen transport.
- Parenteral iron supplements (iron dextran) are only given for severe anemia.

NURSING CONSIDERATIONS: Administer parenteral iron using the Z-track method.

41.1 Sickled blood cells

cross section of a red blood cell

normal red blood cells

cross section of a sickled blood cell

abnormal, sickled, red blood cells

41.2 RBC indices

	NORMAL MCV, MCH, MCHC	DECREASED MCV, MCH, MCHC	INCREASED MCV
CLASSIFICATION	Normocytic, normochromic anemia	Microcytic, hypochromic anemia	Macrocytic anemia
POSSIBLE CAUSES	Acute blood loss Sickle-cell disease	Iron-deficiency anemia Anemia of chronic illness Chronic blood loss	Vitamin B_{12} deficiency Folic acid deficiency

CLIENT EDUCATION
- Instruct to have hemoglobin checked in 4 to 6 weeks to determine efficacy.
- Vitamin C can increase oral iron absorption.
- Instruct the client to take iron supplements between meals to increase absorption, if tolerated.
- Inform the client stools can appear green to black in color while taking iron.

Erythropoietin: epoetin alfa

A hematopoietic growth factor used to increase production of RBCs

NURSING CONSIDERATIONS
- Monitor for an increase in blood pressure.
- Monitor Hgb and Hct twice per week.
- Monitor for a cardiovascular event if Hgb increases too rapidly (greater than 1 g/dL in 2 weeks).

CLIENT EDUCATION: Reinforce the importance of having Hgb and Hct evaluated on a twice-per-week basis until targeted levels are reached.

Vitamin B_{12} supplementation (cyanocobalamin)

- Vitamin B_{12} is necessary to convert folic acid from its inactive form to its active form. All cells rely on folic acid for DNA production.
- Vitamin B_{12} supplementation can be given orally if the deficit is due to inadequate dietary intake. However, if deficiency is due to lack of intrinsic factor being produced by the parietal cells of the stomach or malabsorption syndrome, it must be administered parenterally or intranasally to be absorbed.

NURSING CONSIDERATIONS
- Administer vitamin B_{12} according to appropriate route related to cause of vitamin B_{12} anemia (parenteral vs. oral).
- Administer parenteral forms of vitamin B_{12} IM or deep subcutaneous to decrease irritation. Do not mix other medications in the syringe.

CLIENT EDUCATION
- Clients who lack intrinsic factor or have an irreversible-malabsorption syndrome should be informed that this therapy must be continued for the rest of their life.
- A client should receive vitamin B_{12} injections on a monthly basis.

Folic acid supplements

Folic acid is a water-soluble, B-complex vitamin. It is necessary for the production of new RBCs.

NURSING CONSIDERATIONS: Folic acid can be given orally or parenterally.

CLIENT EDUCATION
- Large doses of folic acid can mask vitamin B_{12} deficiency.
- Large doses of folic acid will turn the client's urine dark yellow.

THERAPEUTIC PROCEDURES

Blood transfusions

- Blood transfusions lead to an immediate improvement in blood-cell counts and manifestations of anemia.
- Typically only used when the client has significant manifestations of anemia, because of the risk of blood-borne infections.

COMPLICATIONS

Heart failure

Heart failure can develop due to the increased demand on the heart to provide oxygen to tissues. A low Hct decreases the amount of oxygen carried to tissues in the body, which makes the heart work harder and beat faster (tachycardia, palpitations).

NURSING ACTIONS
- Administer oxygen, and monitor oxygen saturation.
- Monitor cardiac rhythm.
- Obtain daily weight.
- Administer blood transfusion as prescribed.
- Administer cardiac medications as prescribed (diuretics, antidysrhythmics).
- Administer antianemia medications as prescribed.

Application Exercises

1. A nurse is planning care for a client who has Hgb 7.5 g/dL and Hct 21.5%. Which of the following actions should the nurse include in the plan of care? (Select all that apply.)

   A. Provide assistance with ambulation.

   B. Monitor oxygen saturation.

   C. Weigh the client weekly.

   D. Obtain stool specimen for occult blood.

   E. Schedule daily rest periods.

2. A nurse is teaching a client who has a new prescription for ferrous sulfate. Which of the following information should the nurse include in the teaching?

   A. Stools will be dark red.

   B. Take with a glass of milk if gastrointestinal distress occurs.

   C. Foods high in vitamin C will promote absorption.

   D. Take for 14 days.

3. A nurse is providing discharge teaching to a client who had a gastrectomy for stomach cancer. Which of the following information should the nurse include in the teaching? (Select all that apply.)

   A. "You will need a monthly injection of vitamin B_{12} for the rest of your life."

   B. "Using the nasal spray form of vitamin B_{12} on a daily basis can be an option."

   C. "An oral supplement of vitamin B_{12} taken on a daily basis can be an option."

   D. "You should increase your intake of animal proteins, legumes, and dairy products to increase vitamin B_{12} in your diet."

   E. "Add soy milk fortified with vitamin B_{12} to your diet to decrease the risk of pernicious anemia."

4. A nurse is completing an integumentary assessment of a client who has anemia. Which of the following findings should the nurse expect?

   A. Absent turgor

   B. Spoon-shaped nails

   C. Shiny, hairless legs

   D. Yellow mucous membranes

5. A nurse in a clinic receives a phone call from a client seeking information about a new prescription for erythropoietin. Which of the following information should the nurse review with the client?

   A. The client needs an erythrocyte sedimentation rate (ESR) test weekly.

   B. The client should have his hemoglobin checked twice a week.

   C. Oxygen saturation levels should be monitored.

   D. Folic acid production will increase.

PRACTICE Active Learning Scenario

A nurse educator is presenting a community education program on anemia to a group of clients. What should be included in this presentation? Use the ATI Active Learning Template: System Disorder to complete this item.

PATHOPHYSIOLOGY RELATED TO CLIENT PROBLEM: Describe at least three causes of the disorder.

EXPECTED FINDINGS: Identify at least six.

LABORATORY TESTS: Describe the importance of the total iron-binding capacity (TIBC) test.

Application Exercises Key

1. A. **CORRECT:** The nurse should assist the client when ambulating to prevent a fall because the client who has anemia can experience dizziness.

   B. **CORRECT:** The nurse should monitor oxygen saturation when the client has anemia due to the decreased oxygen-carrying capacity of the blood.

   C. The nurse should weigh the client daily to determine if the client is losing weight from inadequate oral intake or gaining weight, which can indicate a complication of heart failure due to lack of oxygen from low hemoglobin level.

   D. **CORRECT:** The nurse should obtain the client's stool to test for occult blood, which can identify a possible cause of anemia caused from gastrointestinal bleeding.

   E. **CORRECT:** The nurse should schedule the client to rest throughout the day because the client who has anemia can experience fatigue. Rest periods should be planned to conserve energy.

   Ⓝ *NCLEX® Connection: Physiological Adaptation, Illness Management*

2. A. The nurse should teach the client that stools will be dark green to black in color when taking iron.

   B. The nurse should instruct the client that milk binds with iron and decreases its absorption.

   C. **CORRECT:** The nurse should teach the client that vitamin C enhances the absorption of iron by the intestinal tract.

   D. The nurse should instruct the client that iron therapy usually takes 4 to 6 weeks for Hgb and Hct to return to the expected reference range.

   Ⓝ *NCLEX® Connection: Pharmacological and Parenteral Therapies, Medication Administration*

3. A. **CORRECT:** The client who had a gastrectomy will require monthly injections of vitamin B_{12} for the rest of his life due to lack of intrinsic factor being produced by the parietal cells of the stomach.

   B. **CORRECT:** Cyanocobalamin nasal spray used daily is an option for a client who had a gastrectomy.

   C. Oral supplements of vitamin B_{12} will not be absorbed due to the lack of intrinsic factor produced by the parietal cells of the stomach.

   D. Dietary sources of vitamin B_{12} will not be absorbed due to the lack of intrinsic factor produced by the parietal cells of the stomach.

   E. Dietary sources of vitamin B_{12} will not be absorbed due to the lack of intrinsic factor produced by the parietal cells of the stomach.

   Ⓝ *NCLEX® Connection: Physiological Adaptation, Alterations in Body Systems*

4. A. Absent skin turgor is a finding in a client who has dehydration.

   B. **CORRECT:** Deformities of the nails, such as being spoon-shaped, are findings in a client who has anemia.

   C. Shiny, hairless legs are present in a client who has peripheral vascular disease.

   D. Yellow mucous membranes are found in a client who has jaundice. The client who has anemia will have pale nail beds and mucous membranes.

   Ⓝ *NCLEX® Connection: Reduction of Risk Potential, System Specific Assessment*

5. A. The nurse should include in the teaching that the effectiveness of erythropoietin is evaluated by changes in the hematocrit.

   B. **CORRECT:** The nurse should include in the teaching that hemoglobin and hematocrit are monitored twice a week until the targeted levels are reached.

   C. The nurse should monitor the client's blood pressure for an increase and determine if the provider should prescribe an antihypertensive.

   D. The nurse should inform the client that erythropoietin promotes increased production of RBCs.

   Ⓝ *NCLEX® Connection: Pharmacological and Parenteral Therapies, Medication Administration*

PRACTICE Answer

Using the ATI Active Learning Template: System Disorder

PATHOPHYSIOLOGY RELATED TO CLIENT PROBLEM: Anemia is an abnormally low amount of circulating red blood cells, hemoglobin concentration, or both. It can be due to blood loss, inadequate production or increased destruction of red blood cells, and dietary deficiencies of folic acid, iron, erythropoietin, and/or vitamin B_{12}.

EXPECTED FINDINGS
- Shortness of breath and fatigue with exertion
- Tachycardia, palpitations, dizziness, or syncope upon standing or with exertion
- Pallor, pale nail beds, pale mucous membranes, nail bed deformities
- Smooth, sore, bright-red tongue
- Can be asymptomatic, pallor, fatigue, irritability, numbness and tingling of extremities, dyspnea on exertion, sensitivity to cold, pain, and hypoxia with sickle-cell crisis

LABORATORY TESTS: A total iron-binding capacity (TIBC) test is an indirect measurement of serum transferrin, a protein that binds with iron and transports it for storage. Serum transferrin is an indicator of the total iron stores in the body.

Ⓝ *NCLEX® Connection: Physiological Adaptation, Alterations in Body Systems*

UNIT 5   **NURSING CARE OF CLIENTS WHO HAVE HEMATOLOGIC DISORDERS**
SECTION: HEMATOLOGIC DISORDERS

CHAPTER 42 # Coagulation Disorders

Coagulation disorders occur secondary to an alteration in platelets, clotting factors, or both. Coagulopathy is the term for any condition that affects an individual's ability to coagulate. Coagulopathies are suspected when the usual measures used to stop bleeding fail.

Coagulopathy can occur secondary to an autoimmune disorder or extensive blood loss in which platelets and clotting factors are lost. In some cases, the development of microemboli in the circulatory system paradoxically uses up the clotting factors that cause hemorrhages to occur at the same time intravascular clotting occurs.

Idiopathic thrombocytopenic purpura (ITP) is a coagulopathy that is an autoimmune disorder in which the life span of platelets is decreased by antiplatelet antibodies although platelet production is normal. This can result in severe hemorrhage following a cesarean birth or lacerations.

Heparin-induced thrombocytopenia (HIT) is an immunity-mediated clotting disorder that causes unexplained low blood platelet count as a result of treatment with heparin.

Disseminated intravascular coagulation (DIC) is a life-threatening coagulopathy in which clotting and anticlotting mechanisms occur at the same time. A client who has DIC is at risk for both internal and external bleeding, as well as damage to organs resulting from ischemia caused by microclots.

ASSESSMENT

RISK FACTORS

ITP

- Female (ages 20 to 40 years)
- Autoimmune disorder
- Recent virus (children only)

HIT

- Female
- Receiving heparin longer than 1 week
- Exposure to unfractionated heparin
- Postsurgical thromboprophylaxis (prevention of thromboembolic disease)

DIC secondary to other complications

- Septicemia
- Cardiopulmonary arrest
- Trauma (hemorrhage, burns, crush injuries)
- Obstetric complications (toxemia, amniotic fluid embolus, placental abruption)
- Cancer

EXPECTED FINDINGS

- Unusual spontaneous bleeding from the gums and nose (epistaxis)
- Oozing, trickling, or flow of blood from incisions or lacerations
- Petechiae and ecchymoses
- Hematuria
- Excessive bleeding from venipuncture, injection sites, or slight traumas
- Tachycardia, hypotension, and diaphoresis
- Organ failure secondary to microemboli
- Respiratory distress
- Redness, pain, warmth and swelling of lower extremities (HIT)

LABORATORY TESTS

- Hemoglobin (decreased with DIC and ITP): male, 14 to 18 g/dL; female, 12 to 16 g/dL
- Platelet levels (thrombocytopenia; decreased with DIC, HIT, and ITP): 140,000 to 400,000 mm³
- Fibrinogen levels (decreased with DIC): 60 to 100 mg/dL
- Prothrombin time (increased with DIC): 11.0 to 12.5 seconds
- Partial thromboplastin (increased with DIC): aPTT, 30 to 40 seconds; PTT, 60 to 70 seconds
- Thrombin time (increased with DIC): 8 to 11 seconds
- Fibrin split product levels/fibrin degradation products (increased with DIC): less than 10 mcg/mL
- D-dimer (increased with DIC): less than 0.4 mcg/mL
- Blood typing and cross-match

PATIENT-CENTERED CARE

NURSING CARE

DIC

- Nursing interventions for DIC initially focus on assessing for and correcting the underlying cause (sepsis, hemorrhage). Focus then turns to preventing organ damage secondary to microemboli and replacing the blood's clotting components.
- Monitor for signs of microemboli (cyanotic nail beds, pain).

DIC, HIT, and ITP

- Regularly assess vital signs and hemodynamic status.
- Monitor for signs of organ failure or intracranial bleed (oliguria, decreased level of consciousness).
- Monitor laboratory values for clotting factors.
- Administer fluid volume replacement.
- Transfuse blood, platelets, and other clotting products.
- Monitor for complications from administration of blood and blood products.
- Avoid use of NSAIDs.
- Administer supplemental oxygen.
- Provide protection from injury. Qs
- Instruct client to avoid Valsalva maneuver (could cause cerebral hemorrhage).
- Implement bleeding precautions (avoid use of needles).

MEDICATIONS

ITP: Corticosteroids and immunosuppressants

HIT: Anticoagulants with direct thrombin inhibitor (argatroban, lepirudin, bivalirudin)

DIC: Anticoagulants (heparin) can be used to decrease microclots from forming and using up clotting factors

THERAPEUTIC PROCEDURES

ITP: Splenectomy can be performed if the client does not respond to medical management.

Application Exercises

1. A nurse is caring for a client who has disseminated intravascular coagulation (DIC). Which of the following laboratory values indicates the client's clotting factors are depleted? (Select all that apply.)

   A. Platelets 100,000/mm³

   B. Fibrinogen levels 57 mg/dL

   C. Fibrin degradation products 4.3 mcg/mL

   D. D-dimer 0.03 mcg/mL

   E. Sedimentation rate 38 mm/hr

2. A nurse is assessing a client and suspects the client is experiencing DIC. Which of the following physical findings should the nurse anticipate?

   A. Bradycardia

   B. Hypertension

   C. Epistaxis

   D. Xerostomia

3. A nurse is caring for a client who has idiopathic thrombocytopenic purpura (ITP). The nurse should notify the provider and report possible small-vessel clotting when which of the following is assessed?

   A. Petechiae on the upper chest

   B. Hypotension

   C. Cyanotic nail beds

   D. Severe headache

4. A nurse is caring for a client who has DIC. Which of the following medications should the nurse anticipate administering?

   A. Heparin

   B. Vitamin K

   C. Mefoxin

   D. Simvastatin

5. A nurse is teaching a newly licensed nurse about heparin-induced thrombocytopenia. Which of the following risk factors for this disorder should the nurse include in the teaching?

   A. Warfarin therapy for atrial fibrillation

   B. Placental abruption

   C. Systemic lupus erythematosus

   D. Heparin therapy for deep-vein thrombosis

PRACTICE Active Learning Scenario

A nurse is developing a plan of care for a client who has disseminated intravascular coagulation (DIC). What interventions should the nurse include in the plan of care? Use the ATI Active Learning Template: System Disorder to complete this item.

NURSING CARE: Describe five interventions.

Application Exercises Key

1. A. **CORRECT:** In DIC, platelet levels are decreased, causing clotting factors to become depleted. Clotting times are increased, which raises the risk for fatal hemorrhage.

   B. **CORRECT:** In DIC, fibrinogen levels are decreased, causing clotting factors to become depleted. Clotting times are increased, which raises the risk for fatal hemorrhage.

   C. Fibrin degradation products are increased when DIC occurs.

   D. A D-dimer level is increased when DIC occurs.

   E. The sedimentation rate is increased, but it is not an indicator of DIC.

   Ⓝ *NCLEX® Connection: Reduction of Risk Potential, Laboratory Values*

2. A. Tachycardia is a finding that is indicative of DIC.

   B. Hypotension is a finding that is indicative of DIC.

   C. **CORRECT:** Epistaxis is unexpected bleeding of the gums and nose and is a finding indicative of DIC.

   D. Xerostomia is dryness of the mouth and is not indicative of DIC.

   Ⓝ *NCLEX® Connection: Physiological Adaptation, Pathophysiology*

3. A. Petechiae on the upper chest can indicate impaired clotting.

   B. Hypotension can indicate impaired clotting.

   C. **CORRECT:** Cyanotic nail beds indicate microvascular clotting is occurring and should be immediately reported to avoid ischemic loss of the fingers or toes.

   D. Severe headache can indicate cerebral bleeding.

   Ⓝ *NCLEX® Connection: Physiological Adaptation, Unexpected Response to Therapies*

4. A. **CORRECT:** Heparin can be administered to decrease the formation of microclots, which deplete clotting factors.

   B. Vitamin K promotes blood coagulation and is not prescribed for a client who has DIC.

   C. Mefoxin is an antibiotic given to treat bacterial infection and is not a medication that the nurse should anticipate being administered to a client who has DIC.

   D. Simvastatin is an antilipemic given to treat hyperlipidemia and is not a medication that the nurse should anticipate being administered to a client who has DIC.

   Ⓝ *NCLEX® Connection: Physiological Adaptation, Hemodynamics*

5. A. Warfarin therapy and atrial fibrillation are not related to development of HIT.

   B. Placental abruption is a risk factor for development of DIC.

   C. Systemic lupus erythematosus is an autoimmune disorder that places the client at risk for development of ITP.

   D. **CORRECT:** The client who is receiving heparin therapy for longer than 1 week is at increased risk for the development of HIT.

   Ⓝ *NCLEX® Connection: Physiological Adaptation, Hemodynamics*

PRACTICE Answer

Using ATI Active Learning Template: System Disorder

NURSING CARE

- Monitor for signs of microemboli (cyanotic nail beds, pain).
- Regularly assess vital signs and hemodynamic status.
- Monitor for signs of organ failure or intracranial bleed (oliguria, decreased level of consciousness).

- Monitor laboratory values for clotting factors.
- Administer fluid volume replacement.
- Transfuse blood, platelets, and other clotting products.
- Monitor for complications from the administration of blood and blood products.
- Avoid use of NSAIDs.

- Administer supplemental oxygen.
- Provide protection from injury.
- Instruct client to avoid Valsalva maneuver (could cause cerebral hemorrhage).
- Implement bleeding precautions (avoid use of needles).

Ⓝ *NCLEX® Connection: Physiological Adaptation, Hemodynamics*

When reviewing the following chapters, keep in mind the relevant topics and tasks of the NCLEX outline, in particular:

Client Needs: Physiological Adaptation

FLUID AND ELECTROLYTE IMBALANCES: Evaluate the client's response to interventions to correct fluid or electrolyte imbalance.

HEMODYNAMICS: Apply knowledge of pathophysiology to interventions in response to client abnormal hemodynamics.

MEDICAL EMERGENCIES: Evaluate and document the client's response to emergency interventions.

CHAPTER 43 *Fluid Imbalances*

The body maintains homeostasis when the characteristics of body fluid remain in balance: volume, concentration (osmolality), composition (electrolyte concentration), and acidity (pH). In the healthy adult client, 55% to 60% of body weight is comprised of body fluid. This decreases to about 50% to 55% in a healthy older adult client.

Fluid moves between compartments through selectively permeable membranes by a variety of methods (diffusion, active transport, filtration, osmosis) to maintain homeostasis. Diffusion is the passive movement of electrolytes and other particles from higher concentration to lower concentration gradient. Active transport requires energy (ATP) to move electrolytes against the concentration gradient into the cell membrane. Filtration is the movement of fluids across the capillaries. Osmosis is the pulling of water into and out of the cells by osmotic pressure.

Balance is maintained through input and output. Intake is regulated not only by thirst, but social and habit play a role in adequate fluid intake Fluid output occurs in all of the following organs, the kidneys, skin, lungs, and GI tract. The kidneys are the major regulator of fluid output.

BODY FLUIDS

Body fluids are distributed between two compartments.

Intracellular (ICF)
- Two thirds of body water
- Body fluids within the cell

Extracellular (ECF)
- One third of body water
- Body fluids outside of the cell membrane
- Further divided into parts
  - **Intravascular fluid:** The liquid part of blood or the plasma
  - **Interstitial fluid**: Located between the cells and outside of the blood vessels
  - **Transcellular body fluids:** Secreted by epithelial cells (cerebrospinal, pleural, peritoneal, and synovial fluids)

CAUSES OF VOLUME IMBALANCES

Abnormal gastrointestinal (GI) losses: Vomiting, nasogastric suctioning, diarrhea

Abnormal skin losses: Diaphoresis

Abnormal renal losses: Diuretic therapy, diabetes insipidus, kidney disease, adrenal insufficiency, osmotic diuresis

Third spacing: Peritonitis, intestinal obstruction, ascites, burns

Hemorrhage

Altered intake, such as nothing by mouth (NPO)

Fluid volume deficits

- Fluid volume deficits can be divided into two main categories: volume imbalances and osmolality imbalances. When there is an issue with volume imbalance, it relates to a lack of body fluid in the extracellular compartment. Osmolality imbalances occur when there is disturbance in concentration of body fluid.
- Volume imbalances occur when too little or too much isotonic fluid is present.
- Osmolality imbalances occur when body fluid becomes either hypertonic or hypotonic. Hypernatremia (water deficit) and hyponatremia (water excess or intoxication) are good examples of this type of imbalance.

ASSESSMENT

RISK FACTORS

Fluid loss

- Strenuous exercising
- Increased intake of caffeine and alcohol
- Living at high elevations or in dry climates
- The effect of fluid imbalance in older adults is greater due to the loss of elasticity of the skin, decrease in glomerular filtration and concentrating ability of the kidneys, loss of muscle mass (muscle tissue holds more body water), and diminished thirst reflex. ©

EXPECTED FINDINGS

Hypovolemia

VITAL SIGNS: Hyperthermia, tachycardia (in an attempt to maintain a normal blood pressure), thready pulse, hypotension, orthostatic hypotension, decreased central venous pressure, tachypnea (increased respirations to compensate for lack of fluid volume within the body), hypoxia

NEUROMUSCULOSKELETAL: Dizziness, syncope, confusion, weakness, fatigue

GASTROINTESTINAL: Thirst, dry furrowed tongue, nausea, vomiting, anorexia, acute weight loss

RENAL: Oliguria (decreased production and concentration of urine)

OTHER FINDINGS: Diminished capillary refill, cool clammy skin, diaphoresis, sunken eyeballs, flattened neck veins, poor skin turgor and tenting, weight loss, low central venous pressure

Osmolality imbalances or hypernatremia

- Extreme thirst
- Skin that is dry and flushed
- Postural hypotension
- Fever
- Restlessness, confusion, agitation
- Coma and seizures can occur because onset of fluid imbalance is rapid.

LABORATORY TESTS

Hematocrit (Hct): Increased in hypovolemia

BUN: Increased (greater 25 mg/dL) due to hemoconcentration

Urine specific gravity: Greater than 1.030

Serum sodium: Greater than 145 mEq/L

Serum osmolality: Greater than 295 mOsm/kg

PATIENT-CENTERED CARE

NURSING CARE

- Monitor I&O.
- Monitor vital signs. Orthostatic measurements should be assessed as a client is at increased risk of falls when orthostatic hypotension present.
- Monitor for changes in mentation and confusion (an indication of worsening fluid imbalance). Administer IV hydration as prescribed.
- Monitor weight every 8 hr while fluid replacement is in progress.
- Assess level of gait stability. Encourage the client to use call light and ask for assistance. Qs
- Initiate fall precautions.
- Encourage the client to change positions, rolling from side to side or standing up slowly.

INTERPROFESSIONAL CARE

The nurse should collaborate with other members of the health care team to determine appropriate fluid volume replacement and oxygen management.

CLIENT EDUCATION

- Encourage the client to drink plenty of liquids to promote hydration.
- Educate the client regarding causes of dehydration, such as nausea and vomiting.

COMPLICATIONS

Hypovolemic shock

- Occurs with significant loss of body fluid.
- The client's mean arterial pressure decreases (which slows blood flow and perfusion to tissues of the body) and the cells are no longer able to carry oxygen to the blood adequately (due to the loss of red blood cells).

NURSING ACTIONS
- Administer oxygen, and monitor oxygen saturation. Oxygen saturation less than 70% is a medical emergency.
- Stay with an unstable client suffering from hypovolemic shock.
- Monitor vital signs at least every 15 min.
- Provide fluid replacement with the following.
  - **Colloids:** whole blood, packed RBCs, plasma, synthetic plasma expanders
  - **Crystalloids:** lactated Ringer's, normal saline
- Administer vasoconstrictors (dopamine, norepinephrine, phenylephrine), agents to improve myocardial perfusion (sodium nitroprusside), and/or positive inotropic medications (dobutamine, milrinone).
- Perform hemodynamic monitoring.

Fluid volume excesses

Overhydration occurs when there is an excess of fluids in the body. It is a clinical indication that the intake of fluids and the excretion of fluids is not in balance. Another term for this phenomenon is hypervolemia, as there is excess fluid in the extracellular space.

- Fluid overload can also occur when the electrolytes in the body are not in balance. For example, the lack of or excess of serum sodium can result in fluid imbalance. For more information, see **CHAPTER 44: ELECTROLYTE IMBALANCES**.
- Clients who have fluid overload are at risk for developing pulmonary edema or congestive heart failure.

HEALTH PROMOTION AND DISEASE PREVENTION

- In healthy people, the body will compensate for slight changes in fluid imbalance and the excessive intake of electrolytes. In the elderly population, the risk of fluid imbalance is greater due to changes in the body with age (e.g., reduced kidney function).
- When clients have known heart disease and impairment of kidney function, it important for the nurse to instruct the client regarding the following.
  - Consume a diet low in sodium. Consult with the provider regarding diet restrictions.
  - Restrict fluid intake. Consult with provider regarding prescribed restrictions.

ASSESSMENT

RISK FACTORS

Causes of hypervolemia
- Clients who have compromised regulatory systems, such as heart failure, kidney disease, and cirrhosis
- Overdose of sodium concentrated fluids
- Fluid shifts that occur following burns
- Prolonged use of corticosteroids
- Severe stress
- Hyperaldosteronism

EXPECTED FINDINGS

Fluid volume overload

VITAL SIGNS: Tachycardia, bounding pulse, hypertension, tachypnea, increased central venous pressure

NEUROMUSCULAR: Weakness due to excess fluid retained, which depletes energy and increases the workload for the body; headache; altered level of consciousness

GASTROINTESTINAL: Ascites

RESPIRATORY: Crackles, cough, increased respiratory rate, dyspnea caused from an excess of fluids within the body and lungs

OTHER SIGNS: Peripheral edema due to an excess of fluids within the body and lungs, resulting in weight gain, distended neck veins, and increased urine output

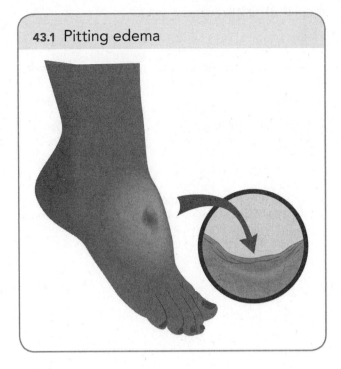

43.1 Pitting edema

LABORATORY TESTS

- Decreased Hct and Hgb
- Decreased serum and urine osmolarity
- Decreased urine sodium and specific gravity
- Decreased BUN due to plasma dilution

DIAGNOSTIC PROCEDURES

Chest x-ray: Reveals possible pulmonary congestion

PATIENT-CENTERED CARE

NURSING CARE

- Monitor I&O.
- Monitor daily weight.
- Assess breath sounds.
- Monitor peripheral edema.
- Maintain sodium-restricted diet as prescribed.
- Maintain fluid restrictions if prescribed.
- Encourage rest.
- Monitor clients receiving diuretics.
- Encourage the client to discuss use of over-the-counter medications with the provider, as some of these contain sodium.
- Position the client in the semi-Fowler's position, and reposition to prevent tissue breakdown in edematous skin.
- Use a pressure-reducing mattress, and assess bony prominence on a regular basis.
- Monitor serum sodium and potassium levels.

INTERPROFESSIONAL CARE

- Respiratory services may be consulted for oxygen management.
- Pulmonology may be consulted if fluid moves into lungs.

CLIENT EDUCATION

- Encourage client to weigh himself daily. Notify the provider if there is a 1- to 2-lb gain in 24 hr, or a 3-lb gain in 1 week. After the first ½-lb weight gain, each addition pound of weight gain is equal to 500 mL retained fluid.
- Instruct the client to consume a low-sodium diet, read food labels to check sodium content, and keep a record of daily sodium intake. Q𝗘𝗕𝗣
- Promote fluid restriction intake. Consult with the provider regarding prescribed restrictions.

COMPLICATIONS

Pulmonary edema

- Pulmonary edema can be caused by severe fluid overload.
- Manifestations include anxiety, tachycardia, increased vein distention, premature ventricular contractions, dyspnea at rest, change in level of consciousness, restlessness, lethargy, ascending crackles (fluid level within lungs), and cough productive of frothy pink-tinged sputum.

NURSING ACTIONS

- Position the client in high-Fowler's to maximize ventilation.
- Administer oxygen, positive airway pressure, and/or possible intubation and mechanical ventilation.
- Administer morphine, nitrates, and diuretic as prescribed if blood pressure is adequate.

1. A nurse is admitting a client who reports nausea, vomiting, and weakness. The client has dry oral mucous membranes. Which of the following findings should the nurse identify as manifestations of fluid volume deficit? (Select all that apply.)

    A. Decreased skin turgor

    B. Concentrated urine

    C. Bradycardia

    D. Low-grade fever

    E. Tachypnea

2. A nurse is admitting an older adult client who is experiencing dyspnea, weakness, weight gain of 2 lb, and 1+ bilateral edema of the lower extremities. The client has temperature 37.2° C (99° F), pulse 96/min, respirations 26/min, oxygen saturation 94% on 3 L oxygen via nasal cannula, and blood pressure 152/96 mm Hg. Which of the following manifestations of fluid volume excess should the nurse expect? (Select all that apply.)

    A. Dyspnea

    B. Edema

    C. Bradycardia

    D. Hypertension

    E. Weakness

3. A nurse is assessing a client who is dehydrated for fluid volume deficit. Which of the following findings should the nurse expect in the client?

    A. Moist skin

    B. Distended neck veins

    C. Increased urinary output

    D. Tachycardia

4. A nurse is caring for an older adult client in a long-term care facility. The client has become weak and confused. He ate 40% of his breakfast and lunch. The client's temperature is 38.3° C (100.9° F), pulse 92/min, respirations 20/min, and blood pressure 108/60 mm Hg. He has lost ¾ lb and reports dizziness when assisted to the bathroom. He also has a nonproductive cough with diminished breath sounds in the right lower lobe. Which of the following actions should the nurse take?

    A. Initiate fluid restrictions to limit intake.

    B. Observe for signs of peripheral edema.

    C. Encourage the client to ambulate to promote oxygenation.

    D. Monitor for orthostatic hypotension

PRACTICE Active Learning Scenario

A nurse is planning care for a client who is experiencing fluid volume excess. What nursing actions should the nurse include in the plan of care? Use the ATI Active Learning Template: System Disorder to complete this item.

NURSING CARE: Describe three interventions the nurse should take.

Application Exercises Key

1. A. **CORRECT:** Decreased skin turgor is a manifestation present with fluid volume deficit. Skin turgor is decreased due to the lack of fluid within the body and results in dryness of the skin.

   B. **CORRECT:** Concentrated urine is a manifestation present with fluid volume deficit. Urine is concentrated due to lack of fluid in the vascular system causing a decreased profusion of the kidneys and resulting in an increased urine specific gravity.

   C. Tachycardia is a manifestation present with fluid volume deficit due to an attempt to maintain a normal blood pressure.

   D. **CORRECT:** Low-grade fever is a manifestation present with fluid volume deficit. Low-grade fever is one of the body's ways to maintain homeostasis to compensate for lack of fluid within the body.

   E. **CORRECT:** Tachypnea is a manifestation present with fluid volume deficit. Increased respirations are the body's way to obtain oxygen due to the lack of fluid volume within the body.

   Ⓝ *NCLEX® Connection: Physiological Adaptation, Fluid and Electrolyte Imbalances*

2. A. **CORRECT:** Dyspnea is a manifestation present with fluid volume excess. Dyspnea is due to an excess of fluids within the body and lungs, and the client is struggling to breathe to obtain oxygen.

   B. **CORRECT:** Edema is a manifestation present with fluid volume excess. Weight gain can be a result of edema.

   C. Tachycardia and bounding pulses are manifestations related to fluid volume excess.

   D. **CORRECT:** Hypertension is a manifestation related to fluid volume excess. Blood pressure rises as the heart must work harder due to the excess fluid.

   E. **CORRECT:** Weakness is a manifestation present with fluid volume excess. Weakness is due to the excess fluid that is retained, which depletes energy and increases the workload for the body.

   Ⓝ *NCLEX® Connection: Physiological Adaptation, Fluid and Electrolyte Imbalances*

3. A. Moist skin is a manifestation of fluid volume excess.

   B. Distended neck veins are a manifestation of fluid volume excess.

   C. Increased urinary output is a manifestation of fluid volume excess.

   D. **CORRECT:** Tachycardia is an attempt to maintain blood pressure, a manifestation of fluid volume deficit.

   Ⓝ *NCLEX® Connection: Physiological Adaptation, Fluid and Electrolyte Imbalances*

4. A. The nurse should offer fluids when the client has manifestations of dehydration.

   B. The nurse should monitor for signs of poor skin turgor when the client has manifestations of fluid volume deficit.

   C. The nurse should keep the client in bed and assist him to the bathroom as needed because he is at risk for falling due to manifestations of dehydration.

   D. **CORRECT:** The nurse should monitor for orthostatic hypotension because he has manifestations of dehydration due to decreased circulatory volume.

   Ⓝ *NCLEX® Connection: Physiological Adaptation, Fluid and Electrolyte Imbalances*

PRACTICE Answer

Using the ATI Active Learning Template: System Disorder

NURSING CARE

- Check ABGs, SaO_2, CBC, and chest x-ray results.
- Position the client in semi-Fowler's.
- Obtain daily weight.
- Monitor intake and output.
- Administer supplemental oxygen as prescribed.
- Reduce IV flow rates.
- Administer diuretics (osmotic, loop) as prescribed.
- Limit fluid and sodium intake as prescribed.
- Monitor and document presence of edema (pretibial, sacral, periorbital).
- Reposition the client at least every 2 hr.
- Support arms and legs to decrease dependent edema as appropriate.
- Monitor vital signs and heart rhythm.
- Auscultate lung sounds for crackles.

Ⓝ *NCLEX® Connection: Physiological Adaptation, Fluid and Electrolyte Imbalances*

CHAPTER 44 # Electrolyte Imbalances

Electrolytes are charged ions dissolved in body fluids. Cations are positively charged, and anions are negatively charged. Electrolytes are distributed between intracellular (ICF) and extracellular (ECF) fluid compartments. The distributions of ions differs in ICF and ECF. The difference in the concentration of electrolytes in the ICF and ECF maintains cell excitability and allows for the transmission of nerve impulses.

Body fluids should be electrically neutral; the negative and positive ions in the body fluids are equal in number. When dissolved in water or another solvent, electrolytes separate into ions and conduct either a positive (cations: magnesium, potassium, sodium, calcium, and hydrogen ions) or negative (anions: phosphate, sulfate, chloride, bicarbonate, and proteinate ions) electrical current.

Healthy people can develop an imbalance of electrolytes from an imbalance of intake and output. Ill and older adult clients are at higher risk of electrolyte imbalance. Although laboratory tests can accurately reflect the electrolyte concentrations in plasma, it is not possible to directly measure electrolyte concentrations within cells.

EXPECTED REFERENCE RANGES

Sodium: 136 to 145 mEq/L

Calcium: 9.0 to 10.5 mg/dL

Potassium: 3.5 to 5.0 mEq/L

Magnesium: 1.3 to 2.1 mEq/L

Chloride: 98 to 106 mEq/L

Phosphorus: 3.0 to 4.5 mg/dL

Sodium imbalances

- Sodium (Na^+) is the major electrolyte (cation) found in ECF, and maintains ECF osmolarity.
- Sodium within ICF is low (14 mEq/L). The difference in ICF and ECF sodium levels is very important in maintaining skeletal muscle contraction, cardiac contraction, and nerve impulse transmission.
- Water flows in the direction of sodium concentration. The ECF sodium level influences fluid retention, excretion, and movement of fluid from one body space to another.
- The kidneys regulate sodium levels with the assistance of aldosterone, antidiuretic hormone (ADH), and natriuretic peptide.
- Decreased sodium levels are known as hyponatremia.
- Elevated sodium levels are known as hypernatremia.

Hyponatremia

Hyponatremia is a net gain of water or loss of sodium-rich fluids that results in sodium levels less than 136 mEq/L.
- Hyponatremia delays and slows the depolarization of membranes.
- Water moves from the ECF into the ICF, causing cells to swell (cellular edema).
- Urine sodium levels helps to differentiate between non-kidney fluid loss (vomiting, diarrhea, and sweating) and kidney salt wasting, which can occur with diuretic use.
- Hyponatremia generally is caused by fluid imbalance, which results in sodium loss.
- Compensatory mechanisms include the kidney excretion of sodium-free water.

ASSESSMENT

RISK FACTORS

Actual sodium deficits
- Excessive sweating
- Diuretics
- Wound drainage (especially gastrointestinal)
- Nasogastric tube suction of isotonic gastric contents
- Decreased secretion of aldosterone
- Hyperlipidemia
- Kidney disease
- Inadequate sodium intake (nothing by mouth [NPO] status)
- Hyperglycemia
- Low-sodium diet
- Cerebral salt wasting syndrome

Relative sodium deficits due to dilution
- Hypotonic fluid excess (PO ingestion)
- Psychogenic polydipsia
- Freshwater submersion accident
- Kidney failure (nephrotic syndrome)
- Heart failure
- Irrigation with hypotonic fluids
- Syndrome of inappropriate ADH secretion
- Anticonvulsant medications, SSRIs, or desmopressin
- Older adult clients are at a greater risk due to increased incidence of chronic illnesses, use of diuretic medications, and risk for insufficient sodium intake. ©

EXPECTED FINDINGS

- Clinical indicators depend on whether it is associated with a normal (euvolemic), decreased (hypovolemic), or increased (hypervolemic) ECF volume.
- If the client is hypervolemic with hyponatremia, palpate the bounding pulse. The client can have normal to high blood pressure.
- Muscle weakness can lead to respiratory compromise.

VITAL SIGNS: Can vary based on state of ECF volume. All due to hypovolemia: Hypothermia, tachycardia, rapid thready pulse, hypotension, orthostatic hypotension, diminished peripheral pulses.

NEUROMUSCULOSKELETAL: Headache, confusion, lethargy, muscle weakness to the point of possible respiratory compromise, fatigue, decreased deep-tendon reflexes (DTRs), seizures, lightheadedness, dizziness.

GASTROINTESTINAL: Increased motility, hyperactive bowel sounds, abdominal cramping, nausea.

LABORATORY TESTS

Serum sodium: Decreased, less than 136 mEq/L

Serum osmolarity: Decreased, less than 270 mOsm/L

PATIENT-CENTERED CARE

NURSING CARE

- Replacement of sodium should not exceed 12 mEq/L in a 24-hr period because rapid rise in sodium level risks development of neurological damage due to demyelination.
- If the client can tolerate PO fluids, sodium can be easily replaced by intake of foods and fluids.
- Administer IV fluids (lactated Ringer's or 0.9% isotonic saline).
- Report abnormal laboratory findings to the provider.
- Fluid overload: Restrict water intake as prescribed by the provider.
- Hypertonic sodium solution may be used to decreased cerebral edema.

Acute hyponatremia

- Administer hypertonic oral and IV fluids as prescribed.
- Administer 3% sodium chloride slowly, and monitor sodium levels frequently. When using hypertonic solutions, the serum sodium level should not be greater than 125 mEq/L.
- The goal is to elevate the serum sodium level enough to decrease neurological manifestations associated with hyponatremia such as lethargy, confusion, and seizures.
- Encourage foods and fluids high in sodium (beef broth, tomato juice).
- Monitor I&O and daily weight.
- Monitor vital signs and level of consciousness. Report abnormal findings to the provider.
- Administer medications as prescribed (such as conivaptan or tolvaptan, which promote excretion of excess fluid).

INTERPROFESSIONAL CARE

- Nephrology may be consulted for electrolyte and fluid replacement.
- Respiratory services may be consulted for oxygen management.
- Nutritional services may be consulted for high-sodium food choices and restricting fluid intake.

CLIENT EDUCATION

- Encourage the client to weigh daily and to notify the provider of a 1- to 2-lb gain in 24 hr, or 3-lb (1.4 kg) gain in 1 week.
- Instruct the client to consume a high-sodium diet, including reading food labels to check sodium content, and keeping a daily record of sodium intake.

COMPLICATIONS

Acute hyponatremia

Complications (coma, seizures, respiratory arrest) can result from acute hyponatremia if not treated immediately.

NURSING ACTIONS
- Maintain an open airway, and monitor vital signs.
- Implement seizure precautions, and take appropriate action if seizures occur.
- Monitor level of consciousness.

Hypernatremia

Increased sodium causes hypertonicity of the serum. This causes a shift of water out of the cells, resulting in dehydrated cells.

- Hypernatremia is a serum sodium level greater than 145 mEq/L.
- Hypernatremia is a serious electrolyte imbalance. It can cause significant neurological, endocrine, and cardiac disturbances.

ASSESSMENT

RISK FACTORS

- Water deprivation (NPO)
- Hypertonic enteral feedings without adequate water supplement
- Diabetes insipidus
- Heatstroke
- Hyperventilation
- Watery stools
- Burns
- Excessive sweating
- Excessive sodium retention: kidney failure, Cushing's syndrome, aldosteronism, some medications (e.g., glucocorticosteroids)
- Excessive intake of oral sodium
- Age-related changes, specifically decreased total body water content and inadequate fluid intake related to an altered thirst mechanism ⓒ
- Compensatory mechanisms, including increased thirst and production of ADH

EXPECTED FINDINGS

Thirst

VITAL SIGNS: Hyperthermia, tachycardia, orthostatic hypotension

NEUROMUSCULOSKELETAL: Restlessness; irritability; muscle twitching to the point of muscle weakness, including respiratory compromise; decreased or absent DTRs; seizures; coma

GASTROINTESTINAL: Thirst, dry mucous membranes, nausea, vomiting, anorexia, occasional diarrhea

LABORATORY TESTS

Serum sodium: Increased to greater than 145 mEq/L

Serum osmolarity: Increased to greater than 300 mOsm/L

Urine sodium: Decreased urine

Urine specific gravity and osmolarity: Increased

PATIENT-CENTERED CARE

NURSING CARE

- Report abnormal laboratory findings to the provider.
- Monitor level of consciousness, and ensure safety.
- Monitor vital signs and heart rhythm.
- Auscultate lung sounds.
- Provide oral hygiene and other comfort measures to decrease thirst.
- Monitor I&O, and alert the provider of inadequate urinary output.

Fluid loss

Based on serum osmolarity and hemodynamic stability
- Administer 5% dextrose and 0.45% sodium chloride solution. It is a hypertonic solution prior to infusion, but once infused the glucose rapidly metabolizes and it becomes a hypotonic solution.
- Administer isotonic nonsaline IV fluids (5% dextrose in water).

Excess sodium

- Encourage water intake, and discourage sodium intake.
- Administer diuretics (loop diuretics) for clients who have poor kidney excretion.

INTERPROFESSIONAL CARE

Nutritional services may be consulted for low-sodium food choices and to restrict fluid intake.

CLIENT EDUCATION

- Encourage the client to weigh daily. Notify the provider of a 1- to 2-lb gain in 24 hr, or 3-lb (1.4 kg) gain in 1 week.
- Encourage the client to consume a low-sodium diet, read food labels for sodium content, and keep a record of daily sodium intake.
- Encourage fluids as prescribed.

COMPLICATIONS

Acute hypernatremia

Complications (seizures, convulsion, death) can result from acute hypernatremia if not treated immediately.

NURSING ACTIONS
- Maintain open airway, and monitor vital signs.
- Implement seizure precautions, and take appropriate action if seizures occur.
- Monitor level of consciousness.

Potassium imbalances

- Potassium (K+) is the major cation in ICF. 98% of the body's potassium within the cells.
- Potassium plays a vital role in cell metabolism; transmission of nerve impulses; functioning of cardiac, lung, and muscle tissues; and acid-base balance.
- Potassium has a reciprocal action with sodium.
- Minor variations in the level of potassium in the body is a significant finding.
- Decreased potassium levels are known as hypokalemia.
- Elevated potassium levels are known as hyperkalemia.

Hypokalemia

Hypokalemia is the result of an increased loss of potassium from the body or movement of potassium into the cells, resulting in a serum potassium less than 3.5 mEq/L.

ASSESSMENT

RISK FACTORS

Actual potassium deficits
- Overuse of diuretics, digitalis, corticosteroids
- Increased secretion of aldosterone
- Cushing's syndrome
- Loss via GI tract-vomiting diarrhea, prolonged nasogastric suctioning, NPO status, and excessive use of laxatives or tap water enema administered repeatedly because tap water is hypotonic, and gastrointestinal losses are isotonic
- Kidney disease, which impairs the reabsorption of potassium

Relative potassium deficit
- Alkalosis
- Hyperinsulinism
- Hyperalimentation
- Total parental nutrition
- Water intoxication
- Older adult clients due to increased use of diuretics and laxatives Ⓒ

EXPECTED FINDINGS

VITAL SIGNS: Decreased blood pressure, thready weak pulse, orthostatic hypotension

NEUROLOGIC: Altered mental status, anxiety, and lethargy that progresses to acute confusion and coma

ECG: Flattened T wave, prominent U waves, ST depression, prolonged PR interval

GASTROINTESTINAL: Hypoactive bowel sounds, nausea, vomiting, constipation, abdominal distention. Paralytic ileus can develop.

MUSCULAR: Weakness. Deep-tendon reflexes can be reduced.

RESPIRATORY: Shallow breathing

LABORATORY TESTS

Serum potassium: Decreased to less than 3.5 mEq/L

DIAGNOSTIC PROCEDURES

Electrocardiogram (ECG): Show findings of dysrhythmias: premature ventricular contractions, ventricular tachycardia, inverted T waves, ST depression.

PATIENT-CENTERED CARE

NURSING CARE

- Report abnormal findings to the provider.
- Assess for phlebitis (tissue irritant).
- Never give potassium via IM or subcutaneous route, which can cause necrosis of the tissues.
- Monitor and maintain adequate urine output.
- Observe for shallow ineffective respirations and diminished breath sounds.
- Monitor cardiac rhythm, and intervene promptly as needed.
- Monitor clients receiving digoxin. Hypokalemia increases the risk for digoxin toxicity.
- Monitor level of consciousness, and maintain client safety.
- Monitor bowel sounds and abdominal distention, and intervene as needed.
- Monitor oxygen saturation levels, which should remain greater than 95%.
- Assess hand grasps for muscle weakness.
- Assess DTRs.

Replacement of potassium

- Encourage foods high in potassium: avocados, broccoli, dairy products, dried fruit, cantaloupe, bananas, juices, melon, lean meats, milk, whole grains, and citrus fruits.
- Provide oral potassium supplementation.

IV potassium supplementation

- Never administer by IV push (high risk of cardiac arrest).
- The maximum recommended rate is 10 mEq/hr.

INTERPROFESSIONAL CARE

- Nephrology may be consulted for electrolyte and fluid management.
- Respiratory services may be consulted for oxygen management.
- Nutritional services may be consulted for food choices and potassium-rich foods.
- Cardiology may be consulted for dysrhythmias.

CLIENT EDUCATION

- Educate the client regarding potassium-rich foods to consume.
- Teach the client ways to prevent a decrease in potassium by excessive use of diuretics and laxatives.

COMPLICATIONS

Respiratory failure

NURSING ACTIONS
- Maintain an open airway, and monitor vital signs.
- Monitor level of consciousness.
- Monitor for hypoxemia and hypercapnia.
- Assist with intubation and mechanical ventilation if indicated.

Cardiac arrest

NURSING ACTIONS
- Perform continuous cardiac monitoring.
- Treat dysrhythmias.

Hyperkalemia

Hyperkalemia is the result of an increased intake of potassium, movement of potassium out of the cells, or inadequate kidney excretion resulting in a serum potassium level greater than 5.0 mEq/L.
- Increased risk of cardiac arrest
- Rare in clients who have normal kidney function

ASSESSMENT

RISK FACTORS

Clients who are chronically ill

Actual potassium excess
- Older adult clients due to decreases in renin and aldosterone, and increased use of salt substitutes, ACE inhibitors, and potassium-sparing diuretics Ⓖ

Relative potassium excess
- Extracellular shift caused from decreased insulin production, acidosis (diabetic ketoacidosis), tissue damage (sepsis, trauma, surgery, fever, myocardial infarction), hyperuricemia

EXPECTED FINDINGS

Vital signs: Slow irregular pulse, hypotension

Neuromusculoskeletal: Restlessness, irritability, weakness to the point of ascending flaccid paralysis, paresthesia

ECG: Premature ventricular contractions, ventricular fibrillation, peaked T waves, widened QRS

Gastrointestinal: Increased motility, diarrhea, hyperactive bowel sounds

Other signs: Oliguria

LABORATORY TESTS

Serum potassium: Increased to greater than 5.0 mEq/L

Hemoglobin and hematocrit
- Increased with dehydration
- Decreased with kidney failure

BUN and creatinine: Increased with kidney failure

Arterial blood gases: Metabolic acidosis (pH less than 7.35) with kidney failure

DIAGNOSTIC PROCEDURES

Electrocardiogram: Will show dysrhythmias (ventricular fibrillation, peaked T waves, widened QRS)

PATIENT-CENTERED CARE

NURSING CARE

Priority nursing care is to prevent falls, assessing for cardiac complications, and health teaching.

- Avoid administering "aged" blood in clients who have impaired kidney function because the deterioration of red blood cells releases potassium into the stored blood.
- Report abnormal findings to the provider.
- Monitor I&O.
- Assess for muscle weakness.
- Observe for GI manifestations, such as nausea and intestinal colic.
- Report abnormal findings in lab work, such as BUN, creatinine, glucose, and arterial blood gases.
- Encourage the client to avoid foods high in potassium, such as citrus fruits, legumes, whole-grain foods, lean meat, milk, eggs, coffee, tea, cocoa, and some cola beverages high in potassium. Encourage the client to read food labels for potassium content.
- Foods with less potassium include, butter, margarine, cranberry juice, ginger ale, hard candy, root beer, sugar, and honey.
- Clients who have impaired kidney function and are taking potassium-conserving diuretics should not receive potassium replacement or salt substitutes.
- For clients who have elevated potassium levels, report and stop IV infusion of potassium, maintain IV access, stop all potassium supplements, and promote a potassium-restricted diet.
- The client may receive furosemide to promote potassium excretion.
- A combination of glucose and insulin administration may be prescribed to promote reduction of potassium levels. This promotes uptake of potassium by the cells, which in turns decreases the extracellular content of potassium.
- Kayexalate (oral or rectal) may be prescribed to promote intestinal potassium excretion.
- Promote movement of potassium from ECF to ICF.
  - Administer IV fluids with dextrose and regular insulin.
  - Administer sodium bicarbonate to reverse acidosis.
- Monitor cardiac rhythm, and intervene promptly as needed.

MEDICATIONS

To increase potassium excretion

Loop diuretics (furosemide)

- Administer if kidney function is adequate.
- Loop diuretics increase the depletion of potassium from the renal system.

NURSING CONSIDERATIONS: Maintain IV access.

CLIENT EDUCATION

- Educate the client on a potassium-restricted diet.
- Instruct the client to withhold oral potassium supplements until further advised by the provider.

Cation exchange resins

Sodium polystyrene sulfonate works as a laxative and excretes excess potassium from the body.

NURSING CONSIDERATIONS: If potassium levels are extremely high, dialysis can be required.

CLIENT EDUCATION

- Educate the client on a potassium-restricted diet.
- Instruct the client to hold oral potassium supplements until advised by the provider.

INTERPROFESSIONAL CARE

- Nephrology may be consulted if dialysis is needed and for electrolyte and fluid management.
- Nutritional services may be consulted for food choices containing potassium-restricted foods.
- Cardiology may be consulted for dysrhythmias.

CLIENT EDUCATION

- Educate the client about potassium-restricted foods to consume.
- Teach the client ways to prevent an increase in potassium by reading food labels and avoiding salt substitutes containing potassium.

COMPLICATIONS

Cardiac arrest

NURSING ACTIONS
- Treat dysrhythmias.
- Perform continuous cardiac monitoring.

Other electrolyte imbalances

CALCIUM: Hypocalcemia, hypercalcemia

CHLORIDE: Hypochloremia. hyperchloremia

MAGNESIUM: Hypomagnesemia, hypermagnesemia

PHOSPHORUS: Hypophosphatemia, hyperphosphatemia

In particular, nurses should be aware of the implications of hypocalcemia and hypomagnesemia.

Hypocalcemia

Hypocalcemia is a total serum calcium less than 9.0 mg/dL.

ASSESSMENT QPCC

RISK FACTORS

- Lactose intolerance
- Malabsorption syndromes (Crohn's disease)
- End-stage kidney disease (ESKD)
- Thyroidectomy
- Hypoparathyroidism
- Inadequate intake of calcium
- Vitamin D deficiency (increasingly common) or lack of 25-hydroxy vitamin D related to ESKD
- Pancreatitis
- Hyperphosphatemia
- Medications that can predispose clients to hypocalcemia include antacids that contain aluminum, caffeine, cisplatin, corticosteroids, mithramycin, phosphates, and loop diuretics.

EXPECTED FINDINGS

Tetany is the most common manifestation seen in clients in a hypocalcemic state. It is caused by neural excitability-spontaneous discharges from both the sensory and motor fibers (peripheral nerves).
- Paresthesia of the fingers and lips (early manifestation)
- Muscle twitches as hypocalcemia progresses
- Seizure due to irritability of the central nervous system
- Frequent, painful muscle spasms at rest in the foot or calf (Charley horses)
- Hyperactive DTRs
- Positive Chvostek's sign (tapping on the facial nerve triggering facial twitching)
- Positive Trousseau's sign (hand/finger spasms with sustained blood pressure cuff inflation)
- History of thyroid surgery or irradiation of the upper chest or neck, which places a client at risk for developing hypocalcemia

CARDIOVASCULAR: Prolonged QT interval as a result of a prolonged ST segment. Risk of torsades de pointes. Decreased myocardial contractility (decreased heart rate and hypotension when hypocalcemia is severe).

GASTROINTESTINAL: Hyperactive bowel sounds, diarrhea, and abdominal cramps

LABORATORY TESTS

Calcium level less than 9.0 mg/dL

DIAGNOSTIC PROCEDURES

Electrocardiogram changes: Prolonged QT and ST interval

PATIENT-CENTERED CARE

NURSING CARE

- Administer oral or IV calcium supplements. Vitamin D supplements enhance the absorption of calcium.
- Implement seizure precautions.
- Avoid overstimulation. Keep the client's room quiet, limit visitors, and use soft lighting in the room.
- Have emergency equipment on standby.
- Encourage foods high in calcium, including dairy products, canned salmon, sardines, fresh oysters, and dark leafy green vegetables.
- The client can require administration of calcium gluconate or calcium chloride (not used as often due to risk of tissue damage if infiltrated). IV administration should be diluted in dextrose 5% and water and given as a bolus infusion (using an infusion pump). If administered too quickly, cardiac arrest could occur.

INTERPROFESSIONAL CARE

- Endocrinology may be consulted for electrolyte and fluid management.
- Respiratory services may be consulted for oxygen management.
- Nutritional services may be consulted for food choices high in calcium.
- Cardiology may be consulted for dysrhythmias.

CLIENT EDUCATION

- Educate the client about consuming foods high in calcium (yogurt, milk).
- Teach the client ways to increase calcium in diet by reading food labels.

Hypomagnesemia

Hypomagnesemia is a serum magnesium level less than 1.3 mg/dL.

ASSESSMENT

RISK FACTORS

Can be seen in Celiac disease or Crohn's disease
- Malnutrition (insufficient magnesium intake)
- Ethanol ingestion (magnesium excretion)
- Diarrhea
- Citrate from blood products
- Steatorrhea

EXPECTED FINDINGS

Possible depressed mood, apathy, or agitation.

Neuromuscular: Increased nerve impulse transmission (hyperactive DTRs, paresthesias, muscle tetany, seizures), positive Chvostek's and Trousseau's signs

Gastrointestinal: Hypoactive bowel sounds, constipation, abdominal distention, paralytic ileus

PATIENT-CENTERED CARE

NURSING CARE

- Discontinue magnesium-depleting medications (e.g., loop diuretics, osmotic diuretics, aminoglycoside antibiotics, and medications that contain phosphorus).
- Administer oral or IV magnesium sulfate following safety protocols. IV route is used because IM can cause pain and tissue damage. Oral magnesium can cause diarrhea and increase magnesium depletion. Monitor DTRs hourly during administration of magnesium sulfate.
- IV magnesium sulfate is given via an infusion pump not to exceed 150 mg/min, or 67 mEq over an 8-hr period.
- Encourage foods high in magnesium, including dark green vegetables, nuts, whole grains, seafood, peanut butter, and cocoa. If there is mild hypomagnesemia, dietary changes may be used to correct it.
- Clients receiving digitalis should be monitored closely if magnesium is low because it predisposes the client to digitalis toxicity.

INTERPROFESSIONAL CARE

- Endocrinology may be consulted for electrolyte and fluid management.
- Respiratory services may be consulted for oxygen management.
- Nutritional services may be consulted for food choices high in magnesium.
- Cardiology may be consulted for dysrhythmias.

CLIENT EDUCATION

- Educate the client regarding foods that are high in magnesium.
- Teach the client ways to increase magnesium in diet by reading food labels.

Application Exercises

1. A nurse is caring for a client who has a serum sodium level 133 mEq/L and serum potassium level 3.4 mEq/L. The nurse should recognize that which of the following treatments can result in these laboratory findings?

   A. Three tap water enemas

   B. 0.9% sodium chloride solution IV at 50 mL/hr

   C. 5% dextrose with 0.45% sodium chloride solution with 20 mEq of K⁺ IV at 80 mL/hr

   D. Antibiotic therapy

2. A nurse is caring for a client who has a serum potassium 5.4 mEq/L. The nurse should assess for which of the following manifestations?

   A. ECG changes

   B. Constipation

   C. Polyuria

   D. Paresthesia

3. A nurse is caring for a client who has a nasogastric tube attached to low intermittent suctioning. The nurse should monitor for which of the following electrolyte imbalances?

   A. Hypercalcemia

   B. Hyponatremia

   C. Hyperphosphatemia

   D. Hyperkalemia

4. A nurse is assessing a client who has hyperkalemia. The nurse should identify which of the following conditions as being associated with this electrolyte imbalance?

   A. Diabetic ketoacidosis

   B. Heart failure

   C. Cushing's syndrome

   D. Thyroidectomy

5. A nurse is assessing a client for Chvostek's sign. Which of the following techniques should the nurse use to perform this test?

   A. Apply a blood pressure cuff to the client's arm.

   B. Place the stethoscope bell over the client's carotid artery.

   C. Tap lightly on the client's cheek.

   D. Ask the client to lower her chin to her chest.

PRACTICE Active Learning Scenario

A nurse is caring for a client who has hypokalemia. Use the ATI Active Learning Template: System Disorder to complete this item.

ALTERATION IN HEALTH (DIAGNOSIS)

NURSING CARE: Describe at least six actions.

INTERPROFESSIONAL CARE: Describe one action.

CLIENT EDUCATION: Describe one teaching point.

COMPLICATIONS: Describe one.

Application Exercises Key

1. A. **CORRECT:** Three tap water enemas can result in a decrease in serum sodium and potassium. Tap water is hypotonic, and gastrointestinal losses are isotonic. This creates an imbalance and solute dilution.

   B. 0.9% sodium chloride is an isotonic solution and will not produce these results.

   C. 5% dextrose with 0.45% sodium chloride is an isotonic solution with 20 mEq of K^+ at 80 mL/hr and would not produce these results.

   D. Antibiotic therapy would not produce these results.

   Ⓝ *NCLEX® Connection: Physiological Adaptation, Fluid and Electrolyte Imbalances*

2. A. **CORRECT:** The nurse should assess for ECG changes. Potassium levels can affect the heart and result in arrhythmias.

   B. Constipation is a manifestation of hypokalemia.

   C. Polyuria is a manifestation of hypokalemia.

   D. Paresthesia is a manifestation of hypokalemia.

   Ⓝ *NCLEX® Connection: Physiological Adaptation, Fluid and Electrolyte Imbalances*

3. A. An increase in calcium is not indicated with nasogastric losses due to suctioning.

   B. **CORRECT:** The nurse should monitor the client for hyponatremia. Nasogastric losses are isotonic and contain sodium.

   C. An increase in phosphatemia is not indicated with nasogastric losses due to suctioning.

   D. A decrease in potassium can occur from nasogastric losses due to suctioning.

   Ⓝ *NCLEX® Connection: Physiological Adaptation, Fluid and Electrolyte Imbalances*

4. A. **CORRECT:** Hyperkalemia, an increase in serum potassium, is a laboratory finding associated with diabetic ketoacidosis.

   B. Hyponatremia, a decrease in serum sodium, is a laboratory finding associated with heart failure.

   C. Hypernatremia, an increase in serum sodium, is a laboratory finding associated with Cushing's syndrome.

   D. Hypocalcemia, a decrease in serum calcium, is a laboratory finding is found in clients following a thyroidectomy.

   Ⓝ *NCLEX® Connection: Physiological Adaptation, Fluid and Electrolyte Imbalances*

5. A. Applying a blood pressure cuff to the client's arm is performed to assess for Trousseau's sign.

   B. Placing the stethoscope bell over the client's carotid artery is performed to auscultate a carotid bruit.

   C. **CORRECT:** The nurse taps the client's cheek over the facial nerve just below and anterior to the ear to elicit Chvostek's sign. A positive response is indicated when the client exhibits facial twitching on this side of her face.

   D. Asking the client to lower her chin to her chest is performed to assess for range of motion of the neck.

   Ⓝ *NCLEX® Connection: Reduction of Risk Potential, Diagnostic Tests*

PRACTICE Answer

Using the ATI Active Learning Template: System Disorder

ALTERATION IN HEALTH (DIAGNOSIS): Hypokalemia is the result of an increased loss of potassium from the body or movement of potassium into the cells, resulting in a serum potassium less than 3.5 mEq/L.

NURSING CARE
- Report abnormal findings to the provider.
- Replacement of potassium
  - Encourage foods high in potassium (avocados, broccoli, dairy products, dried fruit, cantaloupe, bananas, juices, melon, lean meats, milk, whole grains, and citrus fruits).
  - Provide oral potassium supplementation.
- IV potassium supplementation
  - Never administer by IV push (high risk of cardiac arrest).
  - The maximum recommended rate is 10 mEq/hr.
  - Assess for phlebitis (tissue irritant).
- Potassium must never be given by IM or subcutaneous route, which can cause necrosis of the tissues.
- Monitor and maintain adequate urine output.
- Observe for shallow ineffective respirations and diminished breath sounds.
- Monitor cardiac rhythm, and intervene promptly as needed.
- Monitor clients receiving digoxin. Hypokalemia increases the risk for digoxin toxicity.
- Monitor level of consciousness, and maintain client safety.
- Monitor bowel sounds and abdominal distention, and intervene as needed.
- Monitor oxygen saturation levels, which should remain greater than 95%.
- Assess hand grasps for muscle weakness.
- Assess deep-tendon reflexes.

INTERPROFESSIONAL CARE
- Nephrology may be consulted for electrolyte and fluid management.
- Respiratory services may be consulted for oxygen management.
- Nutritional services may be consulted for food choices and potassium-rich foods.
- Cardiology may be consulted for dysrhythmias.

CLIENT EDUCATION
- Educate the client regarding potassium-rich foods to consume.
- Teach the client ways to prevent a decrease in potassium by excessive use of diuretics and laxatives.

COMPLICATIONS
- Respiratory failure
- Cardiac arrest

Ⓝ *NCLEX® Connection: Physiological Adaptation, Fluid and Electrolyte Imbalances*

UNIT 6 NURSING CARE OF CLIENTS WHO HAVE FLUID/ ELECTROLYTE/ACID-BASE IMBALANCES

CHAPTER 45 *Acid-Base Imbalances*

For cells to function optimally, metabolic processes must maintain a steady balance between the acids and bases found in the body. Acid-base balance represents homeostasis of hydrogen (H⁺) ion concentration in body fluids. Hydrogen shifts between the extracellular and intracellular compartments to compensate for acid-base imbalances. Minor changes in hydrogen concentration have major effects on normal cellular function.

Arterial pH is an indirect measurement of hydrogen ion concentration and is a result of respiratory and kidney compensation function. Arterial blood gases (ABGs) are most commonly used to evaluate acid-base balance. The pH is the expression of the balance between carbon dioxide (CO_2), which is regulated by the lungs, and bicarbonate (HCO_3^-), a base regulated by the kidneys. The greater the concentration of hydrogen, the more acidic the body fluids and the lower the pH. The lower the concentration of hydrogen, the more alkaline the body fluids and the higher the pH.

MAINTENANCE OF ACID-BASE BALANCE

Acid–base balance is maintained by chemical, respiratory, and kidney function.

Chemical (bicarbonate and intracellular fluid) and protein buffers (albumin and globulins)
- First line of defense
- Either bind or release hydrogen ions as needed
- Respond quickly to changes in pH

Respiratory buffers
- Second line of defense
- Control the level of hydrogen ions in the blood through the control of CO_2 levels
- When a chemoreceptor senses a change in the level of CO_2, a signal is sent to the brain to alter the rate and depth of respirations.
  - Hyperventilation: Decrease in hydrogen ions (helps to blow of excess hydrogen ions)
  - Hypoventilation: Increase in hydrogen ions

Kidney buffers
- Kidneys are the third line of defense.
- This buffering system is much slower to respond, but it is the most effective buffering system with the longest duration.
- Kidneys control the movement of bicarbonate in the urine. Bicarbonate can be reabsorbed into the bloodstream or excreted in the urine in response to blood levels of hydrogen.
- Kidneys can also produce more bicarbonate when needed.
  - High hydrogen ions: Bicarbonate reabsorption and production
  - Low hydrogen ions: Bicarbonate excretion

COMPENSATION

Compensation refers to the process by which the body attempts to correct changes and imbalances in pH levels.
- Full compensation occurs when the pH level of the blood returns to normal (7.35 to 7.45).
- If the pH level is not able to normalize, it is referred to as partial compensation.

45.1 Insufficient compensation

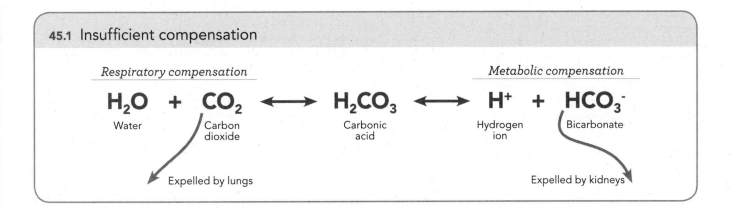

$$H_2O \ + \ CO_2 \ \longleftrightarrow \ H_2CO_3 \ \longleftrightarrow \ H^+ \ + \ HCO_3^-$$

Respiratory compensation — Water, Carbon dioxide, Carbonic acid (Expelled by lungs)

Metabolic compensation — Hydrogen ion, Bicarbonate (Expelled by kidneys)

EXAMPLES

- Metabolic alkalosis, metabolic acidosis, respiratory alkalosis, and respiratory acidosis are examples of acid-base imbalances.
- Acid-base imbalances are a result of insufficient compensation. Respiratory and kidney function play a large role in the body's ability to effectively compensate for acid-base alterations. Organ dysfunction negatively affects acid-base compensation. **(45.1)**

HEALTH PROMOTION AND DISEASE PREVENTION

- Encourage a healthy diet and physical activity.
- Limit the consumption of alcohol.
- Encourage drinking six to eight cups of water daily.
- Maintain an appropriate weight for height and body frame.
- Promote smoking cessation.

ASSESSMENT

RISK FACTORS

Respiratory acidosis: Hypoventilation

RESULTS FROM
- Respiratory depression from opioids, poisons, anesthetics
- Clients who have brain tumors, cerebral aneurysm, stroke or overhydration, trauma, or neurological diseases (myasthenia gravis, Guillain-Barré when respiratory effort is affected)
- Inadequate chest expansion due to muscle weakness, pneumothorax/hemothorax, flail chest, obesity, sleep apnea, tumors, or deformities
- Airway obstruction that occurs in from neck edema, or localized lymph node enlargement, foreign bodies or mucus
- Alveolar-capillary blockage secondary to a pulmonary embolus, thrombus, acute respiratory distress syndrome, chest trauma, drowning, or pulmonary edema
- Inadequate mechanical ventilation

RESULTS IN
- Increased CO_2
- Increased or normal H^+ concentration

MANIFESTATIONS
- **Vital signs:** Initial tachycardia and hypertension; bradycardia and hypotension develop as acidosis worsens
- **Dysrhythmias:** Ventricular fibrillation can be the first indication in a client receiving anesthesia.
- **Neurological:** Initial anxiety, irritability, and confusion; lethargy and possibly coma develop as acidosis worsens
- **Respiratory:** Ineffective, shallow, rapid breathing
- **Skin:** Pale or cyanotic
- Chronic respiratory acidosis can be seen in clients who have pulmonary disease, sleep apnea, and obesity.

NURSING CARE: Oxygen therapy, maintain patent airway, and enhance gas exchange (positioning and breathing techniques, ventilatory support, bronchodilators, mucolytics).

Respiratory alkalosis: Hyperventilation

RESULTS FROM
- Hyperventilation due to fear, anxiety, intracerebral trauma, salicylate toxicity, or excessive mechanical ventilation.
- Hypoxemia from asphyxiation, high altitudes, shock, or early-stage asthma or pneumonia.

RESULTS IN
- Decreased CO_2
- Decreased or normal H^+ concentration

MANIFESTATIONS
- **Vital signs:** Tachypnea
- **Neurological:** Inability to concentrate, numbness, tingling, tinnitus, and possible loss of consciousness
- **Cardiovascular:** Tachycardia, ventricular, and atrial dysrhythmias
- **Respiratory:** Rapid, deep respirations

NURSING CARE: Oxygen therapy, anxiety reduction interventions, and rebreathing techniques

Metabolic acidosis

RESULTS FROM
- Excess production of hydrogen ions
- Diabetic ketoacidosis (DKA)
- Starvation
- Lactic acidosis can result from:
  - Heavy exercise
  - Seizure activity
  - Hypoxia
- Excessive intake of acids
  - Ethyl alcohol
  - Methyl alcohol
  - Acetylsalicylic acid (aspirin)
- Inadequate elimination of hydrogen ions
  - Kidney failure
  - Severe lung problems
- Inadequate production of bicarbonate
  - Kidney failure
  - Pancreatitis
- Impaired liver or pancreatic function: Liver failure
- Excess elimination of bicarbonate: Diarrhea

RESULTS IN
- Decreased HCO_3^-
- Increased H^+ concentration

MANIFESTATIONS
- Dysrhythmias
- **Vital signs:** Bradycardia, weak peripheral pulses, hypotension, tachypnea
- **Neurological:** Headache, drowsiness, confusion
- **Respiratory:** Rapid, deep respirations (Kussmaul respirations)
- **Skin:** Warm, dry, pink

NURSING CARE: Varies with causes. If DKA, administer insulin. If related to GI losses, administer antidiarrheals and provide rehydration. If serum bicarbonate is low, administer sodium bicarbonate 1 mEq/kg.

Metabolic alkalosis

RESULTS FROM
- Base excess
- Oral ingestion of excess amount of bases (antacids)
- Venous administration of bases (blood transfusions, total parenteral nutrition, or sodium bicarbonate)
- Acid deficit
  - Loss of gastric secretions (through prolonged vomiting, nasogastric suction)
  - Potassium depletion (due to thiazide diuretics, laxative overuse, Cushing's syndrome, hyperaldosteronism)
- Increased digitalis toxicity

RESULTS IN
- Increased HCO_3^-
- Decreased H^+ concentration

MANIFESTATIONS
- **Vital signs:** Tachycardia, normotensive or hypotensive
- **Dysrhythmias:** Atrial tachycardia, ventricular issues when pH increases
- **Neurological:** Numbness, tingling, tetany, muscle weakness, hyperreflexia, confusion, convulsion
- **Respiratory:** Depressed skeletal muscles resulting in ineffective breathing

NURSING CARE: Varies with causes (GI losses: administer antiemetics, fluids, and electrolyte replacements). If related to potassium depletion, discontinue causative agent.

DIAGNOSTIC PROCEDURES

To determine the type of imbalance, follow these steps. **(45.2)**

STEP 1: Look at pH.
- If less than 7.35, identify as acidosis.
- If greater than 7.45, identify as alkalosis. Q_{EBP}

STEP 2: Look at PaCO₂ and HCO₃⁻ simultaneously.
- Determine which is in the expected reference range.
- Conclude that the other is the indicator of imbalance.
- Identify $PaCO_2$ less than 35 or greater than 45 mm Hg as respiratory in origin.
- Identify HCO_3^- less than 22 or greater than 26 mEq/L as metabolic in origin.

STEP 3: Combine diagnoses of Steps 1 and 2 to name the type of imbalance.

STEP 4: Evaluate the PaO₂ and SaO₂. If the results are less than the expected reference range, the client is hypoxic.

STEP 5: Determine compensation as follows.
- **Uncompensated:** The pH is outside the expected reference range, and either the HCO_3^- or the $PaCO_2$ is outside the expected reference range.
- **Partially compensated:** The pH, HCO_3^-, and $PaCO_2$ are outside the expected reference range.
- **Fully compensated:** The pH is within the expected reference range, but the $PaCO_2$ and HCO_3^- are both outside the expected reference range. Looking at the pH will provide a clue as to which system initiated the problem, respiratory or metabolic. If the pH is less than 7.40, think "acidosis," and determine which system has the acidosis value. If the pH is greater than 7.40, think "alkalosis," and determine which system has the alkalosis value.

PATIENT-CENTERED CARE

NURSING CARE

For all acid-base imbalances, it is imperative to treat the underlying cause.

INTERPROFESSIONAL CARE

- Respiratory services can be consulted for oxygen therapy, breathing treatments, and ABGs.
- Pulmonology services can be consulted for respiratory management.

CLIENT EDUCATION

- Education can vary in relation to the client's condition.
- Encourage adherence to the prescribed diet and dialysis regimen for clients who have kidney dysfunction.
- Encourage the client to weigh daily and notify the provider if there is a 1- to 2-lb (0.5 to 0.9 kg) gain in 24 hr or a 3-lb (1.4 kg) gain in 1 week.
- Promote smoking cessation if the client is a smoker.
- Teach the client to take medication as prescribed. Encourage adherence to the medication regimen for clients who have COPD.
- Set up referral services (home oxygen).

COMPLICATIONS

Convulsions, coma, and respiratory arrest

NURSING ACTIONS
- Implement seizure precautions, and perform management interventions if necessary.
- Provide life-support interventions if necessary.

45.2 Types of results

The following are the five classic types of ABG results demonstrating balance and imbalance.

Step 1: Look at pH	Step 2: Determine which is in the normal range		Step 3: Combine names
pH	PACO₂	HCO₃⁻	DIAGNOSIS
7.35 to 7.45	35 to 45	21 to 28	Homeostasis
Less than 7.35	Greater than 45	22 to 26	Respiratory acidosis
Less than 7.35	35 to 45	Less than 22	Metabolic acidosis
Greater than 7.45	Less than 35	22 to 26	Respiratory alkalosis
Greater than 7.45	35 to 45	Greater than 26	Metabolic alkalosis

Application Exercises

1. A nurse is caring for a client admitted with confusion and lethargy. The client was found at home unresponsive with an empty bottle of aspirin lying next to her bed. Vital signs reveal blood pressure 104/72 mm Hg, heart rate 116/min with regular rhythm, and respiratory rate 42/min and deep. Which of the following arterial blood gas findings should the nurse expect?

   A. pH 7.68
   PaO_2 96 mm Hg
   $PaCO_2$ 38 mm Hg
   HCO_3^- 28 mEq/L

   B. pH 7.48
   PaO_2 100 mm Hg
   $PaCO_2$ 28 mm Hg
   HCO_3^- 23 mEq/L

   C. pH 6.98
   PaO_2 100 mm Hg
   $PaCO_2$ 30 mm Hg
   HCO_3^- 18 mEq/L

   D. pH 7.58
   PaO_2 96 mm Hg
   $PaCO_2$ 38 mm Hg
   HCO_3^- 29 mEq/L

2. A nurse is caring for a client who was in a motor-vehicle accident. The client reports chest pain and difficulty breathing. A chest x-ray reveals the client has a pneumothorax. Which of the following arterial blood gas findings should the nurse expect?

   A. pH 7.06
   PaO_2 86 mm Hg
   $PaCO_2$ 52 mm Hg
   HCO_3^- 24 mEq/L

   B. pH 7.42
   PaO_2 100 mm Hg
   $PaCO_2$ 38 mm Hg
   HCO_3^- 23 mEq/L

   C. pH 6.98
   PaO_2 100 mm Hg
   $PaCO_2$ 30 mm Hg
   HCO_3^- 18 mEq/L

   D. pH 7.58
   PaO_2 96 mm Hg
   $PaCO_2$ 38 mm Hg
   HCO_3^- 29 mEq/L

3. A nurse is obtaining arterial blood gases for a client who has vomited for 24 hr. The nurse should expect which of the following acid-base imbalances to result from vomiting for 24 hr?

   A. Respiratory acidosis

   B. Respiratory alkalosis

   C. Metabolic acidosis

   D. Metabolic alkalosis

4. A charge nurse is teaching a group of nurses about conditions related to metabolic acidosis. Which of the following statements by a unit nurse indicates the teaching has been effective?

   A. "Metabolic acidosis can occur due to diabetic ketoacidosis."

   B. "Metabolic acidosis can occur in a client who has myasthenia gravis."

   C. "Metabolic acidosis can occur in a client who has asthma."

   D. "Metabolic acidosis can occur due to cancer."

5. A nurse is assessing a client who has pancreatitis. The client's arterial blood gases reveal metabolic acidosis. Which of the following are expected findings? (Select all that apply.)

   A. Tachycardia

   B. Hypertension

   C. Bounding pulses

   D. Hyperreflexia

   E. Dysrhythmia

   F. Tachypnea

PRACTICE Active Learning Scenario

A nurse is caring for a client who has liver cancer. The client's arterial blood gases reveal metabolic acidosis. Use the ATI Active Learning Template: System Disorder to complete this item.

RISK FACTORS: Include three conditions related to metabolic acidosis.

NURSING CARE: Include two nursing actions.

COMPLICATIONS: Identify one.

Application Exercises Key

1. A. These arterial blood gases indicate metabolic alkalosis.

    B. These arterial blood gases indicate respiratory alkalosis.

    C. **CORRECT:** An aspirin overdose would result in arterial blood gas findings of metabolic acidosis.

    D. These arterial blood gases indicate metabolic alkalosis.

    Ⓝ *NCLEX® Connection: Reduction of Risk Potential, Laboratory Values*

2. A. **CORRECT:** A pneumothorax can cause alveolar hypoventilation and increased carbon dioxide levels, resulting in a state of respiratory acidosis.

    B. These ABGs are within the expected reference range and reflect homeostasis.

    C. Metabolic acidosis is not indicated for this client.

    D. Metabolic alkalosis is not indicated for this client.

    Ⓝ *NCLEX® Connection: Reduction of Risk Potential, Laboratory Values*

3. A. Respiratory acidosis is not indicated for this client.

    B. Respiratory alkalosis is not indicated for this client.

    C. Metabolic acidosis is not indicated for this client.

    D. **CORRECT:** Excessive vomiting causes a loss of gastric acids and an accumulation of bicarbonate in the blood, resulting in metabolic alkalosis.

    Ⓝ *NCLEX® Connection: Physiological Adaptation, Fluid and Electrolyte Imbalances*

4. A. **CORRECT:** Metabolic acidosis results from an excess production of hydrogen ions, which occurs in diabetic ketoacidosis.

    B. Respiratory acidosis can occur in a client who has myasthenia gravis.

    C. Respiratory acidosis can occur in a client who has asthma.

    D. Respiratory acidosis can occur due to cancer.

    Ⓝ *NCLEX® Connection: Physiological Adaptation, Fluid and Electrolyte Imbalances*

5. A. Tachycardia is an expected finding for a client who has respiratory acidosis or metabolic alkalosis.

    B. Hypertension is an expected finding of respiratory acidosis.

    C. Bounding pulses is an expected finding for respiratory acidosis due to hypertension.

    D. Hyperreflexia is an expected finding for a client who has metabolic alkalosis.

    E. **CORRECT:** Dysrhythmia is an expected finding in a client who has pancreatitis and metabolic acidosis.

    F. **CORRECT:** Tachypnea is an expected finding in a client who has pancreatitis and metabolic acidosis.

    Ⓝ *NCLEX® Connection: Physiological Adaptation, Illness Management*

PRACTICE Answer

Using ATI Active Learning Template: System Disorder

RISK FACTORS

Metabolic acidosis results from:
- Excess production of hydrogen ions
- Diabetic ketoacidosis (DKA)
- Starvation

Lactic acidosis can result from:
- Heavy exercise
- Seizure activity
- Hypoxia
- Excessive intake of acids such as the following:
  - Ethyl alcohol
  - Methyl alcohol
  - Acetylsalicylic acid (aspirin)
- Inadequate elimination of hydrogen ions
  - Kidney failure
  - Severe lung problems
- Inadequate production of bicarbonate
  - Kidney failure
  - Pancreatitis
  - Impaired liver or pancreatic function
  - Liver failure
- Excess elimination of bicarbonate (diarrhea)

Metabolic acidosis results in:
- Decreased HCO_3^-
- Increased H^+ concentration

NURSING CARE: Varies with causes. If DKA, administer insulin. If related to GI losses, administer antidiarrheals and provide rehydration. If serum bicarbonate is low, administer sodium bicarbonate 1 mEq/kg.

COMPLICATIONS: Convulsions, coma, and respiratory arrest

Nursing Actions
- Implement seizure precautions, and perform management interventions if necessary.
- Provide life-support interventions if necessary.

Ⓝ *NCLEX® Connection: Physiological Adaptation, Fluid and Electrolyte Imbalances*

When reviewing the following chapters, keep in mind the relevant topics and tasks of the NCLEX outline, in particular:

Client Needs: Basic Care and Comfort

ELIMINATION: Assess and manage the client with an alteration in elimination.

NUTRITION AND ORAL HYDRATION: Provide/maintain special diets based on client diagnosis/nutritional needs and cultural considerations.

Client Needs: Pharmacological and Parenteral Therapies

BLOOD AND BLOOD PRODUCTS: Document necessary information on the administration of red blood cells/blood products.

PHARMACOLOGICAL PAIN MANAGEMENT: Assess client need for administration of a PRN pain medication.

TOTAL PARENTERAL NUTRITION: Administer parenteral nutrition and evaluate client response.

Client Needs: Reduction of Risk Potential

DIAGNOSTIC TESTS: Perform diagnostic testing.

POTENTIAL FOR COMPLICATIONS OF DIAGNOSTIC TESTS/TREATMENTS/PROCEDURES
Maintain tube patency.

Intervene to prevent aspiration.

THERAPEUTIC PROCEDURES: Manage client during and/or following a procedure with moderate sedation.

UNIT 7   **NURSING CARE OF CLIENTS WHO HAVE GASTROINTESTINAL DISORDERS**
SECTION: DIAGNOSTIC AND THERAPEUTIC PROCEDURES

CHAPTER 46 # Gastrointestinal Diagnostic Procedures

Gastrointestinal diagnostic procedures often involve endoscopes and x-rays to visualize parts of the gastrointestinal system and to evaluate gastrointestinal contents. Procedures include liver function tests, other blood tests, urine bilinogen, fecal occult blood test (FOBT), stool samples, endoscopy, and gastrointestinal (GI) series.

Liver function tests and other blood tests

- Liver function tests are aspartate aminotransferase (AST), alanine aminotransferase (ALT), alkaline phosphatase (ALP), bilirubin, and albumin.
- Other blood tests that provide information on the functioning of the GI system include amylase, lipase, alpha-fetoprotein, and ammonia.

INDICATIONS

Suspected liver, pancreatic, or biliary tract disorder

CONSIDERATIONS

PREPROCEDURE: Explain to the client how blood is obtained and what information this will provide.

POSTPROCEDURE: Inform the client when and how results are provided.

Urine bilirubin

Also known as urobilinogen, this is a urine test to determine the presence of bilirubin in the urine.

INDICATIONS

Suspected liver or biliary tract disorder

CONSIDERATIONS

PREPROCEDURE

NURSING ACTIONS: The test can be performed by using a dipstick (urine bilirubin) or a 24-hr urine collection (urobilinogen).

CLIENT EDUCATION: Teach the client how to collect urine and provide proper collection container.

POSTPROCEDURE

NURSING ACTIONS: Inform the client when and how results are provided.

INTERPRETATION OF FINDINGS

A positive or elevated finding indicates possible liver disorder (cirrhosis, hepatitis), biliary obstruction, hemolytic anemia, or pernicious anemia.

46.1 Blood tests: Interpretation of findings

BLOOD TEST	EXPECTED REFERENCE RANGE	INTERPRETATION OF FINDINGS
Aspartate aminotransferase	0 to 35 units/L	Elevation occurs with hepatitis or cirrhosis.
Alanine aminotransferase	4 to 36 units/L	
Alkaline phosphatase	30 to 120 units/L	Elevation indicates liver damage.
Amylase	30 to 220 units/L	Elevation occurs with pancreatitis.
Lipase	0 to 160 units/L	
Total bilirubin	0.3 to 1 mg/dL	Elevations indicate altered liver function, bile duct obstruction, or other hepatobiliary disorder.
Direct (conjugated) bilirubin	0.1 to 0.3 mg/dL	
Indirect (unconjugated) bilirubin	0.2 to 0.8 mg/dL	
Albumin	3.5 to 5 g/dL	Decrease can indicate hepatic disease.
Alpha-fetoprotein	Less than 40 mcg/L	Elevated in liver cancer, cirrhosis, hepatitis.
Ammonia	10 to 80 mcg/dL	Elevated in liver disease.

Fecal occult blood test and stool samples

A stool sample is collected and tested for blood, ova and parasites (*Giardia lamblia*), and bacteria (*Clostridium difficile*). Stool also can be collected to assess for DNA changes in the vimentin gene, which can predispose a client to cancer of the intestine.

INDICATIONS

CLIENT PRESENTATION
- GI bleeding
- Unexplained diarrhea

CONSIDERATIONS

PREPROCEDURE

NURSING ACTIONS
- **Occult blood:** Provide the client with cards impregnated with guaiac that can be mailed to provider or with a specimen collection cup. If the cards are used, three samples are usually required.
- **Stool for ova and parasites and bacteria:** Provide the client with a specimen collection cup.

CLIENT EDUCATION
- **Occult blood:** Instruct the client about proper collection technique. The client might also need to be instructed about medication restrictions (anticoagulants, NSAIDs) for 7 days before the testing starts, and dietary restrictions to follow (vitamin C rich foods, red meat, chicken, fish) prior to obtaining samples. Qpcc
- **Stool for ova and parasites and bacteria:** Instruct the client about proper collection technique (time frame for submission to laboratory, need for refrigeration).

POSTPROCEDURE

NURSING ACTIONS: Inform the client when and how the results are provided.

INTERPRETATION OF FINDINGS

- At least three repeats of a positive guaiac FOBT confirms GI bleeding.
- A positive finding for blood is indicative of GI bleeding (ulcer, colitis, cancer).

Stool samples

- A positive finding for ova and parasites is indicative of a GI parasitic infection.
- A positive finding for *Clostridium difficile* is indicative of this opportunistic infection, which usually becomes established secondary to use of broad-spectrum antibiotics.
- A change in the vimentin gene can be an indicator of colorectal cancer.

Endoscopy

- Endoscopic procedures allow direct visualization of body cavities, tissues, and organs through the use of a flexible, lighted tube (endoscope). They are performed for diagnostic and therapeutic purposes.
- Endoscopic procedures are performed in a variety of facilities. The provider can perform biopsies, remove abnormal tissue, and perform minor surgery, such as cauterizing a bleeding ulcer. A contrast medium can be injected to allow visualization of structures beyond the capabilities of the scope.

GASTROINTESTINAL SCOPE PROCEDURES
- Colonoscopy
- Esophagogastroduodenoscopy (EGD)
- Endoscopic retrograde cholangiopancreatography (ERCP)
- Small bowel capsule endoscopy (M2A)
- Sigmoidoscopy

INDICATIONS

POTENTIAL DIAGNOSES: GI bleeding, ulcerations, inflammation, polyps, malignant tumors

CLIENT PRESENTATION
- Anemia (secondary to bleeding)
- Abdominal discomfort
- Abdominal distention or mass

CONSIDERATIONS

General endoscopic procedures

PREPROCEDURE
- NURSING ACTIONS
  - Evaluate the client's understanding of the procedure.
  - Verify that a consent form has been signed.
  - Assess vital signs, and verify the client's allergies.
  - Evaluate baseline laboratory tests and report unexpected findings to the provider (CBC, electrolyte panel, BUN, creatinine, PT, aPTT, and liver function studies). Evaluate chest x-ray, ECG, and ABGs, as indicated.
  - Evaluate the client's medical history for increased risk of complications.
  - **Age** can influence the client's ability to understand the procedures, tolerance of the required positioning, and compliance with pretest preparation. ⓒ
  - **Current health status:** Consider conditions and medications that can affect the client's tolerance of and recovery from the procedure.
  - **Cognitive status:** Determine the client's understanding of the procedure and baseline mental status.
  - **Support system:** Determine whether a support person will assist the client after the procedure.
  - **Recent food or fluid intake:** Can affect the provider's ability to visualize key structures and increase the risk for complications (aspiration). Notify the provider if dietary restrictions were not followed.

- **Medications:** Some medications (NSAIDs, warfarin, aspirin) place the client at risk for complications. Notify the provider if medication restrictions were not followed.
- **Previous radiographic examinations:** Any recent radiographic examinations using barium can affect the provider's ability to view key structures. Notify the provider if contrast has been recently used.
- **Electrolyte and fluid status:** Imbalances secondary to repeated enemas can affect bowel preparation tolerance, especially in older adult clients.
- Ensure that the client followed proper bowel preparation (laxatives, enemas). Inadequate bowel preparation can result in cancellation and delays the examination. This can also lead to the client experiencing extended periods of being NPO or on a liquid diet.
- Ensure that the client is NPO for the prescribed period prior to the examination.
- CLIENT EDUCATION
  - Provide instructions regarding medication and food restrictions.
  - Provide prescriptions for medications used for the bowel prep.
  - Instruct the client about the number and type of enemas, if prescribed.

POSTPROCEDURE
- NURSING ACTIONS
  - Monitor vital signs.
  - Assess for complications.
- CLIENT EDUCATION: If a biopsy was performed, food restrictions may be prescribed. QPCC

Colonoscopy

Use of a flexible fiberoptic colonoscope, which enters through the anus, to visualize the rectum and the sigmoid, descending, transverse, and ascending colon

ANESTHESIA: **Moderate sedation:** Midazolam, an opiate such as fentanyl, and/or propofol are commonly used medications.

POSITIONING: Left side with knees to chest

PREPARATION
- Bowel prep
- Can include laxatives, such as bisacodyl and polyethylene glycol
- Polyethylene glycol is not recommended for older adult clients because it can cause fluid and electrolyte imbalances. Ⓖ
- Polyethylene glycol can inhibit the absorption of some medications. Review the client's medications and consult with the provider.
- Clear liquid diet (avoid red, purple, orange fluids). NPO after midnight.
- The client must avoid medications indicated by the provider, such as aspirin, anticoagulants, and antiplatelet medication.

POSTPROCEDURE
- Notify the provider of severe pain (possible perforation) or indication of hemorrhage.
- Monitor for rectal bleeding.
- Monitor vital signs and respiratory status. Maintain an open airway until the client is awake.
- Resume normal diet as prescribed.
- Encourage increased fluid intake.
- Instruct the client that there can be increased flatulence due to air instillation during the procedure.
- Instruct the client not to drive or use equipment for 12 to 18 hr after the procedure.

EGD

Insertion of endoscope through the mouth into the esophagus, stomach, and duodenum to identify or treat areas of bleeding, dilate an esophageal stricture, and diagnose gastric lesions or celiac disease

ANESTHESIA: **Moderate sedation per IV access:** Topical anesthetic to depress the gag reflex, atropine to decrease secretions

POSITIONING: Left side-lying with head of bed elevated

PREPARATION: NPO 6 to 8 hr. Remove dentures prior to procedure.

POSTPROCEDURE
- Monitor vital signs and respiratory status. Maintain an open airway until the client is awake.
- Notify the provider of bleeding, abdominal or chest pain, and any evidence of infection.
- Withhold fluids until return of gag reflex. Qs
- Discontinue IV fluid therapy when the client tolerates oral fluids without nausea and vomiting.
- Instruct the client not to drive or use equipment for 12 to 18 hr after the procedure.
- Teach the client to use throat lozenges if a sore throat or hoarse voice persists following the procedure.

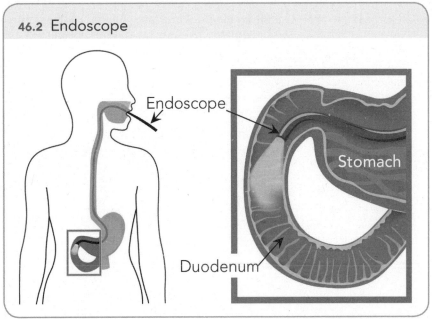

46.2 Endoscope

Endoscope

Stomach

Duodenum

ERCP

Insertion of an endoscope through the mouth into the biliary tree via the duodenum. Allows visualization of the biliary ducts, gall bladder, liver, and pancreas. X-rays are taken after a contrast medium is injected into the common duct.

ANESTHESIA: **Moderate sedation per IV access:** Topical anesthetic to depress the gag reflex, atropine to decrease secretions

POSITIONING: Initially semi-prone with repositioning throughout procedure

PREPARATION
- NPO 6 to 8 hr. Remove dentures prior to procedure.
- Explain the procedure and the need to change positions during the procedure.

POSTPROCEDURE
- Monitor vital signs and respiratory status. Maintain an open airway until the client is awake.
- Notify the provider of bleeding, abdominal or chest pain, and any evidence of infection.
- Withhold fluids until return of gag reflex.
- Discontinue IV fluid therapy when the client tolerates oral fluids without nausea and vomiting.
- Instruct the client not to drive or use equipment for 12 to 18 hr after the procedure.
- Teach the client to use throat lozenges if a sore throat or hoarse voice persists following the procedure.

M2A

Swallow the capsule with a glass of water for a video enteroscopy to visualize the entire small bowel over an 8-hr period. The capsule is not used to view the colon.

ANESTHESIA: None

POSITIONING: Return to normal activity during the study

PREPARATION
- Fast (water only) for 8 to 10 hr before the test and NPO for first 2 hr of the testing. Normal eating 4 hr after swallowing the capsule.
- The abdomen is marked for the location of the sensor. Eight-lead sensors are placed and connected to a data recorder, which captures images of the small intestines. Qℓ

POSTPROCEDURE
- After 8 hr, the client returns the recorder for downloading of the images.
- The client will evacuate the capsule in the stool.

Sigmoidoscopy

Scope is shorter than colonoscope, allowing visualization of the anus, rectum, and sigmoid colon to test for colon cancer, investigate for a GI bleed, diagnose or monitor inflammatory bowel disease.

ANESTHESIA: None required

POSITIONING: On left side

PREPARATION
- Bowel prep, which can include laxatives, such as bisacodyl, cleansing enema or sodium biphosphate enema
- Clear liquid diet at least 24 hr before the procedure
- NPO after midnight
- The client must avoid medications as indicated by the provider.

POSTPROCEDURE
- Monitor vital signs and respiratory status.
- Monitor for rectal bleeding.
- Resume normal diet as prescribed.
- Encourage increased fluid intake.
- Instruct the client that there can be increased flatulence due to air instillation during the procedure.

INTERPRETATION OF FINDINGS

Can indicate a need for medication or surgical removal of a lesion.

COMPLICATIONS

Oversedation

Use of moderate sedation places the client at risk for oversedation. Qs

MANIFESTATIONS: Difficult to arouse, poor respiratory effort, evidence of hypoxemia, tachycardia, and elevated or low blood pressure

NURSING ACTIONS
- Be prepared to administer antidotes for sedatives administered prior to and during the procedure.
- Administer oxygen, and monitor vital signs. Maintain an open airway until awake.
- Notify the provider immediately, and call for assistance.

CLIENT EDUCATION: Driving and major decision-making are restricted until the effects of the sedation have worn off. This varies with the type of agent used.

Hemorrhage

MANIFESTATIONS: Bleeding, cool and clammy skin, hypotension, tachycardia, dizziness, and tachypnea

NURSING ACTIONS
- Assess for hemorrhage from the site. Monitor vital signs.
- Monitor diagnostic test results (particularly Hgb and Hct).
- Notify the provider immediately.

CLIENT EDUCATION: Report fever, pain, and bleeding to the provider.

Aspiration

Using moderate sedation or topical anesthesia can affect the gag reflex.

MANIFESTATIONS: Dyspnea, tachypnea, adventitious breath sounds, tachycardia, and fever

NURSING ACTIONS
- Keep the client NPO until the gag reflex returns. Ensure that the client is awake and alert prior to consuming food or fluid. Encourage the client to deep breathe and cough to promote removal of secretions.
- Notify the provider if there is a delay in gag reflex return.

CLIENT EDUCATION: Report any respiratory congestion or compromise to the provider.

Perforation of the gastrointestinal tract

Manifestations include chest or abdominal pain, fever, nausea, vomiting, and abdominal distention.

NURSING ACTIONS: Monitor diagnostic tests for evidence of infection, including elevated WBC, and notify the provider of unexpected findings.

CLIENT EDUCATION: Report fever, pain, and bleeding to the provider.

Gastrointestinal series

GI studies are done with or without contrast and help define anatomic or functional abnormalities.
- These include radiographic imaging of the esophagus, stomach, and entire intestinal tract.
- Upper GI imaging is done by having the client drink a radiopaque liquid (barium). For small bowel follow-through, barium is traced through the small intestine to the ileocecal junction.
- A barium enema is done by instilling a radiopaque liquid into the rectum and colon.

INDICATIONS

POTENTIAL DIAGNOSES: Gastric ulcers, peristaltic disorders, tumors, varices, and intestinal enlargements or constrictions

CLIENT PRESENTATION: Abdominal pain, altered elimination habits (constipation, diarrhea), or GI bleeding

CONSIDERATIONS

PREPROCEDURE

NURSING CONSIDERATIONS
- Inform the client about medications, food and fluid restrictions (clear liquid and/or low residue diet, NPO after midnight), and avoiding smoking or chewing gum (increases peristalsis).
- Assess the client's understanding of bowel preparation (laxatives, enemas) so the image will not be distorted by feces.
- Barium enema studies must be scheduled prior to upper GI studies. Q EBP
- Assess for contraindications to bowel preparation (possible bowel perforation or obstruction, inflammatory disease).

CLIENT EDUCATION
- Tell the client to restrict food and fluids for bowel preparation.
- Inform the client that if the small intestine is to be visualized, additional radiographs will be done over the next 24 hr.

POSTPROCEDURE

NURSING ACTIONS
- Monitor elimination of contrast material, and administer a laxative if prescribed.
- Increase fluid intake to promote elimination of contrast material.

CLIENT EDUCATION
- Instruct the client to monitor elimination of contrast material and to report retention of contrast material (constipation) or diarrhea accompanied by weakness.
- Discuss the possible need for an over-the-counter medication to prevent constipation resulting from the barium.
- Instruct the client that stools will be white for 24 to 72 hr until barium clears. The client should report abdominal fullness, pain, or delay in return to brown stool.

INTERPRETATION OF FINDINGS

Include altered bowel shape and size, increased motility, or obstruction.

Application Exercises

1. A nurse is reviewing bowel prep using polyethylene glycol with a client scheduled for a colonoscopy. Which of the following instructions should the nurse include in the teaching?

   A. Check with the provider about taking current medications when consuming bowel prep.

   B. Consume a normal diet until starting the bowel prep.

   C. Expect the bowel prep to not begin acting until the day after all the prep is consumed.

   D. Discontinue the bowel prep once feces start to be expelled.

2. A nurse is having difficulty arousing a client following an esophagogastroduodenoscopy (EGD). Which of the following is the priority action by the nurse?

   A. Assess the client's airway.

   B. Allow the client to sleep.

   C. Prepare to administer an antidote to the sedative.

   D. Evaluate preprocedure laboratory findings.

3. A nurse in a clinic is instructing a client about a fecal occult blood test, which requires mailing three specimens. Which of the following statements by the client indicates understanding of the teaching?

   A. "I will continue taking my warfarin while I complete these tests."

   B. "I'm glad I don't have to follow any special diet at this time."

   C. "This test determines if I have parasites in my bowel."

   D. "This is an easy way to screen for colon cancer."

4. A nurse is completing preprocedure teaching for a client who will undergo a sigmoidoscopy. Which of the following information should the nurse include in the teaching? (Select all that apply.)

   A. Increased flatulence can occur following the procedure.

   B. NPO status should be maintained preprocedure.

   C. Conscious sedation is used.

   D. Repositioning will occur throughout the procedure.

   E. Fluid intake is limited the day after the procedure.

5. A nurse is reviewing the health record of a client who has a suspected tumor of the jejunum. The nurse should anticipate a prescription for which of the following tests? (Select all that apply.)

   A. Serum alpha-fetoprotein

   B. Endoscopic retrograde cholangiopancreatography (ERCP)

   C. Gastrointestinal x-ray with contrast

   D. Small bowel capsule endoscopy (M2A)

   E. Colonoscopy

PRACTICE Active Learning Scenario

A nurse in a clinic is reviewing teaching with a client who will undergo a gastrointestinal series of x-rays. What should the nurse include in the teaching? Use the ATI Active Learning Template: Diagnostic Procedure to complete this item.

DESCRIPTION OF PROCEDURE: Describe the procedure and technique involved.

INDICATIONS: Identify at least three potential diagnoses and two manifestations.

CLIENT EDUCATION: Describe three teaching points.

Application Exercises Key

1. A. **CORRECT:** The nurse should instruct the client to check with the provider about taking current medication, because some medications can be withheld when taking polyethylene glycol due to their lack of absorption.

   B. The nurse should instruct the client to consume a clear liquid diet prior to starting the bowel prep.

   C. The nurse should instruct the client that the actions of polyethylene glycol begin within 2 to 3 hr after consumption.

   D. The nurse should instruct the client to consume the full amount prescribed.

   Ⓝ *NCLEX® Connection: Reduction of Risk Potential, Therapeutic Procedures*

2. A. **CORRECT:** When using the airway, breathing, and circulation priority-setting framework, assessing and maintaining an open airway is the priority action the nurse should take.

   B. The nurse should continue to allow the client to rest. However, another action is the priority.

   C. The nurse should prepare to administer an antidote to the sedative used during the procedure. However, another action is the priority.

   D. The nurse should evaluate the preprocedure laboratory findings. However, another action is the priority.

   Ⓝ *NCLEX® Connection: Reduction of Risk Potential, Therapeutic Procedures*

3. A. Clients are instructed to stop taking anticoagulants prior to obtaining stool specimens for fecal occult blood testing because they can interfere with the results.

   B. Clients are instructed to avoid consuming red meat, chicken, and fish prior to obtaining stool specimens for fecal occult blood testing because this can interfere with the results.

   C. Fecal occult blood testing does not identify parasites present in stool.

   D. **CORRECT:** Fecal occult blood testing is a screening procedure for colon cancer.

   Ⓝ *NCLEX® Connection: Reduction of Risk Potential, Therapeutic Procedures*

4. A. **CORRECT:** The nurse should teach the client that increased flatulence can occur due to the instillation of air during the procedure.

   B. **CORRECT:** The nurse should instruct the client to remain NPO after midnight the night before the procedure.

   C. The nurse should inform the client that sedation is not indicated for a sigmoidoscopy.

   D. The nurse should inform the client that the position to lie for the procedure is on the left side.

   E. The nurse should instruct the client to increase, not limit fluid intake following the procedure.

   Ⓝ *NCLEX® Connection: Reduction of Risk Potential, Therapeutic Procedures*

5. A. Serum alpha-fetoprotein is a laboratory test used in cases of suspected liver cancer.

   B. An ERCP is used to visualize the duodenum, biliary ducts, gall bladder, liver, and pancreas.

   C. **CORRECT:** A gastrointestinal x-ray with contrast involves the client drinking barium, which is then traced through the small intestine to the junction with the colon. This would identify a tumor in the jejunum.

   D. **CORRECT:** M2A is a procedure in which the client swallows a capsule with a glass of water for a video enteroscopy to visualize the entire small bowel over an 8-hr period.

   E. A colonoscopy is the use of a flexible fiberoptic colonoscope, which enters through the anus, to visualize the rectum and the sigmoid, descending, transverse, and ascending colon.

   Ⓝ *NCLEX® Connection: Reduction of Risk Potential, Diagnostic Tests*

PRACTICE Answer

Using the ATI Active Learning Template: Diagnostic Procedure

DESCRIPTION OF PROCEDURE:
Radiographic images are used to define anatomic or functional abnormalities of the esophagus, stomach, and intestinal tract. These can include an upper GI image, which includes the client drinking radiopaque barium liquid that is traced through the small intestine. The client can have a barium enema, in which liquid barium is instilled into the rectum and colon.

INDICATIONS
- Diagnoses: Gastric ulcers, peristaltic disorders, tumors, varices, intestinal enlargements or constrictions
- Manifestations: Abdominal pain, altered elimination habits (constipation, diarrhea), gastrointestinal bleeding

CLIENT EDUCATION
- Follow fluid and food restrictions for bowel preparation.
- Additional radiographs can be done over a 24-hr period.
- Monitor elimination of contrast media, and report retention of contrast media (constipation) or diarrhea accompanied by weakness. Over-the-counter medication can be used to prevent constipation.
- Stool can be white for 24 to 72 hr until barium clears the system. Report abdominal fullness, pain, or a delay in a return to brown stool.

Ⓝ *NCLEX® Connection: Reduction of Risk Potential, Therapeutic Procedures*

CHAPTER 47 ## Gastrointestinal Therapeutic Procedures

Gastrointestinal therapeutic procedures are performed for maintenance of nutritional intake, and treatment of gastrointestinal obstructions, obesity, and other disorders.

Gastrointestinal therapeutic procedures nurses should be knowledgeable about include enteral feedings, total parenteral nutrition (TPN), paracentesis, nasogastric decompression, bariatric surgeries, and ostomies.

Enteral feedings

Enteral feedings are instituted when a client is unable take adequate nutrition orally.

INDICATIONS

POTENTIAL DIAGNOSES

- Inability to eat due to a medical condition (comatose, intubated)
- Pathologies that cause difficulty swallowing or increase risk of aspiration (stroke, advanced Parkinson's disease, multiple sclerosis)
- Inability to maintain adequate oral nutritional intake and need for supplementation due to increased metabolic demands (cancer therapy, burns, sepsis)

CLIENT PRESENTATION

- Malnutrition (decreased prealbumin, decreased transferrin or total iron-binding capacity)
- Aspiration pneumonia

COMPLICATIONS

Overfeeding

Overfeeding results from infusion of a greater quantity of feeding than can be readily digested, resulting in abdominal distention, nausea, and vomiting.

NURSING ACTIONS
- Check residual every 4 to 6 hr.
- Follow protocol for slowing or withholding feedings for excess residual volumes. Many facilities hold for residual volumes of 100 to 200 mL and then restart at a lower rate after a period of rest.
- Check pump for proper operation and ensure feeding infused at correct rate.

Diarrhea

Diarrhea occurs secondary to concentration of feeding or its constituents.

NURSING ACTIONS
- Slow the rate of feeding and notify the provider.
- Confer with a dietitian.
- Provide skin care and protection.
- Evaluate for *Clostridium difficile* if diarrhea continues, especially if it has a very foul odor.

Aspiration pneumonia

Pneumonia can occur secondary to aspiration of feeding, and can be a life-threatening complication. Tube displacement is the primary cause of aspiration of feeding.

NURSING ACTIONS
- Stop the feeding. Qs
- Turn the client to his side and suction the airway. Administer oxygen if indicated.
- Monitor vital signs for an elevated temperature.
- Auscultate breath sounds for increased congestion and diminishing breath sounds.
- Notify the provider and obtain a chest x-ray if prescribed.

Refeeding syndrome

Refeeding syndrome is a potentially life-threatening condition that occurs when enteral feeding is started in a client who is in a starvation state and whose body has begun to catabolize protein and fat for energy.

NURSING ACTIONS
- Monitor for new onset of confusion or seizures.
- Assess for shallow respirations.
- Monitor for increased muscular weakness.
- Notify the provider and obtain serum electrolytes if needed.

Total parenteral nutrition

TPN is a hypertonic IV bolus solution. The purpose of TPN administration is to prevent or correct nutritional deficiencies and minimize the adverse effects of malnourishment.

- TPN administration is usually through a central line, such as a tunneled triple lumen catheter or a single- or double-lumen peripherally inserted central (PICC) line.
- TPN contains complete nutrition, including calories in a high concentration (10% to 50%) of dextrose, lipids/essential fatty acids, protein, electrolytes, vitamins, and trace elements. Standard IV bolus therapy is typically no more than 700 calories/day.
- Partial parenteral nutrition or peripheral parenteral nutrition (PPN) is less hypertonic, intended for short-term use, and administered in a large peripheral vein. Usual dextrose concentration is 10% or less. Risks include phlebitis.

INDICATIONS

Any condition that
- Affects the ability to absorb nutrition.
- Has a prolonged recovery.
- Creates a hypermetabolic state.
- Creates a chronic malnutrition.

POTENTIAL DIAGNOSES

- Chronic pancreatitis
- Diffuse peritonitis
- Short bowel syndrome
- Gastric paresis from diabetes mellitus
- Severe burns

CLIENT PRESENTATION

- Weight loss greater than 10% of body weight and NPO or unable to eat or drink for more than 5 days
- Hypermetabolic state
- Muscle wasting, poor tissue healing, burns, bowel disease disorders, acute kidney failure

CONSIDERATIONS

PREPARATION OF THE CLIENT

- Determine the client's readiness for TPN. Qᴘᴄᴄ
- Obtain daily laboratory values, including electrolytes. Solutions are customized for each client according to daily laboratory results.

ONGOING CARE

- The flow rate is gradually increased and gradually decreased to allow body adjustment (usually no more than a 10% hourly increase in rate).

  ! Never abruptly stop TPN. Speeding up/slowing down the rate is contraindicated. An abrupt rate change can alter blood glucose levels significantly. Qs

- Assess vital signs every 4 to 8 hr.
- Follow sterile procedures to minimize the risk of sepsis.
  ○ TPN solution is prepared by the pharmacy using aseptic technique with a laminar flow hood.
  ○ Change tubing and solution bag (even if not empty) every 24 hr.
  ○ A filter is added to the tubing to collect particles from the solution.
  ○ Do not use the line for other IV bolus solutions (prevents contamination and interruption of the flow rate).
  ○ Do not add anything to the solution due to risks of contamination and incompatibility.
  ○ Use sterile procedures, including a mask, when changing the central line dressing (per facility procedure).

INTERVENTIONS

- Check capillary glucose every 4 to 6 hr for at least the first 24 hr.
- Clients receiving TPN frequently need supplemental regular insulin until the pancreas can increase its endogenous production of insulin.
- Keep dextrose 10% in water at the bedside in case the solution is unexpectedly ruined or the next bag is not available. This will minimize the risk of hypoglycemia with abrupt changes in dextrose concentrations.
- If a bag is unavailable and administered late, do not attempt to catch up by increasing the infusion rate because the client can develop hyperglycemia.
- OLDER ADULT CLIENTS have an increased incidence of glucose intolerance. Ⓖ

COMPLICATIONS

Metabolic complications

Metabolic complications include hyperglycemia, hypoglycemia, and vitamin deficiencies.

NURSING ACTIONS
- Daily laboratory tests are prescribed and results obtained before a new solution is prepared.
- Fluid needs are typically replaced with a separate IV bolus to prevent fluid volume excess.
- Monitor for hyperglycemia.

Air embolism

A pressure change during tubing changes can lead to an air embolism.

NURSING ACTIONS
- Monitor for manifestations of an air embolism (sudden onset of dyspnea, chest pain, anxiety, hypoxia).
- Clamp the catheter immediately and place the client on his left side in Trendelenburg position to trap air. Administer oxygen and notify the provider so trapped air can be aspirated.

Infection

Concentrated glucose is a medium for bacteria.

NURSING ACTIONS
- Observe the central line insertion site for local infection (erythema, tenderness, exudate).
- Change the sterile dressing on a central line per protocol (typically every 48 to 72 hr).
- Change IV tubing per protocol (typically every 24 hr).
- Observe the client for manifestations of systemic infection (fever, increased WBC, chills, malaise). Qpcc

> ! Do not use TPN line for other IV bolus fluids and medications (repeated access increases the risk for infection).

Fluid Imbalance

TPN is a hyperosmotic solution (three to six times the osmolarity of blood), which poses a risk for fluid shifts, placing client at increased risk of fluid volume excess.

OLDER ADULT CLIENTS are more vulnerable to fluid and electrolyte imbalances. Ⓖ

NURSING ACTIONS
- Assess lungs for crackles and monitor for respiratory distress.
- Monitor daily weight and I&O.
- Use a controlled infusion pump to administer TPN at the prescribed rate.
- Do not speed up the infusion to catch up.
- Gradually increase the flow rate until the prescribed infusion rate is achieved.

Paracentesis

A paracentesis is performed by inserting a needle or trocar through the abdominal wall into the peritoneal cavity. The therapeutic goal is relief of abdominal ascites pressure.
- A paracentesis can be performed in a provider's office, outpatient center, radiology department, or acute care setting at the bed side.
- Usually preformed with ultrasound as a safety precaution.
- Once drained, ascitic fluid can be sent for laboratory culture.

INDICATIONS

POTENTIAL DIAGNOSES

Abdominal ascites

- Ascites is an abnormal accumulation of protein-rich fluid in the abdominal cavity most often caused by cirrhosis of the liver. The result is increased abdominal girth and distention.
- Respiratory distress is the determining factor in the use of a paracentesis to treat ascites, and in the evaluation of treatment effectiveness.

CLIENT PRESENTATION

Compromised lung expansion, increased abdominal girth, rapid weight gain

CONSIDERATIONS

PREPROCEDURE

NURSING ACTIONS
- Determine the client's readiness for the procedure. Variables such as the age of the client and chronic and acute diseases can influence ability to tolerate and recover from this procedure. Ⓖ
- Assess pertinent lab results (serum albumin, protein, glucose, amylase, BUN, and creatinine).
- Verify that the client has signed the informed consent form.
- Gather equipment for the procedure.
- Have the client void, or insert an indwelling urinary catheter.
- Position the client in an upright position, either on the edge of the bed with feet supported or a high-Fowler's position in the bed. Clients who have ascites are typically more comfortable sitting up.
- Review baseline vital signs, record weight, and measure abdominal girth.
- Administer sedation as prescribed.
- Administer IV bolus fluids or albumin, prior to or after a paracentesis, to restore fluid balance.

CLIENT EDUCATION

- Explain the procedure and its purpose to the client.
- Instruct the client that local anesthetics will be used at the insertion site.
- Explain that there can be pressure or pain with needle insertion.
- Assess the client's knowledge of the procedure.

INTRAPROCEDURE

NURSING ACTIONS

- Monitor vital signs.
- Adhere to standard precautions.
- Label laboratory specimens and send to the laboratory.
- Between 4 and 6 L fluid is slowly drained from the abdomen by gravity. The nurse is responsible for monitoring the amount of drainage and notifying the provider of any evidence of complications.

POSTPROCEDURE

NURSING ACTIONS

- Maintain pressure at the insertion site for several minutes. Apply a dressing to the site.
- If the insertion site continues to leak after holding pressure for several minutes, dry sterile gauze dressings should be applied and changed as often as necessary.
- Check vital signs, record weight, and measure abdominal girth. Document and compare to preprocedure measurements.
- Continue to monitor vital signs and insertion site per facility protocol.
- Monitor temperature every 4 hr for a minimum of 48 hr. Fever can indicate a bowel perforation.
- Assess I&O every 4 hr.
- Administer medication.
  - Diuretics such as spironolactone and furosemide can be prescribed to control fluid volume.
  - Potassium supplements can be necessary when a loop diuretic such as furosemide has been administrated.
- Administer IV bolus fluids or albumin as prescribed.
- Assist the client into a position of comfort with the head of the bed elevated to promote lung expansion.
- Document color, odor, consistency, and amount of fluid removed; location of insertion site; evidence of leakage at the insertion site; manifestations of hypovolemia; and changes in mental status.
- Continue monitoring of serum albumin, protein, glucose, amylase, electrolytes, BUN, and creatinine levels.

CLIENT EDUCATION

- Avoid alcohol, maintain a low-sodium diet, take prescribed medications, and monitor the puncture site for bleeding or leakage of fluid.
- Report changes in mental and cognitive status due to change in fluid and electrolyte balance.
- Change positions slowly to decrease the risk of falls, which can be related to hypovolemia from the removal of ascites fluid.

COMPLICATIONS

Hypovolemia

Albumin levels can drop dangerously low because the peritoneal fluid removed contains a large amount of protein. The removal of this protein-rich fluid can cause shifting of intravascular volume, resulting in hypovolemia.

NURSING ACTIONS

- Preventive measures include slow drainage of fluid and administration of plasma expanders, such as albumin, to counter albumin losses.
- Monitor for evidence of hypovolemia, such as tachycardia, hypotension, pallor, diaphoresis, and dizziness.
- Report unexpected findings the provider.

Bladder perforation

Bladder perforation is a rare but possible complication. Manifestations include hematuria, low or no urine output, suprapubic pain or distention, symptoms of cystitis, and fever. Qs

NURSING ACTIONS: If a bladder perforation is suspected, notify the provider immediately.

CLIENT EDUCATION: Inform the client to report manifestations of bladder perforation.

Peritonitis

Peritonitis can occur as a result of injury to the intestines during needle insertion. Manifestations include sharp, constant abdominal pain, fever, nausea, vomiting, and diminished or absent bowel sounds.

NURSING ACTIONS: Notify the provider immediately.

CLIENT EDUCATION: Inform the client to report findings listed above.

Bariatric surgeries

Bariatric surgeries are a treatment for morbid obesity when other weight control methods have failed. The client may try using pharmacological medication for weight loss before choosing bariatric surgery, including:

- **Orlistat** prevents digestion of fats. Adverse effects are oily discharge, reduced food and vitamin absorption, and decreased bile flow.
- **Lorcaserin** stimulates serotonin receptors in the hypothalamus in the brain to curb appetite. Adverse effects can be headache, dry mouth, fatigue, and nausea.
- **Phentermine-topiramate** suppresses the appetite and induces a feeling of satiety. Adverse effects include dry mouth, constipation, nausea, change in taste, dizziness, insomnia, and numbness and tingling of extremities. Contraindicated if the client has hyperthyroidism, glaucoma, or is taking an MAO inhibitor.

Bariatric surgeries include gastric restrictive and malabsorption.

- **Restrictive surgeries**, such as laparoscopic adjustable gastric band (LAGB) or laparoscopic sleeve gastrectomy (LSG), limit the amount of food eaten at one time due to decreased volume capacity. Weight loss is often regained after a period of time unless the client adheres to stringent weight loss protocols and lifestyle modifications. **(47.1)**
  - LAGB involves the placement of an adjustable band at the proximal portion of the stomach to restrict stomach volume to 10 to 15 mL.
  - LSG involves removal of the portion of the stomach that secretes ghrelin, a hormone that stimulates feelings of hunger. Up to 85% of the stomach is removed.
- **Vertical-banded gastroplasty** involves the creation of a new, smaller stomach pouch using staples to decrease its functional size. **(47.2)**
- **Malabsorption surgeries**, such as Roux-en-Y gastric bypass (RNYGB) or simply gastric bypass, interfere with the absorption of food and nutrients from the GI tract. Most clients maintain 60% to 70% of weight loss even 20 years postprocedure.
  - RNYGB involves restricting the volume of the stomach to 20 to 30 mL, bypassing the majority of the stomach and the duodenum. A section of the jejunum is anastomosed to the smaller section of the stomach, bypassing the majority of the stomach. **(47.3)**
- Some procedures combine more than one of these approaches.

Many clients undergo plastic surgery to remove excess skin following weight loss.

INDICATIONS

DIAGNOSIS

History of morbid obesity with unsuccessful attempts at nonsurgical weight loss

CLIENT PRESENTATION

BMI greater than 40, or BMI greater than 35 with comorbidities

CONSIDERATIONS

PREPROCEDURE

NURSING ACTIONS

- Encourage the client to express emotions about eating behaviors, weight, and weight loss to identify psychosocial factors related to obesity.
- Ensure that the client understands needed diet and lifestyle changes.
- Prepare the client for postoperative course and potential complications.
- Arrange for availability of a bariatric bed and mechanical lifting devices to prevent client/staff injury. Qs
- Assess pertinent lab results (CBC, electrolytes, BUN, creatinine, HbA1C, iron, vitamin B_{12}, thiamine, and folate).
- Apply sequential compression stockings to help prevent deep vein thrombosis.

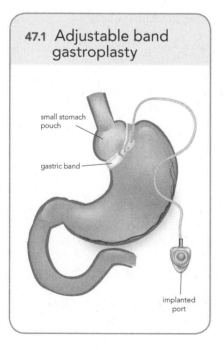

47.1 Adjustable band gastroplasty

small stomach pouch

gastric band

implanted port

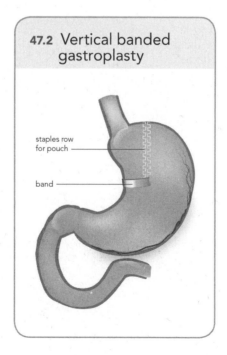

47.2 Vertical banded gastroplasty

staples row for pouch

band

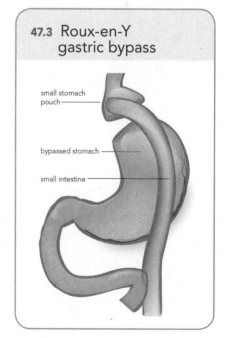

47.3 Roux-en-Y gastric bypass

small stomach pouch

bypassed stomach

small intestine

POSTPROCEDURE

NURSING ACTIONS

- Monitor for leak of anastomosis (increasing back, shoulder, abdominal pain; restlessness; tachycardia; oliguria) and notify the provider immediately. This is a life-threatening emergency.
- Notify the provider for suspected nasogastric (NG) tube displacement. The NG tube is typically sutured in place following stomach surgery; do not attempt to manipulate the tube.
- Provide postoperative care and prevent postoperative complications.
- Monitor for the development of postoperative complications that are at increased risk due to obesity (atelectasis, thromboemboli, skin fold breakdown, incisional hernia, peritonitis).
- Assess the airway and oxygen saturation per facility protocol. Maintain the client in a semi-Fowler's position for lung expansion.
- Monitor bowel sounds.
- Apply an abdominal binder as prescribed to prevent dehiscence if there is an abdominal incision.
- Ambulate the client as soon as possible.
- Resume fluids as prescribed. The first fluids can be restricted to 30 mL and increased in frequency and volume.
- Provide six small meals a day when the client can resume oral nutrients. Observe for indications of dumping syndrome (cramps, diarrhea, tachycardia, dizziness, fatigue).
- Collaborate with case management and mental health resources to assist with long-term behavior modification. Qᴛᴄ

CLIENT EDUCATION

- Instruct the client on limitations regarding liquids or pureed foods for the first 6 weeks, as well as the volume that can be consumed (often not to exceed 1 cup).
- Instruct the client to walk daily for at least 30 min.
- Remind the client that overeating can dilate the surgically created pouch causing weight to be regained.
- Instruct the client to take vitamin and mineral supplements.

COMPLICATIONS

Dehydration

- Warn the client that excessive thirst or concentrated urine can be an indication of dehydration and the surgeon should be notified.
- Work with the client to establish goals and schedule for adequate daily fluid intake.

Malabsorption/malnutrition

Because bariatric surgeries reduce the size of the stomach or bypass portions of the intestinal tract, fewer nutrients are ingested and absorbed.

NURSING ACTIONS

- Monitor the client's tolerance of increasing amounts of food and fluids.
- Refer the client for dietary management.
- Encourage the client to consume meals in a low-Fowler's position and to remain in this position for 30 min after eating to delay stomach emptying and minimize dumping syndrome.

CLIENT EDUCATION

- Instruct the client to eat two servings of protein a day.
- Instruct the client to eat only nutrition-dense foods. Avoid empty calories, such as colas and fruit juice drinks.

Nasogastric decompression

Clients who have an intestinal obstruction require NG decompression. An NG tube is inserted, then suction is applied to relieve abdominal distention. Treatment continues until the obstruction resolves or is removed. The obstruction can be mechanical (tumors, adhesions, fecal impaction) or functional (paralytic ileus).

INDICATIONS

POTENTIAL DIAGNOSES

Any disorder that causes a mechanical or functional intestinal obstruction (e.g., surgery, trauma, GI tract infections, and conditions in which peristalsis is absent)

CLIENT PRESENTATION

- Vomiting (begins with stomach contents and continues until fecal material is also being regurgitated)
- Bowel sounds absent (paralytic ileus) or hyperactive and high-pitched (obstruction)
- Intermittent, colicky abdominal pain and distention
- Hiccups
- Abdominal distention

CONSIDERATIONS

PREPROCEDURE

NURSING ACTIONS: Gather necessary equipment and supplies.

CLIENT EDUCATION: Instruct the client on the purpose of the NG tube and the client's role in its placement.

POSTPROCEDURE

NURSING ACTIONS
- Assess and maintain proper function of the NG tube and suction equipment.
- Maintain accurate I&O.
- Assess bowel sounds and abdominal girth; return of flatus.
- Encourage repositioning and ambulation to help increase peristalsis.
- Monitor tube for displacement (decrease in drainage, increased nausea, vomiting, distention).
- Assess pertinent lab results (electrolytes, hematocrit).
- Provide frequent oral and nares care.

CLIENT EDUCATION: Instruct the client to maintain NPO status.

COMPLICATIONS

Fluid/electrolyte imbalance

NURSING ACTIONS
- Monitor for fluid and electrolyte imbalance (metabolic acidosis: low obstruction; alkalosis: high obstruction).
- Monitor I&O, observing for discrepancies.

Skin breakdown

NURSING ACTIONS: Assess nasal skin for irritation.

Ostomies

An ostomy is a surgical opening from the inside of the body to the outside and can be located in various areas of the body. Ostomies can be permanent or temporary.
- A stoma is the artificial opening created during the ostomy surgery. **(47.4)**
- Main types of ostomies performed in the abdominal area
  - **Ileostomy:** A surgical opening into the ileum to drain stool, which is typically frequent and liquid since large intestine is bypassed
  - **Colostomy:** A surgical opening into the large intestine to drain stool, with the ascending colon producing more liquid stools, the transverse colon producing more formed stools, and the sigmoid colon producing near-normal stool

INDICATIONS

POTENTIAL DIAGNOSES

Ileostomy: when the entire colon must be removed due to disease (Crohn's disease, ulcerative colitis).

Colostomy: when a portion of the bowel must be removed (cancer, ischemic injury) or requires rest for healing (diverticulitis, trauma).

CONSIDERATIONS

PREPROCEDURE

NURSING ACTIONS
- Determine the client's readiness for the procedure. Assess visual acuity, manual dexterity, cognitive status, cultural influences, and support systems. Qpcc
- Initiate a referral to the wound ostomy care nurse (WOCN) for ostomy placement marking and client teaching. Qtc
- Work collaboratively with the WOCN to begin teaching the client and support person about ostomy care and management.

CLIENT EDUCATION: Instruct the client and a support person regarding care and management of an ostomy.

POSTPROCEDURE

NURSING ACTIONS
- Assess the type and fit of the ostomy appliance. Monitor for leakage (risk to skin integrity). Fit the ostomy appliance based on the following.
  - Type and location of the ostomy
  - Visual acuity and manual dexterity of the client
- Assess peristomal skin integrity and appearance of the stoma. The stoma should appear pink and moist.
- Apply skin barriers and creams (adhesive paste) to peristomal skin and allow to dry before applying a new appliance.
- Evaluate stoma output. Output should be more liquid and more acidic the closer the ostomy is to the proximal small intestine.
- Empty the ostomy bag when it is one-fourth to one-half full of drainage.
- Assess for fluid and electrolyte imbalances, particularly with a new ileostomy.
- Evaluate ability of the client or support person to perform ostomy care.

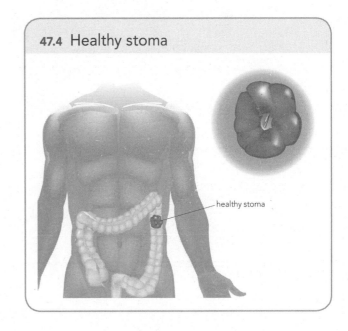

47.4 Healthy stoma

healthy stoma

CLIENT EDUCATION

- Educate the client regarding dietary changes and ostomy appliances that can help manage flatus and odor.
  - Foods that can cause odor include fish, eggs, asparagus, garlic, beans, and dark green leafy vegetables. Buttermilk, cranberry juice, parsley and yogurt help to decrease odor.
  - Foods that can cause gas include dark green leafy vegetables, beer, carbonated beverages, dairy products, and corn. Chewing gum, skipping meals, and smoking can also cause gas. Yogurt, crackers, and toast can be ingested to decrease gas.
  - After an ostomy involving the small intestine is placed, instruct the client to avoid high-fiber foods for the first 2 months after surgery, chew food well, increase fluid intake, and evaluate for evidence of blockage when slowly adding high-fiber foods to the diet.
  - Proper appliance fit and maintenance prevent odor when pouch is not open. Filters, deodorizers, or a breath mint can be placed in the pouch to minimize odor while the pouch is open.
- Provide opportunities for the client to discuss feelings about the ostomy and concerns about its effect on the client's life. Encourage the client to look at and touch the stoma. Qₚcc
- Refer the client to a local ostomy support group. Qₜc

COMPLICATIONS

Stomal ischemia/necrosis

Stomal appearance should normally be pink or red and moist.

- Signs of stomal ischemia are pale pink or bluish purple color and dry appearance.
- If the stoma appears black or purple in color, this indicates a serious impairment of blood flow and requires immediate intervention.

NURSING ACTIONS: Obtain vital signs, oxygen saturation, and current laboratory results. Notify the provider or surgeon of unexpected findings.

CLIENT EDUCATION: Teach the client to watch for indications of stomal ischemia/necrosis.

Intestinal obstruction

Intestinal obstruction can occur for a variety of reasons.

NURSING ACTIONS
- Monitor and record output from the stoma.
- Assess for manifestations of obstruction, including abdominal pain, hypoactive or absent bowel sounds, distention, nausea, and vomiting. Notify the surgeon of unexpected findings.

CLIENT EDUCATION: Note indications of an intestinal obstruction following discharge.

47.5 Changing an ostomy device

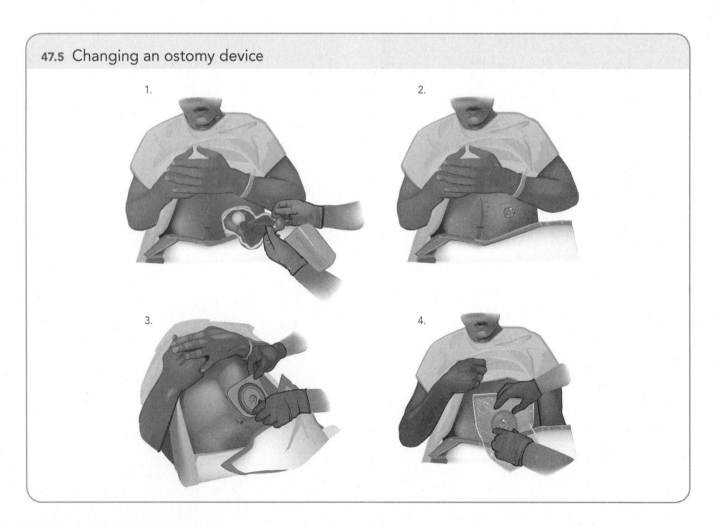

1.
2.
3.
4.

47.6 Expected output for ostomies

ILEOSTOMY	TRANSVERSE COLOSTOMY	SIGMOID COLOSTOMY
Normal postoperative output		
More than 1,000 mL/day Can be bile-colored and liquid	Small semi-liquid with some mucus 2 to 3 days after surgery Blood can be present in the first few days after surgery	Small to moderate amount of mucus with semi-formed stool 4 to 5 days after surgery
Postoperative changes in output		
After several days to weeks, the output decreases to approximately 500 to 1,000 mL/day Becomes more paste-like as the small intestine assumes the absorptive function of the large intestine	After several days to weeks, output becomes more stool-like, semi-formed, or formed	After several days to weeks, output resembles semi-formed stool
Pattern of output		
Continuous output	Resumes a pattern similar to the preoperative pattern	Resumes a pattern similar to the preoperative pattern

Application Exercises

1. A nurse is caring for a client following a paracentesis. Which of the following findings indicate the bowel was perforated during the procedure?

   A. Client report of upper chest pain

   B. Decreased urine output

   C. Pallor

   D. Temperature elevation

2. A nurse is planning care for a client who has a new prescription for total parenteral nutrition (TPN). Which of the following interventions should be included in the plan of care? (Select all that apply.)

   A. Obtain a capillary blood glucose four times daily.

   B. Administer prescribed medications through a secondary port on the TPN IV tubing.

   C. Monitor vital signs three times during the 12-hr shift.

   D. Change the TPN IV tubing every 24 hr.

   E. Ensure a daily aPTT is obtained.

3. A nurse is providing care to a client who is 1 day postoperative following a paracentesis. The nurse observes clear, pale-yellow fluid leaking from the operative site. Which of the following is an appropriate nursing intervention?

   A. Place a clean towel near the drainage site.

   B. Apply a dry, sterile dressing.

   C. Apply direct pressure to the site.

   D. Place the client in a supine position.

4. A nurse is completing discharge teaching with a client who is 3 days postoperative following a transverse colostomy. Which of the following should the nurse include in the teaching?

   A. Mucus will be present in stool for 5 to 7 days after surgery.

   B. Expect 500 to 1,000 mL of semi liquid stool after 2 weeks.

   C. Stoma should be moist and pink.

   D. Change the ostomy bag when it is ¾ full.

5. A nurse is caring for a client who is receiving TPN solution. The current bag of solution was hung 24 hr ago, and 400 mL remains to infuse. Which of the following is the appropriate action for the nurse to take?

   A. Remove the current bag and hang a new bag.

   B. Infuse the remaining solution at the current rate and then hang a new bag.

   C. Increase the infusion rate so the remaining solution is administered within the hour and hang a new bag.

   D. Remove the current bag and hang a bag of lactated Ringer's.

Application Exercises Key

1. A. A report of sharp, constant abdominal pain is associated with bowel perforation.

   B. Decreased urine output is associated with bladder perforation during a paracentesis.

   C. Pallor may indicate hypovolemia related to fluid removal of ascites fluid during the procedure.

   D. **CORRECT:** Fever is an indication of bowel perforation during a paracentesis.

   Ⓝ *NCLEX® Connection: Reduction of Risk Potential, Potential for Complications of Diagnostic Tests/Treatments/Procedures*

2. A. **CORRECT:** The client is at risk for hyperglycemia during the administration of TPN and can require supplemental insulin.

   B. No other medications or fluids should be administered through the IV tubing being used to administer TPN due to the increased risk of infection and disruption of the rate of TPN infusion.

   C. **CORRECT:** Vital signs are recommended every 4 to 8 hr to assess for fluid volume excess and infection.

   D. **CORRECT:** It is recommended to change the IV tubing that is used to administer TPN every 24 hr.

   E. aPTT measures the coagulability of the blood, which is unnecessary during the administration of TPN.

   Ⓝ *NCLEX® Connection: Pharmacological and Parenteral Therapies, Total Parenteral Nutrition (TPN)*

3. A. Sterile dressings should be applied to the operative site to prevent infection and allow for assessment of drainage.

   B. **CORRECT:** Application of a sterile dressing will contain the drainage and allow continuous assessment of color and quantity.

   C. Application of direct pressure can cause discomfort and potential harm to the client. The nurse should apply a sterile dressing to the site and monitor the quantity and characteristic of the drainage.

   D. The client should be placed with the head of the bed elevated to promote lung expansion.

   Ⓝ *NCLEX® Connection: Reduction of Risk Potential, Therapeutic Procedures*

4. A. Mucus and blood can be present for 2 to 3 days after surgery.

   B. Output should become stool-like, semi-formed, or formed within days to weeks.

   C. **CORRECT:** A pink, moist stoma is an expected finding with a transverse colostomy.

   D. The ostomy bag should be changed when it is ¼ to ½ full.

   Ⓝ *NCLEX® Connection: Physiological Adaptation, Alterations in Body Systems*

5. A. **CORRECT:** The current bag of TPN should not hang more than 24 hr due to the risk of infection.

   B. The current bag of TPN should not hang more than 24 hr due to the risk of infection.

   C. The rate of TPN infusion should never be increased abruptly due to the risk of hyperglycemia.

   D. Administration of TPN should never be discontinued abruptly due to the sudden change in blood glucose that can occur.

   Ⓝ *NCLEX® Connection: Pharmacological and Parenteral Therapies, Total Parenteral Nutrition (TPN)*

PRACTICE Active Learning Scenario

A nurse educator is reviewing care of a client who will have bariatric surgery with a group of newly hired nurses. What should the nurse include in this discussion? Use the ATI Active Learning Template: Therapeutic Procedure to complete this item.

DESCRIPTION OF PROCEDURE: Describe three types of bariatric surgery.

NURSING INTERVENTIONS: Describe at least five, to include equipment needed to promote client/staff safety.

CLIENT EDUCATION: Describe postoperative pattern of food and fluid consumption.

PRACTICE Active Learning Scenario

Using the ATI Active Learning Template: Therapeutic Procedure

DESCRIPTION OF PROCEDURE
- Vertical banded gastroplasty involves stapling a portion of the stomach to decrease its functional size.
- Adjustable banded gastroplasty involves constricting the functional size of the stomach.
- Intestinal bypass involves bypassing the stomach and part of the small intestine to decrease the absorption of nutrients and calories.

NURSING INTERVENTIONS
- Encourage client to express emotions related to weight, weight loss, and eating behaviors to identify related psychosocial concerns.
- Ensure the client understands required dietary and lifestyle changes.
- Arrange for availability of a bariatric bed and mechanical lifting device to prevent client/staff injury.
- Monitor for leak of anastomosis and notify provider immediately if this occurs.
- Assess airway and oxygen saturation. Maintain client in semi-Fowler's position for lung expansion.
- Monitor bowel sounds.
- Apply abdominal binder if prescribed.
- Ambulate client as soon as possible.
- Monitor intake and output.
- Monitor NG tube placement and function, as well as function of suction equipment.

CLIENT EDUCATION
- Fluids will be allowed beginning with 30 mL and gradually increase in volume and frequency.
- Food will be allowed beginning with six small meals.
- Volume might be limited to 1 cup of liquid or pureed foods.

Ⓝ *NCLEX® Connection: Reduction of Risk Potential, Therapeutic Procedures*

CHAPTER 48 *Esophageal Disorders*

The esophagus is a muscular tube that leads from the throat to the stomach. The esophagus is about 25 cm (10 in) long. It extends from the base of pharynx to the stomach, about 4 cm (1.6 in) below the diaphragm. Esophageal disorders can affect any part of the esophagus.

There are two sphincters: upper esophageal (UES) also referred to as the oropharyngeal sphincter, and the lower esophageal (LES) also referred to as gastroesophageal sphincter. They prevent the reflux of food and fluids into the mouth or esophagus. **(48.1)**

Common problems in the esophagus, such as structural defects, inflammation, obstruction, and cancer, interfere with nutrition.

48.1 Esophageal sphincters

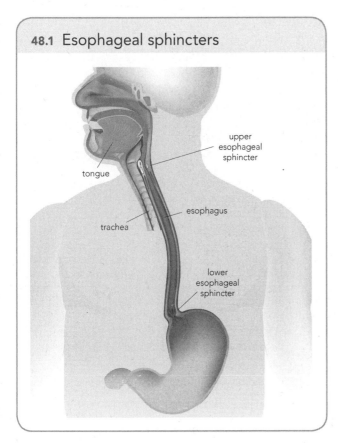

- tongue
- trachea
- upper esophageal sphincter
- esophagus
- lower esophageal sphincter

Contractions of the esophagus propel food and fluids toward the stomach, while relaxation of the lower esophageal sphincter allows passage into the stomach. Following this, the LES contracts, preventing reflux of food back up into the esophagus.

Esophageal disorders include gastroesophageal reflux disease (GERD), hiatal hernia, and esophageal varices.

Gastroesophageal reflux disease

GERD is a common condition characterized by gastric content and enzyme backflow into the esophagus. Some backflow of stomach contents into the esophagus is normal. When the reflux is excessive due to any of the following conditions—an incompetent LES, pyloric stenosis, hiatal hernia, excessive intra-abdominal or intragastric pressure, or motility problems—the corrosive fluids irritate the esophageal tissue, causing delay in their clearance. This further exposes esophageal tissue to the acidic fluids, causing more irritation.

- The primary treatment of GERD is diet and lifestyle changes, advancing to medication use (antacids, H_2-receptor antagonists, proton pump inhibitors) and surgery. Qpcc
- Untreated GERD leads to inflammation, breakdown, and long-term complications, such as Barrett's esophagus or adenocarcinoma of the esophagus.

HEALTH PROMOTION AND DISEASE PREVENTION

- Maintain a weight below BMI of 30.
- Stop smoking.
- Limit or avoid alcohol and tobacco use.
- Eat a low-fat diet.
- Avoid foods that lower the LES pressure.
- Avoid eating or drinking 2 hr before bed.
- Avoid tight-fitting clothes.
- Elevate the head of the bed 6 to 8 inches.

ASSESSMENT

RISK FACTORS

- Obesity
- Older age (delayed gastric emptying and weakened LES tone) ©
- Sleep apnea
- Nasogastric tube

CONTRIBUTING FACTORS

- Excessive ingestion of foods that relax the LES include fatty and fried foods, chocolate, caffeinated beverages (coffee), peppermint, spicy foods, tomatoes, citrus fruits, and alcohol
- Prolonged or frequent abdominal distention (from overeating or delayed emptying)
- Increased abdominal pressure from obesity, pregnancy, bending at the waist, ascites, or tight clothing at the waist
- Medications that relax the LES (theophylline, nitrates, calcium channel blockers, anticholinergics, and diazepam)
- Increased gastric acid caused by medications (NSAIDs) or stress (environmental)
- Debilitation resulting in weakened LES tone
- Hiatal hernia (LES displacement into the thorax with delayed esophageal clearance)
- Lying flat

EXPECTED FINDINGS

- Classic report of dyspepsia after eating an offending food or fluid, and regurgitation
- Radiating pain (neck, jaw, or back)
- Report of a feeling of having a heart attack.
- Pyrosis (burning sensation in the esophagus)
- Dyspepsia (indigestion)
- Dysphagia or odynophagia (pain on swallowing)
- Pain that worsens with position (bending, straining, laying down)
- Pain that occurs after eating and lasts 20 min to 2 hr
- Throat irritation (chronic cough, laryngitis), hypersalivation, bitter taste in mouth (caused by regurgitation). Chronic GERD can lead to dysphagia.
- Increased flatus and eructation (burping).
- Pain is relieved (almost immediately) by drinking water, sitting upright, or taking antacids.
- Manifestations occurring four to five times per week on a consistent basis are considered diagnostic.
- Tooth erosion

PHARYNGITIS DIAGNOSTIC PROCEDURES

Esophagogastroduodenoscopy (EGD)

- EGD is done under moderate sedation to observe for tissue damage and to dilate strictures in the esophagus. The esophageal lining should be pink but is often red with persistent GERD. Biopsies will be done to determine if high-grade dysplasia (HGD) is present.
- HGD is evidenced by squamous mucosa of the esophagus replaced by columnar epithelium (cells seen in the stomach or intestines). When HGD is found, there is a 30% increase in chance of developing cancer.
- EGD allows visualization of the esophagus, revealing esophagitis or Barrett's epithelium (premalignant cells).

NURSING ACTIONS: Verify gag response has returned prior to providing oral fluids or food following the procedure. Qs

Esophageal pH monitoring

A small catheter is placed through the nose and into the distal esophagus, or a small capsule is attached to the esophageal wall during endoscopy. pH readings are taken in relation to food, position, and activity for 24 to 48 hr.
- Most accurate method of diagnosing GERD
- Especially helpful in diagnosis for clients who have atypical manifestations

NURSING ACTIONS: Instruct the client to keep a journal of foods and beverages consumed, symptoms, and activity during the 24-hr test period.

Esophageal manometry

Esophageal manometry records lower esophageal sphincter pressure and peristaltic activity of the esophagus. The client swallows three small tubes, and pressure readings and pH levels are tested.

Barium swallow

Barium swallow identifies a hiatal hernia, strictures, or structural abnormalities, which would contribute to or cause GERD.

NURSING ACTIONS: Instruct the client to use cathartics to evacuate the barium from the GI tract following the procedure. Failure to eliminate the barium places the client at risk for fecal impaction.

PATIENT-CENTERED CARE

MEDICATIONS

Proton pump inhibitors (PPIs)

Pantoprazole, omeprazole, esomeprazole, rabeprazole, and lansoprazole reduce gastric acid by inhibiting the cellular pump of the gastric parietal cells necessary for gastric acid secretion.

NURSING CONSIDERATIONS
- Monitor for electrolyte imbalances and hypoglycemia in clients who have diabetes mellitus.
- Long-term use has been related to the development of community-acquired pneumonia and Clostridium difficile infections.

CLIENT EDUCATION: Long-term use of PPIs places the client at risk for fractures, especially in older adults. Ⓖ

Antacids

Aluminum hydroxide, magnesium hydroxide, calcium carbonate, and sodium bicarbonate neutralize excess acid and increase LES pressure.

NURSING CONSIDERATIONS: Ensure there are no contraindications with other prescribed medications (levothyroxine). Evaluate kidney function in clients taking magnesium hydroxide.

CLIENT EDUCATION: Instruct the client to take antacids when acid secretion is the highest (1 to 3 hr after eating and at bedtime), and to separate from other medications by at least 1 hr.

Histamine₂ receptor antagonists

Ranitidine, famotidine, and nizatidine reduce the secretion of acid. The onset is longer than antacids, but the effect has a longer duration.

NURSING CONSIDERATIONS: Use cautiously in clients who have kidney disease.

CLIENT EDUCATION
- Take with meals and at bedtime.
- Separate dosages from antacids (1 hr before or after taking antacid).

Prokinetics

Metoclopramide increases the motility of the esophagus and stomach.

NURSING CONSIDERATIONS: Monitor the client taking metoclopramide for extrapyramidal side effects.

CLIENT EDUCATION: Instruct the client to report abnormal, involuntary movement.

THERAPEUTIC PROCEDURES

Stretta procedure uses radiofrequency energy, applied by an endoscope, to decrease vagus nerve activity. This causes the LES muscle tissue to contract and tighten.

Fundoplication

Fundoplication can be indicated for clients who fail to respond to other treatments. The fundus of the stomach is wrapped around and behind the esophagus through a laparoscope to create a physical barrier.

NURSING CONSIDERATIONS: Complications following fundoplication include temporary dysphagia (monitor for aspiration), gas bloat syndrome (difficulty belching to relieve distention), and atelectasis/pneumonia (monitor respiratory function).

CLIENT EDUCATION
- **Diet**
  - Avoid offending foods.
  - Avoid large meals.
  - Remain upright after eating.
  - Avoid eating before bedtime.
  - Consume four to six small meals throughout the day.
- **Lifestyle**
  - Avoid clothing that is tight-fitting around the abdomen.
  - Lose weight, if applicable.
  - Elevate the head of the bed 15.2 to 20.3 cm (6 to 8 in) with blocks.

COMPLICATIONS

Aspiration of gastric secretion

CAUSES: Reflux of gastric fluids into the esophagus can be aspirated into the trachea.

RISKS ASSOCIATED WITH ASPIRATION
- Asthma exacerbations from inhaled aerosolized acid
- Frequent upper respiratory, sinus, or ear infections
- Aspiration pneumonia

Barrett's epithelium (premalignant) and esophageal adenocarcinoma

CAUSE: Reflux of gastric fluids leads to esophagitis. In chronic esophagitis, the body continuously heals inflamed tissue, eventually replacing normal esophageal epithelium with premalignant tissue (Barrett's epithelium) or malignant adenocarcinoma.

NURSING ACTIONS: Determine the cause of GERD with the client and review lifestyle changes that can decrease gastric reflux. Monitor nutritional status. Qᴘᴄᴄ

Hiatal hernia

Hiatal hernia (diaphragmatic hernia) is a protrusion of the stomach (in part or in total) above the diaphragm into the thoracic cavity through the hiatus (the opening in the diaphragm). There are two types of hiatal hernia.

Sliding (more common): a portion of the stomach and gastroesophageal junction move above the diaphragm. This generally occurs with increases in intra-abdominal pressure or while the client is in a supine position.

Paraesophageal (rolling) part of the fundus of the stomach moves above the diaphragm although the gastroesophageal junction remains below the diaphragm.

HEALTH PROMOTION AND DISEASE PREVENTION

- Avoid eating immediately prior to going to bed.
- Avoid foods and beverages that decrease LES pressure (fatty and fried foods, chocolate, coffee, peppermint, spicy foods, tomatoes, citrus fruits, and alcohol).
- Exercise regularly.
- Maintain a healthy weight.
- Elevate the head of the bed on 6-inch blocks.
- Avoid straining or excessive vigorous exercise.
- Avoid wearing clothing that is tight around the abdomen.

ASSESSMENT

EXPECTED FINDINGS

Presenting manifestations depend on the type of hiatal hernia and are typically worse following a meal

Sliding: heartburn, reflux, chest pain, dysphagia, belching

Paraesophageal: fullness after eating, sense of breathlessness/suffocation, chest pain, worsening of symptoms when reclining

PHYSICAL ASSESSMENT FINDINGS
- Pharyngitis
- Inspiratory/expiratory wheeze

DIAGNOSTIC PROCEDURES

Barium swallow with fluoroscopy

Allows visualization of the esophagus.

NURSING ACTIONS: Instruct the client to use cathartics to evacuate the barium from the GI tract following the procedure. Failure to eliminate the barium places the client at risk for fecal impaction.

Esophagogastroduodenoscopy (EGD)

Allows visualization of the esophagus and the gastric lining.

NURSING ACTIONS: Verify gag response has returned prior to providing oral fluids or food following the procedure Qs

CT scan of the chest with contrast

Allows visualization of the esophagus and stomach.

NURSING ACTIONS: Assess for iodine allergies if IV contrast is to be used. Encourage fluids following procedure to promote dye excretion and minimize risk of renal injury. Monitor BUN/creatinine

PATIENT-CENTERED CARE

MEDICATIONS

Proton pump inhibitors

Pantoprazole, omeprazole, esomeprazole, rabeprazole, and lansoprazole reduce gastric acid by inhibiting the cellular pump of the gastric parietal cells necessary for gastric acid secretion.

NURSING CONSIDERATIONS
- Monitor for electrolyte imbalances and hypoglycemia in clients who have diabetes mellitus.
- Long-term use has been related to the development of community-acquired pneumonia and *Clostridium difficile* infections.

CLIENT EDUCATION: Long-term use of PPIs places clients at risk for fractures, especially in older adults. ©

Antacids

Aluminum hydroxide, magnesium hydroxide, calcium carbonate, and sodium bicarbonate neutralize excess acid and increase LES pressure.

NURSING CONSIDERATIONS: Ensure there are no contraindications with other prescribed medications (levothyroxine). Evaluate kidney function in clients taking magnesium hydroxide.

CLIENT EDUCATION: Instruct the client to take antacids when acid secretion is the highest (1 to 3 hr after eating and at bedtime), and to separate from other medications by at least 1 hr.

THERAPEUTIC PROCEDURES

Fundoplication: reinforcement of the LES by wrapping a portion of the fundus of the stomach around the distal esophagus

Laparoscopic Nissen fundoplication: minimally invasive with fewer complications

NURSING CONSIDERATIONS: Elevate the head of the bed to promote lung expansion. Instruct the client to support the incision during movement and coughing to minimize strain on the suture lines.

CLIENT EDUCATION: Consume a soft diet for the first week postoperatively. Avoid carbonated beverages. Ambulate, but avoid heavy lifting.

COMPLICATIONS: Temporary dysphagia, gas bloat syndrome (difficulty burping and distention), atelectasis/pneumonia

COMPLICATIONS

Volvulus: twisting of the esophagus and/or stomach

Obstruction (paraesophageal hernia): blockage of food in the herniated portion of the stomach

Strangulation (paraesophageal hernia): compression of the blood vessels to the herniated portion of the stomach

Iron-deficiency anemia (paraesophageal hernia): resulting from bleeding into the gastric mucosa due to obstruction

Esophageal varices

- Esophageal varices are swollen, fragile blood vessels that are generally found in the submucosa of the lower esophagus, but varices can develop higher in the esophagus or extend into the stomach. (48.2)
- Esophageal varices occur as a result of portal hypertension, usually due to cirrhosis of the liver.
- When esophageal varices hemorrhage, it is often a medical emergency associated with a high mortality rate. Reoccurrence of esophageal bleeding is common.

HEALTH PROMOTION AND DISEASE PREVENTION

- Avoid alcohol consumption.
- Avoid heavy lifting.
- Avoid straining with bowel movements.
- Chew food completely, as poorly chewed foods can irritate the area.
- Avoid salicylates and other medications that can irritate the esophagus.

ASSESSMENT

RISK FACTORS

- Portal hypertension (elevated blood pressure in veins that carry blood from the intestines to the liver)
  - Caused by impaired circulation of blood through the liver. Collateral circulation subsequently develops, creating varices in the upper stomach and esophagus. Varices are fragile and can bleed easily.
  - The primary risk factor for development of esophageal varices.
- Alcoholic cirrhosis
- Viral hepatitis
- OLDER ADULT CLIENTS frequently have depressed immune function, decreased liver function, and cardiac disorders that make them especially vulnerable to bleeding. ©

EXPECTED FINDINGS

- The client can experience no manifestations until the varices begin to bleed. Hematemesis, melena, and a general deterioration of the client's physical and mental status.
- Activities that precipitate bleeding are the Valsalva maneuver, lifting heavy objects, coughing, sneezing, and alcohol consumption.

PHYSICAL ASSESSMENT FINDINGS
(BLEEDING ESOPHAGEAL VARICES)
- Shock
- Hypotension
- Tachycardia
- Cool clammy skin

LABORATORY TESTS

Liver function tests indicate a liver disorder.

Hemoglobin and hematocrit tests can indicate anemia secondary to occult bleeding or overt bleeding.

Elevated serum ammonia level indicates an increased nitrogen load from the bleeding varices.

DIAGNOSTIC PROCEDURES

Endoscopy

Therapeutic interventions can be performed during the endoscopy.

NURSING ACTIONS: Administer preprocedure sedation. After the procedure, monitor vital signs and take measures to prevent aspiration.

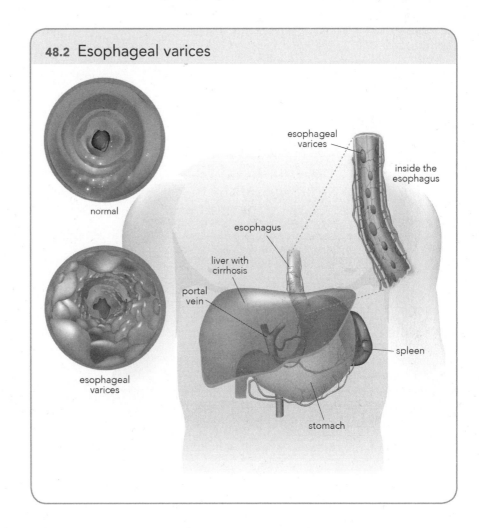

48.2 **Esophageal varices**

normal

esophageal varices

esophageal varices

inside the esophagus

esophagus

liver with cirrhosis

portal vein

spleen

stomach

PATIENT-CENTERED CARE

NURSING CARE Qs

If bleeding is suspected, establish IV access with a large bore needle, monitor vital signs and hematocrit, type and cross-match for possible blood transfusions, and monitor for overt and occult bleeding.

MEDICATIONS

Nonselective beta-blockers

- Propranolol is prescribed to decrease heart rate and consequently reduce hepatic venous pressure.
- Used prophylactically (not for emergency hemorrhage).

Vasoconstrictors

- Octreotide is a synthetic form of the hormone somatostatin decreases the bleeding from the esophageal varices but does not affect the blood pressure.
- Vasopressin causes constriction of the esophageal and proximal gastric veins and reduces portal pressure.

NURSING CONSIDERATIONS

- Vasopressin should not be given to clients who have coronary artery disease due to resultant coronary constriction. Potent vasoconstriction can also cause problems with peripheral and cerebral circulation. If Vasopressin is used in combination with nitroglycerin IV in this client population, it can decrease or prevent the vasoconstriction of the coronary arteries.
- Monitor for fluid retention and hyponatremia, as vasopressin has an antidiuretic effect.

THERAPEUTIC PROCEDURES

Endoscopic variceal ligation (EVL)

Endoscopic variceal ligation (esophageal banding therapy) can be used for acute bleeding.
- During endoscopy, the varices are rubber banded to cut off the circulation to the varices. Necrosis of the tissue occurs with eventual sloughing of the varix.
- There is a significant decrease in re-bleeding as well as decreased mortality postprocedure.

COMPLICATIONS

- Superficial ulceration
- Dysphagia
- Temporary chest discomfort
- Esophageal strictures (rare)

NURSING ACTIONS: Administer preprocedure sedation. After the procedure, monitor vital signs and take measures to prevent aspiration.

Endoscopic sclerotherapy

During endoscopy, a sclerosing agent is injected into the varices resulting in thrombosis of the varicosity.

COMPLICATIONS

- Bleeding
- Perforation of the esophagus
- Aspiration pneumonia
- Esophageal stricture

NURSING ACTIONS

- Administer preprocedure sedation. After the procedure, monitor vital signs and take measures to prevent aspiration.
- Antacids, H_2-receptor blockers, or PPIs can be administered after the procedure to protect the esophagus and prevent acid reflux which is often caused by sclerotherapy.

Transjugular intrahepatic portal-systemic shunt (TIPS)

- TIPS is used to treat an acute episode of bleeding when EVL and pharmacological measures are not controlling the variceal bleeding. It rapidly lowers the portal pressure. The procedure is costly, and therefore is only used when other measures do not work.
- While the client is under sedation or general anesthesia, a catheter is passed into the liver via the jugular vein in the neck. A stent is then placed between the portal and hepatic veins bypassing the liver. Portal hypertension is subsequently relieved.

COMPLICATIONS

- Bleeding
- Sepsis
- Heart failure
- Organ perforation
- Liver failure

NURSING ACTIONS: Monitor vital signs. Keep the head of the bed elevated.

Esophagogastric balloon tamponade

- Rarely used but can be used to temporarily control bleeding until another measure can be implemented.
- Risks: Tube migration, which can lead to airway obstruction; aspiration of gastric contents into lungs.
- Clients are often intubated to protect the airway.
- Can cause necrosis of tissue if left in place for extended period of time. Balloon should be in place no longer than 12 hr.

NURSING ACTIONS

- Check balloons for leaks prior to insertion.
- Monitor placement of the tube and observe for possible obstruction of airway.
- Monitor for aspiration into the lungs and secretions or blood from the esophagus.
- Provide oral suction as needed.
- Maintain balloon pressure at prescribed pressure for prescribed time to decrease risk of esophageal or gastric necrosis from ischemia.
- Monitor the client who has decreased mentation or confusion and who might pull on the tube.

Surgical interventions

- Considered as a last resort. TIPS has replaced many surgical measures. High morbidity and mortality rates continue to be seen with surgical intervention.
- Bypass procedures establish a venous shunt that bypasses the liver, decreasing portal hypertension.
  - Common shunts include **splenorenal** (splenic, left renal veins), **mesocaval** (mesenteric vein, vena cava), and **portacaval** (portal vein, inferior vena cava).
  - Clients commonly have a nasogastric tube inserted during surgery to monitor for hemorrhage.

NURSING ACTIONS (PRE-, POSTPROCEDURE)
- Monitor for an increase in liver dysfunction or encephalopathy.
- Monitor nasogastric tube secretions for bleeding.
- Monitor PT, aPTT, platelets, and INR.

INTERPROFESSIONAL CARE

Alcohol recovery program (varices secondary to alcohol use disorder)

COMPLICATIONS

Hypovolemic shock

Due to hemorrhage from varices

NURSING ACTIONS
- Observe for manifestations of hemorrhage and shock (tachycardia, hypotension).
- Monitor vital signs, Hgb, Hct, and coagulation studies.
- Replace losses and support therapeutic procedures to stop and control bleeding.

Application Exercises

1. A nurse is caring for a client who has a new diagnosis of gastroesophageal reflux disease (GERD). The nurse should anticipate prescriptions for which of the following medications? (Select all that apply.)
   - A. Antacids
   - B. Histamine$_2$ receptor antagonists
   - C. Opioid analgesics
   - D. Fiber laxatives
   - E. Proton pump inhibitors

2. A nurse is admitting a client who has bleeding esophageal varices. The nurse should anticipate a prescription for which of the following medications?
   - A. Propranolol
   - B. Metoclopramide
   - C. Ranitidine
   - D. Vasopressin

3. A nurse is completing an assessment of a client who has GERD. Which of the following is an expected finding?
   - A. Absence of saliva
   - B. Loss of tooth enamel
   - C. Sweet taste in mouth
   - D. Absence of eructation

4. A nurse is teaching a client who has a hiatal hernia. Which of the following client statements indicates an understanding of the teaching?
   - A. "I can take my medications with soda."
   - B. "Peppermint tea will increase my indigestion."
   - C. "Wearing an abdominal binder will limit my symptoms."
   - D. "I will drink hot chocolate at bedtime to help me sleep."
   - E. "I can lift weights as a way to exercise."

5. A nurse is completing discharge teaching to a client who is postoperative following fundoplication. Which of the following statements by the client indicates understanding of the teaching?
   - A. "When sitting in my lounge chair after a meal, I will lower the back of it."
   - B. "I will try to eat three large meals a day."
   - C. "I will elevate the head of my bed on blocks."
   - D. "When sleeping, I will lay on my left side."

PRACTICE Active Learning Scenario

A nurse is preparing a poster on GERD to be displayed at a community health fair. What should be included in the poster? Use the ATI Active Learning Template: System Disorder to complete this item.

ALTERATION IN HEALTH (DIAGNOSIS)

RISK FACTORS: Describe at least eight.

EXPECTED FINDINGS: Describe at least eight.

Application Exercises Key

1. A. **CORRECT:** Antacids neutralize gastric acid which irritates the esophagus during reflux.

    B. **CORRECT:** Histamine$_2$ receptor antagonists decrease acid secretion, which contributes to reflux.

    C. Opioid analgesics are not effective in treating GERD.

    D. Fiber laxatives are not effective in treating GERD.

    E. **CORRECT:** Proton pump inhibitors decrease gastric acid production, which contributes to reflex.

    Ⓝ *NCLEX® Connection: Physiological Adaptation, Alterations in Body Systems*

2. A. Propranolol is not used for clients who are actively bleeding. It can be given prophylactically to decrease portal hypertension.

    B. Metoclopramide decreases motility of the esophagus and stomach.

    C. Histamine$_2$-receptor antagonists are administered following surgical procedures for bleeding esophageal varices.

    D. **CORRECT:** Vasopressin constricts blood vessels and is used to treat bleeding esophageal varices.

    Ⓝ *NCLEX® Connection: Physiological Adaptation, Alterations in Body Systems*

3. A. Hypersalivation is an expected finding in a client who has GERD.

    B. **CORRECT:** Tooth erosion is an expected finding in a client who has GERD.

    C. A client who has GERD would report a bitter taste in the mouth.

    D. Increased burping is an expected finding in a client who has GERD.

    Ⓝ *NCLEX® Connection: Physiological Adaptation, Pathophysiology*

4. A. Carbonated beverages decrease LES pressure and should be avoided by the client who has a hiatal hernia.

    B. **CORRECT:** Peppermint decreases LES pressure and should be avoided by the client who has a hiatal hernia

    C. Tight restrictive clothing or abdominal binders should be avoided by the client who has a hiatal hernia, as this increases intra-abdominal pressure and causes the protrusion of the stomach into the thoracic cavity.

    D. The client should avoid consuming anything immediately prior to bedtime. Additionally, chocolate relaxes the lower esophageal sphincter and should be avoided by a client who has a hiatal hernia

    E. Heavy lifting and vigorous activities are to be avoided in the client who has a hiatal hernia.

    Ⓝ *NCLEX® Connection: Health Promotion and Maintenance, Health Promotion/Disease Prevention*

5. A. The client is instructed to remain upright after eating following a fundoplication.

    B. The client is instructed to avoid large meals after a fundoplication.

    C. **CORRECT:** After a fundoplication, the client is instructed to elevate the head of the bed to limit reflux.

    D After a fundoplication, the client is instructed to sleep on the right side.

    Ⓝ *NCLEX® Connection: Reduction of Risk Potential, Therapeutic Procedures*

PRACTICE Answer

Using the ATI Active Learning Template: System Disorder

ALTERATION IN HEALTH (DIAGNOSIS):
Gastroesophageal reflux disease (GERD) is a common condition characterized by gastric content and enzyme backflow into the esophagus. These fluids are corrosive to esophageal tissue, causing a delay in their clearance. This further exposes esophageal tissue to the acidic fluids, increasing tissue irritation.

RISK FACTORS
- Obesity
- Older age
- Sleep apnea
- Excessive ingestion of foods that relax the lower esophageal sphincter (fatty and fried foods, chocolate, caffeinated beverages, peppermint, spicy foods, tomatoes, citrus fruits, and alcohol)
- Pregnancy
- Bending at the waist, wearing tight clothing at the waist
- Medications (theophylline, nitrates, calcium channel blockers, anticholinergics, NSAIDs)
- Stress
- Hiatal hernia
- Lying flat

EXPECTED FINDINGS
- Dyspepsia after eating and regurgitation (classic)
- Throat irritation (chronic cough, laryngitis)
- Hypersalivation
- Bitter taste in mouth
- Chest pain due to esophageal spasm
- Increased flatus and eructation (burping)
- Pain relieved by drinking water, sitting upright or taking antacids

Ⓝ *NCLEX® Connection: Health Promotion and Maintenance, Health Promotion/Disease Prevention*

CHAPTER 49 *Peptic Ulcer Disease*

A peptic ulcer is an erosion of the mucosal lining of the stomach, esophagus, or duodenum. The most common area for a peptic ulcer is the duodenum. The mucous membranes can become eroded to the point that the epithelium is exposed to gastric acid and pepsin, which can precipitate bleeding and perforation. Perforation that extends through all the layers of the stomach or duodenum can cause peritonitis. An individual who has a peptic ulcer has peptic ulcer disease.

Most peptic ulcers are caused by an infection from gram-negative bacteria *Helicobacter pylori* (*H. pylori*). Contact with the bacteria occurs from food, water, or exposure to body fluids such as saliva. Some people infected with the *H. pylori* bacteria do not develop ulcers. Stress ulcer occurs from an acute period of physiological stressful events, such as burns, shock, severe sepsis, or multiple organ trauma. These ulcers are different clinically from a peptic ulcer and can be present in a ventilated client in the intensive care unit. Curling's ulcer is seen in clients who have burns. Cushing's ulcer can be seen in clients who have head/brain trauma. Bleeding is the primary manifestation of the stress ulcer. Clients experiencing trauma often receive proton-pump inhibitor prophylaxis to prevent the development of stress ulcers.

HEALTH PROMOTION AND DISEASE PREVENTION

- Drink alcohol in moderation.
- Stop smoking and use of tobacco products.
- Use stress management techniques.
- Avoid NSAIDs as indicated.
- Limit caffeine-containing beverages.
- Consume a balanced diet.
- Engage regularly in exercise.

ASSESSMENT

RISK FACTORS

Causes of peptic ulcers
- *Helicobacter pylori* (*H. pylori*) infection
- NSAID and corticosteroid use
- Severe stress
- Familial tendency
- Hypersecretory states
- Gastrin-secreting benign or malignant tumors of the pancreas
- Type O blood
- Excess alcohol consumption
- Chronic pulmonary or kidney disease
- Zollinger–Ellison syndrome (combination of peptic ulcers, hypersecretion of gastric acid, and gastrin-secreting tumors)
- Pernicious anemia

EXPECTED FINDINGS

- Dyspepsia: heartburn, bloating, nausea, and vomiting (vomiting is rare but can be caused by a gastric outlet obstruction). Can be perceived as uncomfortable fullness or hunger.
- Dull, gnawing pain or burning sensation at the midepigastrium or the back

49.1 Ulcer pain

GASTRIC ULCER	DUODENAL ULCER
• Pain most commonly occurs 30 to 60 min after a meal	• Pain occurs 1.5 to 3 hr after a meal.
• Less often pain at night (30% to 40% of clients)	• Awakening with pain during the night
• Pain exacerbated by ingestion of food	• Pain relieved by ingestion of food or antacid
• Malnourishment	• Well-nourished
• Hematemesis	• Melena

PHYSICAL ASSESSMENT FINDINGS
- Pain or epigastric tenderness or abdominal distension
- Bloody emesis (hematemesis) or stools (melena)
- Weight loss

LABORATORY TESTS

H. pylori testing: Gastric samples are collected via an endoscopy to test for *H. pylori*.

Urea breath testing: The client exhales into a collection container (baseline), drinks carbon-enriched urea solution, and is asked to exhale into a collection container. The client should take nothing by mouth (NPO) prior to the test. If *H. pylori* is present, the solution will break down and carbon dioxide will be released. Serologic testing documents the presence of *H. pylori* based on antibody assays.

Stool sample tests for the presence of the *H. pylori* antigen.

Hemoglobin and hematocrit (unexpected findings secondary to bleeding)

Stool sample for occult blood

DIAGNOSTIC PROCEDURES

Esophagogastroduodenoscopy (EGD)

Refer to **CHAPTER 46: GASTROINTESTINAL DIAGNOSTIC PROCEDURES**. An EGD provides a definitive diagnosis of peptic ulcers and can be repeated to evaluate the effectiveness of treatment. Gastric samples are obtained to test for *H. pylori*.

NURSING ACTIONS: Monitor vital signs until sedation wears off. Keep client NPO until return of gag reflex. Monitor for manifestations of perforation: pain, bleeding, fever.

CLIENT EDUCATION: NPO 6 to 8 hr prior to the exam.

PATIENT-CENTERED CARE

NURSING CARE

- Instruct clients to avoid foods that cause distress (e.g., coffee, tea, carbonated beverages).
- Monitor for orthostatic changes in vital signs and tachycardia, as these findings are suggestive of gastrointestinal bleeding or perforation.
- Administer saline lavage via nasogastric tube.
- Administer medication as prescribed.
- Decrease environmental stress.
- Encourage rest periods.
- Encourage smoking cessation and avoiding alcohol consumption.
- Monitor laboratory results (e.g., hemoglobin, hematocrit, coagulation studies).

MEDICATIONS

Antibiotics

Metronidazole, amoxicillin, clarithromycin, and tetracycline eliminate *H. pylori* infection.

NURSING CONSIDERATIONS: A combination of two or three different antibiotics can be administered.

CLIENT EDUCATION: Instruct the client to complete a full course of medication.

Histamine$_2$-receptor antagonists

Ranitidine, famotidine, cimetidine, and nizatidine suppress the secretion of gastric acid by selectively blocking H$_2$ receptors in parietal cells lining the stomach.
- Used in conjunction with antibiotics to treat ulcers caused by *H. pylori*.
- Used to prevent stress ulcers in clients who are NPO after major surgery, have large areas of burns, are septic, or have increased intracranial pressure.

NURSING CONSIDERATIONS
- Ranitidine and famotidine can be administered IV in acute situations.
- Ranitidine can be taken with or without food.
- Treatment of peptic ulcer disease is usually started as an oral dose twice a day until the ulcer is healed, followed by a maintenance dose usually taken once a day at bedtime.

CLIENT EDUCATION
- Instruct clients to notify the provider of obvious or occult GI bleeding (coffee-ground emesis).
- Complete the prescribed regimen, even when symptoms subside.

Proton-pump inhibitors

Pantoprazole, esomeprazole, omeprazole, lansoprazole, and rabeprazole suppress gastric acid secretion by irreversibly inhibiting the enzyme that produces gastric acid, and inhibit basal and stimulated acid production.

NURSING CONSIDERATIONS
- Insignificant adverse effects with short-term treatment.
- Long-term use can increase the risk of fractures, pneumonia, acid rebound, and the possibility of developing *Clostridium difficile*.
- Rabeprazole and pantoprazole are enteric-coated tablets and should not be crushed.

CLIENT EDUCATION
- Instruct the client not to crush, chew, or break sustained-release capsules.
- Instruct the client to take omeprazole and lansoprazole once a day prior to eating the main meal of the day.
- Instruct the client to take rabeprazole after the morning meal.
- Encourage the client to avoid alcohol and irritating medications (NSAIDs).
- Complete the prescribed regimen, even when symptoms subside.

Antacids

- Aluminum hydroxide and magnesium hydroxide neutralize acid in the gut. The medication provides symptomatic relief but generally does not accelerate healing.
- Antacids can be given 7 times per day, 1 to 2 hr after meals and at bedtime, to neutralize gastric acid, which occurs with food ingestion.

NURSING CONSIDERATIONS

- Give 1 to 2 hr apart from other medications to avoid reducing the absorption of other medications.
- Monitor kidney function of clients prescribed aluminum hydroxide and magnesium hydroxide.

CLIENT EDUCATION

- Encourage compliance by reinforcing the intended effect of the antacid (relief of pain, promote healing of ulcer).
- Teach clients to take all medications at least 1 to 2 hr before or after taking an antacid.
- Avoid the use of flavored antacids, which delay emptying of the stomach.

Mucosal protectants

- Sucralfate coats the ulcer and protects it from the actions of pepsin and acid.
- Bismuth subsalicylate prevents *H. pylori* from binding to the mucosal wall.

NURSING CONSIDERATIONS

- Administer on an empty stomach 1 hr before meals and at bedtime.
- Oral suspension is easier for the older adult clients to ingest because the tablet form is large and difficult to swallow.
- Monitor for adverse effect of constipation.

CLIENT EDUCATION

- Clients taking bismuth subsalicylate should avoid aspirin products to avoid salicylate overdose.
- Clients taking bismuth subsalicylate can have black stools. This is temporary and harmless.

THERAPEUTIC PROCEDURES

Esophagogastroduodenoscopy (EGD)

Areas of bleeding can be treated with epinephrine or laser coagulation.

NURSING ACTIONS

- PREPROCEDURE: Initiate two large-bore IV catheters.
- POSTPROCEDURE: Monitor vital signs. Keep client NPO until gag reflex returns.

Surgical interventions

Can be used in clients when ulcers do not heal following 12 to 16 weeks of medical treatment, hemorrhage, perforation, or obstruction.

Gastrectomy: All or part of the stomach is removed with laparoscopic or open approach.
- **Antrectomy:** The antrum portion (lower portion of stomach) of the stomach is removed.
- **Gastrojejunostomy (Billroth II procedure):** The lower portion of the stomach is excised, the remaining stomach is anastomosed to the jejunum, and the remaining duodenum is surgically closed.

Vagotomy: The vagus nerve is cut to decrease gastric acid production in the stomach. Often done laparoscopically to reduce postoperative complications.

Pyloroplasty: The opening between the stomach and small intestine is enlarged to increase the rate of gastric emptying.

NURSING ACTIONS

- Monitor the incision for evidence of infection.
- Place the client in a semi-Fowler's position to facilitate lung expansion.
- Monitor nasogastric tube drainage. Scant blood can be seen in first 12 to 24 hr.
- Notify the provider before repositioning or irrigating the nasogastric tube (disruption of sutures). Qs
- Monitor bowel sounds.
- Advance diet as tolerated to avoid undesired effects (abdominal distention, diarrhea).
- Administer medication as prescribed (analgesics, stool softeners).

CLIENT EDUCATION

- Teach the client to take vitamin and mineral supplements due to decreased absorption after a gastrectomy, including vitamin B_{12}, vitamin D, calcium, iron, and folate.
- Tell the client to consume small, frequent meals while avoiding large quantities of carbohydrates as directed.

INTERPROFESSIONAL CARE

Nutrition consult: Diet that restricts acid-producing foods: milk products, caffeine, decaffeinated coffee, spicy foods, medications (NSAIDs)

COMPLICATIONS

Perforation/hemorrhage

When peptic ulcers perforate or bleed, it is an emergency situation.

- Perforation presents as severe epigastric pain spreading across the abdomen. The pain can radiate into the shoulders, especially the right shoulder due to irritation of the phrenic nerve. The abdomen can become tender and rigid (boardlike). Hyperactive to diminished bowel sounds can be auscultated, and there is rebound tenderness. The client will display symptoms of shock, hypotension, and tachycardia. Perforation is a surgical emergency.
- Gastrointestinal bleeding in the form of hematemesis or melena can cause manifestations of shock (hypotension, tachycardia, dizziness, confusion), and decreased hemoglobin.

NURSING ACTIONS

- Perform frequent assessments of pain and vital signs to detect subtle changes that can indicate perforation or bleeding. Qs
- Provide oxygen and ventilator support as needed.
- Start two large-bore IV lines for replacement of blood and fluids.
- Report findings, prepare the client for endoscopic or surgical intervention, replace fluid and blood losses to maintain blood pressure, insert nasogastric tube, and provide saline lavages.

Pernicious anemia

- Occurs due to a deficiency of the intrinsic factor normally secreted by the gastric mucosa.
- Manifestations include pallor, glossitis, fatigue, and paresthesias.

CLIENT EDUCATION: Lifelong monthly vitamin B_{12} injections will be necessary.

Dumping syndrome

This can occur following gastrectomy surgery, and is a group of manifestations that occur following eating. A shift of fluid to the abdomen is triggered by rapid gastric emptying or high-carbohydrate ingestion. The rapid release of metabolic peptides following ingestion of a food bolus causes dumping syndrome.

- The client can report a full sensation, weakness, diaphoresis, palpitations, dizziness, and diarrhea. Vasomotor symptoms that can occur 10 to 90 min following a meal are pallor, perspiration, palpitations, headache, feeling of warmth, dizziness, and drowsiness.
- Late symptoms of dumping syndrome can be related to the rapid release of blood glucose, followed by an increase in insulin production resulting in hypoglycemia.

NURSING ACTIONS

- Monitor for vasomotor manifestations.
- Assist/instruct the client to lie down when vasomotor manifestations occur.
- Administer medications.
  - Octreotide subcutaneously can be prescribed if manifestations are severe and not effectively controlled with dietary measures. Octreotide blocks gastric and pancreatic hormones, which can lead to findings of dumping syndrome.
  - Acarbose slows the absorption of carbohydrates.
- Malnutrition and fluid electrolyte imbalances can occur due to altered absorption. Monitor I&O, laboratory values, and weight.

49.2 Vasomotor manifestations

	EARLY MANIFESTATIONS	LATE MANIFESTATIONS
ONSET	Within 30 min after eating	1.5 to 3 hr after eating
CAUSE	Rapid emptying	Excessive insulin release
SYMPTOMS	Nausea, vomiting, sweating, and dizziness	Dizziness and sweating
		Tachycardia and palpitations
	Tachycardia	Shakiness and feelings of anxiety
	Palpitations	Confusion

CLIENT EDUCATION

- Lying down after a meal slows the movement of food within the intestines.
- Limit the amount of fluid ingested at one time.
- Eliminate liquids with meals, for 1 hr prior to, and following a meal.
- Consume a high-protein, high-fat, low-fiber, and low- to moderate-carbohydrate diet.
- Avoid milk and sugars (sweets, fruit juice, sweetened fruit, milk shakes, honey, syrup, jelly).
- Consume small, frequent meals rather than large meals.

Pyloric obstruction

- Pyloric obstruction occurs due to scarring, edema, or spasm of the area distal to the pyloric sphincter and prevents emptying of the stomach.
- Manifestations include feeling of fullness, distention, nausea after eating, and emesis consisting of undigested food.

NURSING ACTIONS

- Insert an NG tube for gastric decompression.
- Monitor fluid and electrolyte status.

Application Exercises

1. A nurse in the emergency department is completing an assessment of a client who has suspected stomach perforation due to a peptic ulcer. Which of the following findings should the nurse expect? (Select all that apply.)

   A. Rigid abdomen

   B. Tachycardia

   C. Elevated blood pressure

   D. Circumoral cyanosis

   E. Rebound tenderness

2. A nurse is teaching a client who has a new diagnosis of dumping syndrome following gastric surgery. Which of the following information should the nurse include in the teaching?

   A. Eat three moderate-sized meals a day.

   B. Drink at least one glass of water with each meal.

   C. Eat a bedtime snack that contains a milk product.

   D. Increase protein in the diet.

3. A nurse is completing discharge teaching for a client who has an infection due to *Helicobacter pylori (H. pylori)*. Which of the following statements by the client indicates understanding of the teaching?

   A. "I will continue my prescription for corticosteroids."

   B. "I will schedule a CT scan to monitor improvement."

   C. "I will take a combination of medications for treatment."

   D. "I will have my throat swabbed to recheck for this bacteria."

4. A nurse is completing an assessment of a client who has a gastric ulcer. Which of the following findings should the nurse expect? (Select all that apply.)

   A. Client reports pain relieved by eating.

   B. Client states that pain often occurs at night.

   C. Client reports a sensation of bloating.

   D. Client states that pain occurs 30 min to 1 hr after a meal.

   E. Client experiences pain upon palpation of the epigastric region.

5. A nurse is teaching a client who has a duodenal ulcer and a new prescription for esomeprazole. Which of the following information should the nurse include in the teaching? (Select all that apply.)

   A. Take the medication 1 hr before a meal.

   B. Limit NSAIDs when taking this medication.

   C. Expect skin flushing when taking this medication.

   D. Increase fiber intake when taking this medication.

   E. Chew the medication thoroughly before swallowing.

PRACTICE Active Learning Scenario

A nurse is preparing a poster about peptic ulcer disease to be displayed at a community health fair. What should be included in the poster? Use the ATI Active Learning Template: System Disorder to complete this item.

ALTERATION IN HEALTH (DIAGNOSIS): Include the types of ulcers.

HEALTH PROMOTION AND DISEASE PREVENTION: Describe at least three prevention activities.

RISK FACTORS: Describe four risk factors for peptic ulcers.

Application Exercises Key

1. A. **CORRECT:** Manifestations of perforation include a rigid, board-like abdomen.

   B. **CORRECT:** Tachycardia occurs due to gastrointestinal bleeding that accompanies a perforation.

   C. Hypotension is an expected finding in a client who has a perforation and bleeding.

   D. Circumoral cyanosis is not a manifestation of perforation.

   E. **CORRECT:** Rebound tenderness is an expected finding in a client who has a perforation.

   Ⓝ *NCLEX® Connection: Physiological Adaptation, Unexpected Response to Therapies*

2. A. The client should consume small, frequent meals rather than moderate-sized meals.

   B. The client should eliminate liquids with meals and for 1 hr prior to and following meals.

   C. The client should avoid milk products.

   D. **CORRECT:** The client should eat a high-protein, high-fat, low-fiber, and moderate- to low-carbohydrate diet.

   Ⓝ *NCLEX® Connection: Basic Care and Comfort, Nutrition and Oral Hydration*

3. A. Corticosteroid use is a contributing factor to an infection caused by *H. pylori*.

   B. An esophagogastroduodenoscopy is done to evaluate for the presence of *H. pylori* and to evaluate effectiveness of treatment.

   C. **CORRECT:** A combination of antibiotics and a histamine₂ receptor antagonist is used to treat an infection caused by *H. pylori*.

   D. *H. pylori* is evaluated by obtaining gastric samples, not a throat swab.

   Ⓝ *NCLEX® Connection: Physiological Adaptation, Alterations in Body Systems*

4. A. A client who has a duodenal ulcer will report that pain is relieved by eating.

   B. Pain that rarely occurs at night is an expected finding.

   C. **CORRECT:** A client report of a bloating sensation is an expected finding.

   D. **CORRECT:** A client who has a gastric ulcer will often report pain 30 to 60 min after a meal.

   E. **CORRECT:** Pain in the epigastric region upon palpation is an expected finding.

   Ⓝ *NCLEX® Connection: Physiological Adaptation, Pathophysiology*

5. A. **CORRECT:** The client is instructed to take the medication 1 hr before meals.

   B. **CORRECT:** The client is instructed to limit taking NSAIDs when on this medication.

   C. Skin flushing is not an adverse effect of this medication.

   D. Fiber intake does not need to be increased when taking this medication.

   E. The client is instructed to swallow the capsule whole. It should not be crushed or chewed.

   Ⓝ *NCLEX® Connection: Pharmacological and Parenteral Therapies, Medication Administration*

PRACTICE Answer

Using the ATI Active Learning Template: System Disorder

ALTERATION IN HEALTH (DIAGNOSIS):
An erosion of the mucosal lining of the stomach or duodenum. Mucous membranes can become eroded to the point that the epithelium is exposed to gastric acid and pepsin, which can precipitate bleeding and perforation. Types of ulcers include gastric, duodenal, and stress ulcers.

HEALTH PROMOTION AND DISEASE PREVENTION
- Drink alcohol in moderation.
- Stop smoking and use of tobacco products.
- Use stress management strategies.
- Avoid NSAIDs.
- Limit caffeine-containing beverages.

RISK FACTORS
- *Helicobacter pylori (H. pylori)*
- NSAID and corticosteroid use
- Severe stress
- Hypersecretory conditions
- Blood type O
- Excess alcohol ingestion
- Chronic pulmonary or kidney disease
- Zollinger-Ellison syndrome

Ⓝ *NCLEX® Connection: Health Promotion and Maintenance, Health Promotion/Disease Prevention*

CHAPTER 50   *Acute and Chronic Gastritis*

Cyclooxygenase (COX) is an enzyme that produces mucosal prostaglandins, decreases gastric acid, increases secretion of bicarbonate and cytoprotective mucus, and provides maintenance of submucosal blood flow to protect the gastric mucosa.

Gastritis is an inflammation in the lining of the stomach, either erosive or nonerosive, and can be acute or chronic.

TYPES OF GASTRITIS

Nonerosive gastritis (acute or chronic) is most often caused by an infection, *Helicobacter pylori*.

Erosive gastritis is likely caused by NSAIDs, alcohol use disorder, or recent radiation treatment.

Acute gastritis has sudden onset, is of short duration, and can result in gastric bleeding if severe. A severe form of acute gastritis is caused by the ingestion of an irritant, (such as a strong acid or alkali) and can result in the development of gangrenous tissue or perforation. Scarring can result leading to pyloric stenosis.

Chronic gastritis can be related to autoimmune disease, such as pernicious anemia, and *H. pylori*.

Extensive gastric mucosal wall damage can cause **erosive gastritis (ulcers)** and increase the risk of stomach cancer.

HEALTH PROMOTION AND DISEASE PREVENTION

- Assist in the reduction of anxiety related to gastritis.
- Follow a prescribed diet.
- Decrease or eliminate alcohol use.
- The client who has pernicious anemia will need vitamin B_{12} injections due to a decrease of the intrinsic factor by the stomach parietal cells.
- Watch for indications of GI bleeding.
- Follow the prescribed medication regimen.
- Eat small, frequent meals, avoiding foods and beverages that cause irritation.
- Report constipation, nausea, vomiting, or bloody stools.
- Stop smoking.

ASSESSMENT

RISK FACTORS

- Family member who has *H. pylori* infection
- Family history of gastritis
- Prolonged use of NSAIDs, corticosteroids (stops prostaglandin synthesis)
- Excessive alcohol use
- Bile reflux disease
- Advanced age
- Radiation therapy
- Smoking
- Caffeine
- Excessive stress
- Exposure to contaminated food or water

BACTERIAL INFECTION: *Helicobacter pylori*, *Salmonella*, *Streptococci*, *Staphylococci*, or *Escherichia coli*

AUTOIMMUNE DISEASES: Systemic lupus, rheumatoid arthritis, and pernicious anemia

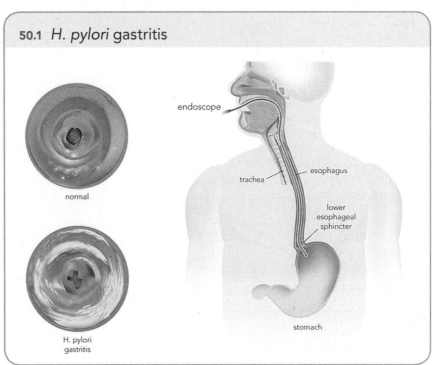

50.1 *H. pylori* gastritis

normal

H. pylori gastritis

endoscope

trachea

esophagus

lower esophageal sphincter

stomach

EXPECTED FINDINGS

PHYSICAL ASSESSMENT FINDINGS
- Dyspepsia, general abdominal discomfort, indigestion
- Headache
- Hiccupping that can last for a few hours to several days
- Upper abdominal pain or burning can increase or decrease after eating
- Nausea and vomiting
- Reduced appetite and weight loss
- Abdominal bloating or distention
- Hematemesis (bloody emesis) and stools that test positive for occult blood

> Manifestations can have rapid onset with acute gastritis.

Erosive gastritis
- Black, tarry stools; coffee-ground emesis
- Acute abdominal pain

LABORATORY TESTS

Noninvasive tests

CBC to check for anemia
- Women, Hgb less than 12 g/dL and RBC less than 4.2 cells/mcL
- Men, Hgb less than 14 g/dL and RBC less than 4.7 cells/mcL

Serum and stool antibody/antigen test for presence of *H. pylori*

C13 urea breath test: Used to measure *H. pylori*

DIAGNOSTIC PROCEDURES

Upper endoscopy

A small flexible scope is inserted through the mouth into the esophagus, stomach, and duodenum to visualize the upper digestive tract. This procedure allows for a biopsy, cauterization, removal of polyps, dilation, or diagnosis. (See **CHAPTER 46: GASTROINTESTINAL DIAGNOSTIC PROCEDURES**.)

CLIENT EDUCATION
- Instruct the client to maintain NPO status 6 to 8 hr prior to procedure.
- Advise the client to have a ride home available after the procedure.
- Inform the client that a local anesthetic will be sprayed onto the back of the throat, but throat can be sore following the procedure. Qs
- Instruct the client to monitor for indications of perforation (chest or abdominal pain, fever, nausea, vomiting, and abdominal distention) and have emergency contact numbers available.

PATIENT-CENTERED CARE

NURSING CARE
- Monitor fluid intake and urine output.
- Administer IV fluids as prescribed.
- Monitor electrolytes. (Diarrhea and vomiting can deplete electrolytes and cause dehydration.)
- Assist the client in identifying foods that are triggers.
- Provide small, frequent meals and encourage the client to eat slowly.
- Advise the client to avoid alcohol, caffeine, and foods that can cause gastric irritation.
- Assist the client in identifying ways to reduce stress.
- Monitor for indications of gastric bleeding (coffee-ground emesis; black, tarry stools).
- Monitor for findings of anemia (tachycardia, hypotension, fatigue, shortness of breath, pallor, feeling lightheaded or dizzy, chest pain).

MEDICATIONS

Histamine₂ antagonists

ACTION: Decreases gastric acid output by blocking gastric histamine$_2$ receptors

MEDICATIONS
- Nizatidine
- Famotidine
- Ranitidine
- Cimetidine

NURSING INTERVENTIONS
- Allow 1 hr before or after to administer antacid. Antacids can decrease the effectiveness of H$_2$ receptor antagonists.
- Monitor for neutropenia and hypotension.
- Dilute and administer slowly when given IV; rapid administration can cause bradycardia and hypotension.

CLIENT EDUCATION
- Advise clients not to smoke or drink alcohol.
- Advise clients to take oral dose with meals. Take famotidine 1 hr before meals to decrease heartburn, acid indigestion, and sour stomach.
- Advise clients to wait 1 hr prior to or following H$_2$ receptor antagonist to take an antacid.
- Advise clients to monitor for indications of GI bleeding (black stools, coffee-ground emesis).

Antacids

ACTION
- Increases gastric pH and neutralizes pepsin
- Improves mucosal protection

MEDICATIONS
- Aluminum hydroxide
- Magnesium hydroxide with aluminum hydroxide

NURSING INTERVENTIONS
- Do not give to clients who have acute kidney injury or chronic kidney failure.
- Monitor aluminum antacids for aluminum toxicity and constipation. Monitor magnesium antacids for diarrhea or hypermagnesemia.

CLIENT EDUCATION
- Advise clients to take antacids on an empty stomach.
- Advise clients to wait 1 hr to take other medications.

Proton pump inhibitors

ACTION: Reduces gastric acid by stopping the hydrogen/potassium ATPase enzyme system in parietal cells, blocking acid production

MEDICATIONS
- Omeprazole
- Lansoprazole
- Rabeprazole sodium
- Pantoprazole
- Esomeprazole

NURSING INTERVENTIONS
- Can cause nausea, vomiting, and abdominal pain.
- Use filter for IV administration for pantoprazole and lansoprazole. Qs

CLIENT EDUCATION
- Advise clients to allow 60 min before eating when taking esomeprazole.
- Do not to crush or chew if any of the medications are enteric-coated or sustained-release.
- It can take up to 4 days to see the effects.
- Advise clients to take medication with or without food according to the instructions.

Prostaglandins

ACTION: Replacement for endogenous prostaglandins that stimulates mucosal protection. Reduces gastric acid secretion.

MEDICATIONS: Misoprostol

NURSING INTERVENTIONS
- May be given with NSAIDs to prevent gastric mucosal damage.
- Can cause abdominal pain and diarrhea.

CLIENT EDUCATION
- Advise clients to use contraceptives.
- Advise clients not to take if there is a chance of becoming pregnant. Qs
- Advise clients to take with food to reduce gastric effects.

Anti-ulcer/mucosal barriers

ACTION: Inhibits acid and forms a protective coating over mucosa

MEDICATIONS: Sucralfate

NURSING INTERVENTIONS: Allow 30 min before or after to give antacid.

CLIENT EDUCATION
- Advise to take on an empty stomach.
- Advise not to smoke or drink alcohol.
- Advise to continue to take medication even if manifestations subside.

Antibiotics

ACTION: Eliminates *H. pylori* infection

MEDICATIONS
- Clarithromycin
- Amoxicillin
- Tetracycline
- Metronidazole

NURSING INTERVENTIONS
- Monitor for increased abdominal pain and diarrhea.
- Monitor electrolytes and hydration if fluid is depleted.
- Should be administered with meals to decrease GI upset.
- Use cautiously in clients who have kidney or hepatic impairment.

CLIENT EDUCATION
- Advise clients to complete prescribed dosage.
- Advise clients to notify the provider of persistent diarrhea, which can indicate superinfection of the bowel.

THERAPEUTIC PROCEDURES

Upper endoscopy: Surgery is prescribed for clients who have ulcerations or significant bleeding, or when nonsurgical interventions are ineffective. (See **CHAPTER 49: PEPTIC ULCER DISEASE.**)

Vagotomy or highly selective vagotomy: A highly selective vagotomy severs only the nerve fibers that control gastric acid secretion, and often is done laparoscopically to reduce postoperative complications. Pyloroplasty is usually done at the same time as the vagotomy.

Partial gastrectomy: Removal of the involved portion of the stomach.

INTERPROFESSIONAL CARE

- A nutritionist can assist in alterations to diet.
- Supportive care might be needed to reduce stress, increase exercise, and stop smoking. QTC

COMPLICATIONS

Gastric bleeding

CAUSES
- Severe acute gastritis with deep tissue inflammation extending into the stomach muscle.
- In chronic erosive gastritis, bleeding can be slow or profuse as in a perforation of the stomach wall.

NURSING ACTIONS
- Monitor vital signs and airway.
- Provide fluid replacement and blood products.
- Monitor CBC and clotting factors.
- Insert a nasogastric (NG) tube for gastric lavage (irrigate with normal saline or water to stop active gastric bleed) as indicated. Obtain an x-ray to confirm placement of NG tube prior to fluid instillation to prevent aspiration. Qᴇʙᴘ
- Monitor NG tube for absence or presence of blood, assess the amount of bleeding, and prevent gastric dilation.
- Administer IV medications (proton-pump inhibitors, H_2-receptor antagonists) as prescribed.

CLIENT EDUCATION: Instruct the client to monitor for indications of slow gastric bleeding (coffee-ground emesis; black, tarry stools). Seek immediate medical attention with severe abdominal pain or vomiting blood. Take medications as directed.

Gastric outlet obstruction

CAUSE: Severe acute gastritis with deep tissue inflammation extending into the stomach muscle

NURSING ACTIONS
- Monitor fluids and electrolytes because continuous vomiting results in loss of chloride (metabolic alkalosis) and severe fluid and electrolyte depletion.
- Provide fluid and electrolyte replacement. Monitor I&O.
- Prepare to insert a NG tube to empty stomach contents.
- Prepare for a diagnostic endoscopy.

CLIENT EDUCATION: Instruct the client to seek medical attention for continuous vomiting, bloating, and nausea.

Dehydration

CAUSE: Loss of fluid due to vomiting or diarrhea

NURSING ACTIONS
- Monitor fluid intake and urine output.
- Provide IV fluids if needed.
- Monitor electrolytes.

CLIENT EDUCATION: Instruct the client to contact a provider for vomiting and diarrhea.

Pernicious anemia

CAUSES
- Chronic gastritis can damage the parietal cells. This can lead to reduced production of intrinsic factor, which is necessary for the absorption of vitamin B_{12}.
- Insufficient vitamin B_{12} can lead to pernicious anemia.

NURSING ACTIONS: Instruct the client of the need for monthly vitamin B_{12} injections.

Dumping syndrome

CAUSES: The rapid release of metabolic peptides following the ingestion of a food bolus.

MANIFESTATIONS
- Early manifestations: Feeling of fullness, weakness, dizziness, palpitations, sweating, abdominal cramping, and diarrhea
- Manifestations resolve after having a bowel movement. However, late or residual vasomotor manifestations can occur 10 min to 3 hr after eating.

NURSING ACTIONS
- Instruct client to lay down following meals to slow movement of food through intestine and prevent injury. Qs
- Instruct the client to eat a high-protein, high-fat, low to moderate carbohydrate diet
- Instruct to eat small meals and limit taking liquids with meals.
- Instruct client on self-administration of octreotide subcutaneous injection two to three times daily before meals, as prescribed.

Application Exercises

1. A nurse is teaching about pernicious anemia with a client who has chronic gastritis. Which of the following information should the nurse include in the teaching?

   A. Pernicious anemia is caused when the cells producing gastric acid are damaged.

   B. Expect a monthly injection of vitamin B_{12}.

   C. Plan to take vitamin K supplements.

   D. Pernicious anemia is caused by an increased production of intrinsic factor.

2. A nurse is providing discharge teaching to a client who has a new prescription for aluminum hydroxide. Which of the following information should the nurse include in the teaching?

   A. Take the medication with food.

   B. Monitor for diarrhea.

   C. Wait 1 hr before taking other oral medications.

   D. Maintain a low-fiber diet.

3. A nurse is planning care for a client who has acute gastritis. Which of the following nursing interventions should the nurse include in the plan of care? (Select all that apply.)

   A. Evaluate intake and output.

   B. Monitor laboratory reports of electrolytes.

   C. Provide three large meals a day.

   D. Administer ibuprofen for pain.

   E. Observe stool characteristics.

4. A nurse is teaching a client who has a new prescription for famotidine. Which of the following statements by the client indicates understanding of the teaching?

   A. "The medicine coats the lining of my stomach."

   B. "The medication should stop the pain right away."

   C. "I will take my pill 1 hr before meals."

   D. "I will monitor for bleeding from my nose."

5. A charge nurse is teaching a group of unit nurses about a client who has chronic gastritis and is scheduled for a selective vagotomy. Which of the following statements by a unit nurse indicates understanding of the purpose of the procedure?

   A. "The client will have increased duodenal gastric emptying."

   B. "The client will have a reduction of gastric acid secretions."

   C. "The client will have an increase of gastric mucus secretion."

   D. "The client will have an increased secretion of hydrogen/potassium ATPase enzymes."

PRACTICE Active Learning Scenario

A nurse is reviewing acute and chronic gastritis with a group of clients. What should the nurse include in this discussion? Use the ATI Active Learning Template: System Disorder to complete this item.

ALTERATION IN HEALTH (DIAGNOSIS)
- Describe gastritis.
- Compare/contrast acute vs. chronic gastritis.

PATHOPHYSIOLOGY RELATED TO CLIENT
PROBLEM: Describe as related to client problem.

RISK FACTORS: Describe six.

Application Exercises Key

1. A. Damage to parietal cells has occurred, which leads to pernicious anemia and causes a decrease of the intrinsic factor by the stomach parietal cells.

   B. **CORRECT:** The nurse should include in the information that the client will receive a monthly injection of vitamin B_{12} to treat pernicious anemia due to a decrease of the intrinsic factor by the stomach parietal cells.

   C. Vitamin K supplements are given to clients who have a bleeding disorder.

   D. Parietal cell damage results in insufficient production of intrinsic factor by the stomach parietal cells.

   Ⓝ *NCLEX® Connection: Physiological Adaptation, Alterations in Body Systems*

2. A. The nurse should advise the client to take aluminum hydroxide on an empty stomach.

   B. The nurse should include in the teaching that aluminum hydroxide can cause constipation.

   C. **CORRECT:** The nurse should advise the client not to take oral medications within 1 hr of an antacid.

   D. The nurse should include in the teaching for the client to increase dietary fiber due to the constipating effect of the medication.

   Ⓝ *NCLEX® Connection: Pharmacological and Parenteral Therapies, Medication Administration*

3. A. **CORRECT:** The nurse should evaluate the client's intake and output to prevent electrolyte loss and dehydration.

   B. **CORRECT:** The nurse should monitor the client's electrolyte laboratory values to prevent fluid loss and dehydration.

   C. The nurse should instruct the client to eat small, frequent meals.

   D. The nurse should instruct the client to avoid taking ibuprofen, an NSAID, because of its erosive capabilities.

   E. **CORRECT:** The nurse should instruct the client to report to the provider any indication of the presence of blood in the stools, which can indicate gastrointestinal bleeding.

   Ⓝ *NCLEX® Connection: Physiological Adaptation, Illness Management*

4. A. Famotidine decreases gastric acid output. It does not have a protective coating action.

   B. The client might need to take famotidine for several days before pain relief occurs when starting this therapy.

   C. **CORRECT:** The client should take famotidine 1 hr before meals to decrease heartburn, acid indigestion, and sour stomach.

   D. The nurse should instruct the client to monitor for GI bleeding when taking famotidine.

   Ⓝ *NCLEX® Connection: Pharmacological and Parenteral Therapies, Medication Administration*

5. A. Pyloroplasty will increase gastric emptying, which is performed to widen the opening from the stomach to the duodenum.

   B. **CORRECT:** Selective vagotomy will reduce gastric acid secretions.

   C. Prostaglandin analog medication will stimulate mucosal protection and decrease gastric acid secretions.

   D. A histamine₂ antagonist medication will inhibit gastric secretion by inhibiting hydrogen/potassium ATPase enzyme system in the gastric parietal cells.

   Ⓝ *NCLEX® Connection: Physiological Adaptation, Alterations in Body Systems*

PRACTICE Answer

Using the ATI Active Learning Template: System Disorder

ALTERATION IN HEALTH (DIAGNOSIS): Gastritis is an inflammation of the lining of the stomach as a result of irritation to the mucosa.
- Acute: Sudden onset, short duration, can result in gastric bleeding.
- Chronic: Slow onset; when profuse, it can damage parietal cells, resulting in pernicious anemia.

PATHOPHYSIOLOGY RELATED TO CLIENT PROBLEM: Gastric acid overwhelms the production of COX 1 enzymes, which provide mucosal prostaglandins that line the stomach. This results in an erosion of the mucosa and increases the risk for ulcers and stomach cancer.

RISK FACTORS
- Bacterial infection (*H. pylori, Salmonella, Streptococci, Staphylococci, E. coli*)
- Family history of *H. pylori*
- Prolonged use of NSAIDs or corticosteroids
- Excessive alcohol use
- Bile reflux disease
- Autoimmune diseases
- Advanced age
- Radiation therapy
- Smoking
- Caffeine
- Excessive stress
- Exposure to contaminated food or water

Ⓝ *NCLEX® Connection: Physiological Adaptation, Alterations in Body Systems*

CHAPTER 51 ## Noninflammatory Bowel Disorders

Noninflammatory bowel disorders can cause pain, changes in bowel pattern, bleeding, and malabsorption. This group of disorders includes hemorrhoids, cancer, hernia, irritable bowel syndrome (IBS), and intestinal obstruction.

Hemorrhoids are distended or edematous intestinal veins resulting from increased intra-abdominal pressure (straining, obesity, prolonged sitting or standing, constipation, weight lifting). Pregnancy increases the risk of hemorrhoids.

Cancer of the small or large intestine can be caused by age-related changes (older than 50 is a greater risk), genetic influence, or chronic bowel disease, such as Crohn's disease or ulcerative colitis.

Nurses should be knowledgeable about noninflammatory bowel disorders and treatments. Topics to be reviewed include hernia, irritable bowel syndrome, and intestinal obstruction.

Hernia

Bowel herniation is the displacement of the bowel through a weakness of the abdominal muscle into other areas of the abdominal cavity.

Incisional hernias can occur as a postsurgical complication due to inadequate healing of the incisional site from malnutrition, infection, or obesity.

A hernia that cannot be moved back into place with gentle palpation is considered irreducible and requires immediate surgical evaluation.

In a hernia that is strangulated, blood supply is cut off to a portion of the bowel, increasing the risk for obstruction, necrosis, and perforation. Findings include abdominal distention, tachycardia, vomiting, and abdominal pain. Surgical intervention is necessary.

ASSESSMENT

RISK FACTORS

- Male sex (indirect inguinal hernia can be large and descend into the scrotum)
- Advanced age (direct hernia) Ⓖ
- Increased intra-abdominal pressure due to pregnancy or obesity (femoral, adult-acquired umbilical hernia)
- Genetics (congenital umbilical hernia)

EXPECTED FINDINGS

Protrusion or lump at involved site (groin area, umbilicus, healed incision)

51.1 Hernia

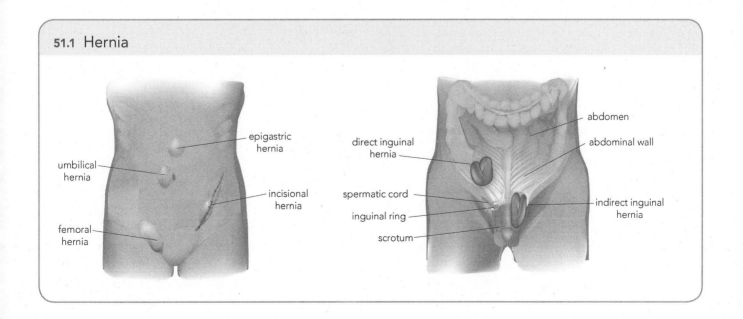

PATIENT-CENTERED CARE

NURSING ACTIONS: If the hernia does not require surgery, instruct the client to wear a truss pad with hernia belt during waking hours to prevent the abdominal contents from bulging into the hernia sac. Inspect skin under the pad daily.

POSTOPERATIVE CLIENT EDUCATION

- Instruct the client to avoid increased intra-abdominal pressure for 2 to 3 weeks (avoid coughing, straining, and lifting objects greater than 10 lb).
- Instruct the client to apply ice as prescribed and inspect and report redness or swelling at the incisional site.
- Instruct the client to prevent constipation by increasing dietary fiber and fluids.
- Instruct the client to rest for several days and return to work when recommended by the surgeon, usually 1 to 2 weeks postoperatively.

Irritable bowel syndrome

IBS is a disorder of the gastrointestinal system that causes changes in bowel function (chronic diarrhea, constipation, bloating, and/or abdominal pain).

- The etiology of IBS is uncertain, but it is thought that environmental, immunological, genetic, hormonal, and stress influence the development and course of the disease. Food intolerances worsen the manifestations.
- **Environmental factors:** Dairy products, caffeinated beverages, infectious agents
- **Immunological factors:** Cytokine genes (pro-inflammatory interleukins), tumor necrosis factor (TNF) alpha
- **Stress-related factors:** Anxiety, depression

HEALTH PROMOTION AND DISEASE PREVENTION

- Avoid foods that trigger exacerbation, such as dairy, wheat, corn, fried foods, alcohol, spicy foods, and aspartame.
- Avoid alcoholic and caffeinated beverages, and other fluids containing fructose and sorbitol.
- Consume 2 to 3 L fluid per day from food and fluid sources.
- Increase fiber intake (approximately 30 to 40 g/day).

ASSESSMENT

RISK FACTORS

- Female sex
- Stress
- Eating large meals containing a large amount of fat
- Caffeine intake
- Alcohol intake

EXPECTED FINDINGS

- Cramping pain in abdomen
- Abdominal pain (left lower quadrant) due to changes in bowel pattern and consistency
- Nausea with meals or passing stool
- Anorexia
- Abdominal bloating
- Belching
- Diarrhea (diarrhea-predominant IBS)
- Constipation (constipation-predominant IBS)
- Hyperactive or hypoactive bowel sounds

LABORATORY TESTS

CBC, serum albumin, erythrocyte sedimentation rate (ESR), and occult stools are all typically within the expected reference range.

DIAGNOSTIC TESTS

- IBS is difficult to diagnose with specific tests and is usually based on the presence of specific characteristic, including abdominal pain accompanied by changes in bowel patterns, abdominal distention, feeling that defecation is not complete, and presence of mucus with stools.
- Other criteria can include recurrent abdominal pain for 3 days during a month in the past 3 months, and two or more of the following.
  - Improvement when the client moves his or her bowels
  - Onset when there is a change in frequency of stools
  - Onset when there is a change in appearance of stools

Hydrogen breath test

The client is asked to exhale into a hydrogen analyzer before and after ingesting test sugar. Positive test results indicate excess hydrogen in the bloodstream from bacterial overgrowth or malabsorption.

CLIENT EDUCATION: Instruct client to remain NPO at least 12 hr prior to test, except for sips of water.

PATIENT-CENTERED CARE

NURSING CARE

- Review strategies to reduce stress.
- Instruct the client to limit the intake of irritating agents (gas-forming foods, caffeine, alcohol).
- Encourage a diet high in fiber and fluids.
- Instruct client to keep a food diary to record intake and bowel patterns (to adjust diet to prevent exacerbations).

MEDICATIONS

Diarrhea-predominant IBS (IBS-D)

Loperamide
- Decreases peristalsis and increases bulk.
- Can cause drowsiness.
- Discontinue if no response after 48 hr.

Psyllium
- Bulk-forming laxative.
- Discontinue for abdominal cramping, rectal bleeding, and vomiting.
- Monitor for electrolyte imbalance.

Alosetron
- An IBS-specific medication that selectively blocks 5-HT3 receptors that innervate the viscera. The expected result is increased firmness in stools, and decreased urgency and frequency of defecation.
- Indicated for IBS-D in women that has lasted more than 6 months and is resistant to conventional management. Use with caution in women and only as a last resort.

NURSING CONSIDERATIONS: Contraindicated for clients who have a history of bowel obstruction, Crohn's disease, ulcerative colitis, impaired intestinal circulation, or thrombophlebitis.

CLIENT EDUCATION
- Instruct the client that manifestations should resolve within 1 to 4 weeks. Discontinue medication after 4 weeks if manifestations persist.
- The client should avoid concurrent use of psychoactive drugs and antihistamines.
- Instruct the client to report constipation, fever, increasing abdominal pain, fatigue, dark urine, bloody urine, or rectal bleeding immediately because alosetron can cause ischemic colitis. Discontinue medication if these manifestations occur. Qs

Constipation-predominant IBS (IBS-C)

Lubiprostone: An IBS-specific medication that increases fluid secretion in the intestine to promote intestinal motility. This is indicated for IBS-C in women.
- NURSING CONSIDERATIONS
  - Contraindicated for clients who have known or possible bowel obstruction.
  - Not effective for treatment of men who have IBS.
- CLIENT EDUCATION: Instruct the client to take with food and water.

Linaclotide
- Increases fluid and motility in the intestine
- Can relieve pain and cramps
- CLIENT EDUCATION: Instruct the client to take daily about 30 min before breakfast.

Intestinal obstruction

Intestinal obstruction can result from mechanical or nonmechanical causes. Manifestations vary according to type.
- Mechanical obstruction occurs when the bowel is blocked by something outside or inside the intestines (e.g., adhesions, tumors, hernias, fecal impactions, strictures due to Crohn's disease, and diverticulitis). Complete mechanical obstructions should be addressed surgically.
- Non-mechanical obstructions are caused by diminished peristalsis within the bowel (paralytic ileus). This can occur postoperatively due to the handling of the intestines during surgery.
- Treatment focuses on fluid and electrolyte balance, decompressing the bowel, and relief/removal of the obstruction.

ASSESSMENT

RISK FACTORS

Mechanical obstructions

Result from the following.
- Encirclement or compression of intestine by adhesions, tumors, fibrosis (endometriosis), or strictures (Crohn's disease, radiation)
  - Postsurgical adhesions are often the cause of small bowel obstructions.
  - Carcinomas are often the cause of large intestine obstructions.
  - OLDER ADULT CLIENTS: Diverticulitis, fecal impaction, and tumors are common causes of obstruction. Bowel regimens can be effective in preventing impactions. Ⓖ
- Hernia (bowel becomes trapped in weakened area of abdominal wall) **(51.1)**
- Volvulus (twisting) or intussusception (telescoping) of bowel segments **(51.3)**

Nonmechanical obstructions

- Nonmechanical obstructions (paralytic ileus) result from decreased peristalsis secondary to the following.
  - Neurogenic disorders (manipulation of the bowel during major surgery and spinal fracture)
  - Vascular disorders (vascular insufficiency and mesenteric emboli)
  - Electrolyte imbalances (hypokalemia)
  - Inflammatory responses (peritonitis or sepsis)
- Manifestations of nonmechanical obstructions include diffuse, constant pain; significant abdominal distention; and frequent vomiting.

EXPECTED FINDINGS

Manifestations vary depending on the location of the obstruction.

Small bowel and large intestine obstructions

- Obstipation: the inability to pass a stool and/or flatus for more than 8 hr despite feeling the urge to defecate
- Abdominal distention
- High-pitched bowel sounds above site of obstruction (borborygmi) with hypoactive bowel sounds below, or overall hypoactive; absent bowel sounds later in process

Small bowel obstructions

- Severe fluid and electrolyte imbalance
- Metabolic alkalosis
- Visible peristaltic waves (possible)
- Epigastric or upper abdominal distention
- Abdominal pain, discomfort
- Profuse, sudden projectile vomiting with fecal odor

Large intestine obstructions

- Minor fluid and electrolyte imbalance
- Metabolic acidosis (possible)
- Significant lower abdominal distention
- Intermittent abdominal cramping
- Infrequent vomiting
- Diarrhea or ribbon-like stools around an impaction

LABORATORY TESTS

- Increased hemoglobin, BUN, creatinine, and hematocrit can indicate dehydration.
- Increased serum amylase and WBC count can occur with strangulating obstructions.
- Arterial blood gases (ABGs) indicate metabolic imbalance, depending on obstruction type.
- Chemistry profiles reveal decreased sodium, chloride, and potassium.

DIAGNOSTIC PROCEDURES

X-ray: Flat plate and upright abdominal x-rays evaluate the presence of free air and gas patterns.

Endoscopy determines the cause of obstruction.

CT scan determines the cause and exact location of the obstruction.

PATIENT-CENTERED CARE

NURSING CARE

Nonmechanical cause of obstruction

- Nothing by mouth with bowel rest.
- Assess bowel sounds.
- Provide oral hygiene.
- Administer IV fluid and electrolyte replacement (particularly potassium).
- Manage pain (once diagnosis identified).
- Encourage ambulation.
- Place in semi-Fowler's position.

Mechanical cause of obstruction

- Prepare for surgery and provide preoperative nursing care.
- Withhold intake until peristalsis resumes.

MEDICATIONS

Prokinetics to promote gastric motility (octreotide) in paralytic ileus or partial obstruction.

Broad-spectrum antibiotics, especially with suspected bowel strangulation.

THERAPEUTIC PROCEDURES

Nasogastric (NG) tube with a vent (to prevent damage to the stomach mucosa during continuous suctioning) is inserted to decompress the bowel.

NURSING ACTIONS
- Maintain intermittent suction as prescribed.
- Assess NG tube patency and placement. Irrigate every 4 hr, or as prescribed.
- Monitor and assess gastric output.
- Monitor nasal area for skin breakdown.
- Provide oral hygiene every 2 hr.
- Monitor vital signs, skin integrity, weight, and I&O.

51.2 Bowel intussusception

colon

intussusceptum

ileum

cecum

Surgical interventions

Procedure varies based on cause of obstruction. Can include lysis of adhesions, colon resection, colostomy creation (temporary or permanent), embolectomy, thrombectomy, resection of gangrenous intestinal tissue, or complete colectomy

Exploratory laparotomy

To determine the cause of obstruction and rectify if possible.

NURSING ACTIONS
- Ensure the client understands the type of procedure (open or laparoscopic).
- Monitor for hemodynamic instability.
- Administer IV fluid replacement and maintenance as prescribed.
- Monitor bowel sounds.
- Maintain NG tube patency and measure output.
- Clamp NG tube as prescribed to assess the client's tolerance prior to removal.
- Advance diet as tolerated when prescribed, beginning with clear liquids. Clamp tube after eating for 1 to 2 hr.
- Instruct client to report intolerance of intake following NG tube removal (nausea, vomiting, increasing distention).

COMPLICATIONS

Dehydration (small bowel obstruction)

CAUSE: Persistent vomiting

NURSING ACTIONS
- Assess hydration through evaluation of hematocrit, BUN, orthostatic vital signs, skin turgor/mucous membranes, urine output, and specific gravity. Notify the provider of a fluid imbalance.
- Administer IV fluids as prescribed.

Electrolyte imbalance (small bowel obstruction)

CAUSE: Persistent vomiting

NURSING ACTIONS
- Monitor electrolytes, especially potassium levels. Qs
- Notify the provider of an electrolyte imbalance.
- Administer IV fluids as prescribed to replace electrolytes.

Metabolic alkalosis (small intestinal obstruction)

CAUSE: Persistent vomiting, leading to a loss of gastric hydrochloride.

NURSING ACTIONS
- Monitor for hypoventilation (confusion, hypercarbia), which is a compensatory action by the lungs.
- Obtain arterial blood gas.
- Notify the provider of unexpected laboratory findings.
- Replace fluid and electrolytes as prescribed.
- Provide oral hygiene to alleviate increased thirst response. Thirst response is decreased in the older adult. Provide oral hygiene routinely to ensure maintenance of moist mucous membranes. Ⓒ

Metabolic acidosis (large bowel obstructions)

CAUSE: A lower level obstruction

NURSING ACTIONS
- Monitor for deep, rapid respirations (compensatory action by the lungs), confusion, hypotension, and flushed skin.
- Obtain arterial blood gas.
- Notify the provider of unexpected laboratory findings.

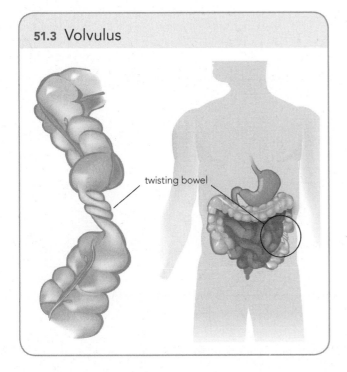

51.3 Volvulus

twisting bowel

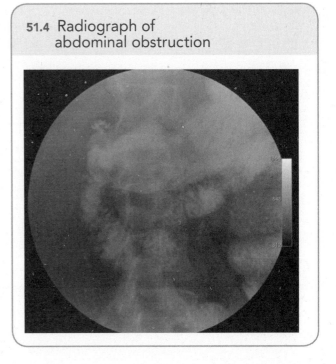

51.4 Radiograph of abdominal obstruction

Application Exercises

1. A nurse is completing an admission assessment for a client who has a small bowel obstruction. Which of the following findings should the nurse report to the provider? (Select all that apply.)

   A. Emesis prior to insertion of the nasogastric tube

   B. Urine specific gravity 1.040

   C. Hematocrit 60%

   D. Serum potassium 3.0 mEq/L

   E. WBC 10,000/uL

2. A nurse is planning care for a client who has a small bowel instruction and a nasogastric (NG) tube in place. Which of the following interventions should the nurse include in the plan of care? (Select all that apply.)

   A. Document the NG drainage with the client's output.

   B. Irrigate the NG tube every 8 hr.

   C. Assess bowel sounds.

   D. Provide oral hygiene every 2 hr.

   E. Monitor NG tube for placement.

3. A nurse is caring for a client who has a small bowel obstruction from adhesions. Which of the following findings are consistent with this diagnosis? (Select all that apply.)

   A. Emesis greater than 500 mL with a fecal odor

   B. Report of spasmodic abdominal pain

   C. High-pitched bowel sounds

   D. Abdomen flat with rebound tenderness to palpation

   E. Laboratory findings indicating metabolic acidosis

4. A nurse is assessing an older adult client in an extended care facility. The nurse should recognize which of the following findings is a manifestation of an obstruction of the large intestine due to a fecal impaction?

   A. The client reports he had a bowel movement yesterday.

   B. The client is having small, frequent liquid stools.

   C. The client is flatulent.

   D. The client indicates he vomited once this morning.

5. A nurse is completing discharge teaching with a client who has irritable bowel syndrome (IBS). Which of the following instructions should the nurse include in the teaching?

   A. Avoid foods that trigger exacerbation.

   B. Consume 15 to 20 g of fiber daily.

   C. Plan three moderate to large meals per day.

   D. Limit fluid intake to 1L each day.

PRACTICE Active Learning Scenario

A nurse is preparing a poster on caring for a client who has a bowel obstruction. What information should the nurse include on the poster? Use the ATI Active Learning Template: System Disorder to complete this item.

RISK FACTORS: Identify at least two for each form of obstruction.

EXPECTED FINDINGS: Compare and contrast the types of obstructions.

DIAGNOSTIC PROCEDURES: Identify at least two.

Application Exercises Key

1. A. Profuse emesis is an expected finding for a client who has a small bowel obstruction. The nurse does not need to report this finding to the provider.

   B. **CORRECT:** This urine specific gravity is greater than the expected reference range of 1.005 to 1.030. An increased urine specific gravity is an indication of dehydration. The nurse should report this finding to the provider.

   C. **CORRECT:** The Hct is greater than the expected reference range of 42% to 52% for men and 37% to 47% for women. An elevated HCT indicates hemoconcentration, which is due to dehydration.

   D. **CORRECT:** This serum potassium is below the expected reference range of 3.5 to 5.0 mEq/L caused by potassium loss from vomiting. Hypokalemia can cause dysrhythmias, muscle weakness, and lethargy, and requires potassium replacement. The nurse should report this finding to the provider

   E. This WBC is within the expected reference range of 5,000 to 10,000/mm³. The nurse does not need to report this finding to the provider.

   (N) *NCLEX® Connection: Reduction of Risk Potential, Laboratory Values*

2. A. **CORRECT:** The nurse should document the NG drainage as output. This helps determine the amount of fluid replacement needed.

   B. The NG tube is irrigated every 4 hr to maintain patency.

   C. **CORRECT:** Bowel sounds should be assessed to evaluate treatment and resolution of the obstruction.

   D. **CORRECT:** An NG tube promotes mouth breathing. The nurse should provide frequent oral hygiene to provide comfort.

   E. **CORRECT:** The nurse should check the placement of the NG tube prior to irrigation to prevent aspiration and periodically to prevent an increase in abdominal distention.

   (N) *NCLEX® Connection: Reduction of Risk Potential, Therapeutic Procedures*

3. A. **CORRECT:** Large emesis with a fecal odor is a finding in a client who has a small bowel obstruction.

   B. **CORRECT:** Report of abdominal pain is a finding in a client who has a small bowel obstruction.

   C. **CORRECT:** High-pitched bowel sounds are a manifestation of a small- or large-bowel obstruction.

   D. Abdominal distention is a finding in a client who has a small bowel obstruction.

   E. Metabolic alkalosis due to the loss of gastric acid is a finding in a client who has a small bowel obstruction.

   (N) *NCLEX® Connection: Physiological Adaptation, Pathophysiology*

4. A. A report of a bowel movement yesterday does not indicate a mechanical obstruction of the large intestine due to a fecal impaction.

   B. **CORRECT:** Small, frequent liquid stools can be passed around a fecal impaction. Other manifestations include constipation and rectal pain.

   C. The presence of flatus does not indicate a mechanical obstruction of the large intestine due to a fecal impaction.

   D. A report of a single episode of vomiting does not indicate a mechanical obstruction of the large intestine due to a fecal impaction. Frequent vomiting is a manifestation of a small-bowel obstruction.

   (N) *NCLEX® Connection: Physiological Adaptation, Pathophysiology*

5. A. **CORRECT:** The client should eliminate foods that trigger exacerbation.

   B. A client who has IBS should increase daily fiber intake to 30 to 40 g.

   C. A client who has IBS should eat small frequent meals.

   D. A client who has IBS should drink 2 to 3 L fluids per day to promote a consistent bowel pattern.

   (N) *NCLEX® Connection: Basic Care and Comfort, Nutrition and Oral Hydration*

PRACTICE Answer

Using the ATI Active Learning Template: System Disorder

RISK FACTORS
- Mechanical
  - Encirclement or compression of intestines by adhesions, tumors, fibrosis, or strictures
  - Volvulus, intussusception
  - Hernia, fecal impaction
- Nonmechanical: decreased peristalsis due to neurogenic or vascular disorders, electrolyte imbalances, and inflammatory responses
  - Small bowel: postsurgical adhesions
  - Large bowel: carcinoma

EXPECTED FINDINGS
- Mechanical: mild, colicky, intermittent pain
- Nonmechanical: vague, diffuse, constant pain; significant abdominal distention
  - Small bowel obstruction
    - Visible peristaltic waves possible
    - Profuse, sudden projectile vomiting with fecal odor, which relieves pain
    - Severe fluid and electrolyte imbalance, metabolic alkalosis
  - Large bowel obstruction
    - Significant abdominal distention, infrequent vomiting, diarrhea or "ribbon-like" stools around an impaction, minor fluid and electrolyte imbalance, metabolic acidosis (possible)
    - Bowel sounds: hyperactive above and hypoactive below the obstruction, inability to pass a stool, and/or flatus for more than 8 hr despite urge to defecate

DIAGNOSTIC PROCEDURES
- X-rays (flat plate, upright abdominal)
- Endoscopy
- CT scan

(N) *NCLEX® Connection: Physiological Adaptation, Alterations in Body Systems*

CHAPTER 52 *Inflammatory Bowel Disease*

Inflammatory bowel disease (IBD) can affect structures or segments along the gastrointestinal tract. The term includes both acute and chronic disorders.

Acute and chronic IBD can result in nutritional deficits, altered bowel elimination, infection, pain, and fluid or electrolyte imbalances. The nurse needs to be knowledgeable about acute and chronic IBD in order to collaborate with the client and the interprofessional team in treating and managing these disorders.

ACUTE INFLAMMATORY BOWEL DISEASE

Appendicitis

Inflammation of the appendix
- Caused by an obstruction of the lumen or opening of the appendix.
- Fecaliths, or hard pieces of stool, can be the initial cause of the obstruction.
- Adolescents and young adults are at increased risk.
- Refer to the **NURSING CARE OF CHILDREN REVIEW MODULE, CHAPTER 23: GASTROINTESTINAL STRUCTURAL AND INFLAMMATORY DISORDERS**.

Peritonitis

Inflammation of the peritoneum
- Results from infection of the peritoneum due to puncture (surgery or trauma), septicemia, or rupture of part of the gastrointestinal tract.
- This can lead to septicemia, and is a life-threatening event.

Gastroenteritis

Inflammation of the stomach and small intestine
- Triggered by infection (either bacterial or viral).
- Vomiting and frequent, watery stools place the client at increased risk for fluid and electrolyte imbalance and impaired nutrition.

CHRONIC INFLAMMATORY BOWEL DISEASE

Ulcerative colitis and Crohn's disease are characterized by frequent stools, crampy abdominal pain, exacerbations, and remissions.

Ulcerative colitis

Edema and inflammation primarily in the rectum and rectosigmoid colon.
- In severe cases, it can involve the entire length of the colon. Mucosa and submucosa become hyperemic (increase in blood flow), and the colon will become edematous and reddened. It can lead to abscess formation.
- Edema and thickened bowel mucosa can cause partial bowel obstruction. Intestinal mucosal cell changes can lead to colon cancer or insufficient production of intrinsic factor, resulting in insufficient absorption of vitamin B_{12} (pernicious anemia).
- Classified as either mild, moderate, severe, and fulminant

Crohn's disease

Inflammation and ulceration of the gastrointestinal tract, often at the distal ileum.
- All bowel layers can become involved; lesions are sporadic. Fistulas are common.
- Can involve the entire GI tract from the mouth to the anus.
- Malabsorption and malnutrition can develop when the jejunum and ileum become involved. Requires supplemental vitamins and minerals, possibly including vitamin B_{12} injections.

Diverticulitis

Diverticulitis is inflammation and infection of the bowel mucosa caused by bacteria, food, or fecal matter trapped in one or more diverticula (pouch-like herniations in the intestinal wall). Diverticulitis is not to be confused with diverticulosis, which is the presence of many small diverticula in the colon without inflammation.
- Not all clients who have diverticulosis develop diverticulitis.
- Diverticula can perforate and cause peritonitis, and or severe bleeding.

ASSESSMENT

Etiology of ulcerative colitis and Crohn's disease is unknown but possibly due to a combination of genetic, environmental, and immunological causes.

RISK FACTORS

Genetics: Ulcerative colitis and Crohn's disease

Culture: Caucasians (ulcerative colitis), Jewish heritage (ulcerative colitis and Crohn's disease), and African Americans (diverticular disease)

Gender and age: The incidence of ulcerative colitis peaks at adolescence to young adulthood (more often in females) and older adulthood (more often in males). Crohn's disease usually develops in adolescents and young adults, but can occur at any age. Diverticulitis occurs more often in older adults and affects men more frequently than women. ©

Tobacco use: Crohn's disease

EXPECTED FINDINGS

Ulcerative colitis

- Abdominal pain/cramping: often left-lower quadrant pain
- Anorexia and weight loss

PHYSICAL ASSESSMENT FINDINGS
- Fever
- Diarrhea: up to 15 to 20 liquid stools/day
- Stools can contain mucus, blood, or pus.
- Abdominal distention, tenderness, and/or firmness upon palpation
- High-pitched bowel sounds
- Rectal bleeding

Crohn's disease

- Abdominal pain/cramping: often right-lower quadrant pain
- Anorexia and weight loss

PHYSICAL ASSESSMENT FINDINGS
- Fever
- Diarrhea: five loose stools/day with mucus or pus
- Abdominal distention, tenderness and/or firmness upon palpation
- High-pitched bowel sounds
- Steatorrhea

Diverticulitis

- Acute onset of abdominal pain often in left-lower quadrant
- Nausea and vomiting

PHYSICAL ASSESSMENT FINDINGS
- Fever
- Chills
- Tachycardia

LABORATORY TESTS

Ulcerative colitis

Hematocrit and hemoglobin: Decreased

Erythrocyte sedimentation rate (ESR): Increased

WBC: Increased

C-reactive protein: Increased

Serum albumin: Decreased

Stool for occult blood: Can be positive

K+, Mg, and Ca: Decreased

Crohn's disease

Hematocrit and hemoglobin: Decreased

ESR: Increased

WBC: Increased

C-reactive protein: Increased

Serum albumin: Decreased

Folic acid and B$_{12}$: Decreased

Anti-glycan antibodies: Increased

Stool for occult blood: Can be positive

Urinalysis: WBC

K+, Mg, and Ca: Decreased

Diverticulitis

Hematocrit and hemoglobin: Decreased

ESR: Increased

WBC: Increased

Stool for occult blood: Can be positive

DIAGNOSTIC PROCEDURES

Magnetic resonance enterography: Used with all IBD

CLIENT EDUCATION: Instruct clients to maintain NPO for 4 to 6 hr prior to the exam, and they will need to drink a contrast medium.

Ulcerative colitis

Sigmoidoscopy or colonoscopy: Can diagnose ulcerative colitis.

Barium enema: Helpful to distinguish ulcerative colitis from other disease processes.

CT scan or MRI: Can identify the presence of abscesses.

Stool examination: For the presence of parasites or microbes.

Crohn's disease

Endoscopy
- Newer diagnostic tools such as video capsule endoscopy are being used.
- **Proctosigmoidoscopy**: Performed to identify inflamed tissue.
- **Colonoscopy and sigmoidoscopy**: A lighted, flexible scope is inserted into the rectum to visualize the rectum and large intestine.

Abdominal ultrasound, x-ray, and CT scan: CT scans can show bowel thickening.

Barium enema: Barium is inserted into the rectum as a contrast medium for x-rays. This allows for the rectum and large intestine to be visualized, and is used to diagnose ulcerative colitis. A barium enema can show the presence of diverticulosis and is contraindicated in the presence of diverticulitis due to the risk of perforation.

NURSING ACTIONS: Monitor postprocedure for manifestations of bowel perforations (rectal bleeding, firm abdomen, tachycardia, hypotension). **Qs**

FINDINGS
- Small intestine ulcerations and narrowing is consistent with Crohn's disease.
- Ulcerations and inflammation of the sigmoid colon and rectum is significant for ulcerative colitis.

CLIENT EDUCATION
- Instruct the client to remain NPO as required, and provide bowel preparation instructions.
- Inform the client of possible abdominal discomfort and cramping during the barium enema.

PATIENT-CENTERED CARE

NURSING CARE

Ulcerative colitis and Crohn's disease
- Instruct the client to seek emergency care for indications of bowel obstruction or perforation (fever, severe abdominal pain, vomiting). **Qs**
- The client should receive instructions regarding the usual course of the disease process.
- The client should receive instructions regarding medication therapy and vitamin supplements.
- The client will need monitoring by colonoscopy due to the increased risk of colon cancer.
- Instruct clients who have extreme or long exacerbations that NPO status and administration of total parenteral nutrition promotes bowel rest while providing adequate nutrition.
- Educate the client to eat high-protein, high-calories, low-fiber foods.
- Assist the client in identifying foods that trigger manifestations.
- Instruct the client to avoid caffeine and alcohol, and to take a multivitamin that contains iron.
- Advise the client that small frequent meals can reduce the occurrence of manifestations.
- Inform the client that dietary supplements that are high in protein and low in fiber (elemental and semi-elemental products, canned nutrition beverages) can be used.
- Monitor for electrolyte imbalance, especially potassium. Diarrhea can cause a loss of fluids and electrolytes.
- Monitor I&O, and assess for dehydration.
- Educate the client regarding the use of vitamin supplements and B_{12} injections, if needed.

Diverticulitis
- For severe manifestations (severe pain, high fever), the client is hospitalized, NPO, and receives nasogastric suctioning, IV fluids, IV antibiotics, and opioid analgesics for pain.
- Instruct the client who has mild diverticulitis about self-care at home. The client should take medications as prescribed (antibiotics, analgesics, antispasmodics) and get adequate rest.
- Educate the client to consume a clear liquid diet until manifestations subside. The client can progress to a low-fiber diet as tolerated.
- Instruct the client to add fiber to the diet once solid foods are tolerated without other manifestations. The client should slowly advance to a high-fiber diet as tolerated when inflammation resolves.
- Teach the client to avoid seeds or indigestible material, which can block diverticulum (nuts, popcorn, seeds).
- Instruct client to avoid foods or drinks that can irritate the bowel. (Avoid alcohol. Limit fat to 30% of daily calorie intake.)
- Provide the client with instructions to promote normal bowel function and consistency. (Can take bulk-forming laxatives. Drink adequate fluids. Avoid use of enemas.)

MEDICATIONS FOR ULCERATIVE COLITIS, CROHN'S DISEASE

5-aminosalicylic acid: Anti-inflammatory

Reduces inflammation of the intestinal mucosa and inhibits prostaglandins

Sulfonamides: Sulfasalazine
- NURSING CONSIDERATIONS
  - These medications are contraindicated if the client has a sulfa allergy.
  - Monitor CBC, and kidney and hepatic function.
  - Sulfasalazine is given orally.
  - Adverse effects include nausea, fever, and rash.
  - Monitor for the development of agranulocytosis, hemolytic anemia, and macrocytic anemia.
  - Can take up to 2 to 4 weeks for therapeutic effects.
- CLIENT EDUCATION
  - Advise the client to take the medication with a full glass of water after meals.
  - Tell the client to avoid sun exposure.
  - Teach the client to increase fluid intake to 2 L/day.
  - Tell the client this medication can cause urine, skin, and contact lenses to have a yellow-orange color.
  - Tell the client to notify the provider if nausea, vomiting, anorexia, sore throat, rash, bruising, or fever occur.
  - The client should take medication as directed. The usual maintenance dose of sulfasalazine is 2 to 4 g/day.

Nonsulfonamides
- Mesalamine
- Balsalazide
- Olsalazine (for clients intolerant to sulfasalazine, rarely used)
- NURSING CONSIDERATIONS
  - The adverse effects are not as serious as sulfasalazine.
  - These medications can be contraindicated if the client has a salicylate or sulfa allergy.
  - Monitor for kidney toxicity.
  - Inform the client to report headache or gastrointestinal problems (abdominal discomfort, diarrhea).

Corticosteroids

Reduces inflammation and pain

MEDICATIONS
- Prednisone
- Prednisolone
- Hydrocortisone
- Budesonide

NURSING CONSIDERATIONS
- For rectal inflammation, topical steroids can be administered by a retention enema.
- Used to induce remission.
- Not for long-term use due to adverse effects.
- Prolonged use can lead to adrenal suppression, osteoporosis, risk of infection, and cushingoid syndrome. Use corticosteroids in low doses to minimize adverse effects.
- Monitor blood pressure.
- Reduce systemic dose slowly.
- Monitor electrolytes and glucose.
- Can slow healing.

CLIENT EDUCATION
- Advise the client to take the oral dose with food.
- Warn the client to avoid discontinuing dose suddenly.
- Tell the client to report unexpected increase in weight or other indications of fluid retention.
- Teach the client to avoid crowds and other exposures to infectious diseases.
- Instruct the client to report evidence of infection (clients who have Crohn's disease; can mask infection).

Immunosuppressants

Mechanism of action in treatment of IBD is unknown.

MEDICATIONS
- Cyclosporine
- Methotrexate
- Azathioprine
- Mercaptopurine

NURSING CONSIDERATIONS
- Monitor for pancreatitis and neutropenia.
- Can take up to 6 months to see therapeutic effects.
- Not used as monotherapy.
- Reserved for refractory disease due to toxicity.

CLIENT EDUCATION
- Teach clients to avoid crowds and other chances of exposures to infectious diseases and to report evidence of infection.
- Advise the client to monitor for indications of bleeding, bruising, or infection.

Immunomodulators

- Suppresses the immune response
- Inhibits tumor necrosis factor, an antibody found in Crohn's disease

MEDICATIONS
- Infliximab
- Adalimumab (self-administered by subcutaneous injection)
- Natalizumab (can cause progressive multi-focal leukoencephalopathy a deadly brain infection)
- Certolizumab

NURSING CONSIDERATIONS
- Follow directions for IV use with care and in accordance with facility policy; can require pretreatment to reduce infusion reactions. Q EBP
- Many adverse effects are possible, including chills, fever, hypotension/hypertension, dysrhythmias, and blood dyscrasias.
- Monitor liver enzymes, coagulation studies, and CBC.

CLIENT EDUCATION
- Teach clients to avoid crowds and other chances of exposures to infectious diseases and to report evidence of infection. The client is at risk for development or reactivation of tuberculosis.
- Advise the client to monitor and report evidence of bleeding, bruising, or infection, and transfusion or allergic reaction.

Antidiarrheals

Suppress the number of stools

MEDICATIONS
- Diphenoxylate and atropine
- Loperamide

NURSING CONSIDERATIONS
- Used to decrease risk of fluid volume deficit and electrolyte imbalance. They also reduce discomfort.
- Use of antidiarrheals can lead to toxic megacolon (massive dilation of the colon with a risk of the development of gangrene and peritonitis). Use cautiously. Qs
  - Observe for manifestations of toxic megacolon that can result in gangrene and peritonitis (hypotension, fever, abdominal distention, decrease or absence of bowel sounds).
- Observe for indications of respiratory depression, especially in older adult clients.

CLIENT EDUCATION: Due to the central nervous system effects, teach the client to avoid hazardous activities until the response to the medication is established.

MEDICATION FOR DIVERTICULITIS

Antimicrobials

Treat infection (decrease inflammation in Crohn's disease, ineffective for ulcerative colitis)

MEDICATIONS
- Ciprofloxacin
- Metronidazole
- Sulfamethoxazole-trimethoprim

NURSING CONSIDERATIONS
- Can cause a superinfection. Instruct client to observe for manifestations of thrush or vaginal yeast infection.
- Discontinue ciprofloxacin for tendon pain. Can cause tendon rupture.
- Decreased dose should be used for clients who have impaired kidney function.
- Monitor kidney and hepatic studies.

CLIENT EDUCATION
- Instruct client that urine can darken (expected, harmless effect).
- Teach client to monitor for manifestations of CNS effects (numbness of extremities, ataxia, and seizures) and to notify the provider immediately.

THERAPEUTIC PROCEDURES

Clients who do not have success with medical treatment or who have complications (bowel perforation, colon cancer) are candidates for surgery.

Ulcerative colitis: Colectomy with or without ileostomy

Crohn's disease
- Laparoscopic stricturoplasty to increase the diameter of the bowel for bowel strictures
- Surgical repair of fistulas or in response to other complications related to the disease (perforation)

Diverticulitis (dependent on problem)
- Required for rupture of the diverticulum that results in peritonitis, bowel obstruction, uncontrolled bleeding, or abscess
- Colon resection with or without colostomy

PREOPERATIVE CARE
- Preoperative care is similar to care for clients who have other abdominal surgeries.
- Provide preoperative teaching.
- If the creation of a stoma is planned, collaborate with an enterostomal therapy nurse regarding care related to the stoma. Qᴛᴄ
- Administer antibiotic bowel prep (neomycin), if prescribed.
- Administer cleansing enema or laxative, if prescribed.

POSTOPERATIVE CARE
- Postoperative care is similar to care for clients who have other types of abdominal surgery.
- The client should be NPO and have a nasogastric tube to suction, unless the surgery was performed laparoscopically.
- An ileostomy can drain as much as 1,000 mL/day. Prevent fluid volume deficit. Replace fluid loss with IV fluids if the client is NPO. Oral hydration is slowly introduced in 1 to 2 days. Qs

CARE AFTER DISCHARGE: Refer the client who has an ostomy to an enterostomal therapist and an ostomy support group.

INTERPROFESSIONAL CARE
- Refer the client for nutritional counseling.
- The client might benefit from complementary therapy (biofeedback, massage, yoga).
- Recommend community support groups or a mental health referral for assistance with coping. Qᴘᴄᴄ

COMPLICATIONS

Complications of ulcerative colitis, Crohn's disease, and diverticulitis include bleeding and fluid and electrolyte imbalance. Peritonitis can occur due to perforation of the bowel. Abscess formation can occur as a complication of diverticular disease and Crohn's disease.

Peritonitis

- A life threatening inflammation of the peritoneum and lining of the abdominal cavity.
- It is often caused by bacteria in the peritoneal cavity.

ASSESSMENT FINDINGS
- Rigid, board-like abdomen (hallmark indication)
- Abdominal distention
- Nausea, vomiting
- Rebound tenderness
- Tachycardia
- Fever

NURSING ACTIONS
- Place the client in Fowler's or semi-Fowler's position to promote drainage of peritoneal fluid and improve lung expansion. Q EBP
- Monitor respiratory status and administer oxygen as prescribed. Turn, cough, deep breathe. Provide mechanical ventilation if needed.
- Maintain and monitor nasogastric suction.
- Keep the client NPO.
- Monitor fluid and electrolyte status.
- Monitor for hypovolemia.
- Administer IV antibiotics as prescribed.
- Collaborate with case management to determine home care and wound management needs. Q TC
- If surgery is performed:
  - Closely monitor postoperative vital signs.
  - Monitor I&O every hour immediately after surgery.
  - Monitor surgical dressing for bleeding.
  - If the client requires wound irrigation postoperatively, use sterile technique, and monitor irrigation intake and output to prevent fluid retention.

CLIENT EDUCATION
- Instruct the client to maintain adequate rest and resume home activity slowly, as tolerated. No heavy lifting for at least 6 weeks.
- Teach the client to monitor for evidence of return infection. Notify the provider immediately.

Bleeding due to deterioration of the bowel

NURSING ACTIONS
- Observe for indications of rectal bleeding.
- Monitor vital signs.
- Check laboratory values, especially hematocrit, hemoglobin, and coagulation factors.

CLIENT EDUCATION
- Instruct the client to report rectal bleeding.
- Explain to the client the importance of bed rest.

Fluid and electrolyte imbalance

Occurs due to loss of fluid through diarrhea, vomiting, and nasogastric suctioning.

NURSING ACTIONS
- Monitor laboratory values, and provide replacement therapy.
- Monitor weight.
- Assess for indications of fluid volume deficit (loss or absence of skin turgor).

CLIENT EDUCATION
- Instruct the client to record and report the number of loose stools.
- Encourage the client to maintain adequate fluid intake.
- Advise the client to follow the prescribed diet.

Abscess and fistula formation

Occurs due to the destruction of the bowel wall, leading to an infection

NURSING ACTIONS
- Monitor fluid and electrolytes.
- Observe for manifestations of dehydration.
- Provide a diet high in protein and calories (at least 3,000 calories/day), and low in fiber.
- Administer a vitamin supplement.
- Consult with an enterostomal therapist to develop a plan to prevent skin breakdown and promote wound healing. Q TC
- Monitor for evidence of infection, which can indicate abdominal abscesses or sepsis.
- Ensure the function of drainage devices if used.

Toxic megacolon

Occurs due to inactivity of the colon. Massive dilation of the colon occurs, and the client is at risk for perforation.

NURSING ACTIONS
- Maintain nasogastric suction.
- Administer IV fluids and electrolytes.
- Administer prescribed medications (antibiotics, corticosteroids).
- Prepare the client for surgery (usually an ileostomy) if the client does not begin to show improvement within 72 hr.

Application Exercises

1. A nurse is reviewing the serum laboratory data of a client who has an acute exacerbation of Crohn's disease. Which of the following laboratory tests should the nurse expect to be elevated? (Select all that apply.)

   A. Hematocrit

   B. Erythrocyte sedimentation rate

   C. WBC

   D. Folic acid

   E. Albumin

2. A nurse is assessing a client who has been taking prednisone following an exacerbation of inflammatory bowel disease. The nurse should recognize which of the following findings as the priority?

   A. Client reports difficulty sleeping.

   B. The client's urine is positive for glucose.

   C. Client reports having an elevated body temperature.

   D. Client reports gaining 4 lb in the last 6 months.

3. A nurse is teaching a client who has a new prescription for sulfasalazine. Which of the following instructions should the nurse include in the teaching?

   A. "Take the medication 2 hr after eating."

   B. "Discontinue this medication if your skin turns yellow-orange."

   C. "Notify the provider if you experience a sore throat."

   D. "Expect your stools to turn black."

4. A nurse is completing discharge teaching with a client who has Crohn's disease. Which of the following instructions should the nurse include in the teaching?

   A. Decrease intake of calorie-dense foods.

   B. Drink canned protein supplements.

   C. Increase intake of high fiber foods.

   D. Take a bulk-forming laxative daily.

5. A nurse in a clinic is teaching a client who has ulcerative colitis. Which of the following statements by the client indicates understanding of the teaching?

   A. "I will plan to limit fiber in my diet."

   B. "I will restrict fluid intake during meals."

   C. "I will switch to black tea instead of drinking coffee."

   D. "I will try to eat three moderate to large meals a day."

PRACTICE Active Learning Scenario

A nurse is teaching a client who has diverticulitis. What should the nurse include in the teaching? Use the ATI Active Learning Template: System Disorder to complete this item.

PATHOPHYSIOLOGY RELATED TO CLIENT PROBLEM

RISK FACTORS: Identify two.

EXPECTED FINDINGS: Identify two expected findings.

DIAGNOSTIC PROCEDURES: Identify three.

CLIENT EDUCATION: Describe dietary teaching.

Application Exercises Key

1. A. Hematocrit is decreased as a result of chronic blood loss.

   B. **CORRECT:** Increased erythrocyte sedimentation rate is a finding in a client who has Crohn's disease as a result of inflammation.

   C. **CORRECT:** Increased WBC is a finding in a client who has Crohn's disease.

   D. A decrease in folic acid level is indicative of malabsorption due to Crohn's disease.

   E. A decrease in serum albumin is indicative of malabsorption due to Crohn's disease.

   Ⓝ *NCLEX® Connection: Physiological Adaptation, Pathophysiology*

2. A. The client is at risk for sleep deprivation because prednisone can cause anxiety and insomnia. However, another finding is the priority.

   B. The client is at risk for hyperglycemia because prednisone can cause glucose intolerance. However, another finding is the priority.

   C. **CORRECT:** The greatest risk to the client is infection because prednisone can cause immunosuppression. Therefore, the nurse should identify indications of an infection, such as an elevated body temperature, as the priority finding.

   D. The client is at risk for weight gain because prednisone can cause fluid retention. However, another finding is the priority.

   Ⓝ *NCLEX® Connection: Pharmacological and Parenteral Therapies, Adverse Effects/Contraindications/Side Effects/Interactions*

3. A. Sulfasalazine should be taken right after meals and with a full glass of water to reduce gastric upset and prevent crystalluria.

   B. Yellow-orange coloring of the skin and urine is a harmless effect of sulfasalazine.

   C. **CORRECT:** Sulfasalazine can cause blood dyscrasias. The client should monitor and report any manifestations of infection, such as a sore throat.

   D. Sulfasalazine can cause thrombocytopenia and bleeding. Black stools are a manifestation of gastrointestinal bleeding, and the client should report this to the provider.

   Ⓝ *NCLEX® Connection: Pharmacological and Parenteral Therapies, Medication Administration*

4. A. A high-protein diet is recommended for the client who has Crohn's disease.

   B. **CORRECT:** A high-protein diet is recommended for the client who has Crohn's disease. Canned protein supplements are encouraged.

   C. A low-fiber diet is recommended for the client who has Crohn's disease to reduce inflammation.

   D. Bulk-forming laxatives are recommended for the client who has diverticulitis.

   Ⓝ *NCLEX® Connection: Physiological Adaptation, Illness Management*

5. A. **CORRECT:** A low-fiber diet is recommended for the client who has ulcerative colitis to reduce inflammation.

   B. A client who has dumping syndrome should avoid fluids with meals.

   C. Caffeine can increase diarrhea and cramping. The client should avoid caffeinated beverages, such as black tea.

   D. Small, frequent meals are recommended for the client who has ulcerative colitis.

   Ⓝ *NCLEX® Connection: Basic Care and Comfort, Nutrition and Oral Hydration*

PRACTICE Answer

Using the ATI Active Learning Template: System Disorder

PATHOPHYSIOLOGY RELATED TO CLIENT PROBLEM: Inflammation and infection of the bowel mucosa caused by bacteria or fecal matter trapped in one or more diverticula (pouches in the intestine)

RISK FACTORS
- Older adult clients
- Male gender

EXPECTED FINDINGS
- Decreased hemoglobin and hematocrit.
- Stool can be positive for occult blood.

DIAGNOSTIC PROCEDURES
- Abdominal x-ray
- CT scan
- Colonoscopy
- Sigmoidoscopy

CLIENT EDUCATION
- Consume clear liquid until manifestations subside. Progress to a low fiber diet as tolerated. Add fiber once solid foods are tolerated. Slowly advance to a high-fiber diet.
- Avoid seeds or indigestible material (nuts, popcorn, seeds).
- Avoid alcohol. Limit fat to 30% of daily caloric intake.

Ⓝ *NCLEX® Connection: Physiological Adaptation, Illness Management*

CHAPTER 53 *Cholecystitis and
Cholelithiasis*

Cholecystitis is an inflammation of the gallbladder wall. Cholecystitis is most often caused by gallstones (cholelithiasis) obstructing the cystic and/or common bile ducts (bile flows from the gallbladder to the duodenum) causing bile to back up and the gall bladder to become inflamed.

Cholelithiasis is the presence of stones in the gallbladder related to the precipitation of either bile or cholesterol into stones. Bile is used for the digestion of fats. It is produced in the liver and stored in the gall bladder. Cholecystitis can be acute or chronic, and can obstruct the pancreatic duct, causing pancreatitis. It can also cause the gallbladder to rupture, resulting in secondary peritonitis.

HEALTH PROMOTION AND DISEASE PREVENTION

- Consume a low-fat diet rich in HDL sources (seafood, nuts, olive oil).
- Participate in a regular exercise program.
- Do not smoke.

ASSESSMENT

RISK FACTORS

- More common in females (hormone therapy and use of some oral contraceptives)
- High-fat diet
- Obesity (impaired fat metabolism, high cholesterol)
- Genetic predisposition
- Older adults (decreased contractility, more likely to develop gallstones) Ⓖ
- Type 2 diabetes mellitus (high triglycerides) or Crohn's disease
- Low-calorie, liquid protein diets
- Rapid weight loss (increases cholesterol)
- Native American or Mexican ethnicity

EXPECTED FINDINGS

- Sharp pain in the right upper quadrant, often radiating to the right shoulder
- Pain with deep inspiration during right subcostal palpation (Murphy's sign)
- Intense pain (increased heart rate, pallor, diaphoresis) with nausea and vomiting after ingestion of high-fat food caused by biliary colic
- Rebound tenderness (Blumberg's sign performed by the provider or advanced practice nurse)
- Dyspepsia, eructation (belching), and flatulence
- Fever

PHYSICAL ASSESSMENT FINDINGS

- Jaundice, clay-colored stools, steatorrhea (fatty stools), dark urine, and pruritus (accumulation of bile salts in the skin) in clients who have chronic cholecystitis (due to biliary obstruction).
- OLDER ADULT CLIENTS who have diabetes mellitus can have atypical presentation of cholecystitis (absence of pain or fever). Ⓖ

LABORATORY TESTS

- Increased WBC indicates inflammation.
- Direct, indirect, and total serum bilirubin increased if bile duct obstructed.
- Amylase and lipase increased with pancreatic involvement.
- Aspartate aminotransferase (AST), lactate dehydrogenase (LDH), and alkaline phosphatase (ALP) (increased with liver dysfunction) can indicate the common bile duct is obstructed.

DIAGNOSTIC PROCEDURES

Ultrasound visualizes gallstones and a dilated common bile duct.

Abdominal x-ray or CT scan can visualize calcified gallstones and an enlarged gallbladder.

Hepatobiliary scan (HIDA) assesses the patency of the biliary duct system after an IV injection of contrast.

Endoscopic retrograde cholangiopancreatography allows for direct visualization using an endoscope that is inserted through the esophagus and into the common bile duct via the duodenum. A sphincterotomy with gallstone removal can be done during this procedure. (Refer to **CHAPTER 46: GASTROINTESTINAL DIAGNOSTIC PROCEDURES.**)

Magnetic resonance cholangiopancreatography combines the use of oral/IV contrast with an MRI. This test assists the provider in determining the cause of cholecystitis or cholelithiasis.

PATIENT-CENTERED CARE

NURSING CARE

Administer analgesics as needed and prescribed.

MEDICATIONS

Analgesics

- Opioid analgesics, such as morphine sulfate or hydromorphone, are preferred for acute biliary pain.
- An NSAID, such as ketorolac, is used for mild to moderate pain. Monitor for GI bleeding.

Bile acid

Bile acid (chenodiol, ursodiol) gradually dissolves cholesterol-based gall stones

NURSING CONSIDERATIONS: Use caution in clients who have liver conditions or disorders with varices.

CLIENT EDUCATION: Teach clients to report abdominal pain, diarrhea, or vomiting. The medication is limited to 2 years of administration and requires a gallbladder ultrasound every 6 months during the first year to determine effectiveness.

THERAPEUTIC PROCEDURES

Extracorporeal shock wave lithotripsy

Shock waves are used to break up stones. This can be used more on nonsurgical candidates of normal weight who have small, cholesterol-based stones.

NURSING ACTIONS
- Instruct and assist client to lay on fluid-filled pad for delivery of shock waves.
- Administer analgesia, as prescribed.

CLIENT EDUCATION: Inform the client that several procedures can be required to break up all stones. The client might have pain intraprocedure due to gallbladder spasms or movement of the stones.

Cholecystectomy

- Removal of the gallbladder with a laparoscopic, minimally invasive, or open approach
- The client usually is discharged within 24 hr if a laparoscopic approach is used. An open approach can require hospitalization for 1 to 2 days.

NURSING ACTIONS
- **Laparoscopic approach:** Provide immediate postoperative care.
- **Minimally invasive approach:** Natural orifice transluminal endoscopic surgery. Explain to the client that this surgical procedure is performed through entry of the mouth, vagina, or rectum. This approach eliminates visible incisions and decreases the risk of complications for the client.
- **Open approach:** The provider may place a Jackson-Pratt drain in the gallbladder bed or a T-tube in the common bile duct.

- Though used less commonly, clients can have a T-tube placed in the common bile duct to drain bile if there were intraoperative complications involving the bile duct.
- **Care of the drainage tube**
  - Clients can have a Jackson-Pratt drain or other drainage tube placed intraoperatively to prevent accumulation of fluid in the gallbladder bed.
  - Monitor and record drainage (initially serosanguineous stained with green-brown bile).
  - Antibiotics are often prescribed to decrease the risk for infection.
- **Care of the T-tube**
  - Instruct client to report an absence of drainage with manifestations of nausea and pain (can indicate obstruction in the T-tube).
  - Inspect the surrounding skin for evidence of infection or bile leakage.
  - If prescribed, elevate the T-tube above the level of the abdomen to prevent the total loss of bile.
  - Monitor and record the color and amount of drainage.
  - Clamp the tube 1 hr before and after meals to provide the bile necessary for food digestion.
  - Assess stools for color (stools clay-colored until biliary flow is reestablished).
  - Monitor for bile peritonitis (pain, fever, jaundice).
  - Monitor and document response to food.
  - Expect removal of the tube in 1 to 3 weeks.

CLIENT EDUCATION
- **Laparoscopic or NOTES approach**
  - Instruct the client to ambulate frequently to minimize free air pain, common following laparoscopic surgery (under the right clavicle, shoulder, scapula).
  - Tell the client to monitor the incision for evidence of infection or wound dehiscence (laparoscopic approach).
  - Educate the client regarding pain control.
  - Teach the client to report indications of bile leak (pain, vomiting, abdominal distention) to the provider.
  - Teach the client to resume activity gradually and as tolerated, and to resume the preoperative diet.
- **Open approach**
  - Instruct the client to resume activity gradually. Avoid heavy lifting for 4 to 6 weeks.
  - Tell the client to begin with clear liquids and advance to solid foods as peristalsis returns.
  - Remind the client to report sudden increase in drainage, foul odor, pain, fever, or jaundice. **Qs**
  - Teach the client to take showers instead of baths until drainage tube is removed.
  - Instruct the client that the color of stools should return to brown in about a week, and diarrhea is common.
- **Dietary counseling**
  - Encourage a low-fat diet (reduce dairy products and avoid fried foods, chocolate, nuts, gravies). The client can have increased tolerance of small, frequent meals.
  - Tell the client to avoid gas-forming foods (beans, cabbage, cauliflower, broccoli).
  - Promote weight reduction.
  - Instruct the client to take fat-soluble vitamins or bile salts as prescribed to enhance absorption and aid with digestion.

COMPLICATIONS

Obstruction of the bile duct

This can cause ischemia, gangrene, and a rupture of the gallbladder wall. A rupture of the gallbladder wall can cause a local abscess or peritonitis (rigid, board-like abdomen, guarding), which requires a surgical intervention and administration of broad spectrum antibiotics.

Bile peritonitis

This can occur if adequate amounts of bile are not drained from the surgical site. This is a rare but potentially fatal complication.

NURSING ACTIONS
- Monitor for pain, fever, and jaundice.
- Report findings to the provider immediately.

Postcholecystectomy syndrome

Manifestations of gallbladder disease can continue after surgery. The client will report findings similar to those experienced prior to surgery related to pain and nausea. Manifestations can recur immediately or months later.

NURSING ACTIONS
- Assess pain characteristics and other reported findings.
- Instruct client on the need for possible further diagnostic evaluation.

PRACTICE Active Learning Scenario

A nurse is presenting a program on gallbladder disease to a group of clients at a health fair. What information should the nurse include in the program? Use the ATI Active Learning Template: System Disorder to complete this item.

RISK FACTORS: Describe at least four.

EXPECTED FINDINGS: Describe at least eight findings.

CLIENT EDUCATION: Describe three preventative activities.

Application Exercises

1. A nurse is providing discharge teaching to a client who is postoperative following open cholecystectomy with T-tube placement. Which of the following instructions should the nurse include in the teaching? (Select all that apply.)

   A. Take baths rather than showers.

   B. Clamp T-tube for 1 hr before and after meals.

   C. Keep the drainage system above the level of the abdomen.

   D. Expect to have the T-tube removed 3 days postoperatively.

   E. Report brown-green drainage to the provider.

2. A nurse is reviewing nutrition teaching for a client who has cholecystitis. The nurse should identify that which of the following food choices can trigger cholecystitis?

   A. Brownie with nuts

   B. Bowl of mixed fruit

   C. Grilled turkey

   D. Baked potato

3. A nurse is completing preoperative teaching for a client who is scheduled for a laparoscopic cholecystectomy. Which of the following should be included in the teaching?

   A. "The scope will be passed through your rectum."

   B. "You might have shoulder pain after surgery."

   C. "You will have a Jackson-Pratt drain in place after surgery."

   D. "You should limit how often you walk for 1 to 2 weeks."

4. A nurse is reviewing a new prescription for ursodiol with a client who has cholelithiasis. Which of the following information should the nurse include in the teaching?

   A. This medication is used to decrease acute biliary pain.

   B. This medication requires thyroid function monitoring every 6 months.

   C. This medication is not recommended for clients who have diabetes mellitus.

   D. This medication dissolves gallstones gradually over a period of up to 2 years.

5. A nurse in a clinic is reviewing the laboratory reports of a client who has suspected cholelithiasis. Which of the following is an expected finding?

   A. Serum amylase 80 units/L

   B. WBC 9,000/mm³

   C. Direct bilirubin 2.1 mg/dL

   D. Alkaline phosphatase 25 units/L

Application Exercises Key

1. A. Soaking in bath water is not recommended while the T-tube is in place due to the increased risk for introduction of organisms and infection.

   B. **CORRECT:** The T-tube is clamped 1 hr before and after meals to provide the bile needed for digestion of food.

   C. **CORRECT:** The provider may prescribe elevation of the T- above the level of the abdomen to prevent the total loss of bile.

   D. The T-tube usually remains in place for 1 to 3 weeks postoperatively.

   E. The purpose of the T-tube is to drain bile from the common bile duct. Bile is brown-green, so this is an expected finding.

   (N) *NCLEX® Connection: Reduction of Risk Potential, Therapeutic Procedures*

2. A. **CORRECT:** Foods that are high in fat, such as a brownie with nuts, can cause cholecystitis.

   B. Fruits are low in fat and not associated with cholecystitis.

   C. Turkey is low in fat and not associated with cholecystitis.

   D. Baked potatoes are low in fat and not associated with cholecystitis.

   (N) *NCLEX® Connection: Basic Care and Comfort, Nutrition and Oral Hydration*

3. A. Surgery is possibly performed through the rectum during the natural orifice transluminal endoscopic surgery (NOTES) approach.

   B. **CORRECT:** Shoulder pain is expected postoperatively due to free air that is introduced into the abdomen during laparoscopic surgery.

   C. A Jackson-Pratt may be placed during the open surgery approach.

   D. The client is instructed to ambulate frequently following a laparoscopic surgical approach to minimize the free air that has been introduced.

   (N) *NCLEX® Connection: Reduction of Risk Potential, Therapeutic Procedures*

4. A. Opioid analgesics are preferred for the treatment of acute biliary pain.

   B. The client should have an ultrasound of the gallbladder every 6 months during the first year of treatment to determine effectiveness of the medication.

   C. Ursodiol is used cautiously in clients who have liver conditions or disorders with varices.

   D. **CORRECT:** Ursodiol is a bile acid that gradually dissolves cholesterol-based gall stones. The medication can be taken for up to 2 years.

   (N) *NCLEX® Connection: Pharmacological and Parenteral Therapies, Medication Administration*

5. A. The nurse should expect the client who has cholelithiasis to have an elevated serum amylase level if pancreatic involvement is present. A serum amylase of 80 units/L is within the expected reference range.

   B. The nurse should expect the client who has cholelithiasis to have an elevated WBC level due to inflammation. A WBC of 9,000/mm³ is within the expected reference range.

   C. **CORRECT:** The nurse should expect the client who has cholelithiasis to have an elevated direct bilirubin level if the bile duct is obstructed. A direct bilirubin level of 2.1 mg/dL is greater than the expected reference range.

   D. The nurse should expect the client who has cholelithiasis to have an elevated alkaline phosphatase (ALP) level if the common bile duct is obstructed. An ALP of 25 units/L is less than the expected reference range.

   (N) *NCLEX® Connection: Reduction of Risk Potential, Laboratory Values*

PRACTICE Answer

Using the ATI Active Learning Template: System Disorder

RISK FACTORS

- Female sex (hormone therapy, and some oral contraceptives)
- High-fat or low-calorie, liquid protein diets
- Obesity
- Genetic predisposition
- Age over 60 years
- Type 2 diabetes mellitus
- Rapid weight loss
- Native American or Mexican ethnicity

EXPECTED FINDINGS

- Sharp pain in the right upper quadrant that often radiates to the right shoulder
- Pain upon deep inspiration during right subcostal palpation
- Intense pain with nausea and vomiting after ingestion of high-fat food
- Dyspepsia
- Eructation (belching)
- Flatulence
- Fever
- Jaundice
- Clay-colored stools
- Steatorrhea (fatty stools)
- Dark urine
- Pruritus

CLIENT EDUCATION

- Get regular exercise.
- Stop smoking.
- Consume a low-fat diet rich in HDL sources (seafood, nuts, olive oil).

(N) *NCLEX® Connection: Physiological Adaptation, Pathophysiology*

CHAPTER 54 *Pancreatitis*

The islets of Langerhans in the pancreas secrete insulin and glucagon. The pancreatic tissues secrete digestive enzymes that break down carbohydrates, proteins, and fats.

Pancreatitis is an autodigestion of the pancreas by pancreatic digestive enzymes that activate prematurely before reaching the intestines. The mechanism of action is unclear. Inflammation of the pancreatic tissue causes duct obstruction, which can lead to increased pressure and duct rupture, causing the release of pancreatic enzymes into the pancreatic tissue. Pancreatitis can result in pancreatic inflammation, necrosis, and hemorrhage. Classic presentation of an acute attack includes severe, constant, knifelike pain (left upper quadrant, midepigastric, and/or radiating to the back).

Acute pancreatitis is an inflammatory process due to activated pancreatic enzymes autodigesting the pancreas ranging from mild to necrotizing hemorrhagic pancreatitis (widespread bleeding and necrosis).

Chronic pancreatitis is a progressive, destructive disease of inflammation and fibrosis of the pancreas. Chronic pancreatitis is classified as chronic calcifying pancreatitis (often associated with alcohol use disorder), chronic obstructive pancreatitis (often associated with cholelithiasis), autoimmune pancreatitis, and idiopathic and hereditary pancreatitis.

HEALTH PROMOTION AND DISEASE PREVENTION

- Avoid excessive alcohol consumption.
- Eat a low-fat diet.

ASSESSMENT

RISK FACTORS

- Biliary tract disease: Gallstones can cause a blockage where the common bile duct and pancreatic duct meet.
- Alcohol use: The primary cause of chronic pancreatitis is alcohol use disorder. Times of increased alcohol consumption, such as vacations or holidays, are associated with acute pancreatitis.
- Increased age: Pancreatitis is more common in older adults. Ⓖ
- Endoscopic retrograde cholangiopancreatography (ERCP) (postprocedure complication)
- Gastrointestinal surgery
- Metabolic disturbances (hyperlipidemia, hyperparathyroidism, hypercalcemia)
- Kidney failure or transplant
- Genetic predisposition
- Trauma
- Penetrating ulcer (gastric or duodenal)
- Medication toxicity
- Viral infections: coxsackievirus B and human immunodeficiency virus
- Cigarette smoking

EXPECTED FINDINGS

- Sudden onset of severe, boring pain (goes through the body)
  - Epigastric, radiating to back, left flank, or left shoulder
  - Worse when lying down
- Pain relieved somewhat by fetal position or sitting upright, bending forward
- Nausea and vomiting
- Weight loss

PHYSICAL ASSESSMENT FINDINGS

- Seepage of blood-stained exudates into tissue as a result of pancreatic enzyme actions
  - Ecchymoses on the flanks: Turner's sign (54.1)
  - Bluish-gray periumbilical discoloration: Cullen's sign (54.2)
- Generalized jaundice
- Absent or decreased bowel sounds (possible paralytic ileus)
- Warm, moist skin; fruity breath (evidence of hyperglycemia)
- Ascites
- Tetany due to hypocalcemia
  - Trousseau's sign: hand spasm when blood pressure cuff is inflated
  - Chvostek's sign: facial twitching when facial nerve is tapped

LABORATORY TESTS

- **Serum amylase** increases within 12 to 24 hr, and remains increased for 2 to 3 days (continued elevation can indicate pancreatic abscess or pseudocyst).
  Serum lipase increases slowly but remains increased for up to 2 weeks.
  - Urine amylase remains increased for up to 2 weeks.
  - Increases in enzymes indicate pancreatic cell injury.

  > MEMORY AID: In pancreatitis, the "ases" (aces) are high.

- **WBC count:** Increased due to infection and inflammation
- **Platelets:** Decreased
- **Serum calcium and magnesium:** Decreased due to fat necrosis with pancreatitis
- **Serum liver enzymes and bilirubin:** Increased with associated biliary dysfunction
- **Serum glucose:** Increased due to a decrease in insulin production by the pancreas
- **Erythrocyte sedimentation rate:** Elevated

DIAGNOSTIC PROCEDURES

Computed tomography scan with contrast is reliably diagnostic of acute pancreatitis.

PATIENT-CENTERED CARE

NURSING CARE

- Rest the pancreas.
  - NPO: No food until pain-free
  - For severe pancreatitis: Total parenteral nutrition or jejunal feedings (contraindicated if paralytic ileus develops, less risk of hyperglycemia)
  - When diet is resumed: Bland, high protein, low-fat diet with no stimulants (caffeine); small, frequent meals ⓆEBP
  - Administer antiemetic as needed, as prescribed
  - Nasogastric tube: Gastric decompression (for severe vomiting or paralytic ileus)
  - No alcohol consumption
  - No smoking
  - Limit stress
  - Pain management
- Position the client for comfort (fetal, side-lying, head of the bed elevated, sitting up or leaning forward).
- Administer analgesics and other medications as prescribed.
- Monitor blood glucose, and provide insulin as needed (potential for hyperglycemia).
- Monitor hydration status (orthostatic blood pressure, I&O, laboratory values).
- Administer IV fluids and electrolyte replacement as prescribed.

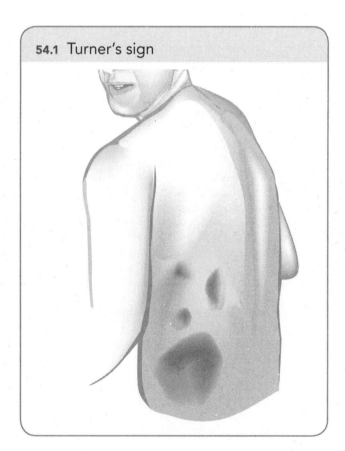

54.1 Turner's sign

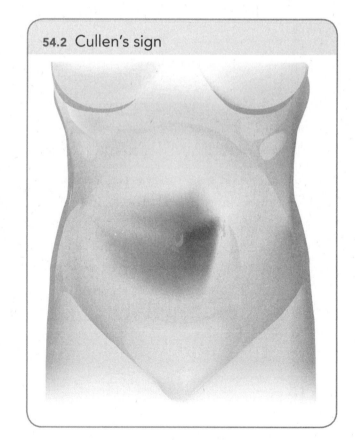

54.2 Cullen's sign

MEDICATIONS

Opioid analgesics

Morphine or hydromorphone for acute pain

NURSING CONSIDERATIONS: Meperidine is discouraged due to the risk of seizures, especially in older adult clients. Ⓖ

Antibiotics: Imipenem

Antibiotics can be used, but are generally indicated for clients who have acute necrotizing pancreatitis.

NURSING CONSIDERATIONS
- Monitor for evidence of infection.
- Monitor for seizures.

Histamine receptor antagonists: Ranitidine

Decreases gastric acid secretion.

CLIENT EDUCATION: Take 1 hr before or 1 hr after antacid.

Proton pump inhibitors: Omeprazole

Decreases gastric acid secretion.

NURSING CONSIDERATIONS: Monitor for hypomagnesemia.

Pancreatic enzymes: Pancrelipase

Aid with digestion of fats and proteins when taken with meals and snacks.

NURSING CONSIDERATIONS
- The client can sprinkle contents of capsules on nonprotein foods.
- The client should drink a full glass of water following pancrelipase.
- Clients should wipe lips and rinse mouth after taking (to prevent skin breakdown or irritation).
- Instruct the client to take pancrelipase after antacid or histamine receptor antagonists.
- Teach the client to take pancrelipase with every meal and snack.

THERAPEUTIC PROCEDURES

- ERCP to create an opening in the sphincter of Oddi if pancreatitis is caused by gallstones
- Cholecystectomy if pancreatitis is a result of cholecystitis and gallstones
- Sphincterotomy to enlarge the pancreatic duct sphincter
- Endoscopic pancreatic necrosectomy and natural orifice transluminal endoscopic surgery to remove necrotic tissue
- Pancreaticojejunostomy (Roux-en-Y) reroutes drainage of pancreatic secretions into jejunum

INTERPROFESSIONAL CARE

- Dietary referral for postpancreatitis diet and nutritional supplements can be indicated when oral intake is resumed.
- Home health services can be indicated for clients regarding nutritional needs, possible wound care, and assistance with ADLs. Ⓠᴛᴄ
- Alcoholics Anonymous (AA) can be indicated for a client or family member who has an alcohol use disorder.

CLIENT EDUCATION

Chronic pancreatitis due to alcohol use: Encourage the client to avoid alcohol intake and caffeinated beverages, and to participate in support groups for individuals who have alcohol use disorder. Ⓠᴘᴄᴄ

COMPLICATIONS

Hypovolemia

Up to 6 L of fluid can be third-spaced; caused by retroperitoneal loss of protein-rich fluid from proteolytic digestion. The client can develop hypovolemic shock.

NURSING ACTIONS: Monitor for vital signs, electrolytes, and for hypotension and tachycardia. Provide IV fluid and electrolyte replacement.

Pancreatic infection

Pseudocyst (outside pancreas); abscess (inside pancreas)

CAUSE: Leakage of fluid out of damaged pancreatic duct

MANIFESTATIONS: Fever, epigastric mass, nausea, vomiting, jaundice

NURSING ACTIONS
- Monitor for rupture and hemorrhage.
- Maintain sump tube if placed for drainage of cyst.
- Monitor skin around tube for breakdown secondary to corrosive enzymes.

Type 1 diabetes mellitus

CAUSE: Lack or absence of insulin (due to destruction of pancreatic beta cells)

NURSING ACTIONS
- Monitor blood glucose.
- Administer insulin as prescribed.

CLIENT EDUCATION: Inform the client about long-term diabetes management.

Left lung effusion and atelectasis

- More common complication in older adults Ⓒ
- Can precipitate pneumonia

CAUSES
- Splinting of chest due to pain upon coughing and deep breathing
- Pancreatic ascites

NURSING ACTIONS: Monitor for hypoxia, and provide ventilatory support.

Coagulation defects

Disseminated intravascular coagulopathy

CAUSES: Release of thromboplastic endotoxins secondary to necrotizing hemorrhagic pancreatitis

NURSING ACTIONS: Monitor coagulation studies and for bleeding.

Multi-system organ failure

Inflammation of pancreas is believed to trigger systemic inflammation.

CAUSE: Necrotizing hemorrhagic pancreatitis

NURSING ACTIONS
- Administer treatments as prescribed.
- Monitor for evidence of organ failure (respiratory distress, jaundice, oliguria). Qs
- Report unexpected findings to provider.

Application Exercises

1. A nurse is completing the admission assessment of a client who has acute pancreatitis. Which of the following findings is the priority to report?

    A. History of cholelithiasis

    B. Elevated serum amylase level

    C. Decrease in bowel sounds upon auscultation

    D. Hand spasms present when blood pressure is checked

2. A nurse is preparing to administer pancrelipase to a client who has pancreatitis. Which of the following actions should the nurse take?

    A. Instruct the client to chew the medication before swallowing.

    B. Offer a glass of water following medication administration.

    C. Administer the medication 30 min before meals.

    D. Sprinkle the contents on peanut butter.

3. A nurse is completing an admission assessment of a client who has pancreatitis. Which of the following findings should the nurse expect?

    A. Pain in right upper quadrant radiating to right shoulder

    B. Report of pain being worse when sitting upright

    C. Pain relieved with defecation

    D. Epigastric pain radiating to the left shoulder

4. A nurse is assessing a client who has pancreatitis. Which of the following actions should the nurse take to assess the presence of Cullen's sign.

    A. Tap lightly at the costovertebral margin on the client's back.

    B. Palpate the right lower quadrant.

    C. Inspect the skin around the umbilicus.

    D. Auscultate the area below the scapula.

5. A nurse is completing nutrition teaching for a client who has pancreatitis. Which of the following statements by the client indicates an understanding of the teaching? (Select all that apply.)

    A. "I plan to eat small, frequent meals."

    B. "I will eat easy-to-digest foods with limited spice."

    C. "I will use skim milk when cooking."

    D. "I plan to drink regular cola."

    E. "I will limit alcohol intake to two drinks per day."

PRACTICE Active Learning Scenario

A nurse is reviewing the plan of care for a client who has pancreatitis. What should the nurse include in the plan? Use the ATI Active Learning Template: System Disorder to complete this item.

ALTERATION IN HEALTH (DIAGNOSIS): Describe the classic presentation of pancreatitis.

LABORATORY TESTS: Describe four tests and expected findings.

NURSING CARE: Describe at least six nursing actions.

Application Exercises Key

1. A. The client is at risk for chronic obstructive pancreatitis from cholelithiasis. However, another finding is the priority to report.

    B. The client is at risk for pancreatic abscess or pseudocyst, which a continuous elevation of amylase can indicate. Increased serum amylase is expected for 2 to 3 days with acute pancreatitis. However, another finding is the priority to report.

    C. The client is at risk for paralytic ileus from acute pancreatitis. However, another finding is the priority to report.

    D. **CORRECT:** The greatest risk to the client is ECG changes and hypotension from hypocalcemia. Hand spasms when taking blood pressure is a manifestation of hypocalcemia.

    Ⓝ *NCLEX® Connection: Physiological Adaptation, Medical Emergencies*

2. A. Pancrelipase should be swallowed without chewing to reduce irritation and slow the release of the medication.

    B. **CORRECT:** The client should drink a full glass of water following administration of pancrelipase.

    C. Pancrelipase should be administered with every meal and snack.

    D. The contents of the pancrelipase capsule may be sprinkled on nonprotein foods, and peanut butter is a protein food.

    Ⓝ *NCLEX® Connection: Pharmacological and Parenteral Therapies, Medication Administration*

3. A. A client who has cholecystitis will report pain in the right upper quadrant radiating to the right shoulder.

    B. A client who has pancreatitis will report pain being worse when lying down.

    C. A client who has pancreatitis will report that pain is relieved by assuming the fetal position.

    D. **CORRECT:** A client who has pancreatitis will report severe, boring epigastric pain that radiates to the back, left flank, or left shoulder.

    Ⓝ *NCLEX® Connection: Physiological Adaptation, Pathophysiology*

4. A. This action assesses for pain, which can indicate pyelonephritis.

    B. This action assesses for the presence of rebound tenderness.

    C. **CORRECT:** Cullen's sign is indicated by a bluish-gray discoloration in the periumbilical area.

    D. Lung sounds are assessed by auscultating the area below the scapula.

    Ⓝ *NCLEX® Connection: Reduction of Risk Potential, System Specific Assessments*

5. A. **CORRECT:** Small, frequent meals are recommended for the client who has pancreatitis.

    B. **CORRECT:** Bland, easy-to-digest foods are recommended for the client who has pancreatitis.

    C. **CORRECT:** Low-fat foods are recommended for the client who has pancreatitis.

    D. Caffeine-free beverages are recommended for the client who has pancreatitis. Regular cola contains caffeine.

    E. The client who has pancreatitis should avoid any alcohol intake.

    Ⓝ *NCLEX® Connection: Basic Care and Comfort, Nutrition and Oral Hydration*

PRACTICE Answer

Using the ATI Active Learning Template: System Disorder

ALTERATION IN HEALTH (DIAGNOSIS): Severe, constant, knifelike pain (left upper quadrant, midepigastric, and/or radiating to the back)

LABORATORY TESTS
- Serum amylase (increases within 12 hr, remains increased for 4 days)
- Serum lipase value (increases slowly and remains increased for up to 2 weeks)
- Urine amylase remains increased for up to 2 weeks
- Increased WBC count due to inflammation/infection
- Decreased serum calcium and magnesium
- Serum liver enzymes and bilirubin increased with associated biliary dysfunction
- Serum glucose increased

NURSING CARE
- Maintain NPO status until the client is pain-free.
- Administer total parenteral nutrition or jejunal feedings (contraindicated if paralytic ileus develops).
- Maintain NG tube (for severe vomiting or paralytic ileus).
- Resume diet beginning with bland, high protein, low-fat foods, and no caffeine.
- Plan small, frequent meals.
- Administer antiemetics as needed.
- Limit stress.
- Provide pain management.
- Remind the client to not consume alcohol or smoke.

Ⓝ *NCLEX® Connection: Physiological Adaptation, Alterations in Body Systems*

CHAPTER 55 *Hepatitis and
Cirrhosis*

Hepatitis is an inflammation of liver cells.
Hepatitis can be caused by a viral or toxic agent,
or as a secondary infection in conjunction with
another virus. It is classified as acute or chronic.

Cirrhosis is permanent scarring of the liver that
is usually caused by chronic inflammation.

Hepatitis

- Viral hepatitis is the most common type of hepatitis.
- Toxic and drug-induced hepatitis occurs secondary to
  an exposure to a chemical or medication agent such as
  alcohol, industrial toxins, ephedra, or acetaminophen.
- Hepatitis can occur in conjunction with other
  viruses such as varicella-zoster, cytomegalovirus, or
  herpes simplex.
- After exposure to a virus or toxin, the liver becomes
  enlarged from the inflammatory process. As the disease
  progresses, there is an increase in inflammation and
  necrosis, interfering with blood flow to the liver.
- Individuals can be infected with hepatitis and remain
  free of manifestations, and therefore are unaware that
  they could be contagious.

Major categories of viral hepatitis
- Hepatitis A virus (HAV)
- Hepatitis B virus (HBV)
- Hepatitis C virus (HCV)
- Hepatitis D virus (HDV)
- Hepatitis E virus (HEV)

HEALTH PROMOTION AND
DISEASE PREVENTION

- Provide community health education interventions on
  transmission and exposure.
- Follow vaccination recommendations according to
  the CDC.
- Follow isolation precautions according to the CDC.
- Reinforce and use safe injection practices. Qs
  - Aseptic technique for preparation and administration
    of parenteral medications
  - Sterile, single-use, disposable needle and syringe for
    each injection
  - Single-dose vials whenever possible
  - Needleless systems or safety caps
- Use personal protective equipment, such as gown,
  gloves, and goggles, appropriate to the type of exposure.
  - Hepatitis A: Clients who are incontinent of stool
  - Hepatitis B or C: Exposure to blood
- Use proper hand hygiene (before preparing and eating
  food, after using the toilet or changing a diaper).
- When traveling to underdeveloped countries, drink
  purified water, and avoid sharing eating utensils and
  bed linens.

ASSESSMENT

RISK FACTORS

Hepatitis A

ROUTE OF TRANSMISSION: Fecal-oral

RISK FACTORS
- Ingestion of contaminated food or water,
  especially shellfish
- Close personal contact with an infected individual

Hepatitis B

ROUTE OF TRANSMISSION: Blood

RISK FACTORS
- Unprotected sex with infected individual
- Infants born to infected mothers
- Contact with infected blood
- Substance use disorder (injectable substances)

Hepatitis C

ROUTE OF TRANSMISSION: Blood

RISK FACTORS
- Substance use disorder (injectable substances)
- Blood, blood products, or organ transplants
- Contaminated needle sticks, unsanitary tattoo equipment
- Sexual contact

Hepatitis D

ROUTE OF TRANSMISSION: Coinfection with HBV

RISK FACTORS
- Substance use disorder (injectable substances)
- Unprotected sex with infected individual

Hepatitis E

ROUTE OF TRANSMISSION: Fecal-oral

RISK FACTORS: Ingestion of food or water contaminated with fecal waste

Additional risk factors

- Unscreened blood transfusions (prior to 1992)
- Hemodialysis
- Percutaneous exposure (dirty needles, sharp instruments, body piercing, tattooing, use of another person's substance use paraphernalia or personal hygiene tools)
- Unprotected sexual intercourse with a hepatitis-infected person, sex with multiple partners, anal sex
- Ingestion of food prepared by a hepatitis-infected person who does not practice proper sanitation precautions
- Travel/residence in underdeveloped country (using tap water to clean food products, drinking contaminated water)
- Eating or living in crowded environments (correctional facilities, dormitories, universities, long-term care facilities, military base housing)

EXPECTED FINDINGS

- Failure to take personal precautions with blood and body fluid
- Influenza-like manifestations
  - Fatigue
  - Decreased appetite with nausea
  - Abdominal pain
  - Joint pain

PHYSICAL ASSESSMENT FINDINGS
- Fever
- Vomiting
- Dark-colored urine
- Clay-colored stool
- Jaundice

LABORATORY TESTS Q_{EBP}

Hepatitis A

Alanine aminotransferase (ALT): Elevated; expected reference range 4 to 36 units/L.

Aspartate aminotransferase (AST): Elevated; expected reference range 0 to 35 units/L.

Alkaline phosphatase (ALP): Normal or elevated; expected reference range 30 to 120 units/L.

Total bilirubin level: Elevated; expected reference range 0.3 to 1.0 mg/dL.

Hepatitis A virus antibodies (anti-HAV): Presence indicates the presence of hepatitis A.

Immunoglobulin M antibodies (IgM): Presence indicates inflammation of the liver.

Immunoglobulin G antibodies (IgG): Presence indicates permanent immunity to hepatitis A.

Hepatitis B

ALT: Elevated

AST: Elevated

ALP: Normal or elevated

Total bilirubin level: Elevated

Hepatitis B surface antigen (HBsAg): Presence indicates that the individual is infectious. However, a client who is vaccinated against HBV will have a positive HBsAg, indicating immunity to the disease.

Hepatitis B surface antibody (anti-HBs): Presence indicates recovery and immunity from HBV infection.

Hepatitis B core antibody (anti-HBc): Presence indicates previous or ongoing infection.

IgM antibody to hepatitis B core antigen (IgM anti-HBc): Presence indicates acute infection.

Hepatitis B e antigen (HBeAg): Presence indicates that the virus is replicating.

Hepatitis B e antibody (anti-HBe): Presence is a predictor of long-term clearance of the virus.

Antibodies to HBsAb: Presence indicates recovery and immunity to hepatitis B.

Hepatitis C

ALT: Elevated

AST: Elevated

ALP: Normal or elevated

Total bilirubin level: Elevated

Hepatitis C virus antibodies (anti-HCV): Detects presence of antibodies to hepatitis C infection.

Enzyme immunoassay (EIA): Detects presence of antigens or antibodies to hepatitis C infection.

Enhanced chemiluminescence immunoassay (CIA): Detects presence of antibody to hepatitis C infection.

Recombinant immunoblot assay (RIBA): Detects presence of antibody to hepatitis C infection.

HCV RNA polymerase chain reaction (PCR): Qualitative test to detect the presence and amount of HCV.

Hepatitis D

Identification of intrahepatic delta antigen

Hepatitis D virus antibodies (anti-HDV): Presence indicates the presence of HDV.

Hepatitis E

Hepatitis E virus antibodies (anti-HEV): Presence indicates the presence of HEV.

DIAGNOSTIC PROCEDURES

Liver biopsy

This is the most definitive diagnostic approach, and it is used to identify the intensity of the infection, and the degree of liver damage.

PREPROCEDURE NURSING ACTIONS
- Explain the procedure.
- Witness informed consent.
- Ensure the client fasts starting at midnight on the day of the procedure in case surgery is needed due to a complication. Qs
- Administer medications as prescribed.

INTRAPROCEDURE NURSING ACTIONS
- Assist the client into the supine position with the upper right quadrant of the abdomen exposed.
- Assist the client with relaxation techniques.
- Instruct the client to exhale and hold for at least 10 seconds while the needle is inserted. Qs
- Instruct the client to resume breathing once the needle is withdrawn.
- Apply pressure to the puncture site.

POSTPROCEDURE NURSING ACTIONS
- Assist the client to a right side-lying position and maintain for several hours.
- Monitor vital signs.
- Assess for abdominal pain.
- Assess for bleeding from the puncture site.
- Assess for manifestations of pneumothorax (dyspnea, cyanosis, restlessness) due to accidental puncture of the pleura or lung.

PATIENT-CENTERED CARE

NURSING CARE

- Most clients will be cared for in the home unless they are acutely ill.
- Enforce contact precautions if indicated.
- Provide a high-carbohydrate, high-calorie, low- to moderate-fat, and low- to moderate-protein diet, and small, frequent meals to promote nutrition and healing.
- Promote hepatic rest and the regeneration of tissue.
  - Administer only necessary medications.
  - Avoid over-the-counter medications or herbal supplements.
  - Avoid alcohol.
  - Limit physical activity.
- Educate the client and family regarding measures to prevent the transmission of the disease to others at home. Qpcc
  - Avoid sexual intercourse until hepatitis antibody testing is negative.
  - Use proper hand hygiene.
- Provide culturally sensitive care.

MEDICATIONS

Hepatitis A

- Hepatitis A immunization is recommended for post-exposure protection.
- Immunoglobulin is recommended for post-exposure protection for clients older than 40 years, younger than 12 months, who have chronic liver disease, who are immunosuppressed, or who are allergic to the vaccine.

Hepatitis B, D

Acute infection: No medications; supportive care

Chronic infection: Antiviral medications: adefovir dipivoxil, interferon alfa-2b, peginterferon alfa-2a, lamivudine, entecavir, and telbivudine

Hepatitis C

Combination therapy with peginterferon alfa-2a and ribavirin is the preferred treatment.

Hepatitis E

No medications; supportive care

INTERPROFESSIONAL CARE

Possible consults with infection control, social worker, primary care provider, and/or community resources

COMPLICATIONS

Chronic hepatitis
- Ongoing inflammation of the liver cells
- Results from hepatitis B, C, or D
- Increases the client's risk for liver cancer

Fulminating hepatitis
- Extremely severe and potentially fatal form of viral hepatitis.
- Clients develop manifestations of viral hepatitis, then within hours or days develop severe liver failure.
- No medications, supportive care.

Cirrhosis of the liver: Permanent scarring of the liver that is usually caused by chronic inflammation

Liver cancer

Liver failure: Irreversible damage to liver cells, with decreased ability to function adequately to meet the body's needs

Cirrhosis

- Cirrhosis is extensive scarring of the liver caused by necrotic injury or a chronic reaction to inflammation over a prolonged period of time. Normal liver tissue is replaced with fibrotic tissue that lacks function.
- Portal and periportal areas of the liver are primarily involved, affecting the liver's ability to handle the flow of bile by nodules blocking the bile ducts and normal blood flow throughout the liver. The development of new bile channels causes an overgrowth of tissue and liver scarring/enlargement. Jaundice is often the result.

HEALTH PROMOTION AND DISEASE PREVENTION

- Stay current on immunizations.
- Encourage the client to avoid drinking alcohol, and to engage in an alcohol recovery program if needed. Q_{PCC}

Types of cirrhosis

Postnecrotic: Caused by viral hepatitis, or some medications or toxins

Laennec's: Caused by chronic alcohol use disorder

Biliary: Caused by chronic biliary obstruction or autoimmune disease

ASSESSMENT

RISK FACTORS

- Alcohol use disorder
- Chronic viral hepatitis (hepatitis B, C, or D)
- Autoimmune hepatitis (destruction of the liver cells by the immune system)
- Steatohepatitis (fatty liver disease causing chronic inflammation)
- Damage to the liver caused by medications, substances, toxins, and infections
- Chronic biliary cirrhosis (bile duct obstruction, bile stasis, hepatic fibrosis)
- Cardiac cirrhosis resulting from severe right heart failure inducing necrosis and fibrosis due to lack of blood flow

EXPECTED FINDINGS

- Fatigue
- Weight loss, abdominal pain, distention
- Pruritus (severe itching of skin)
- Confusion or difficulty thinking (due to the buildup of waste products in the blood and brain that the liver is unable to get rid of)
- Personality and mentation changes, emotional lability, euphoria, depression

PHYSICAL ASSESSMENT FINDINGS

- Cognitive changes
- Altered sleep/wake pattern
- Gastroesophageal bleeding (enlarged esophageal veins [varices] develop and burst, causing vomiting and passing of blood in bowel movements) or portal hypertensive gastropathy, which is bleeding of gastric mucosa
- Splenomegaly caused from backup of blood into the spleen, which can cause thrombocytopenia and platelet destruction
- Ascites (bloating or swelling due to fluid buildup in abdomen and legs)
- Jaundice (yellowing of skin) and icterus (yellowing of the eyes) from decreased excretion of bilirubin, resulting in an increase of circulating bilirubin levels
- Petechiae (round, pinpoint, red–purple lesions), ecchymoses (large yellow and purple-blue bruises), nosebleeds, hematemesis, melena (decreased synthesis of prothrombin, deteriorating hepatic function)
- Palmar erythema (redness, warmth of the palms of the hands)
- Spider angiomas (red lesions, vascular in nature with branches radiating on the nose, cheeks, upper thorax, shoulders)
- Dependent peripheral edema of extremities and sacrum
- Asterixis (liver flapping tremor): coarse tremor characterized by rapid, nonrhythmic extension and flexion of the wrists and fingers
- Fetor hepaticus (liver breath): fruity or musty odor

LABORATORY TESTS Q_{EBP}

Serum liver enzymes: Elevated initially

Lactate dehydrogenase (LDH), ALT and AST are elevated due to hepatic inflammation. ALT and AST return to normal when liver cells are no longer able to create an inflammatory response. ALP increases in cirrhosis due to intrahepatic biliary obstruction.

ALT: Expected reference range 4 to 36 units/L

AST: Expected reference range 0 to 35 units/L

ALP: Expected reference range 30 to 120 units/L

Serum bilirubin: Elevated

Bilirubin levels are elevated in cirrhosis due to the inability of the liver to excrete bilirubin.

Bilirubin, indirect (unconjugated): Elevated; expected reference range 0.2 to 0.8 mg/dL

Bilirubin, total: Elevated; expected reference range 0.3 to 1.0 mg/dL

Serum protein

- Decreased due to the lack of hepatic synthesis
- Expected reference range 6.4 to 8.3 g/dL

Serum albumin

- Decreased due to the lack of hepatic synthesis
- Expected reference range 3.5 to 5 g/dL

Hematological tests

RBC: Decreased
- Expected reference range, females 4.2 to 5.4 million/uL
- Expected reference range, males 4.7 to 6.1 million/uL

Hemoglobin: Decreased
- Expected reference range, females 12 to 16 g/dL
- Expected reference range, males 14 to 18 g/dL

Hematocrit: Decreased
- Expected reference range, females 37% to 47%
- Expected reference range, males 42% to 52%

Platelet count: Decreased; expected reference range 150,000 to 400,000 mm³

PT/INR

- Prolonged due to decreased synthesis of prothrombin
- Expected reference range PT 11 to 12.5 sec
- Expected reference range INR 0.8 to 1.1

Ammonia levels

- Increase when hepatocellular injury (cirrhosis) prevents the conversion of ammonia to urea for excretion.
- Expected reference range 6 to 47 µmol/L (10 to 80 mcg/dL)

Serum creatinine levels

- Can increase due to deteriorating kidney function, which can occur as a result of advanced liver disease
- Expected reference range, females 0.5 to 1.1 mg/dL
- Expected reference range, males 0.6 to 1.2 mg/dL

DIAGNOSTIC PROCEDURES

Ultrasound: Used to detect ascites, hepatomegaly, splenomegaly, biliary stones, or biliary obstruction

Abdominal x-rays and CT scan: Used to visualize possible hepatomegaly, ascites, and splenomegaly

MRI: Used to visualize mass lesions and determine whether the liver is malignant or benign

Liver biopsy (most definitive)
- A liver biopsy identifies the progression and extent of the cirrhosis.
- To minimize the risk of hemorrhage, a radiologist may perform the biopsy through the jugular vein, which is threaded to the hepatic vein to obtain tissue for a microscopic evaluation.
- This is done under fluoroscopy for safety because this procedure can be problematic for cirrhosis clients due to an increased risk for bleeding complications. Qs

Esophagogastroduodenoscopy: This is performed under moderate (conscious) sedation to detect the presence of esophageal varices, ulcerations in the stomach, or duodenal ulcers and bleeding.

Endoscopic retrograde cholangiopancreatography: Used to view the biliary tract to assist in removing stones, to collect specimens for biopsy, and for stent placement

PATIENT-CENTERED CARE

NURSING CARE QPCC

Respiratory status: Monitor oxygen saturation levels and distress. Provide comfort measures by positioning the client to ease respiratory effort (can be compromised by plasma volume excess and ascites). Have the client sit in a chair or elevate the head of the bed to 30° with feet elevated.

Skin integrity: Monitor closely for skin breakdown. Implement measures to prevent pressure ulcers. Pruritus, which is associated with jaundice, will cause the client to scratch. Encourage washing with cold water and applying lotion to decrease the itching.

Fluid balance: Monitor for indications of fluid volume excess. Keep strict I&O, obtain daily weights, and assess ascites and peripheral edema. Restrict fluids and sodium if prescribed.

Vital signs: Monitor vital signs and pain level as prescribed.

Neurological status: Monitor for deteriorating mental status and dementia consistent with hepatic encephalopathy. Monitor for asterixis (coarse tremor of wrists and fingers) and fetor hepaticus (fruity breath odor). Lactulose can be given to aid in excretion of ammonia.

Nutritional status: High-carbohydrate, high-protein, moderate-fat, and low-sodium diet with vitamin supplements such as thiamine, folate, and multivitamins

Gastrointestinal status: In the presence of ascites, measure abdominal girth daily over the largest part of the abdomen. Mark the location of tape for consistency. Observe for potential bleeding complications.

Pain status: Assess pain, and administer analgesics and gastrointestinal antispasmodics as needed.

MEDICATIONS QEBP

Because the metabolism of most medications is dependent upon a functioning liver, general medications are administered sparingly, especially opioids, sedatives, and barbiturates.

Diuretics: Decrease excessive fluid in the body.

Beta-blocking agent: Used for clients who have varices to prevent bleeding.

Lactulose: Used to promote excretion of ammonia from the body through the stool.

Nonabsorbable antibiotic: Can be used in place of lactulose.

THERAPEUTIC PROCEDURES

Paracentesis

Used to relieve ascites.

PREPROCEDURE NURSING CARE
- Explain the procedure.
- Witness informed consent.
- Obtain vital signs and weight.
- Assist the client to void to reduce the risk of injury to the bladder. Qs
- Weigh client.

INTRAPROCEDURE NURSING CARE
- Position the client supine with head of bed elevated.
- Assist the client with relaxation techniques.
- Apply dressing over puncture site.

POSTPROCEDURE NURSING CARE
- Monitor vital signs as prescribed.
- Maintain bed rest as prescribed.
- Measure the fluid, and document amount and color.
- Send specimen to the laboratory.
- Access puncture site dressing for drainage.
- Weigh client.

Endoscopic variceal ligation/ endoscopic sclerotherapy

- Varices are either sclerosed or banded endoscopically.
- There is a decreased risk of hemorrhage with banding.

Transjugular intrahepatic portosystemic shunt

Performed in interventional radiology for clients who require further intervention with ascites or hemorrhage.

Surgical bypass shunting procedures

This is a last resort for clients who have portal hypertension and esophageal varices. Ascites is shunted from the abdominal cavity to the superior vena cava.

Liver transplantation

- Portions of healthy livers from deceased donors (most commonly trauma victims) or living donors can be used for transplant.
- The transplanted liver portion will regenerate and grow in size based on the needs of the body.
- The client must meet the transplant criteria to be eligible.
- Clients who have severe cardiac and respiratory disease, metastatic malignant liver cancer, or alcohol/substance use disorder are not candidates for liver transplantation.

PREPROCEDURE NURSING ACTIONS
- Use a multidisciplinary approach.
- Witness informed consent.

POSTPROCEDURE NURSING ACTIONS Qpcc
- Provide close monitoring during the immediate postoperative period in an intensive care unit.
- Monitor vital signs frequently.
- Monitor neurological status.
- Monitor for acute graft rejection: tachycardia, fever, right upper quadrant pain, change in bile color or increased jaundice, increased ALT and AST levels.
- Monitor for infection: fever or excessive, foul-smelling drainage.
- Monitor for clotting problems: blood in drainage tubes, petechiae.
- Monitor for hepatic complications: decreased bile drainage, increased right upper quadrant pain with distention, nausea and vomiting, increased jaundice.
- Monitor for acute kidney injury: change in urine output, increased BUN and creatinine levels and electrolyte imbalance.
- Administer immunosuppressant agents.
- Administer antibiotic prophylaxis.
- Obtain blood cultures as prescribed.
- Keep T-tube in dependent position, and empty frequently, documenting amount and description.

INTERPROFESSIONAL CARE

- A dietary consult can assist with specific diet needs.
- Initiate appropriate referrals (social services, Alcoholics Anonymous, Al-Anon).

CLIENT EDUCATION Qpcc

- Encourage the client to abstain from alcohol and engage in an alcohol recovery program if needed.
  - Helps prevent further scarring and fibrosis of liver
  - Allows healing and regeneration of liver tissue
  - Prevents irritation of the stomach and esophagus lining
  - Helps decrease the risk of bleeding
  - Helps prevent other life-threatening complications
- Consult with the provider prior to taking any over-the-counter medications or herbal supplements. Qs
- Follow diet guidelines.
  - High-calorie, moderate-fat diet
  - Low-sodium diet (if the client has excessive fluid in the peritoneal cavity)
  - Low-protein (if encephalopathy, elevated ammonia)
  - Small, frequent, well-balanced nutritional meals
  - Supplemental vitamin-enriched liquids
  - Replacement and administration of vitamins due to the inability of the liver to store them
  - Fluid intake restrictions if serum sodium is low

COMPLICATIONS

Portal systemic encephalopathy

Clients who have a poorly functioning liver are unable to convert ammonia and other waste products to a less toxic form. These products are carried to the brain and cause neurological manifestations. Clients are treated with medications such as lactulose to reduce the ammonia levels in the body via intestinal excretion. Reductions in dietary protein are indicated as ammonia is formed when protein is broken down by intestinal flora.

NURSING ACTIONS
- Administer lactulose as prescribed.
- Monitor laboratory findings, including potassium, because clients can become hypokalemic with increased stools from the lactulose therapy.
- Assess for changes in the level of consciousness and orientation.
- Report asterixis (flapping of the hands) and fetor hepaticus (liver breath) immediately to the provider. These are clinical indications that encephalopathy is worsening.

CLIENT EDUCATION: Instruct the client about the prescribed diet.

Esophageal varices

CAUSES: Portal hypertension (elevated blood pressure in veins that carry blood from the intestines to the liver) is caused by impaired circulation of blood through the liver. Collateral circulation is subsequently developed, creating varices in the upper stomach and esophagus. Varices are fragile and can bleed easily.

NURSING ACTIONS
- Assist with saline lavage (vasoconstriction), esophagogastric balloon tamponade, blood transfusions, ligation and sclerotherapy, and shunts to stop bleeding and reduce the risk for hypovolemic shock.
- Monitor hemoglobin level and vital signs.
- Monitor for any bleeding.

Acute graft rejection post liver transplantation

This typically occurs between 4 and 10 days after surgery.

INDICATIONS OF REJECTION
- Tachycardia
- Upper right flank pain
- Jaundice
- Laboratory findings indicative of liver failure

CAUSES: Graft vs. host disease (recipient's bone marrow creates T-cells to attack the new organ).

NURSING ACTIONS
- Early diagnosis of graft rejection is necessary to successfully prevent total rejection of the liver.
- Administer immunosuppressants as prescribed.
- Monitor laboratory findings.

CLIENT EDUCATION
- Inform the client of the importance of taking immunosuppressants and monitoring white blood cell count.
- Instruct the client to report indications of rejection to the provider immediately.

Application Exercises

1. A nurse on a medical-surgical unit is admitting a client who has hepatitis B with ascites. Which of the following actions should the nurse include in the plan of care?
   A. Initiate contact precautions.
   B. Weigh the client weekly.
   C. Measure abdominal girth 7.5 cm (3 in) above the umbilicus.
   D. Provide a high-calorie, high-carbohydrate diet.

2. A nurse is caring for a client who has a new diagnosis of hepatitis C. Which of the following laboratory findings should the nurse expect?
   A. Presence of immunoglobulin G antibodies (IgG)
   B. Positive EIA test
   C. Aspartate aminotransferase (AST) 35 units/L
   D. Alanine aminotransferase (ALT) 15 IU/L

3. A nurse is assessing a client who has advanced cirrhosis. The nurse should identify which of the following findings as indicators of hepatic encephalopathy? (Select all that apply.)
   A. Anorexia
   B. Change in orientation
   C. Asterixis
   D. Ascites
   E. Fetor hepaticus

4. A nurse is caring for a client who has cirrhosis. Which of the following medications can the nurse expect to administer to this client? (Select all that apply.)
   A. Diuretic
   B. Beta-blocking agent
   C. Opioid analgesic
   D. Lactulose
   E. Sedative

5. A nurse is teaching a client who has hepatitis B about home care. Which of the following instructions should the nurse include in the teaching? (Select all that apply.)
   A. Limit physical activity.
   B. Avoid alcohol.
   C. Take acetaminophen for comfort.
   D. Wear a mask when in public places.
   E. Eat small frequent meals.

Application Exercises Key

1.   A. Hepatitis B is transmitted via blood. Standard precautions are adequate.

     B. Daily weights are obtained to monitor fluid status.

     C. The client's abdominal girth is measured over the largest part of the abdomen, which will vary by client.

     D. **CORRECT:** The client who has hepatitis B should have a diet high in calories and carbohydrates.

     Ⓝ *NCLEX® Connection: Physiological Adaptation, Illness Management*

2.   A. The presence of IgG is an expected laboratory finding in a client who has hepatitis A infection.

     B. **CORRECT:** A positive EIA test is an expected laboratory finding in a client who has a new diagnosis of hepatitis C.

     C. AST is elevated in clients who have hepatitis C infection; 35 units/L is within the expected reference range.

     D. ALT is elevated in clients who have hepatitis C infection; 15 units/L is within the expected reference range.

     Ⓝ *NCLEX® Connection: Reduction of Risk Potential, Laboratory Values*

3.   A. Anorexia is present in a client who has liver dysfunction, but it is not an indication of hepatic encephalopathy.

     B. **CORRECT:** A change in orientation indicates hepatic encephalopathy in a client who has advanced cirrhosis.

     C. **CORRECT:** Asterixis, a coarse tremor of the wrists and fingers, is observed as a late complication in a client who has cirrhosis and hepatic encephalopathy.

     D. Ascites can be present in a client who has liver dysfunction, but it is not an indication of hepatic encephalopathy.

     E. **CORRECT:** Fetor hepaticus, a fruity breath odor, is a finding of hepatic encephalopathy in the client who has advanced cirrhosis.

     Ⓝ *NCLEX® Connection: Physiological Adaptation, Pathophysiology*

4.   A. **CORRECT:** Diuretics facilitate excretion of excess fluid from the body in a client who has cirrhosis.

     B. **CORRECT:** Beta-blocking agents are prescribed for a client who has cirrhosis to prevent bleeding from varices.

     C. Opioid analgesics are metabolized in the liver. They should not be administered to a client who has cirrhosis.

     D. **CORRECT:** Lactulose is prescribed for a client who has cirrhosis to aid in the elimination of ammonia in the stool.

     E. Sedatives are metabolized in the liver. They should not be administered to a client who has cirrhosis.

     Ⓝ *NCLEX® Connection: Pharmacological and Parenteral Therapies, Medication Administration*

5.   A. **CORRECT:** Limiting physical activity and taking frequent rest breaks conserves energy and assists in the recovery process for a client who has hepatitis B.

     B. **CORRECT:** Alcohol is metabolized in the liver and should be avoided by the client who has hepatitis B.

     C. Acetaminophen is metabolized in the liver and should be avoided by the client who has hepatitis B.

     D. Hepatitis B is a blood-borne disease. Wearing a mask is not necessary to prevent transmission to others.

     E. **CORRECT:** The client who has hepatitis B should eat small frequent meals to promote improved nutrition due to the presence of anorexia.

     Ⓝ *NCLEX® Connection: Physiological Adaptation, Illness Management*

PRACTICE Active Learning Scenario

A nurse is caring for a client who has hepatitis C and will undergo liver biopsy. Use the ATI Active Learning Template: Diagnostic Procedure to complete the following.

DESCRIPTION OF PROCEDURE

NURSING INTERVENTIONS (PRE, INTRA, POST): One preprocedure, one intraprocedure, and one postprocedure.

POTENTIAL COMPLICATIONS: Identify one potential complication of the procedure.

PRACTICE Answer

Using the ATI Active Learning Template: Diagnostic Procedure

DESCRIPTION OF PROCEDURE: A liver biopsy is a procedure to collect a sample of liver tissue for diagnostic testing. A needle is inserted in the intercostal space between the two right lower ribs and into the liver. An aspirate of liver tissue is then collected.

NURSING ACTIONS (PRE, INTRA, POST)
Preprocedure
- Explain the procedure to the client/family.
- Witness informed consent.
- Ensure the client has been fasting since midnight.
- Administer medication as prescribed.

Intraprocedure
- Assist the client into the supine position with the upper right quadrant of the abdomen exposed.
- Assist the client with relaxation techniques.
- Instruct the client to exhale and hold for at least 10 seconds while the needle is inserted.
- Instruct the client to resume breathing once the needle is withdrawn.
- Apply pressure to the puncture site.

Postprocedure
- Assist the client to a right side-lying position and maintain for several hours.
- Monitor vital signs.
- Assess for abdominal pain.
- Assess for bleeding from puncture site.

POTENTIAL COMPLICATIONS
- Bleeding
- Bile peritonitis
- Pneumothorax

Ⓝ *NCLEX® Connection: Reduction of Risk Potential, Diagnostic Tests*

NCLEX® Connections

When reviewing the following chapters, keep in mind the relevant topics and tasks of the NCLEX outline, in particular:

Client Needs: Basic Care and Comfort

ELIMINATION: Assess and manage client with an alteration in elimination.

NON-PHARMACOLOGICAL COMFORT INTERVENTIONS: Provide non-pharmacological comfort measures.

NUTRITION AND ORAL HYDRATION: Provide/maintain special diets based on the client diagnosis/nutritional needs and cultural considerations.

Client Needs: Reduction of Risk Potential

DIAGNOSTIC TESTS: Apply knowledge of related nursing procedures and psychomotor skills when caring for clients undergoing diagnostic testing.

LABORATORY VALUES: Educate client about the purpose and procedure of prescribed laboratory tests.

POTENTIAL FOR COMPLICATIONS OF DIAGNOSTIC TESTS/TREATMENTS/PROCEDURES: Intervene to manage potential circulatory complications.

Client Needs: Physiological Adaptation

ALTERATIONS IN BODY SYSTEMS: Perform and manage care of client receiving peritoneal dialysis.

HEMODYNAMICS: Manage the care of a client receiving hemodialysis or continuous renal replacement therapy.

UNEXPECTED RESPONSE TO THERAPIES
Recognize signs and symptoms of complications and intervene appropriately when providing client care.

Promote the recovery of the client from unexpected response to therapy.

CHAPTER 56 *Renal Diagnostic Procedures*

Renal diagnostic procedures and laboratory assessments evaluate kidney function. By testing kidney function, providers can diagnose disease and evaluate the efficacy of treatment.

LABORATORY TESTS

Serum creatinine

Results from protein and muscle breakdown.
- Kidney disease is the only condition that increases serum creatinine levels.
- Kidney function loss of at least 50% causes an elevation of serum creatinine values.
- Serum creatinine values remain constant in older adults unless they have kidney disease.

Blood urea nitrogen (BUN)

Results from the breakdown of protein in the liver, creating the byproduct urea nitrogen excreted by the kidneys.
- Factors affecting BUN are dehydration, infection, chemotherapy, steroid therapy, and reabsorption of blood in the liver from damaged tissue.
- Elevated BUN suggests kidney disease.

Urinalysis

Evaluates waste products from the kidney and detects urologic disorders.
- Collection of an early-morning specimen provides a more concentrated sample.
- Urinalysis identifies color; clarity; concentration or dilution; specific gravity; acidity or alkalinity; and presence of drug metabolites, glucose, ketone bodies, and protein.
- Glucose, ketone bodies, and protein, including leukocyte esterase and nitrites, are not usually present in urine and can indicate diabetes mellitus; fat metabolism; infection; or, after a cytology analysis, cancer.
- Urine for culture and sensitivity identifies bacteria and determines the type of antibiotic to treat the infection.
- A 24-hr urine collection measures creatinine, urea nitrogen, sodium, chloride, calcium, catecholamines, and proteins.
- A 24-hr collection for creatinine clearance measures the glomerular filtration rate for clients who have impaired kidney function.

RENAL DIAGNOSTIC PROCEDURES

Radiography (x-ray)

- An x-ray of the kidneys, ureters, and bladder (KUB or a "flat plate")
- Allows for visualization of structures and to detect renal calculi, strictures, calcium deposits, or obstructions.

NURSING CONSIDERATIONS
- Ask female clients if they are pregnant.
- Tell clients to remove clothes over the area and all jewelry and metal objects.

COMPLICATIONS: No known complications

CT scan

- Provides three-dimensional imaging of the renal/urinary system to assess for kidney size and obstruction, cysts, or masses.
- IV contrast dye (iodine-based) enhances images.

NURSING CONSIDERATIONS
- Same as KUB without contrast dye
- Same as excretory urography with contrast dye (exclude bowel preparation)

COMPLICATIONS: Dye can cause acute kidney injury.

MRI

Useful for staging cancer, similar to CT.

NURSING CONSIDERATIONS: Clients lie down and have to remain still for the test.

COMPLICATIONS: Poor imaging if a client is unable to lie still

Ultrasound

Assesses the size of kidneys; images the ureters, bladder, masses, cysts, calculi, and obstructions of the lower urinary tract.

NURSING CONSIDERATIONS
- Provide skin care by removing gel after the procedure.
- Good alternative to excretory urography.

COMPLICATIONS: Minimal risk for the client.

Cystography, cystourethrography, voiding cystourethrogram (VCUG)

- Detects urethral or bladder injury after instillation of contrast dye through a urinary catheter to provide an image of the bladder (cystography) and the ureters (cystourethrography).
- VCUG detects via an x-ray during urination whether urine refluxes into the ureters.

NURSING CONSIDERATIONS
- Monitor for infection for the first 72 hr after the procedure.
- Encourage increased fluid intake to dilute urine and minimize burning on urination.
- Monitor urine output (less than 30 mL/hr) if suspected pelvic or urethral trauma.
- Contrast dye does not reach the bloodstream or the kidneys and is not nephrotoxic.

COMPLICATIONS
- Urinary tract infection due to catheter placement
- Cloudy, foul-smelling urine
- Urgency
- Urine positive for leukocyte esterase and nitrites, sediment, and RBCs

Kidney biopsy

Removal of a sample of tissue by excision or needle aspiration for cytological (histological) examination

NURSING CONSIDERATIONS
- Clients receive sedation and ongoing monitoring.
- PREPROCEDURE
  - Review coagulation studies.
  - Nothing by mouth for 4 to 6 hr.
- POSTPROCEDURE
  - Monitor vital signs following sedation.
  - Assess dressings and urinary output (hematuria).
  - Review Hgb and Hct values.
  - Administer PRN pain medication.

COMPLICATIONS
- Hemorrhage
- Infection
- Cloudy, foul-smelling urine
- Urgency
- Urine positive for leukocyte esterase and nitrites, sediment, and RBCs

Cystoscopy, cystourethroscopy

Used to discover abnormalities of bladder wall (cystoscopy) and/or occlusions of ureter or urethra (cystourethroscopy).

NURSING CONSIDERATIONS
- Clients receive anesthesia for the procedure.
- Check for signs of bleeding and infection. Monitor for infection for the first 72 hr after the procedure.
- PREPROCEDURE
  - NPO after midnight.
  - Administer laxative or enemas for bowel preparation the night before the procedure.
- INTRAPROCEDURE
  - Monitor vital signs.
  - General and local anesthesia are options.
  - Place the client in lithotomy position.
- POSTPROCEDURE
  - Monitor vital signs and urine output.
  - Document the color of urine (can be pink-tinged).
  - Irrigate urinary catheter with 0.9% sodium chloride irrigation if blood clots are present or the urine output is decreased or absent.
  - Encourage oral fluids to increase urine output and reduce any burning sensation with urination.

COMPLICATIONS
- Possible urinary tract infection from instrumentation
- Cloudy, foul-smelling urine
- Urgency
- Urine positive for leukocyte esterase, nitrites, sediment, and RBCs

Retrograde pyelogram, cystogram, urethrogram

- Identifies obstruction or structural disorders of the ureters and renal pelvis of the kidneys (pyelogram) by instilling contrast dye during a cystoscopy.
- Identifies fistulas, diverticula, and tumors in the bladder (cystogram) and urethra (urethrogram) by instilling contrast dye during a cystoscopy.

NURSING CONSIDERATIONS: Same as a cystoscopy

COMPLICATIONS: Same as a cystoscopy

Renal scan

Assesses renal blood flow and estimates glomerular filtration rate (GFR) after IV injection of radioactive material to produce a scanned image of the kidneys.

POSTPROCEDURE NURSING CONSIDERATIONS
- Assess blood pressure frequently during and after the procedure if the client receives captopril during the procedure to change the blood flow to the kidneys.
- Alert clients about possible orthostatic hypotension following the procedure if they received captopril.
- Increase fluid intake if hypotension occurs and also to promote excretion of the radioisotope.

COMPLICATIONS
- Radioactive material does not cause nephrotoxicity.
- Clients are not at risk from radioactive material they excrete in the urine.

Excretory urography

Detects obstruction and parenchymal masses, and assesses the size of the kidneys. IV contrast dye (iodine-based) enhances the images.

NURSING CONSIDERATIONS: Same as KUB
- PREPROCEDURE
  - Encourage increased fluids the day before procedure.
  - Bowel cleansing with a laxative or an enema to remove fecal contents, fluid, and gas from the colon for a clearer visualization.
  - NPO after midnight.
  - Determine allergies to iodine, seafood, eggs, milk, or chocolate, or if the client has asthma.
  - Check creatinine and BUN levels.
  - Withhold metformin for 24 hr before the procedure (risk for lactic acidosis from contrast dye with iodine).
- POSTPROCEDURE
  - Administer parenteral fluid, or encourage oral fluids to flush dye through the renal system and prevent complications.
  - Diuretics can increase dye excretion.
  - Check creatinine and BUN serum levels before resuming metformin.

COMPLICATIONS: Dye can cause acute kidney injury.

GERONTOLOGICAL CONSIDERATIONS ©

- Kidney size and function decrease with aging.
- Blood flow adaptability decreases, especially during a hypotensive or hypertensive crisis.
- GFR decreases by half the rate of a young adult.
- Diabetes mellitus, hypertension, and heart failure can affect GFR.
- Kidney injury can occur more easily from contrast dyes and medication due to decreased kidney size, blood flow, and GFR.
- Tubular changes can cause urgency and nocturnal polyuria.
- A weak urinary sphincter muscle and a shorter urethra in women can cause incontinence and urinary tract infections.
- An enlarged prostate in men can cause urinary retention and infection.

PRACTICE Active Learning Scenario

A nurse is developing a plan of care for a client who will undergo a cystoscopy with retrograde pyelogram. What information should the nurse include in the plan of care? Use the ATI Active Learning Template: Diagnostic Procedure to complete this item.

DESCRIPTION OF PROCEDURE: Define the procedure.

INDICATIONS: Identify one indication for cystoscopy and two for retrograde pyelogram.

NURSING INTERVENTIONS (PRE, INTRA, POST): Describe two nursing actions for preprocedure and two for postprocedure.

Application Exercises

1. A nurse is teaching a client who will have an x-ray of the kidneys, ureters, and bladder. Which of the following statements should the nurse include in the teaching?

   A. "You will receive contrast dye during the procedure."

   B. "An enema is necessary before the procedure."

   C. "You will need to lie in a prone position during the procedure."

   D. "The procedure determines whether you have a kidney stone."

2. A nurse is monitoring a client who had a kidney biopsy for postoperative complications. Which of the following complications should the nurse identify as causing the greatest risk to the client?

   A. Infection

   B. Hemorrhage

   C. Hematuria

   D. Pain

3. A nurse is caring for a client who has type 2 diabetes mellitus and will have excretory urography. Prior to the procedure, which of the following actions should the nurse take? (Select all that apply.)

   A. Identify an allergy to seafood.

   B. Withhold metformin for 24 hr.

   C. Administer an enema.

   D. Obtain a serum coagulation profile.

   E. Assess for asthma.

4. A nurse administered captopril to a client during a renal scan. Which of the following actions should the nurse take?

   A. Assess for hypertension.

   B. Limit the client's fluid intake.

   C. Monitor for orthostatic hypotension.

   D. Encourage early ambulation.

5. A nurse is reviewing the results of a client's urinalysis. The findings indicate the urine is positive for leukocyte esterase and nitrites. Which of the following actions should the nurse take?

   A. Repeat the test early the next morning.

   B. Start a 24-hr urine collection for creatinine clearance.

   C. Obtain a clean-catch urine specimen for culture and sensitivity.

   D. Insert an indwelling catheter urinary catheter to collect a urine specimen.

Application Exercises Key

1. A. Clients do not receive any contrast dye for this procedure, as they would for excretory urography.

   B. Clients do not receive an enema before this procedure, because it does not affect the gastrointestinal system.

   C. The client will lie supine, not prone.

   D. **CORRECT:** The nurse should explain to the client that a KUB can identify renal calculi, strictures, calcium deposits, and obstructions of the urinary system.

   Ⓝ *NCLEX® Connection: Reduction of Risk Potential, Diagnostic Tests*

2. A. The client is at risk for infection of the kidney because a biopsy is an invasive procedure. However, another complication is the priority.

   B. **CORRECT:** The greatest risk to the client following a kidney biopsy is hemorrhage due to a lack of clotting at the puncture site. The nurse should report this finding to the provider immediately.

   C. The client is at risk for hematuria, which is a common complication the first 48 to 72 hr after the biopsy. However, another complication is the priority.

   D. The client is at risk for pain after a kidney biopsy because blood in and around the kidney causes pressure on the nerves in the area; however, another complication is the priority.

   Ⓝ *NCLEX® Connection: Reduction of Risk Potential, Diagnostic Tests*

3. A. **CORRECT:** Clients who have an allergy to seafood are at higher risk for an allergic reaction to the contrast dye they will receive during the procedure.

   B. **CORRECT:** Clients who take metformin are at risk for lactic acidosis from the contrast dye with iodine they will receive during the procedure.

   C. **CORRECT:** Clients should receive an enema to remove fecal contents, fluid, and gas from the colon for a more clear visualization.

   D. A serum coagulation profile is essential for a client prior to a kidney biopsy because of the risk of hemorrhage from the procedure.

   E. **CORRECT:** Clients who have asthma have a higher risk of an exacerbation as an allergic response to the contrast dye they will receive during the procedure.

   Ⓝ *NCLEX® Connection: Reduction of Risk Potential, Diagnostic Tests*

4. A. Captopril is an antihypertensive medication. The nurse should assess the client for hypotensive effects.

   B. Increasing the client's fluid intake can help resolve hypotensive effects following the administration of captopril.

   C. **CORRECT:** The nurse should monitor for orthostatic hypotension because this is an adverse effect of captopril. This results in a change in blood flow to the kidneys after the initial dose.

   D. The client is at risk for falls when ambulating due to the hypotensive effects of captopril. The nurse should encourage the client to remain in bed.

   Ⓝ *NCLEX® Connection: Pharmacological and Parenteral Therapies, Medication Administration*

5. A. Repeating the test early the next morning will not change the urinalysis results.

   B. A 24-hr urine collection for creatinine helps to determine kidney function.

   C. **CORRECT:** The nurse should obtain a clean-catch urine specimen for culture and sensitivity. This test will identify which antibiotic will be most effective for treating the client's urinary tract infection.

   D. The nurse should insert a urinary catheter to collect urine when a client cannot empty his bladder.

   Ⓝ *NCLEX® Connection: Reduction of Risk Potential, Diagnostic Tests*

PRACTICE Answer

Using ATI Active Learning Template: Diagnostic Procedure

DESCRIPTION OF PROCEDURE
- Cystoscopy is instrumentation into the urinary tract to inspect the bladder wall.
- Retrograde pyelogram is the injection of dye up the ureters to inspect the ureters and pelvis of the kidney.

INDICATIONS
- Cystoscopy discovers abnormalities of the bladder wall (cysts, tumors, stones).
- Retrograde pyelogram discovers obstructions or structural disorders of the ureters and kidney pelvis (strictures, stones, mass).

NURSING INTERVENTIONS (PRE, INTRA, POST)
Preprocedure
- Clients must be NPO after midnight.
- Administer a laxative the night before the procedure.

Postprocedure
- Monitor vital signs.
- Encourage an increase in oral fluid intake to reduce the burning sensation when voiding.
- Document the color of urine.
- For clients who have a urinary catheter, irrigate it with 0.9% sodium chloride irrigation for active bleeding, clots, or decreased or absent urine output.

Ⓝ *NCLEX® Connection: Reduction of Risk Potential, Diagnostic Tests*

CHAPTER 57 *Hemodialysis and Peritoneal Dialysis*

Dialysis can sustain life for clients who have acute or chronic kidney failure. Dialysis does not replace the hormonal functions of the kidneys. Two types of dialysis are hemodialysis and peritoneal dialysis.

FUNCTIONS OF DIALYSIS

- Rids the body of excess fluid and electrolytes
- Achieves acid-base balance
- Eliminates waste products
- Restores internal homeostasis by osmosis, diffusion, and ultrafiltration

Hemodialysis

Hemodialysis shunts blood from the body through a dialyzer and back into circulation. Hemodialysis requires vascular access.

INDICATIONS

POTENTIAL DIAGNOSES

- Renal insufficiency
- Acute kidney injury
- Chronic kidney disease
- Drug overdose
- Persistent hyperkalemia
- Hypervolemia that does not respond to diuretics

CLIENT PRESENTATION

- Fluid volume changes, electrolyte and pH imbalances, and nitrogenous wastes.
- Hemodialysis is based on symptoms, not the glomerular filtration rate.
- Manifestations include fluid overload, neurological changes, bleeding, and uremia (cognitive impairment, pruritus, nausea, vomiting).

CONSIDERATIONS

PREPROCEDURE

NURSING ACTIONS

- Check for informed consent.
- Use a temporary hemodialysis dual-lumen catheter or subcutaneous device until the provider inserts a long-term device and it is available for access.
- Assess the patency of a long-term device: arteriovenous (AV) fistula or AV graft (presence of bruit, palpable thrill, distal pulses, and circulation).
- Avoid measuring blood pressure, administering injections, performing venipunctures, or inserting IV catheters on or into an arm with an access site. Elevate the extremity following surgical creation of an AV fistula to reduce swelling.
- Assess vital signs, laboratory values (BUN, serum creatinine, electrolytes, Hct), and weight.
- Discuss with the provider medications to withhold until after dialysis. Withhold any dialyzable medications and medications that lower blood pressure.

CLIENT EDUCATION: Inform clients that they will need hemodialysis three times per week, for 3- to 5-hr sessions. The provider will insert two needles, one into an artery and the other into a vein.

INTRAPROCEDURE

NURSING ACTIONS

- Monitor for complications during dialysis.
  - Dialysis circuit clotting, air bubbles in blood tubing, temperature of the dialysate (37.8° C [100° F]), regulation of the ultrafiltration
  - Hypotension, cramping, vomiting, bleeding at the access site, contamination of equipment
- Monitor vital signs and coagulation studies during dialysis. Monitor for bleeding, such as oozing from insertion site.
  - Administer anticoagulants.
  - Heparin prevents clotting of the blood.
  - Monitor aPTT to assess the risk of hemorrhage.
- Have protamine sulfate ready to reverse heparin. Qs
- Provide emotional support and offer activities (books, magazines, music, cards, or television).

CLIENT EDUCATION

- Advise the client to notify the nurse of headache, nausea, or dizziness during dialysis.
- Advise the client not to eat during dialysis.

POSTPROCEDURE

NURSING ACTIONS

- Monitor vital signs and laboratory values (BUN, serum creatinine, electrolytes, Hct). Decreases in blood pressure and changes in laboratory values are common following dialysis.
- Compare the client's preprocedure weight with the postprocedure weight as a way to estimate the amount of fluid the procedure removed.

  1 L fluid equals 1 kg (2.2 lb).

- Assess for the following.
  - Complications (hypotension, clotting of vascular access, headache, muscle cramps, bleeding)
  - Indications of bleeding or infection at the access site
  - Signs of disequilibrium syndrome
  - Signs of hypovolemia (hypotension, dizziness, tachycardia)
- Avoid invasive procedures for 4 to 6 hr after dialysis due to the risk of bleeding as a result of anticoagulation.

CLIENT EDUCATION

- Reinforce AV fistula or AV graft precautions. **Qs**
- Teach the client to perform the following.
  - Alert the nurse of early signs of disequilibrium syndrome, such as nausea and headache.
  - Check the access site at intervals following dialysis. Apply light pressure if bleeding.
  - Check the graft for patency by checking for a thrill or bruit.
  - Monitor the access site for signs of an infection, such as fever, redness, drainage, or swelling.
  - Contact the provider if bleeding from the insertion site lasts longer than 30 min following dialysis, for no thrill/bruit, or signs of infection.
  - Take medications and supplements to replace folate loss.
  - Eat well-balanced meals to include foods high in folate (beans, green vegetables), and take supplements. Each exchange during dialysis depletes protein, requiring the client to increase protein intake over predialysis limitations, but it still might require some restriction.
  - Avoid lifting heavy objects with the access-site arm.
  - Avoid carrying objects that compress or constrict the extremity.
  - Avoid sleeping on top of the extremity with the access device.
  - Perform hand exercises that promote fistula maturation.

COMPLICATIONS

Clotting/infection of the access site

- Anticoagulants prevent blood clots from forming. Monitor for hemorrhage at the insertion site.
- Cannulation can introduce infections at the access site.
  - Immunosuppressive disorders increase the risk for infection.
  - Advanced age is a risk factor for dialysis-induced hypotension and access site complications due to chronic illnesses or fragile veins. **Ⓒ**

NURSING ACTIONS

- Use surgical aseptic technique during cannulation.
- Avoid compression of the access site.
- Avoid venipuncture or blood pressure measurements on the extremity with the access site.
- Administer anticoagulants.
- Assess the graft site for a palpable thrill or audible bruit indicating vascular flow.
- Assess the access site for redness, swelling, or drainage. Monitor for fever.

Disequilibrium syndrome

Disequilibrium syndrome results from too rapid a decrease of BUN and circulating fluid volume. It can result in cerebral edema and increased intracranial pressure.

- Early recognition of disequilibrium syndrome is essential. Manifestations include nausea, vomiting, changes in level of consciousness, seizures, and agitation.
- Advanced age is a risk factor for dialysis disequilibrium and hypotension due to rapid changes in fluid and electrolyte status. **Ⓒ**

NURSING ACTIONS

- Use a slow dialysis exchange rate, especially for older adult clients and first-time hemodialysis.
- Administer anticonvulsants or barbiturates if the client requires them.

Hypotension

Antihypertensive therapy and rapid fluid depletion during dialysis can cause hypotension.

NURSING ACTIONS

- Carefully replace fluid volume by infusing IV fluids or colloid. Slow the dialysis exchange rate.
- Lower the head of the client's bed.
- For severe hypotension that does not respond to fluid replacement, discontinue the dialysis.

Anemia

Blood loss and removal of folate during dialysis can contribute to the anemia that often accompanies chronic kidney disease (from decreased RBC production due to decreased erythropoietin secretion).

NURSING ACTIONS

- Administer erythropoietin to stimulate the production of RBC.
- Monitor Hgb and RBC level.
- Monitor for hypotension and tachycardia.
- Transfuse blood products.

Infectious diseases

Blood transfusions and frequent blood access due to hemodialysis pose a risk for transmission of bloodborne infections such as HIV and hepatitis B and C.

NURSING ACTIONS

- Use sterile equipment and skin antisepsis.
- Use standard precautions.

Peritoneal dialysis

- Peritoneal dialysis involves instillation of hypertonic dialysate solution into the peritoneal cavity and subsequent dwell times. Drain the dialysate solution that includes the waste products. The peritoneum serves as the filtration membrane.
- The client should have an intact peritoneal membrane, without adhesions from infection or multiple surgeries.

INDICATIONS

- Peritoneal dialysis is the treatment of choice for the older adults who require dialysis.
- Peritoneal dialysis treats clients requiring dialysis who:
  - Are unable to tolerate anticoagulation.
  - Have difficulty with vascular access.
  - Have chronic infections or are unstable.
  - Have chronic diseases, such as diabetes mellitus, heart failure, or severe hypertension.

CONSIDERATIONS

PREPROCEDURE

NURSING ACTIONS

- Assess dry weight (without dialysate instillation), vital signs, serum electrolytes, creatinine, BUN, and blood glucose.
- Determine the client's ability to self-perform peritoneal dialysis and follow sterile technique.
  - Level of alertness
  - Past experience with dialysis
  - Understanding of procedure

CLIENT EDUCATION

- Instruct the client about the procedure. The client can feel fullness when the dialysate is dwelling. There can be discomfort initially with dialysate infusion.
- Continuous ambulatory peritoneal dialysis (CAPD) requires 7 days/week for 4 to 8 hr. Clients can continue normal activities during CAPD.
- Continuous-cycle peritoneal dialysis (CCPD) is a 24-hr dialysis. The exchange occurs at night while the client is sleeping. The final exchange is left in to dwell during the day.
- Automated peritoneal dialysis (APD) is a 30-min exchange repeated over 8 to 10 hr while the client is sleeping.

INTRAPROCEDURE

NURSING ACTIONS

- Monitor vital signs frequently during initial dialysis of clients in a hospital setting.
- Monitor serum glucose level (dialysate contains glucose, a hypertonic solution).
- Record the amount of inflow compared to outflow of dialysate.
- Monitor the color (should be clear, light yellow) and amount (should equal or exceed the amount of dialysate inflow) of outflow.
- Monitor for signs of infection (fever; bloody, cloudy, or frothy dialysate return; drainage at access site) and for complications (respiratory distress, abdominal pain, insufficient outflow, discolored outflow).
- Check the access site dressing for wetness (risk of dialysate leakage) and exit-site infections.
- Warm the dialysate prior to instilling. Avoid the use of microwave ovens, which cause uneven heating.
- Adhere to the times for infusion, dwell, and outflow.
- Maintain surgical asepsis of the catheter insertion site and when accessing the catheter.
- Keep the outflow bag lower than the client's abdomen (drain by gravity, prevent reflux).
- Reposition the client if inflow or outflow is inadequate.
- Carefully milk the peritoneal dialysis catheter if a fibrin clot has formed.
- Provide emotional support to the client and family.

POSTPROCEDURE

NURSING ACTIONS: Monitor weight, serum electrolytes, creatinine, BUN, and blood glucose.

CLIENT EDUCATION

- Teach the client home care of the access site.
- Instruct the client and family how to perform peritoneal dialysis exchanges at home. Provide support for home peritoneal dialysis with home visits. Q PCC
- Seek additional information from the National Kidney Foundation for local support groups.
- Teach the client to follow instructions carefully and to take all medications.
- Instruct the client to take essential minerals and vitamins with supplements of phosphorus, calcium, sodium, and potassium.
- Older adult clients can be unable to care for a peritoneal access site due to cognitive or physical deficits. Ⓒ
- Body image changes from bloating can be a concern for clients.

COMPLICATIONS

Peritonitis

Peritoneal dialysis can allow micro-organisms into the peritoneum and cause peritonitis.

NURSING ACTIONS
- Maintain surgical asepsis during the procedure.
- Monitor for infection, such as fever, purulent drainage, redness, swelling, and cloudy or discolored drained dialysate.

CLIENT EDUCATION
- Educate the client to use strict sterile technique during exchanges.
- Instruct the client to notify the provider about any indications of infection.

Infection at the access site

- Infection at the access site can result from leakage of dialysate. Access-site infections can cause peritonitis.
- Advanced age is a risk factor for access site complications due to chronic illnesses and/or fragile veins. Ⓖ

NURSING ACTIONS
- Maintain surgical asepsis at the access site.
- Assess the site for wetness from a leaking catheter.
- Monitor for infection, such as fever, purulent drainage, redness, or swelling.

CLIENT EDUCATION
- Educate the client to use strict sterile technique during exchanges.
- Instruct the client to notify the provider of any indications of infection. Ⓠⓢ
- Advise the client to assess the site for leaks, and prevent tugging or twisting of the tubing.

Protein loss

Peritoneal dialysis can remove protein from the blood as well as excess fluid, wastes, and electrolytes.

NURSING ACTIONS
- Increase the client's dietary intake of protein over predialysis restrictions.
- Monitor serum albumin levels.

CLIENT EDUCATION: Instruct the client to follow the renal diet with an increase in dietary protein.

Hyperglycemia and hyperlipidemia

- Hyperglycemia can result from the hyperosmolarity of the dialysate.
- The blood can absorb glucose from the dialysate.
- Hyperlipidemia can also occur from long-term therapy and lead to hypertension.

NURSING ACTIONS
- Monitor serum glucose.
- Administer insulin for glycemic control.
- Administer antilipemic medication for triglyceride control.

CLIENT EDUCATION
- Instruct the client to check serum glucose.
- Instruct the client to follow the diet the provider recommends.
- Instruct the client to take antihypertensive medication for elevated blood pressure.

Poor dialysate inflow or outflow

- Obstruction or twisting of the tubing can decrease the flow.
- Constipation is a common cause of poor inflow or outflow.

NURSING ACTIONS
- Reposition the client if inflow or outflow is inadequate.
- Milk the tubing to break up fibrin clots.
- Check the tubing for kinks or closed clamps.
- Tell the client to avoid constipation by using stool softeners and consuming a diet high in fiber.

CLIENT EDUCATION
- Advise the client to check the tubing for kinks, and teach the client how to remove a fibrin clot.
- Remind the client to monitor the inflow and outflow, and to change position or lower or raise the dialysate bag to improve flow.
- Advise the client to prevent constipation with diet and stool softeners.
- Encourage the client to lie supine with head slightly elevated during CCPD and APD treatment.

Application Exercises

1. A nurse is teaching a client who has chronic kidney disease and is to begin hemodialysis. Which of the following information should the nurse include in the teaching?

   A. Hemodialysis restores kidney function.

   B. Hemodialysis replaces hormonal function of the renal system.

   C. Hemodialysis allows an unrestricted diet.

   D. Hemodialysis returns a balance to serum electrolytes.

2. A nurse is preparing to initiate hemodialysis for a client who has acute kidney injury. Which of the following actions should the nurse take? (Select all that apply.)

   A. Review the medications the client currently takes.

   B. Assess the AV fistula for a bruit.

   C. Calculate the client's hourly urine output.

   D. Measure the client's weight.

   E. Check serum electrolytes.

   F. Use the access site area for venipuncture.

3. A nurse is planning postprocedure care for a client who received hemodialysis. Which of the following interventions should the nurse include in the plan of care? (Select all that apply.)

   A. Check BUN and serum creatinine.

   B. Administer medications the nurse withheld prior to dialysis.

   C. Observe for signs of hypovolemia.

   D. Assess the access site for bleeding.

   E. Evaluate blood pressure on the arm with AV access.

4. A nurse is caring for a client who develops disequilibrium syndrome after receiving hemodialysis. Which of the following actions should the nurse take?

   A. Administer an opioid medication.

   B. Monitor for hypertension.

   C. Assess level of consciousness.

   D. Increase the dialysis exchange rate.

5. A nurse is planning care for a client who will undergo peritoneal dialysis. Which of the following actions should the nurse take? (Select all that apply.)

   A. Monitor serum glucose levels.

   B. Report cloudy dialysate return.

   C. Warm the dialysate in a microwave oven.

   D. Assess for shortness of breath.

   E. Check the access site dressing for wetness.

   F. Maintain medical asepsis when accessing the catheter insertion site.

PRACTICE Active Learning Scenario

A nurse is reviewing complications that a client can develop when receiving peritoneal dialysis. What complications and nursing actions should the nurse include in the review? Use the ATI Active Learning Template: Diagnostic Procedure to complete this item.

DESCRIPTION OF PROCEDURE: Write out the name, and define the diagnostic test.

POTENTIAL COMPLICATIONS: List three.

NURSING INTERVENTIONS: List two nursing actions for each of the three complications.

Application Exercises Key

1. A. Hemodialysis does not restore kidney function, but it sustains the life of a client who has kidney disease.

    B. Hemodialysis does not replace hormonal function of the renal system due to tissue damage causing dysfunction of the renin-angiotensin-aldosterone system.

    C. Hemodialysis does not allow an unrestricted diet. It requires a diet high in folate and more protein than predialysis restrictions allowed, and low in sodium, potassium, and phosphorus.

    D. **CORRECT:** The nurse should explain to the client that hemodialysis restores electrolyte balance by removing excess sodium, potassium, fluids, and waste products, and also restores acid-base balance.

    Ⓝ *NCLEX® Connection: Physiological Adaptation, Hemodynamics*

2. A. **CORRECT:** By reviewing the medications the client currently takes, the nurse can determine which medications to withhold until after dialysis.

    B. **CORRECT:** Assessing the AV fistula for a bruit determines the patency of the fistula for dialysis.

    C. The client's hourly urine output can vary with the remaining kidney function and does not determine the need for dialysis.

    D. **CORRECT:** Measuring the client's weight before dialysis is essential for comparing it with the client's weight after dialysis.

    E. **CORRECT:** Checking the serum electrolytes determines the need for dialysis.

    F. The nurse should never use the access site area for venipuncture because compression from the tourniquet can cause loss of the vascular access.

    Ⓝ *NCLEX® Connection: Physiological Adaptation, Alterations in Body Systems*

3. A. **CORRECT:** The nurse should check the BUN and serum creatinine to determine the presence and degree of uremia or waste products that remain following dialysis.

    B. **CORRECT:** The nurse should withhold medications the treatment can partially dialyze. After the treatment, the nurse should administer the medications.

    C. **CORRECT:** A client who is post-dialysis is at risk for hypovolemia due to a rapid decease in fluid volume.

    D. **CORRECT:** The nurse should assess the access site for bleeding because the client receives heparin during the procedure to prevent clotting of blood.

    E. The nurse should never measure blood pressure on the extremity that has the AV access site because it can cause collapse of the AV fistula or graft.

    Ⓝ *NCLEX® Connection: Physiological Adaptation, Hemodynamics*

4. A. An altered level of consciousness is a manifestation of disequilibrium syndrome. The nurse should not administer an opioid medication. The provider may prescribe medication to decrease seizure activity.

    B. The nurse should monitor for hypotension due to rapid change in fluids and electrolytes causing disequilibrium syndrome.

    C. **CORRECT:** The nurse should assess the client's level of consciousness. A change in urea levels can cause increased intracranial pressure. Subsequently, the client's level of consciousness decreases.

    D. The nurse should decrease the dialysis exchange rate to slow the rapid changes in fluid and electrolyte status when a client develops disequilibrium syndrome.

    Ⓝ *NCLEX® Connection: Physiological Adaptation, Unexpected Response to Therapies*

5. A. **CORRECT:** The nurse should monitor serum glucose levels because the dialysate solution contains glucose.

    B. **CORRECT:** The nurse should monitor for cloudy dialysate return, which indicates an infection. Clear, light-yellow solution is typical during the outflow process.

    C. The nurse should avoid warming the dialysate in a microwave oven, which causes uneven heating of the solution.

    D. **CORRECT:** The nurse should assess for shortness of breath, which can indicate inability to tolerate a large volume of dialysate.

    E. **CORRECT:** The nurse should check the access site dressing for wetness and look for kinking, pulling, clamping, or twisting of the tubing, which can increase the risk for exit-site infections.

    F. The nurse should maintain surgical, not medical, asepsis when accessing the catheter insertion site to prevent infection from contamination.

    Ⓝ *NCLEX® Connection: Physiological Adaptation, Alterations in Body Systems*

PRACTICE Answer

Using ATI Active Learning Template: Diagnostic Procedure

DESCRIPTION OF PROCEDURE: Peritoneal dialysis to instill a hypertonic dialysate solution into the peritoneal cavity, allow the solution to dwell for prescribed amount of time, and drain the solution that includes the waste products.

POTENTIAL COMPLICATIONS
- Peritonitis
- Protein loss from protein wasting
- Hyperglycemia
- Poor dialysate inflow or outflow

NURSING INTERVENTIONS
Peritonitis
- Maintain surgical asepsis.
- Monitor color of outflow solution, and for pain or fever.

Protein loss
- Increase dietary intake of protein.
- Monitor albumin level.

Hyperglycemia
- Monitor serum glucose level.
- Administer insulin.

Poor dialysate inflow or outflow
- Reposition the client.
- Milk the tubing to break up fibrin clots.
- Check the tubing for kinks or closed clamps.
- Encourage stool softeners and high-fiber diet to prevent constipation.

Ⓝ *NCLEX® Connection: Physiological Adaptation, Alterations in Body Systems*

CHAPTER 58 *Kidney Transplant*

End-stage kidney disease, when the kidneys no longer function, can be treated with a kidney transplant a life-sustaining treatment option other than dialysis. Transplantation can greatly improve the quality of life for a person who is otherwise dependent on dialysis.

The recipient's tissue must be matched with a donor's. Donors for kidney transplantation can be living, non-heart-beating, or cadaver donors. In-depth tissue typing includes assessment of blood type (ABO) compatibility and histocompatibility, including human leukocytic antigen and other minor antigens. Clients receiving a donor kidney from a living, related donor with matching tissue type have the greatest chance of graft survival. Kidneys used from cadaver or non-heart-beating donors must be sufficiently perfused to maintain viability of the organ. The donated kidney is surgically implanted in the client.

INDICATIONS

POTENTIAL DIAGNOSES

INDICATIONS OF END-STAGE KIDNEY DISEASE
- Anuria
- Proteinuria
- Marked azotemia (elevated blood urea nitrogen [BUN] and serum creatinine)
- Severe electrolyte imbalance (hyperkalemia, hypernatremia)
- Fluid volume excess conditions (heart failure, pulmonary edema)
- Uremic lung

CLIENT PRESENTATION

EXPECTED FINDINGS OF END-STAGE KIDNEY DISEASE
- Anorexia
- Fatigue
- Numbness and tingling of extremities
- Shortness of breath
- Dry itchy skin
- Metallic taste in the mouth
- Muscle cramping
- Decreased attention span
- Seizures
- Tremor
- Heart failure
- Edema of hands and feet
- Dyspnea
- Distended jugular veins
- Anemia
- Vomiting
- Pulmonary edema
- Hypertension
- Cardiac dysrhythmias
- Pallor
- Bruising
- Halitosis
- Diminished or dark–colored urine

LABORATORY DATA
- Proteinuria
- Hematuria
- Elevated BUN levels
- Elevated serum creatinine
- Decreased glomerular filtration rate, either estimated from serum or urine creatinine 24 hr values
- Decreased hemoglobin and hematocrit
- Elevated potassium and phosphorus levels
- Sodium within expected reference range, increased, or decreased
- Metabolic acidosis

CONSIDERATIONS

RISK FACTORS

Conditions that increase the risks involved in kidney transplantation surgery, lifelong immunosuppression, and organ rejection
- Age younger than 2 years
- Age older than 70 years: Older adult clients are at risk for developing advanced heart disease and malignancies, which increases the risk for complications with kidney transplantation surgery. Ⓖ
- Advanced, untreatable cardiac disease
- Active cancer
- Chemical dependency
- Chronic infections or systemic diseases (HIV, hepatitis B or C)
- Coagulopathies and certain immune disorders
- Morbid obesity
- Diabetes mellitus
- Chronic pulmonary disease
- Untreated gastrointestinal diseases, such as peptic ulcer disease

PREPROCEDURE

NURSING ACTIONS

- Schedule preoperative laboratory assessments, including blood chemistry studies, CBC and differential, bleeding times, urine culture, blood type, and crossmatch.
- Administer preoperative medications as prescribed.
  - Prophylactic antibiotics
  - Immunosuppressant therapy
    - Methylprednisolone: an anti-inflammatory and immunosuppressant to decrease the immune system response of inflammation and rejection of the donor kidney. Q EBP
    - Cyclosporine: an immunosuppressant medication to prevent rejection of the donor kidney.
    - Mammalian target of rapamycin (mTOR) inhibitors to interrupt the stimulation of T-cell signals
    - Everolimus: used to prevent activation of B cells and T cells to prevent rejection of the donor kidney
  - Monoclonal antibodies: Basiliximab or daclizumab are antibodies that bind with T cells to reduce T-cell growth and activation at the receptor site to prevent rejection of the donor kidney.
- The client usually receives dialysis within 24 hr of surgery.
- To increase the chance of graft survival, blood from the live kidney donor is often transfused into the client receiving the transplant.

CLIENT EDUCATION

- Prepare the client mentally and emotionally for the procedure.
- Inform the client of the interprofessional transplant team involved in the procedure. This includes nurses, provider, transplant surgeon, anesthesiologists and nephrologists, and clinical nurse specialist and other interprofessional health care workers. Q PCC
- Advise the client that compliance with the post-transplant interventions (lifelong immunosuppression) and risk factor reduction (smoking cessation, blood pressure and blood glucose control) are crucial to the success of the transplantation.

INTRAPROCEDURE

NURSING ACTIONS

- Provide padding to the bony prominences to provide comfort and prevent skin breakdown.
- Communicate surgical progress to the client's family members, if available.
- Assist in monitoring urine output and blood loss.
- Document surgical events.
- Assist in arranging postoperative unit placement and communicate postoperative needs of the client.

POSTPROCEDURE

NURSING ACTIONS

- Assess vital signs every 15 min initially and advance to every hour (follow institutional protocol). Maintain blood pressure within prescribed parameters.
- Assess intake and output at least hourly.
  - Urine output should be greater than 30 mL/hr. Notify the provider of oliguria evidenced by urine output less than 30 mL/hr. Q PCC
  - Monitor for abrupt decrease in urine output, indicating rejection, tissue injury, thrombosis of the renal artery, or obstruction in the renal system.
  - Assess urine appearance and odor hourly (initially pink and bloody, gradually returning to clear in a few days to several weeks).
  - Monitor daily urinalysis to check for protein, WBCs, RBCs, ketones, glucose, specific gravity, and pH.
- Daily weight assists in monitoring fluid status.
- Monitor for fluid and electrolyte imbalances, such as hypervolemia, hypovolemia, hypokalemia, and hyponatremia.
- Monitor for manifestations of infection, such as dyspnea, fever, incisional drainage, and redness.
- Monitor for early manifestations of organ rejection (fever, hypertension, pain at the transplant site).
- Assess surgical dressing for bloody drainage, which can indicate hemorrhage or hematoma formation.
- Administer intravenous fluids as prescribed, usually calculated to replace hourly urine output.
- Administer oral fluids and discontinue IV fluid once bowel function returns and fluids are tolerated.
- Encourage the client to turn, cough, and deep breathe to prevent atelectasis and pneumonia.
- Provide urinary catheter care.
  - Attach the large indwelling urinary catheter to dependent bedside drainage.
  - Maintain continuous bladder irrigation as prescribed to prevent obstruction from blood clot formation, which can cause damage to the transplanted kidney.
  - Remove the urinary catheter as soon as possible to decrease the risk of infection.
- Intervene for oliguria as prescribed. Diuretics and/or dialysis can be necessary until kidney function is satisfactory.
  - Mannitol, an osmotic diuretic, preserves urine flow and reduces the risk of acute kidney injury. Filtered mannitol draws water into the nephrons of the kidney and promotes diuresis.
  - Thiazides and loop diuretics are less effective when filtration rate is lower causing less diuresis.
- Monitor for excessive diuresis, which can result in hypovolemia and hypotension, and cause reduced blood flow to the graft. Notify the provider immediately.
- Administer immunosuppressive medications to prevent rejection (prednisone, cyclosporines, or other prescribed medication, and monoclonal antibodies [basiliximab or daclizumab]).
- Monitor for complications, such as infection, hypovolemia, and fluid retention.
- Immediately notify the surgeon if any manifestations of organ rejection appear.

- Administer stool softeners to prevent straining and constipation (risk associated with bowel manipulation during abdominal surgery and the effects of general anesthetics and analgesics).
- Arrange for counseling for the client and family if necessary.
- Arrange for post-transplant follow-up appointments and interventions.

CLIENT EDUCATION
- Instruct the client to monitor and report manifestations of infection, such as fever, incisional drainage, and redness.
- Instruct the client to adhere to the pharmacological regimen (corticosteroids, antilymphocyte preparations, cyclosporine, monoclonal antibodies).
- Instruct the client and family about the prescribed diet and activity level.

DIET RECOMMENDATIONS
- Low-fat to decrease cholesterol
- High-fiber to avoid constipation
- Increased protein to promote healing, and rebuild and maintain muscle mass
- Adequate intake of potassium, calcium, and phosphorus.
- Restricted sodium intake to prevent fluid retention and hypertension especially when taking prednisone
- Avoidance of concentrated sugars or carbohydrates to control glycemic factors when on prednisone
- Magnesium supplements because cyclosporine can reduce magnesium levels

 ! Avoid grapefruit, which causes increased cyclosporine blood levels, when taking cyclosporine. Qs

ACTIVITY RECOMMENDATIONS
- Avoid contact sports that can cause an injury to the transplanted kidney.
- Increase activity as tolerated.

COMPLICATIONS

Organ rejection

NURSING ACTIONS: Monitor for and report manifestations of rejection immediately.

Hyperacute: Occurs within 48 hr after surgery
- ETIOLOGY: An antibody-mediated response causing small blood clots to form in the transplanted kidney that occlude vessels and result in massive cellular destruction. The process is not reversible.
- FINDINGS: Fever, hypertension, pain at the transplant site
- TREATMENT: Immediate removal of the donor kidney

Acute: Occurs 1 week to 2 years after surgery
- ETIOLOGY: An antibody mediated response causing vasculitis in the donor kidney, and cellular destruction starts with inflammation that causes lysis of the donor kidney
- FINDINGS: Oliguria, anuria, low-grade fever, hypertension, tenderness over the transplanted kidney, lethargy, azotemia, and fluid retention
- TREATMENT: Involves increased doses of immunosuppressive medications

Chronic: Occurs gradually over months to years
- ETIOLOGY: Blood vessel injury from overgrowth of the smooth muscles of the blood vessels causing fibrotic tissue to replace normal tissue resulting in a nonfunctioning donor kidney
- FINDINGS: Gradual return of azotemia, fluid retention, electrolyte imbalance, and fatigue
- TREATMENT: Conservative (monitor kidney status, continue immunosuppressive therapy) until dialysis is required

CLIENT EDUCATION
- Teach the client to monitor for manifestations of rejection and to contact the provider immediately.
- Instruct the client that rejection is diagnosed through a kidney scan and kidney biopsies.
- Instruct the client to adhere to the pharmacological regimen.

Ischemia

A delay in transplanting the donor kidney after harvesting can result in hypoxic injury of the donor kidney.

NURSING ACTIONS
- Monitor urine output, serum creatinine, and BUN levels to detect failure of the transplanted kidney. Qpcc
- Report hourly output volumes less than 30 mL/hr.
- Assist the client with dialysis as indicated.
- Prepare the client for a kidney biopsy to distinguish ischemia from organ rejection.

CLIENT EDUCATION: Advise the client that dialysis might be needed until the donor kidney heals.

Renal artery stenosis

Renal artery stenosis is due to scarring of surgical anastomosis.

NURSING ACTIONS
- Monitor for and report hypertension, bruit over artery anastomosis site, and decreased kidney function, such as oliguria and elevated BUN and creatinine. Qpcc
- Prepare the client for a kidney scan to verify the status of renal blood flow.
- Angioplasty and/or surgical intervention might be necessary.

CLIENT EDUCATION: Advise the client to monitor for peripheral edema and have blood pressure checked often.

Thrombosis

A blood clot can form in a major vessel of the transplanted kidney.

NURSING ACTIONS
- Monitor for and report a sudden decrease in urine output.
- Prepare the client for emergency surgery requiring an emergency transplant nephrectomy (removal of the transplant kidney).

CLIENT EDUCATION
- Keep the client informed about the risk of a blood clot.
- Advise the client to inform the provider of a sudden decrease in urine output.

Infection

- Infection is a common cause of first-transplant-year morbidity and mortality.
- Detection of early manifestations of infection are difficult when the client receives immunosuppressive therapy. Vague symptoms include low-grade fevers, mild reports of discomfort, and mental status changes.

NURSING ACTIONS

- Give high priority to infection control measures, such as frequent hand hygiene.
- Monitor for and report manifestations of a localized (wound) or systemic infection (pneumonia, sepsis).

CLIENT EDUCATION

- Instruct the client to monitor for and report manifestations of infection, such as fever, incisional drainage, and redness. Later indications of infection can include fatigue and discomfort. Report any manifestations of infection to the provider.
- Educate the client and family about the increased risk for infection during immunosuppressant therapy and infection control measures, such as frequent hand hygiene and avoiding crowds and people who have a communicable disease. The client might need to wear a face mask when out in public.
- Instruct the client to adhere to the pharmacological regimen.

Application Exercises

1. A nurse is assessing a client who has end-stage kidney disease. Which of the following findings should the nurse expect? (Select all that apply.)

   A. Anuria

   B. Marked azotemia

   C. Crackles in the lungs

   D. Increased calcium level

   E. Proteinuria

2. A nurse is planning postoperative care for a client following a kidney transplant surgery. Which of the following actions should the nurse include in the plan of care? (Select all that apply.)

   A. Obtain daily weights.

   B. Assess dressings for bloody drainage.

   C. Replace hourly urine output with IV fluids.

   D. Expect oliguria in the first 4 hr.

   E. Monitor serum electrolytes.

3. A nurse is teaching a client who is postoperative following a kidney transplant and is taking cyclosporine. Which of the following instructions should the nurse include?

   A. "Decrease your intake of protein-rich foods."

   B. "Take this medication with grapefruit juice."

   C. "Monitor for and report a sore throat to your provider."

   D. "Expect your skin to turn yellow."

4. A client who is scheduled for kidney transplantation surgery is assessed by the nurse for risk factors of surgery. Which of the following findings increase the client's risk of surgery? (Select all that apply.)

   A. Age older than 70 years

   B. BMI of 41

   C. Administering NPH insulin each morning

   D. Past history of lymphoma

   E. Blood pressure averaging 120/70 mm Hg

5. A nurse is preoperative teaching with a client who is scheduled for a kidney transplant about rejection of a transplanted kidney. Which of the following statements should the nurse include in the teaching? (Select all that apply.)

   A. "Expect an immediate removal of the donor kidney for a hyperacute rejection."

   B. "You may need to begin dialysis to monitor your kidney function for a hyperacute rejection."

   C. "A fever is a manifestation of an acute rejection."

   D. "Fluid retention is a manifestation of an acute rejection."

   E. "Your provider will increase your immunosuppressive medications for a chronic rejection."

PRACTICE Active Learning Scenario

A nurse is planning catheter care for a client who is postoperative following kidney transplantation surgery. To maintain indwelling urinary catheter patency and avoid complications, What actions should the nurse take?

Use the ATI Active Learning Template: Nursing Skill to complete this item.

INDICATIONS: List two reasons for an indwelling urinary catheter.

POTENTIAL COMPLICATIONS: Indicate three risk factors.

NURSING INTERVENTIONS: List three postoperative actions.

Application Exercises Key

1. A. **CORRECT:** Anuria is a manifestation of end-stage kidney disease.

   B. **CORRECT:** Marked azotemia is elevated BUN and serum creatinine, is a manifestation of end-stage kidney disease.

   C. **CORRECT:** Crackles in the lungs can indicate the client has pulmonary edema, caused from hypervolemia due to end-stage kidney disease.

   D. Calcium levels are decreased due to increase in serum phosphate levels when the client has end-stage kidney disease.

   E. **CORRECT:** Proteinuria is a manifestation of end-stage kidney disease.

   Ⓝ *NCLEX® Connection: Physiological Adaptation, Pathophysiology*

2. A. **CORRECT:** Daily weights are obtained to assess fluid status.

   B. **CORRECT:** Drainage on the dressing is assessed to monitor for hemorrhage or hematoma.

   C. **CORRECT:** Hourly urine output with IV fluid replacement is monitored to detect abrupt decrease in urine output, which can indicate rejection or other serious conditions of the transplant kidney.

   D. Oliguria can indicate ischemia, acute kidney injury, rejection, or hypovolemia. Report oliguria immediately to the provider.

   E. **CORRECT:** Serum electrolytes is monitored because electrolytes loss can occur with postoperative diuresis.

   Ⓝ *NCLEX® Connection: Physiological Adaptation, Illness Management*

3. A. The client should not decrease protein-rich foods in the diet, which promote healing and rebuilds muscle. There are no restrictions of protein intake for a client taking cyclosporine following a kidney transplant.

   B. The client should not drink grapefruit juice, which can reduce cyclosporine metabolism and cause increased cyclosporine levels.

   C. **CORRECT:** The client should report any manifestations of an infection because this medication causes immunosuppression.

   D. The client should report manifestations of hepatotoxicity, such as jaundice, and abdominal pain.

   Ⓝ *NCLEX® Connection: Pharmacological and Parenteral Therapies, Medication Administration*

4. A. **CORRECT:** A client older than 70 years has an increased risk for complications from surgery, lifelong immunosuppression, and organ rejection.

   B. **CORRECT:** A client who has a BMI of 41 is morbidly obese and is at an increased risk for complications of surgery, lifelong immunosuppression, and organ rejection.

   C. **CORRECT:** A client who requires NPH insulin for type 1 diabetes mellitus is at an increased risk from complication of surgery, lifelong immunosuppression, and organ rejection.

   D. **CORRECT:** A client who has a history of cancer, such as lymphoma, is at an increased risk for complications of surgery, lifelong immunosuppression, and organ rejection.

   E. Blood pressure averaging 120/70 mm Hg is within the expected reference range does not place the client at a greater risk for complication of surgery, lifelong immunosuppression, and organ rejection.

   Ⓝ *NCLEX® Connection: Health Promotion and Maintenance, Health Promotion/Disease Prevention*

5. A. **CORRECT:** Immediate removal of the donor kidney is treatment for hyperacute rejection.

   B. Dialysis can be required as a conservative treatment to monitor the client's kidney function for the progression of chronic kidney failure following kidney transplant.

   C. **CORRECT:** Fever is a manifestation of an acute rejection.

   D. **CORRECT:** Fluid retention is a manifestation of an acute rejection.

   E. Immunosuppressants are increased to treat an acute rejection.

   Ⓝ *NCLEX® Connection: Reduction of Risk Potential, System Specific Assessments*

PRACTICE Answer

Using the ATI Active Learning Template: Nursing Skill

INDICATIONS
- Monitor hourly urinary output.
- Monitor color of urine and clots.

POTENTIAL COMPLICATIONS
- Oliguria
- Infection from an indwelling urinary catheter
- Blood clot formation

NURSING INTERVENTIONS
- Regulate IV fluids according to urinary output, as prescribed.
- Connect the indwelling urinary catheter to the bed lower than the client to promote gravity drainage.
- Remove the indwelling urinary catheter within a few days postprocedure.
- Implement continuous bladder irrigation as prescribed to remove blood clots that can obstruct the indwelling urinary catheter and cause damage to the donor kidney.

Ⓝ *NCLEX® Connection: Reduction of Risk Potential, Potential for Complications of Diagnostic Tests/Treatments/Procedures*

CHAPTER 59
Polycystic Kidney Disease, Acute Kidney Injury, and Chronic Kidney Disease

There are several disorders that affect the renal system and its ability to function. These disorders include acute kidney injury, chronic kidney disease, and polycystic kidney disease.

The kidneys regulate fluid, acid-base, and electrolyte balance, and eliminate wastes from the body.

Kidney failure is diagnosed as acute kidney injury or chronic kidney disease. Without aggressive treatment, or when complicating preexisting conditions exist, acute kidney injury can result in chronic kidney disease.

Acute kidney injury

Acute kidney injury (AKI) is the sudden cessation of renal function that occurs when blood flow to the kidneys is significantly compromised. Manifestations occur abruptly.

PHASES

- **Onset:** Begins with the onset of the event, ends when oliguria develops, and lasts for hours to days.
- **Oliguria:** Begins with the kidney insult; urine output is 100 to 400 mL/24 hr with or without diuretics; and lasts for 1 to 3 weeks.
- **Diuresis:** Begins when the kidneys start to recover; diuresis of a large amount of fluid occurs; and can last for 2 to 6 weeks.
- **Recovery:** Continues until kidney function is fully restored and can take up to 12 months.

CLASSES

AKI is classified as one of three classes.
- **Stage 1 (risk stage):** Serum creatinine 1.5 times baseline and urine output less than 0.5 mL/kg/hr for 6 hr or more.
- **Stage 2 (injury stage):** Serum creatinine 2 times baseline and urine output less than 0.5 mL/kg/hr for 12 hr or more.
- **Stage 3 (failure stage):** Serum creatinine 3 times baseline and urine output less than 0.3 mL/kg/hr for 12 hr or more.

TYPES

- **Prerenal**: Occurs as a result of volume depletion and prolonged reduction of blood flow to the kidneys, which leads to ischemia of the nephrons. Occurs before damage to the kidney. Early intervention restoring fluid volume deficit can reverse AKI and prevent chronic kidney disease (CKD).
- **Intrarenal**: Occurs as a result of direct damage to the kidney from lack of oxygen (acute tubular necrosis).
- **Postrenal**: Occurs as a result of bilateral obstruction of structures leaving the kidney.

HEALTH PROMOTION AND DISEASE PREVENTION

- Drink at least 2 L daily. Consult with the provider regarding prescribed fluid restriction if needed.
- Stop smoking.
- Maintain a healthy weight.
- Use NSAIDs and other prescribed medications cautiously.
- Control diabetes and hypertension to prevent complications.
- Instruct clients to take all antibiotics prescribed for infections.

ASSESSMENT

RISK FACTORS

Prerenal acute kidney injury

- Renal vascular obstruction
- Shock
- Decreased cardiac output causing decreased renal profusion
- Sepsis
- Hypovolemia
- Peripheral vascular resistance
- Use of aspirin, ibuprofen, or NSAIDs
- Liver failure

Intrarenal acute kidney injury

- **Physical injury:** trauma
- **Hypoxic injury:** renal artery or vein stenosis or thrombosis
- **Chemical injury:** acute nephrotoxins (e.g., antibiotics, contrast dye, heavy metals, blood transfusion reaction, alcohol, cocaine)
- **Immunologic injury:** infection, vasculitis, acute glomerulonephritis

Postrenal acute kidney injury

- Stone, tumor, bladder atony
- Prostate hyperplasia, urethral stricture
- Spinal cord disease or injury

EXPECTED FINDINGS

In most cases, the findings of AKI are related to waste buildup and decreased urine output. However, almost every body system can be affected.
- CARDIOVASCULAR: fluid overload (dependent and generalized edema), dysrhythmia (hyperkalemia)
- RESPIRATORY: crackles, decreased oxygenation, shortness of breath
- RENAL: scant to normal or excessive urine output, depending on the phase; possible hematuria
- NEUROLOGICAL: lethargy, muscle twitching, seizures
- INTEGUMENTARY: dry skin and mucous membranes

The nurse should also assess for findings associated with the underlying cause.

LABORATORY TESTS

- Serum creatinine gradually increases 1 to 2 mg/dL every 24 to 48 hr, or 1 to 6 mg/dL in 1 week or less.
- Blood urea nitrogen (BUN) can increase to 80 to 100 mg/dL within 1 week.
- Urine specific gravity varies in postrenal type; can be elevated up to 1.030 in prerenal type or diluted as low as 1.000 in intrarenal type.
- Serum electrolytes: Sodium can be decreased (prerenal azotemia) or increased (intrarenal azotemia); hyperkalemia, hyperphosphatemia, hypocalcemia.
- Hematocrit: decreased
- Urinalysis: presence of sediment (RBC, casts)
- ABG: metabolic acidosis

DIAGNOSTIC PROCEDURES

- X-ray of the pelvis, or kidneys, urethra, and bladder (KUB) to detect calculi and hydronephrosis and to determine size of kidneys
- Ultrasound to detect an obstruction in the urinary tract
- CT scan without contrast dye or MRI to detect anatomical changes, tumors, or other obstruction; patency of ureters; and renal perfusion.
- Kidney biopsy to detect immunological disease or determine kidney dysfunction reversibility and need for dialysis therapy
- Nuclear medicine tests (cystography, retrograde pyelography)

PATIENT-CENTERED CARE

NURSING CARE

- Identify and assist with correcting the underlying cause.
- Monitor central venous pressure (CVP) and for hypotension and tachycardia.
- Monitor fluid intake and output strictly.
- Review laboratory values (BUN, creatinine, electrolytes, hematocrit).
- Avoid using nephrotoxic medications. If necessary, give these medications sparingly and decrease the medication dosage.
- Assess for edema and manifestations of heart failure or pulmonary edema.
- Restrict fluid intake as prescribed.
- Assess for flank pain, nausea, and vomiting (nephrolithiasis).
- Monitor for ECG dysrhythmias and changes (tall T waves).
- Monitor daily weights.
- Assess for changes in urination stream or difficulty starting the stream of urine.
- Assess the urine for blood or particles.
- Treat fever or infection promptly to prevent increase in the client's metabolic rate.
- Provide skin care to prevent injury (bathe with cool water, reposition frequently, provide adequate moisture).
- Provide psychosocial support to the client and family. Teach the client and family about prescribed treatments.
- Teach the client to perform coughing and deep breathing exercises, if lethargic.

NUTRITION

- Implement potassium, phosphate, sodium, and magnesium restrictions, if prescribed (depending on the stage of injury).
- Restrict fluid intake, if prescribed.
- High-protein diet to replace the high rate of protein breakdown due to stress from the illness. Possible total parenteral nutrition (TPN).

MEDICATIONS

- Administer IV fluid therapy as a fluid challenge to promote kidney perfusion, or as fluid replacement if the client is in the diuretic phase.
- Administer diuretics (furosemide, mannitol, ethacrynic acid) to promote increased filtration of blood by kidney.
- For AKI caused by medication nephrotoxicity, administer calcium channel blocker to prevent the movement of calcium into the kidney cells and to maintain cell integrity and increase the glomerular filtration rate (GFR).
- Sodium polystyrene sulfonate replaces sodium with potassium in the intestinal tract to promote potassium excretion.
- Sorbitol induces a bowel movement to promote excretion of excess potassium.
- In an emergency, IV medications (dextrose, insulin and calcium) can be required to reduce potassium.
- Administer sodium bicarbonate if the client has severe metabolic acidosis.
- For hyperphosphatemia, administer phosphate-binding agents.

THERAPEUTIC PROCEDURES

Continuous renal replacement therapy, hemodialysis, peritoneal dialysis

INTERPROFESSIONAL CARE

- Dietitian to calculate protein, calorie, and fluid needs
- Nephrology services to monitor kidney function

Chronic kidney disease

CKD is a progressive, irreversible kidney disease.
- A client who has CKD can be asymptomatic except during periods of stress (infection, surgery, and trauma). As kidney dysfunction progresses, manifestations become apparent.
- Older adult clients are at an increased risk for chronic kidney disease related to the aging process (decreased number of functioning nephrons, decreased GFR). ©
- Older adults clients who are on bed rest, confused, have a lack of thirst, and do not have easy access to water are at a higher risk for dehydration leading to chronic kidney disease.

STAGES

CKD is comprised of five stages.
- **Stage 1:** Minimal kidney damage when GFR within expected reference range (greater than 90 mL/min)
- **Stage 2:** Mild kidney damage with mildly decreased GFR (60 to 89 mL/min)
- **Stage 3:** Moderate kidney damage with moderate decrease in GFR (30 to 59 mL/min)
- **Stage 4:** Severe kidney damage with severe decrease in GFR (15 to 29 mL/min)
- **Stage 5:** Kidney failure and end-stage kidney disease with little or no glomerular filtration (less than 15 mL/min)

HEALTH PROMOTION AND DISEASE PREVENTION

- Drink at least 2 L water daily. Consult with the provider regarding any restrictions.
- Stop smoking.
- Limit alcohol intake.
- Use diet and exercise to manage weight and prevent or control diabetes and hypertension.
- Adhere to medication prescription guidelines to prevent kidney damage.
- Test for albumin in the urine yearly (clients who have diabetes or hypertension).
- Take all antibiotics until completed.
- Limit over-the-counter NSAIDs. Qs

ASSESSMENT

- End-stage kidney disease exists when 90% of the functioning nephrons are destroyed and are no longer able to maintain fluid, electrolyte, and acid–base homeostasis.
- Dialysis or kidney transplantation can maintain life, but neither is a cure for CKD.

RISK FACTORS

- Acute kidney injury
- Diabetes mellitus
- Chronic glomerulonephritis
- Nephrotoxic medications (gentamicin, NSAIDs) or chemicals
- Hypertension, especially in African American clients
- Autoimmune disorders (systemic lupus erythematosus)
- Polycystic kidney disease
- Pyelonephrosis
- Renal artery stenosis
- Recurrent severe infections

EXPECTED FINDINGS

Nausea, fatigue, lethargy, involuntary movement of legs, depression, intractable hiccups

In most cases, findings of chronic kidney disease are related to fluid volume overload and include the following.

NEUROLOGIC: lethargy, decreased attention span, slurred speech, tremors or jerky movements, ataxia, seizures, coma

CARDIOVASCULAR: fluid overload (jugular distention; sacrum, ocular, or peripheral edema), hypertension, dysrhythmias, heart failure, orthostatic hypotension, peaked T wave on ECG (hyperkalemia)

RESPIRATORY: uremic halitosis with deep sighing, yawning, shortness of breath, tachypnea, hyperpnea, Kussmaul respirations, crackles, pleural friction rub, frothy pink sputum

HEMATOLOGIC: anemia (pallor, weakness, dizziness), ecchymoses, petechiae, melena

GASTROINTESTINAL: ulcers in mouth and throat, foul breath, blood in stools, vomiting

MUSCULOSKELETAL: osteodystrophy (thin fragile bones)

RENAL: urine contains protein, blood, particles; change in the amount, color, concentration

SKIN: decreased skin turgor, yellow cast to skin, dry, pruritus, urea crystal on skin (uremic frost)

REPRODUCTIVE: erectile dysfunction

LABORATORY TESTS

Urinalysis: Hematuria, proteinuria, and decrease in specific gravity.

Serum creatinine: Gradual increase over months to years for CKD exceeding 4 mg/dL. Can increase to 15 to 30 mg/dL.

BUN: Gradual increase with elevated serum creatinine over months to years for CKD. Can increase 10 to 20 times the creatinine finding.

Serum electrolytes: Decreased sodium (dilutional) and calcium; increased potassium, phosphorus, and magnesium.

CBC: Decreased hemoglobin and hematocrit from anemia secondary to the loss of erythropoietin in CKD.

DIAGNOSTIC PROCEDURES

Radiologic procedures to detect disease processes, obstruction, and arterial defects
- Ultrasound
- Kidneys, ureter, and bladder (KUB)
- Computerized tomography (CT)
- Magnetic resonance imaging (MRI) without contrast dye
- Aortorenal angiography
- Cystoscopy
- Retrograde pyelography
- Kidney biopsy

PATIENT-CENTERED CARE

NURSING CARE

- Report and monitor irregular findings
  - URINARY ELIMINATION PATTERNS: amount, color, odor, and consistency
  - VITAL SIGNS: blood pressure may be increased or decreased
  - WEIGHT: 1 kg (2.2 lb) daily weight increase is approximately 1 L of fluid retained.
- Assess and monitor vascular access or peritoneal dialysis insertion site.
- Obtain a detailed medication and herb history to determine the client's risk for continued kidney injury.
- Control protein intake based on the client's stage of chronic kidney disease and type of dialysis prescribed.
- Restrict dietary sodium, potassium, phosphorous, and magnesium.
- Provide a diet that is high in carbohydrates and moderate in fat.
- Restrict intake of fluids (based on urinary output).
- Monitor for weight gain trends.
- Adhere to meticulous cleaning of areas on skin not intact and access sites to control infections.
- Balance the client's activity and rest.
- Prepare the client for hemodialysis, peritoneal dialysis, and hemofiltration if indicated.
- Provide skin care in order to increase comfort and prevent breakdown.
- Protect the client from injury. Qs
- Provide emotional support to the client and family.
- Encourage the client to ask questions and discuss fears.
- Administer medications as prescribed.

MEDICATIONS

See the **RN PHARMACOLOGY REVIEW MODULE** for detailed information on these medications.

> ❗ Avoid administering antimicrobial medications (e.g., aminoglycosides and amphotericin B), NSAIDs, angiotensin-converting enzyme inhibitors, angiotensin-receptor blockers, and IV contrast dye, which are nephrotoxic.

Digoxin: a cardiac glycoside that increases contractility of the myocardium and promotes cardiac output
- Monitor digoxin laboratory levels and expect dosages to be reduced due to slow excretion of the medication with CKD.
- Monitor carefully for manifestations of digoxin toxicity, such as nausea, vomiting, anorexia, and visual changes. Monitor potassium level. Qs
- Administer digoxin after dialysis.

Sodium polystyrene: increases elimination of serum potassium.
- Restrict sodium intake. Sodium polystyrene contains sodium and can cause fluid retention and hypertension, a complication of CKD.

Epoetin alfa: stimulates production of red blood cells; given for anemia

Ferrous sulfate: an iron supplement to prevent severe iron deficiency

Calcium carbonate
- Taken with meals to bind phosphate in food and stop phosphate absorption.
- Take 2 hr before or after other medications
- Can cause constipation, so clients can require a stool softener.

Furosemide: a loop-diuretic administered to excrete excess fluids
- Avoid administering to a client who has end-stage kidney disease.
- Clients can also receive thiazide diuretics, potassium-sparing diuretics, and osmotic diuretics.

THERAPEUTIC PROCEDURES

- Peritoneal dialysis
- Hemodialysis
- Kidney transplantation

INTERPROFESSIONAL CARE

- Nephrology services to manage dialysis or kidney failure
- Nutritional services to manage the nutritional needs

CLIENT EDUCATION Q_EBP

- Instruct the client to monitor the daily intake of carbohydrates, proteins, sodium, and potassium, according to the provider's prescription.
- Instruct the client to monitor fluid intake according to fluid restriction prescribed by the provider.
- Instruct the client to avoid antacids containing magnesium.
- Encourage the client to take rest periods from activity.
- Educate the client who is receiving hemodialysis or peritoneal dialysis on an outpatient basis.
- Educate the client on how to measure blood pressure and weight at home.
- Encourage the client to ask questions and discuss fears.
- Encourage the client to diet, exercise, and take medication as prescribed.
- Advise the client to notify the provider if she observes skin breakdown.

CARE AFTER DISCHARGE
- Nephrology services is indicated if the client is to receive outpatient dialysis.
- Refer the client to a community support group relating to the disease.
- Consult nutritional services for the client's dietary needs.
- Refer the client to a smoking-cessation support group and counseling if needed.

COMPLICATIONS

Potential complications include electrolyte imbalance, dysrhythmias, fluid overload, hypertension, metabolic acidosis, secondary infection, and uremia.

Polycystic kidney disease

- Polycystic kidney disease (PKD) is a congenital disorder where clusters of fluid-filled cysts develop in the nephrons. Healthy kidney tissue is replaced by multiple non-functioning cysts.
- PKD is hereditary and is caused by a genetic mutation.
- PKD is more common in Caucasian clients.

FORMS: There are two forms of PKD.
- **Autosomal dominant trait:** Most common form. Cysts begin to multiply when the client reaches age 30.
- **Autosomal recessive trait:** Multiple cysts are present at birth.

ASSESSMENT

EXPECTED FINDINGS

- Familial history of PKD
- Anxiety, guilt
- Abdominal and/or flank pain
  - Dull pain indicates increased kidney size or possible cyst infection
  - Sharp pain indicates ruptured cyst or possible renal lithiasis (kidney stone)
- Headaches
- Hypertension caused by kidney ischemia from the enlarging cysts
- Enlarged abdominal girth
- Constipation
- Bloody and/or cloudy urine
- Renal lithiasis
- Hyponatremia
- Nocturia (excessive urination at night)
- Progressive kidney failure

LABORATORY TESTS

- Urinalysis
- Hematuria, proteinuria, and bacteria indicating infection
- Gradual increase of serum creatinine, BUN, creatinine clearance

DIAGNOSTIC PROCEDURES

Radiologic procedures to detect disease processes and cysts: ultrasound, CT, and MRI.

PATIENT-CENTERED CARE

NURSING CARE

HYPERTENSION CONTROL
- Controlling blood pressure is the highest nursing priority for clients who have PKD.
- Manage hypertension with prescribed medication.
- Teach the client and family how to measure and record blood pressure readings and daily weights.

PAIN MANAGEMENT
- Provide prescribed pain medications and nonpharmacological pain methods, such as relaxation, deep breathing, guided imagery, and distraction. Use NSAIDs cautiously in clients who have kidney disease.
- Apply dry heat to abdomen or flank areas to reduce discomfort.

INFECTION PREVENTION
- Administer antibiotics, such as ciprofloxacin and trimethoprim/sulfamethoxazole. Monitor for antibiotic-induced nephrotoxicity by evaluating serum creatinine levels and urinary output.
- Monitor urine specific gravity to assess renal function and hydration status.

CONSTIPATION PREVENTION
- Provide adequate oral fluid intake (as allowed per prescribed fluid restrictions), increase dietary fiber, and encourage client to ambulate.
- Assess bowel sounds and bowel movements.
- Administer stool softeners as prescribed.

THERAPEUTIC PROCEDURE

Needle aspiration and drainage of cysts

CLIENT EDUCATION

- Instruct the client to monitor blood pressure and weight daily.
- Instruct the client to notify the provider if she experiences an elevated temperature.
- Provide the client information on a low-sodium diet.
- Instruct the client to inform the provider if there are any changes in urine or bowel movements.
- Instruct the client to take all medications as prescribed.

CARE AFTER DISCHARGE
- Refer the client to a community support group related to the disease.
- Consult nutritional services for the client's dietary needs.

Application Exercises

1. A nurse is planning care for a client who has prerenal acute kidney injury (AKI) following abdominal aortic aneurysm repair. Urinary output is 60 mL in the past 2 hr, and blood pressure is 92/58 mm Hg. The nurse should anticipate which of the following interventions?

   A. Prepare the client for a CT scan with contrast dye.

   B. Plan to administer nitroprusside.

   C. Prepare to administer a fluid challenge.

   D. Plan to position the client in Trendelenburg.

2. A nurse is planning care for a client who has postrenal AKI due to metastatic cancer. The client has a serum creatinine of 5 mg/dL. Which of the following interventions should the nurse include in the plan? (Select all that apply.)

   A. Provide a high-protein diet.

   B. Assess the urine for blood.

   C. Monitor for intermittent anuria.

   D. Weight the client once per week.

   E. Provide NSAIDs for pain.

3. A nurse is planning care for a client who has Stage 4 chronic kidney disease. Which of the following actions should the nurse include in the plan of care? (Select all that apply.)

   A. Assess for jugular vein distention.

   B. Provide frequent mouth rinses.

   C. Auscultate for a pleural friction rub.

   D. Provide a high-sodium diet.

   E. Monitor for dysrhythmias.

4. A nurse is reviewing client laboratory data. The nurse should recognize that which of the following findings is expected for a client who has Stage 4 chronic kidney disease?

   A. Blood urea nitrogen (BUN) 15 mg/dL

   B. Glomerular filtration rate (GFR) 20 mL/min

   C. Serum creatinine 1.1 mg/dL

   D. Serum potassium 5.0 mEq/L

5. A nurse is assessing a client who has prerenal AKI. Which of the following findings should the nurse expect? (Select all that apply.)

   A. Reduced BUN

   B. Elevated cardiac enzymes

   C. Reduced urine output

   D. Elevated serum creatinine

   E. Elevated serum calcium

PRACTICE Active Learning Scenario

A nurse is preparing to administer medication to a client who has chronic kidney disease (CKD). What information should the nurse consider when administering medication? Use the ATI Active Learning Template: Medication to complete this item.

MEDICATION: Identify three.

THERAPEUTIC USES: Describe how the medication is used to treat CKD.

NURSING INTERVENTIONS: Describe two for each medication.

Application Exercises Key

1. A. The nurse should not plan for a CT scan. Contrast dye is contraindicated for a client who has possible acute kidney injury.

   B. Nitroprusside is a rapid-acting vasodilator used to rapidly reduce blood pressure for clients who have hypertensive crisis. It is contraindicated for clients who have hypotension.

   C. **CORRECT:** The nurse should plan to administer a fluid challenge for hypovolemia, which is indicated by the client's low urinary output and blood pressure.

   D. The nurse should position the client in reverse Trendelenburg, with the head down and feet up, to treat hypotension.

   Ⓝ *NCLEX® Connection: Physiological Adaptation, Fluid and Electrolyte Imbalances*

2. A. **CORRECT:** The nurse should provide a high-protein diet due to the high rate of protein breakdown that occurs with acute kidney injury.

   B. **CORRECT:** The nurse should assess urine for blood, stones, and particles indicating an obstruction of the urinary structures that leave the kidney.

   C. **CORRECT:** The nurse should assess for intermittent anuria due to obstruction or damage to kidneys or urinary structures.

   D. The nurse should weigh the client daily to monitor for fluid retention due to acute kidney injury.

   E. The nurse should not administer NSAIDs, which are toxic to the nephrons in the kidney.

   Ⓝ *NCLEX® Connection: Physiological Adaptation, Alterations in Body Systems*

3. A. **CORRECT:** The nurse should assess for jugular vein distention, which can indicate fluid overload and heart failure.

   B. **CORRECT:** The nurse should provide frequent mouth rinses due to uremic halitosis caused by urea waste in the blood.

   C. **CORRECT:** The nurse should auscultate for a pleural friction rub related to respiratory failure and pulmonary edema caused by acid base imbalances and fluid retention.

   D. The nurse should monitor serum sodium and reduce the client's dietary sodium intake.

   E. **CORRECT:** The nurse should monitor for dysrhythmias related to increased serum potassium caused by Stage 4 chronic kidney disease.

   Ⓝ *NCLEX® Connection: Physiological Adaptation, Alterations in Body Systems*

4. A. The nurse should expect the BUN to be above the expected reference range, about 10 to 20 times the BUN finding.

   B. **CORRECT:** The GFR is severely decreased to approximately 20 mL/min, which is indicative of stage 4 chronic kidney disease.

   C. In stage 4 chronic kidney disease, a creatinine level can be as high as 15 to 30 mg/dL.

   D. A client in stage 4 chronic kidney disease would have a potassium level greater than 5.0 mEq/L.

   Ⓝ *NCLEX® Connection: Reduction of Risk Potential, Laboratory Values*

5. A. A manifestation of prerenal AKI is an elevated BUN caused by the retention of nitrogenous wastes in the blood.

   B. Elevated cardiac enzymes is a manifestation of cardiac tissue injury, not AKI.

   C. **CORRECT:** A manifestation of prerenal AKI is reduced urine output.

   D. **CORRECT:** A manifestation of prerenal AKI is elevated serum creatinine.

   E. A manifestation of prerenal AKI is reduced calcium level.

   Ⓝ *NCLEX® Connection: Physiological Adaptation, Illness Management*

PRACTICE Answer

Using the ATI Active Learning Template: Medication

MEDICATION
- Digoxin
- Sodium polystyrene
- Furosemide

THERAPEUTIC USES
- Digoxin: A cardiac glycoside: increases contractility of the myocardium and promotes cardiac output.
- Sodium polystyrene: Increases elimination of potassium.
- Calcium carbonate : Binds to phosphate in food and stops phosphate absorption.
- Furosemide: A loop diuretic that causes diuresis of excess fluids.

NURSING INTERVENTIONS
- Digoxin
  - Monitor serum digoxin and potassium levels.
  - Monitor for manifestations of toxicity (nausea, vomiting, anorexia, visual changes).
- Sodium polystyrene
  - Monitor for hypokalemia.
  - Restrict sodium intake.
- Furosemide
  - Monitor intake and output and blood pressure.
  - Avoid administering to a client who has end-stage kidney disease.

Ⓝ *NCLEX® Connection: Physiological Adaptation, Illness Management*

UNIT 8   NURSING CARE OF CLIENTS WHO
HAVE RENAL DISORDERS
SECTION: RENAL SYSTEM DISORDERS

CHAPTER 60 *Infections of the Renal and Urinary System*

The renal system includes the kidneys and the urinary system. The function of the renal system includes maintaining fluid volume, removing waste, regulating blood pressure, maintaining acid-base balance, producing erythropoietin, and activating vitamin D.

There are three components to the urinary system: the ureter, bladder, and urethra. The function of the urinary system is to store and remove urine.

Urinary tract infections are infections of the urinary system, and pyelonephritis is an infection of the kidney and renal pelvis. Acute and chronic glomerulonephritis can develop from a systemic infection and involves the glomeruli of the kidney or the area responsible for filtering particles from the blood to make urine.

Urinary tract infection

- A urinary tract infection (UTI) refers to any portion of the lower urinary tract (ureters, bladder, urethra, prostate). UTIs include the following.
  - Cystitis
  - Urethritis
  - Prostatitis
- An upper UTI refers to conditions such as pyelonephritis (inflammation of the kidney pelvis).
- UTIs are often caused by *Escherichia coli*. Other organisms include enterobacteriaceae micro-organisms (klebsiella, proteus), pseudomonas, and *Staphylococcus saprophyticus*.
- Untreated UTIs can lead to pyelonephritis and urosepsis, which can result in septic shock and death.

ASSESSMENT

RISK FACTORS

- **FEMALE GENDER**
  - Short urethra predisposes women to UTIs
  - Close proximity of the urethra to the rectum
  - Decreased estrogen in aging women promotes atrophy of the urethral opening toward the rectum (increases the risk of urosepsis in women) Ⓖ
  - Sexual intercourse
  - Frequent use of feminine hygiene sprays, tampons, sanitary napkins, and spermicidal jellies
  - Pregnancy
  - Poorly fitted diaphragm
  - Hormonal influences within the vaginal flora
  - Synthetic underwear and pantyhose
  - Wet bathing suits
  - Frequent submersion into baths or hot tubs
- Alkaline urine promotes bacterial growth.
- Indwelling urinary catheters (significant source of infection in clients who are hospitalized)
- Stool incontinence
- Bladder distention
- Urinary conditions (anomalies, stasis, calculi, residual urine)
- Possible genetic links
- Disease (diabetes mellitus)
- **OLDER ADULT CLIENTS** Ⓖ
  - Increased risk of bacteremia, sepsis, and shock
  - Incomplete bladder emptying caused by an enlarged prostate or prostatitis in males
  - Bladder prolapse in females
  - Inability to empty bladder (neurogenic bladder) as a result of a stroke or Parkinson's disease
  - Fecal incontinence with poor perineal hygiene
  - Hypoestrogen in females affecting the mucosa of the vagina and urethra, causing bacteria to adhere to the mucosal surface
  - Renal complications increase due to decreased number of functioning nephrons and fluid intake

EXPECTED FINDINGS

- Lower back or lower abdominal discomfort and tenderness over the bladder area
- Nausea
- Urinary frequency and urgency
- Dysuria, bladder cramping, spasms
- Feeling of incomplete bladder emptying or retention of urine
- Perineal itching
- Hematuria (red-tinged, smoky, coffee-colored urine)
- Pyuria (WBCs in the urine sample)
- Fever
- Vomiting
- Voiding in small amounts
- Nocturia
- Urethral discharge
- Cloudy or foul-smelling urine

OLDER ADULT MANIFESTATIONS ⓖ
- Confusion
- Incontinence
- Loss of appetite
- Nocturia and dysuria
- Hypotension, tachycardia, tachypnea, and fever (indications of urosepsis)

LABORATORY TESTS

Urinalysis and urine culture and sensitivity

NURSING ACTIONS
- Instruct the client regarding proper technique for the collection of a clean-catch urine specimen.
- Collect catheterized urine specimens using sterile technique.

EXPECTED FINDINGS
- Bacteria, sediment, white blood cells (WBC), and red blood cells (RBC)
- Positive leukocyte esterase and nitrates (68% to 88% positive results indicates UTI)

WBC count and differential

- If urosepsis is suspected
- White blood cell count equal to or greater than 10,000/uL with a shift to the left, indicating an increased number of immature cells (neutrophils) in response to infection

Rule out sexually transmitted infections

- STIs can cause manifestations of a UTI.
- *Chlamydia trachomatis*, *Neisseria gonorrhoeae*, and herpes simplex can cause acute urethritis.
- Trichomonas or candida can cause acute vaginal infections.

DIAGNOSTIC PROCEDURES

- Cystoscopy is used for complicated UTIs.
- Cystourethroscopy to detect strictures, calculi, tumors, cystitis.
- Computed tomography (CT) scan to detect pyelonephritis.
- Ultrasonography to detect cysts, tumors, calculi, and abscesses.
- Transrectal ultrasonography to detect prostate and bladder conditions in males.

PATIENT-CENTERED CARE

NURSING CARE

- Promote fluid intake up to 3 L daily.
- Consult with the provider regarding prescribed fluid restrictions if needed.
- Administer antibiotic medications as prescribed.
- Encourage clients to urinate every 3 to 4 hr instead of waiting until the bladder is completely full.
- Recommend warm sitz bath two or three times a day to provide comfort.
- Encourage clients to shower daily to promote good body hygiene.
- Avoid the use of indwelling catheters if possible. This reduces the risk for infection.
- Women who are pregnant require immediate and effective treatment to prevent pyelonephritis that can result in preterm labor. Ⓠs

MEDICATIONS

Fluoroquinolones, nitrofurantoin, trimethoprim, or sulfonamides

Antibiotics used to treat urinary infections by directly killing bacteria and inhibiting bacterial reproduction. ⓆEBP
- Penicillins and cephalosporins are administered less frequently because the medication is less effective and tolerated.
- Nitrofurantoin is an antibacterial medication where therapeutic levels are achieved in the urine only.

NURSING CONSIDERATIONS: If a sulfonamide is prescribed, ask the client about allergy to sulfa.

CLIENT EDUCATION
- Educate the client regarding the need to take all of the prescribed antibiotics even if manifestations subside.
- Encourage the client to take the medication with food.
- Advise clients taking fluoroquinolones or sulfonamides that sun-sensitivity is increased and sunburn is a risk for even dark-skinned individuals. These medications can precipitate in the renal tubules, so advise client to take these medications with a full glass of water and to increase fluid intake.
- Advise clients to monitor and report watery diarrhea that can indicate pseudomembranous colitis.

Phenazopyridine

Bladder analgesic used to treat UTIs

NURSING CONSIDERATIONS: The medication will not treat the infection, but it will help relieve bladder discomfort.

CLIENT EDUCATION
- Inform the client that the medication will turn urine orange.
- Encourage the client to take the medication with food.

INTERPROFESSIONAL CARE

Consult with urology services for managing UTIs.

CLIENT EDUCATION

- Instruct the client to drink at least 3 L fluid daily.
- Instruct the client to bathe daily to promote good body hygiene.
- Advise the client to empty bladder every 3 to 4 hr instead of waiting until the bladder is completely full.
- Advise the client to urinate before and after intercourse.
- Advise the client to drink cranberry juice to decrease the risk of infection. Q EBP
  - The compound in cranberries might stop certain bacteria from adhering to the mucosa of the urinary tract.
  - Clients who have chronic cystitis should avoid cranberry juice, which irritates the bladder.
- Advise the client to empty the bladder as soon as there is an urgency to void.
- Instruct female clients to do the following.
  - Wipe the perineal area from front to back.
  - Avoid using bubble baths, and feminine products and toilet paper containing perfumes.
  - Avoid sitting in wet bathing suits.
  - Avoid wearing pantyhose with slacks or tight clothing.

CARE AFTER DISCHARGE: Urology services can be consulted for management of long-term antibiotic therapy for chronic UTIs.

COMPLICATIONS

Urethral obstruction, pyelonephritis, chronic kidney disease, urosepsis, septic shock, and death

Pyelonephritis

- Pyelonephritis is an infection and inflammation of the kidney pelvis, calyces, and medulla. The infection usually begins in the lower urinary tract with organisms ascending into the kidney pelvis.
- *Escherichia coli* organisms are frequently the cause of acute pyelonephritis.
- Repeated infections can create scarring that changes the blood flow to the kidney, glomerulus, and tubular structure.
- Filtration, reabsorption, and secretion are impaired, which results in a decrease in kidney function.
- **Acute pyelonephritis** is an active bacterial infection that can cause the following.
  - Interstitial inflammation
  - Tubular cell necrosis
  - Abscess formation in the capsule, cortex, or medulla
  - Temporarily altered kidney function (this rarely progresses to chronic kidney disease)
- **Chronic pyelonephritis** is the result of repeated infections that cause progressive inflammation and scarring.
  - This can result in the thickening of the calyces and postinflammatory fibrosis with permanent renal tissue scarring.
  - It is more common with obstructions, urinary anomaly, and vesicoureteral urine reflux.
  - Reflux of urine occurs at the junction where the ureter connects to the bladder.

ASSESSMENT

RISK FACTORS

- Men over age 65 years who have prostatitis and hypertrophy of the prostate Ⓖ
- Chronic urinary stone disorders (stones harbor bacteria)
- Spinal cord injury (clients have a higher incidence of reflux)
- Pregnancy
- Congenital malformations
- Bladder tumors
- Chronic illness (diabetes mellitus, hypertension, chronic cystitis)
- Alkaline urine promotes bacterial growth.
- Incomplete bladder emptying is more common among older adult clients. Ⓖ
- Older adult clients can exhibit gastrointestinal or pulmonary manifestations instead of febrile responses because their temperature can vary at a lower-than-normal state. Causes are inadequate diet, loss of adipose tissue, lack of exercise, and reduction in the client's thermoregulator. Ⓖ

EXPECTED FINDINGS

- Chills
- Colicky-type abdominal pain
- Nausea
- Malaise, fatigue
- Burning, urgency, and frequency with urination
- Costovertebral tenderness
- Flank and back pain
- Nocturia
- Fever
- Tachycardia
- Tachypnea
- Hypertension
- Vomiting
- Inability to concentrate urine or conserve sodium (chronic pyelonephritis)
- Asymptomatic bacteremia

LABORATORY TESTS

- Urinalysis and urine culture and sensitivity same as for a UTI (positive leukocyte esterase and nitrites, WBCs, and bacteria).
- WBC count and differential: same as for a UTI.
- Blood cultures will be positive for the presence of bacteria if a systemic infection is present.
- Serum creatinine and blood urea nitrogen (BUN) are elevated during acute episodes and consistently elevated with chronic infection.
- C-reactive protein is elevated during exacerbating inflammatory processes of the kidneys. Erythrocyte sedimentation rate (ESR) is elevated during acute or chronic inflammation.

DIAGNOSTIC PROCEDURES

- An x-ray of the kidneys, ureters, and bladder (KUB) can demonstrate calculi or structural abnormalities.
- Ultrasonography to detect cysts, tumors, calculi, and abscesses.
- Gallium scan: a nuclear medicine test that uses injectable radioactive dye to visualize organs, glands, bones, and blood vessels that have infection and inflammation.
- Intravenous pyelogram can demonstrate calculi, structural, or vascular abnormalities.

PATIENT-CENTERED CARE

NURSING CARE

Nonsurgical

- Assess/monitor the following.
  - Nutritional status
  - Intake and output
  - Fluid and electrolyte balance
  - Temperature
  - Onset, quality, duration, and severity of pain
- Increase fluid intake to 2 L/day unless contraindicated.
- Administer antipyretic, such as acetaminophen, as needed for fever and opioid analgesics for pain associated with pyelonephritis.
- Provide emotional support.
- Assist with personal hygiene.

Surgical

- Includes all the above information.
- Assess the dressings and incision.
- Balance rest and activities.
- Instruct the client on monitoring for indications of infection.
- Instruct the client on the role of nutritious meals and adequate fluid intake.

MEDICATIONS

See the **RN PHARMACOLOGY REVIEW MODULE** for more detailed information.

Opioid analgesics (opioid agonists), morphine sulfate, and morphine: for moderate to severe pain

Antibiotics Q EBP
- Mild to moderate pyelonephritis treated at home for 14 days with the following.
  - Anti-infective: trimethoprim, sulfamethoxazole/trimethoprim
  - Quinolone antibiotic: ciprofloxacin levofloxacin
- Severe pyelonephritis treated in the hospital for 24 to 48 hr with IV medication
  - Quinolone antibiotic: ciprofloxacin
  - Cephalosporin antibiotic: ceftriaxone, ceftazidime
  - Aminopenicillin antibiotic: ampicillin, ampicillin/sulbactam
  - Aminoglycoside antibiotic: gentamicin, tobramycin

THERAPEUTIC PROCEDURES

Provide preoperative teaching.

Intravenous antibiotics and analgesics are usually administered for each procedure.

Pyelolithotomy: The removal of a large stone from the kidney that causes infections and blocks the flow of urine from the kidney

Nephrectomy: The removal of the kidney when all procedures to clear the client of infection were unsuccessful

Ureteroplasty: Done to repair or revise the ureter and can involve reimplantation of the ureter in the bladder wall to preserve the function of the kidney and eliminate infection

INTERPROFESSIONAL CARE

- Urology services to manage pyelonephritis
- Nutritional services to promote adequate calories

CLIENT EDUCATION

- Educate the client regarding adequate nutritional status.
- Encourage the client to drink at least 2 L fluids daily unless otherwise indicated by the provider.
- Instruct the client to take medications as prescribed.
- Instruct the client to notify the provider if acute onset of pain occurs or a fever is present.
- Encourage the client and family to express their fears and anxiety related to the disease.
- Encourage the client to take rest periods from activity as needed.

CARE AFTER DISCHARGE

- Home care services can be indicated if the client needs assistance with medications or nutritional therapy.
- Follow up with the provider as directed.

COMPLICATIONS

- **Septic shock** (hypotension, tachycardia, fever) due to bacterial organism entering the blood stream
- **Chronic kidney disease** (elevated BUN, creatinine, electrolytes) from inflammation and infection that causes fibrosis of the kidney pelvis and calyx, scarring, and changes in the blood vessels and the glomerular and tubular filtration system
- **Hypertension** (related to fluid and sodium retention) indicating chronic kidney disease caused by destruction of the filtration system of the kidney due to infection

Glomerulonephritis

Immunologic kidney disorder that can start in the kidneys (genetic basis and immune-inducing inflammation) or be a result of other health disorders (lupus erythematosus, diabetic nephropathy) and results in glomerular injury
- Can lead to end-stage kidney disease (ESKD).
- Acute glomerulonephritis often occurs following an infection.
- Chronic glomerulonephritis develops over a period of 20 to 30 years.

ASSESSMENT

RISK FACTORS

- Recent infection particularly of the skin or upper respiratory tract
- Recent travel or other possible exposure to bacteria, viruses, fungi or parasites
- Presence of systemic diseases (systemic lupus erythematosus, Goodpasture syndrome)
- Recent surgery or illness

EXPECTED FINDINGS

- Anorexia
- Nausea
- Dysuria
- Oliguria
- Fatigue
- Hypertension
- Difficulty breathing
- Crackles
- S3 heart sound
- Weight gain
- Reddish-brown or cola-colored urine
- Older adult clients are likely to have the less common manifestations related to circulatory overload, which can be confused with congestive heart failure. ©

LABORATORY TESTS

- Urinalysis shows red blood cells and protein.
- Glomerular filtration rate is decreased.
- Blood, skin or throat cultures (if indicated).
- 24-hr urine collection for protein assay (increased in acute glomerulonephritis and decreased in chronic glomerulonephritis).
- Serum blood urea nitrogen and creatinine are increased.
- Antistreptolysin-O titers are increased after group A beta hemolytic streptococcus infection.
- C3 complement levels decreased.
- Cryoglobulins present.
- Anti-nuclear antibody (ANA) presence.
- Altered electrolytes: Hyperkalemia, hyperphosphatemia, hypocalcemia.

DIAGNOSTIC PROCEDURES

Kidney biopsy will diagnose the condition, determine prognosis, and treatment.

PATIENT-CENTERED CARE

NURSING CARE

- Coordinate care to conserve client energy.
- Consult with provider to determine if fluid restriction is needed.
- Administer antibiotics as prescribed.
- Teach relaxation exercises to decrease stress.
- Monitor blood pressure.
- Monitor respiratory status.
- Monitor fluid and electrolytes.

MEDICATIONS

Antibiotics: Penicillin, erythromycin, or azithromycin is prescribed for glomerulonephritis infection due to streptococcal infection. Ⓠ**EBP**

Antihypertensives: To control hypertension

INTERPROFESSIONAL CARE

- Collaborate with provider and nutritional support regarding any potassium or protein restriction in diet.
- Dialysis or plasmapheresis if necessary.

CLIENT EDUCATION

- Advise client to complete full course of antibiotics.
- Monitor weight daily and report increases to provider.
- Provide instruction on dietary and fluid restrictions.
- Stress basic infection control practices, such as hand hygiene.

CARE AFTER DISCHARGE

- Refer to home care services for continued dialysis or plasmapheresis if needed.
- Follow up with the provider as directed.

Application Exercises

1. A nurse is planning care for a client who has chronic pyelonephritis. Which of the following actions should the nurse plan to take? (Select all that apply.)

   A. Provide a referral for nutrition counseling.

   B. Encourage daily fluid intake of 1 L.

   C. Palpate the costovertebral angle.

   D. Monitor urinary output.

   E. Administer antibiotics.

2. A nurse is caring for a client who has a urinary tract infection (UTI). Which of the following is the priority intervention by the nurse?

   A. Offer a warm sitz bath.

   B. Recommend drinking cranberry juice.

   C. Encourage increased fluids.

   D. Administer an antibiotic.

3. A nurse is preparing educational material to present to a female client who has frequent urinary tract infections. Which of the following information should the nurse include? (Select all that apply.)

   A. Avoid sitting in a wet bathing suit.

   B. Wipe the perineal area back to front following elimination.

   C. Empty the bladder when there is an urge to void.

   D. Wear synthetic fabric underwear.

   E. Take a shower daily.

4. A nurse is caring for several clients. Which of the following clients are at risk for developing pyelonephritis? (Select all that apply.)

   A. A client who is at 32 weeks of gestation

   B. A client who has kidney calculi

   C. A client who has a urine pH of 4.2

   D. A client who has a neurogenic bladder

   E. A client who has diabetes mellitus

5. A nurse is reviewing urinalysis results for four clients. Which of the following urinalysis results indicates a urinary tract infection?

   A. Positive for hyaline casts

   B. Positive for leukocyte esterase

   C. Positive for ketones

   D. Positive for crystals

PRACTICE Active Learning Scenario

A nurse is educating a client who has chronic pyelonephritis. What information should the nurse include in the teaching? Use the ATI Active Learning Template: System Disorder to complete this item.

ALTERATION IN HEALTH (DIAGNOSIS)

COMPLICATIONS: List three, and explain why these occur.

CLIENT EDUCATION: Include three teaching points.

Application Exercises Key

1. A. **CORRECT:** The client requires adequate nutrition to promote healing.

   B. The nurse should encourage fluid intake of 2 L daily to maintain dilute urine.

   C. **CORRECT:** The nurse should gently palpate the costovertebral angle for flank tenderness, which can indicate inflammation and infection.

   D. **CORRECT:** The nurse should monitor urinary output to determine that 1 to 3 L of urine is excreted daily.

   E. **CORRECT:** The nurse should administer antibiotics to treat the bacteriuria and decrease progressive damage to the kidney.

   Ⓝ *NCLEX® Connection: Physiological Adaptation, Illness Management*

2. A. The nurse should offer a warm sitz bath to provide temporary relief of the manifestations of the UTI. However, another action is the priority.

   B. The nurse should recommend that the client drink cranberry juice to prevent a UTI in the future. However, another action is the priority.

   C. The nurse should encourage the client to increase fluid intake to dilute the urine, and flush the kidneys to relieve the manifestations of the UTI. However, another action is the priority.

   D. **CORRECT:** The greatest risk to the client is injury to the renal system and sepsis from the UTI. The priority intervention is to administer antibiotics.

   Ⓝ *NCLEX® Connection: Physiological Adaptation, Unexpected Response to Therapies*

3. A. **CORRECT:** The client should avoid sitting in a wet bathing suit, which can increase the risk for a UTI by colonization of bacteria in a moist, warm environment.

   B. The client should wipe the perineal area from front to back after elimination to prevent contaminating the urethra with bacteria.

   C. **CORRECT:** The client should empty the bladder when there is an urge to void rather than retain urine for an extended period of time, which increases the risk for a UTI.

   D. The client should wear cotton underwear that absorbs moisture and keeps the perineal area drier, thus decreasing colonization of bacteria that can cause a UTI.

   E. **CORRECT:** The client should take a shower daily to promote good body hygiene and decrease colonization of bacteria in the perineal area that can cause a UTI.

   Ⓝ *NCLEX® Connection: Health Promotion and Maintenance, Health Promotion/Disease Prevention*

4. A. **CORRECT:** A client who is at 32 weeks of gestation is at risk for developing pyelonephritis because of increased pressure on the urinary system during pregnancy causing reflux or retention of urine.

   B. **CORRECT:** A client who has kidney calculi is at risk for pyelonephritis because stones harbor bacteria.

   C. The expected reference range for urine pH is 4.6 to 8.0. Alkaline urine promotes bacteria growth. The client who has a urine pH of 4.2 has acidic urine.

   D. **CORRECT:** The client who has a neurogenic bladder can retain urine, promoting bacterial growth and causing pyelonephritis.

   E. **CORRECT:** The client who has diabetes mellitus is at risk of pyelonephritis because glucose that can be in the urine promotes bacterial growth.

   Ⓝ *NCLEX® Connection: Health Promotion and Maintenance, Health Promotion/Disease Prevention*

5. A. Hyaline casts in the urine can indicate proteinuria and can occur following exercise.

   B. **CORRECT:** A positive leukocyte esterase indicates a urinary tract infection.

   C. Ketones in the urine is a manifestation of poorly controlled diabetes mellitus or starvation.

   D. Crystals in the urine can indicate a potential for kidney stone formation.

   Ⓝ *NCLEX® Connection: Reduction of Risk Potential, Laboratory Values*

PRACTICE Answer

Using the ATI Active Learning Template: System Disorder

ALTERATION IN HEALTH (DIAGNOSIS):
Chronic pyelonephritis is a repetitive infection and inflammation of the kidney pelvis, calyces, and medulla, which generally begins from bacteria that ascends from a lower urinary tract infection.

COMPLICATIONS
- Septic shock caused by micro-organisms entering the bloodstream from the infected kidney
- Chronic kidney disease caused by inflammation, fibrosis, and scarring of the kidney filtration structure
- Hypertension (related to fluid and sodium retention) indicating chronic kidney disease caused by destruction of the filtration system of the kidney from infection

CLIENT EDUCATION
- Encourage at least 2 L of fluids daily.
- Instruct the client to take all medications as prescribed.
- Instruct the client to notify the provider of acute, rapid onset of pain.
- Encourage verbalization of fears and anxiety.
- Encourage a balance of rest and activity.

Ⓝ *NCLEX® Connection: Physiological Adaptation, Illness Management*

CHAPTER 61   *Renal Calculi*

Urolithiasis is the presence of calculi (stones) in the urinary tract. The majority of calculi are composed of calcium phosphate or calcium oxalate, but they can contain other substances (uric acid, struvite, cystine).

A diet high in calcium is not believed to increase the risk of calculi formation unless there is a preexisting metabolic disorder or renal tubular defect. Reoccurrence is increased in individuals who have a family history or whose first occurrence of renal calculi is prior to the age of 25.

Most clients can expel calculi without invasive procedures. Factors that influence whether a calculus will pass spontaneously or not include the composition, size, and location of the calculus.

ASSESSMENT

RISK FACTORS

- Cause is unknown
- Increased incidence in males
- Urinary tract lining that is damaged
- Urine flow that is decreased, concentrated, and contains particles (calcium)
- Metabolic defects
  - Increased intestinal absorption or decreased renal excretion of calcium
  - Increased oxalate production (genetic) or inability to metabolize oxalate from foods (black tea, spinach, beets, Swiss chard, chocolate, and peanuts)
  - Increased production or decreased clearance of purines (contributing to increased uric-acid levels)
- High alkalinity or acidity of urine
- Urinary stasis, urinary retention, immobilization, and dehydration
- Decreased fluid intake or increased incidence of dehydration among older adult clients ⊙

EXPECTED FINDINGS

- Severe pain (renal colic)
  - Pain intensifies as the calculus moves through the ureter.
  - Flank pain suggests calculi are located in the kidney or ureter.
  - Flank pain that radiates to the abdomen, scrotum, testes, or vulva suggests calculi in the ureter or bladder.
- Urinary frequency or dysuria (calculi in the bladder)
- Fever
- Diaphoresis
- Pallor
- Nausea/vomiting
- Tachycardia, tachypnea, increased blood pressure (pain), or decreased blood pressure (shock)
- Oliguria/anuria occurs with calculi that obstruct urinary flow. Urinary tract obstruction is a medical emergency and needs to be treated to preserve kidney function.
- Hematuria (rusty or smoky-looking urine) Q𝐄𝐁𝐏

LABORATORY TESTS

Urinalysis

- Altered odor of the urine and increased urine turbidity if infection is present
- Increased RBCs, WBCs, and bacteria (presence of infection)
- Crystals noted on microscopic exam
- Abnormal serum calcium, phosphate, and uric-acid levels in the presence of metabolic disorders/defects

DIAGNOSTIC PROCEDURES

Radiology examination

X-ray of kidney, ureters, bladder (KUB), or intravenous pyelogram (IVP) is used to confirm the presence and location of calculi. IVP is contraindicated if there is a urinary obstruction.

CT or MRI

A CT (noncontrast helical scan) or MRI is used to identify cystine or uric-acid calculi, which cannot be seen on standard x-rays.

Renal ultrasound or cystoscopy

These can confirm the diagnosis.

PATIENT-CENTERED CARE

NURSING CARE

- Report laboratory and diagnostic findings to the provider.
- Provide preoperative and postoperative care as indicated.
- Administer prescribed medications.
- Strain all urine to check for passage of the calculus, and save the calculus for laboratory analysis.
- Encourage increased oral intake to 3 L/day unless contraindicated.
- Administer IV fluids as prescribed.
- Encourage ambulation to promote passage of the calculus.

ASSESS/MONITOR
- Pain status
- Intake and output
- Urinary pH

MEDICATIONS

Analgesics

Opioids
- Morphine sulfate is used in the first 24 to 36 hr with the acute onset of calculi.
- Opioid agents are used to treat moderate to severe pain. These drugs act on the mu and kappa receptors that help alleviate pain. Activation of these receptors produces analgesia (pain relief), respiratory depression, euphoria, sedation, and a decrease in GI motility.
- Use cautiously with clients who have asthma or emphysema due to the risk of respiratory depression.
- NURSING CONSIDERATIONS
  ○ Assess the client frequently.
  ○ Watch for evidence of respiratory depression, especially in older adult clients. If respirations are 12/min or less, stop the medication and notify the provider immediately. Ⓖ
  ○ Monitor vital signs for hypotension and decreased respirations.
  ○ Assess level of sedation (drowsiness, level of consciousness).
- CLIENT EDUCATION: Encourage the client to drink plenty of fluids to prevent constipation.

NSAIDs
- Ketorolac is used to treat mild to moderate pain, fever, and inflammation.
- NURSING CONSIDERATIONS: Observe for indications of bleeding.
- CLIENT EDUCATION
  ○ Instruct the client to watch for bleeding (dark stools, blood in stools).
  ○ Instruct the client to notify the provider if abdominal pain occurs, which can be due to gastric ulceration.

Spasmolytic medications

Oxybutynin alleviates pain by decreasing bladder spasms that can result due to renal calculi.

NURSING CONSIDERATIONS
- Assess for history of glaucoma, as this medication increases intraocular pressure. Ⓠᴘᴄᴄ
- Monitor for dizziness and tachycardia.
- Monitor for urinary retention.

CLIENT EDUCATION
- Instruct the client to report palpitations and problems with voiding or constipation.
- Inform the client that dizziness and dry mouth are common with the medication.
- Encourage the client to suck on hard candies to alleviate dry mouth.

Antibiotics

Gentamicin and cephalexin are used to treat UTIs.

NURSING CONSIDERATIONS
- Administer medication with food to decrease GI distress.
- Monitor for nephrotoxicity and ototoxicity for clients taking gentamicin.

CLIENT EDUCATION
- Inform the client that urine can have foul odor related to the antibiotic.
- Instruct the client to report loose stools related to the medication.

INTERPROFESSIONAL CARE

Urology services can be consulted for management of urolithiasis.

Nutritional services can be consulted for dietary modifications concerning foods related to calculi formation.

THERAPEUTIC PROCEDURES

Extracorporeal shock wave lithotripsy (ESWL)

- Uses sound, laser, or shock-wave energies to break calculi into fragments.
- Requires moderate (conscious) sedation and ECG monitoring during the procedure.

NURSING ACTIONS
- Educate the client regarding the procedure.
- Assess for gross hematuria and strain urine following the procedure.
- Administer analgesics as prescribed.

CLIENT EDUCATION
- Inform the client that bruising is normal at the site where waves are applied.
- Explain to the client that there will be hematuria postprocedure.

Surgical interventions

Stenting is the placement of a small tube in the ureter during a ureteroscopy to dilate the ureter and allow passage of a calculus.

Retrograde ureteroscopy uses a basket, forceps, or loop on the end of the ureteroscope to grasp and remove the calculus.

Percutaneous ureterolithotomy/ nephrolithotomy is the insertion of an ultrasonic or laser lithotripter into the ureter or kidney to grasp and extract the calculus.

Open surgery uses a surgical incision to remove the calculus. This surgery is used for large or impacted calculi (staghorn calculi) or for calculi not removed by other approaches.
- **Ureterolithotomy:** into the ureter
- **Pyelolithotomy:** into the kidney pelvis
- **Nephrolithotomy:** into the kidney

CARE AFTER DISCHARGE: Nutritional services can be consulted for dietary modifications concerning foods related to calculi formation.

CLIENT EDUCATION
Educate the client regarding the role of diet and medications in the treatment and prevention of renal calculi.
- **Calcium phosphate**
  - Limit intake of food high in animal protein (reduction of protein intake decreases calcium precipitation).
  - Limit sodium intake.
  - Reduced calcium intake (dairy products) is individualized.
  - MEDICATIONS
    - Thiazide diuretics (hydrochlorothiazide) are used to increase calcium reabsorption.
    - Orthophosphates are used to decrease urine saturation of calcium oxalate.
    - Sodium cellulose phosphate is used to reduce the intestinal absorption of calcium.
- **Calcium oxalate**
  - Avoid oxalate sources: spinach, black tea, rhubarb, cocoa, beets, pecans, peanuts, okra, chocolate, wheat germ, lime peel, and Swiss chard. ⓆPCC
  - Limit sodium intake.

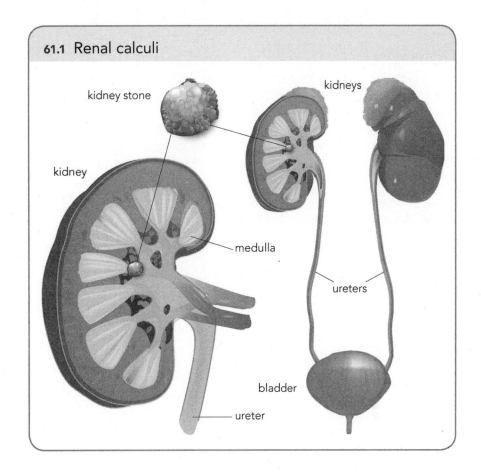

61.1 Renal calculi

kidney stone
kidneys
kidney
medulla
ureters
bladder
ureter

- **Struvite** (magnesium ammonium phosphate): Avoid high-phosphate foods: dairy products, red and organ meats, whole grains.
- **Uric acid** (urate)
  - Decrease intake of purine sources: organ meats, poultry, fish, gravies, red wine, sardines.
  - MEDICATIONS
    - Allopurinol is used to prevent the formation of uric acid.
    - Potassium or sodium citrate or sodium bicarbonate is used to alkalinize the urine.
- **Cystine**
  - Limit animal protein intake.
  - MEDICATIONS
    - Alpha mercaptopropionylglycine (AMPG) is used to lower urine cystine.
    - Captopril is used to lower urine cystine.

COMPLICATIONS

Urosepsis

Occurs when a urinary tract infection spreads to the client's bloodstream. This complication is potentially life-threatening due to organ failure and shock.

NURSING ACTIONS
- Administer antibiotics prophylactically (especially prior to invasive treatment) or to treat an existing infection. Q EBP
- Monitor culture and sensitivity results.
- Monitor for indications of a urinary tract infection (fever, tachycardia, increased urine turbidity, urine odor, elevated serum WBC count, client report of pain with urination).
- Monitor for shock.
- Encourage adequate fluid intake.
- Encourage adequate nutrition.

Obstruction

A calculus can block the passage of urine into the kidney, ureter, or bladder. Urinary output can be diminished or absent.

NURSING ACTIONS
- Notify the provider immediately.
- Prepare the client for removal of the calculus.

Hydronephrosis

Occurs when a calculus has blocked a portion of the urinary tract. The urine backs up and causes distention of the kidney.

NURSING ACTIONS
- Notify the provider immediately.
- Prepare the client for removal of the calculus.

Application Exercises

1. A nurse is completing the admission assessment of a client who has renal calculi. Which of the following findings should the nurse expect?

   A. Bradycardia

   B. Diaphoresis

   C. Nocturia

   D. Bradypnea

2. A nurse is reviewing discharge instructions with a client who had spontaneous passage of a calcium phosphate renal calculus. Which of the following instructions should the nurse include in the teaching? (Select all that apply.)

   A. Limit intake of food high in animal protein.

   B. Reduce sodium intake.

   C. Strain urine for 48 hr.

   D. Report burning with urination to the provider.

   E. Increase fluid intake to 3 L/day.

3. A nurse is teaching a client who is scheduled for extracorporeal shock wave lithotripsy (ESWL). Which of the following statements by the client indicates understanding of the teaching?

   A. "I will be fully awake during the procedure."

   B. "Lithotripsy will reduce my chances of having stones in the future."

   C. "I will report any bruising that occurs to my doctor."

   D. "Straining my urine following the procedure is important."

4. A nurse is caring for a client who has a left renal calculus and an indwelling urinary catheter. Which of the following assessment findings is the priority for the nurse to report to the provider?

   A. Flank pain that radiates to the lower abdomen

   B. Client report of nausea

   C. Absent urine output for 1 hr

   D. Serum WBC count 15,000/mm^3

5. A nurse is completing discharge instructions with a client who has spontaneously passed a calcium oxalate calculus. To decrease the chance of recurrence, the nurse should instruct the client to avoid which of the following foods? (Select all that apply.)

   A. Red meat

   B. Black tea

   C. Cheese

   D. Whole grains

   E. Spinach

PRACTICE Active Learning Scenario

A nurse is planning care for a client who has renal calculi and prescriptions for morphine and oxybutynin for pain control. What should the nurse take into consideration when administering these medications? Use the ATI Active Learning Template: Medication to complete this item.

THERAPEUTIC USES: Identify the rationale for administering morphine and oxybutynin.

COMPLICATIONS: Identify adverse effects the nurse should monitor for when administering each of these medications.

NURSING INTERVENTIONS: Identify nursing considerations and client education the nurse should plan to provide when administering each of these medications.

Application Exercises Key

1. A. Tachycardia is a manifestation associated with a client who has renal calculi.

   B. **CORRECT:** Diaphoresis is a manifestation associated with a client who has renal calculi.

   C. Oliguria is a manifestation associated with a client who has renal calculi.

   D. Tachypnea is a manifestation associated with a client who has renal calculi.

   Ⓝ *NCLEX® Connection: Physiological Adaptation, Pathophysiology*

2. A. **CORRECT:** The client should limit the intake of food high in animal protein, which contains calcium phosphate.

   B. **CORRECT:** The client should limit intake of sodium, which affects the precipitation of calcium phosphate in the urine.

   C. The client does not need to continue straining urine once the calculus has passed.

   D. **CORRECT:** The client should report burning with urination to the provider because this can indicate a urinary tract infection.

   E. **CORRECT:** The client should increase fluid intake to 2 to 3 L/day. A decrease in fluid intake can cause dehydration, which increases the risk of calculi formation.

   Ⓝ *NCLEX® Connection: Reduction of Risk Potential, Therapeutic Procedures*

3. A. The client receives moderate (conscious) sedation for this procedure. The client is not fully awake.

   B. Lithotripsy does not decrease the recurrence rate of renal calculi. The procedure breaks the calculi into fragments so they will pass into urine.

   C. Bruising is an expected finding following lithotripsy and does not need to be reported to the provider.

   D. **CORRECT:** A client is instructed to strain urine following lithotripsy to verify that the calculi have passed.

   Ⓝ *NCLEX® Connection: Basic Care and Comfort, Nutrition and Oral Hydration*

4. A. Flank pain radiating to the lower abdomen is a finding associated with renal calculi, but there is another finding that is a greater risk to the client.

   B. Client report of nausea is a finding associated with renal calculi, but there is another finding that is a greater risk to the client.

   C. **CORRECT:** The greatest risk to this client is damage to the kidney resulting from obstruction of urine flow by the renal calculus. Therefore, the priority finding for the nurse to report to the provider is anuria.

   D. An elevated serum WBC is a finding associated with renal calculus and can indicate a urinary tract infection, but there is another finding that is a greater risk to the client.

   Ⓝ *NCLEX® Connection: Physiological Adaptation, Unexpected Response to Therapies*

5. A. A client who has renal calculi composed of calcium phosphate, struvite, uric acid, or cysteine should limit intake of animal protein.

   B. **CORRECT:** A client who has renal calculi composed of calcium oxalate should avoid intake of black tea because it is a source of oxalate.

   C. A client who has renal calculi composed of calcium phosphate or struvite should limit intake of dairy products.

   D. A client who has renal calculi composed of struvite should limit intake of whole grains.

   E. **CORRECT:** A client who has renal calculi composed of calcium oxalate should avoid intake of spinach because it is a source of oxalate.

   Ⓝ *NCLEX® Connection: Reduction of Risk Potential, Therapeutic Procedures*

PRACTICE Answer

Using the ATI Active Learning Template: Medication

THERAPEUTIC USES

- Morphine sulfate, an opioid, is administered during the first 24 hr to treat moderate to severe pain associated with acute renal calculi.
- Oxybutynin, a spasmolytic, is administered to provide pain relief by decreasing bladder spasms resulting from renal calculi.

COMPLICATIONS

- Morphine sulfate: respiratory depression, euphoria, sedation, decreased GI motility
- Oxybutynin: dizziness, tachycardia, urinary retention, dry mouth, constipation

NURSING INTERVENTIONS

- Morphine sulfate
  - Administer cautiously with clients who have asthma or emphysema due to the risk of respiratory depression.
  - Monitor frequently for respiratory depression, especially in older adults. If respirations are 12/min or less, stop the medication and notify the provider immediately.
  - Monitor vital signs frequently for hypotension.
  - Encourage the client to drink plenty of fluids to prevent constipation.

- Oxybutynin
  - Determine prior to administration if the client has a history of glaucoma, as this medication increases intraocular pressure
  - Monitor for dizziness and tachycardia.
  - Monitor for urinary retention.
  - Instruct the client to report palpitations and problems with voiding or constipation.
  - Inform the client that dizziness and dry mouth are common with the medication.
  - Encourage the client to such on hard candies to alleviate dry mouth.

Ⓝ *NCLEX® Connection: Reduction of Risk Potential, Therapeutic Procedures*

When reviewing the following chapters, keep in mind the relevant topics and tasks of the NCLEX outline, in particular:

Client Needs: Basic Care and Comfort

ELIMINATION
Assess and manage client with an alteration in elimination.

Perform irrigations.

Client Needs: Reduction of Risk Potential

DIAGNOSTIC TESTS: Compare client diagnostic findings with pre-test results.

LABORATORY VALUES: Educate the client about the purpose and procedure of prescribed laboratory tests.

POTENTIAL FOR ALTERATIONS IN BODY SYSTEMS:
Monitor client output for changes from baseline.

Client Needs: Physiological Adaptation

ALTERATIONS IN BODY SYSTEMS: Assess client for signs and symptoms of adverse effects of radiation therapy.

ILLNESS MANAGEMENT: Identify client data that needs to be reported immediately.

PATHOPHYSIOLOGY: Understand general principles of pathophysiology.

CHAPTER 62 # Diagnostic and Therapeutic Procedures for Female Reproductive Disorders

Diagnostic procedures are used to evaluate the structure, condition, and function of a female client's reproductive tissues and organs. Biopsies can also serve as therapeutic purposes in removing abnormal tissue. Another therapeutic procedure that nurses should be knowledgeable about is a hysterectomy.

Pelvic exam with Papanicolaou and human papilloma virus tests

Bimanual examination of the cervix, uterus, fallopian tubes, and ovaries is performed by the provider. The provider inserts two gloved fingers into the vagina and traps the reproductive structures between the fingers of the one hand and the fingers of the opposite hand that is on the abdomen. Palpation of the structures is done during this time.

Two tests are used for cervical cancer screening, the Papanicolaou (Pap) test and the test for human papilloma virus (HPV). Both can be performed prior to the pelvic examination.
- **The Pap test** is use to identify precancerous and cancerous cells of the cervix.
- **The HPV test** is used to identify HPV infections that can lead to cervical cancer.

CONSIDERATIONS

PREPROCEDURE Qpcc

NURSING ACTIONS
- Advise the client that she should schedule the test when she is not menstruating.
- Inform the client that use of vaginal medications, douching, or sexual intercourse within the past 24 hr can alter test results.
- Have the client empty her bladder.
- Place the client in the lithotomy position and drape appropriately.
- Explain to the client how the procedure will be carried out.
- Have all necessary equipment available (cervical scraping tools, glass slides, fixative, perineal pad).

INTRAPROCEDURE

NURSING ACTIONS
- Remain with the client and provide support.
- Have ready the necessary equipment for the provider during procedure.
- Transfer specimens to slides and apply fixative to slides.

POSTPROCEDURE

NURSING ACTIONS: Provide the client with perineal pad and tissues.

CLIENT EDUCATION
- Inform the client that minimal bleeding can occur from the cervix.
- Inform the client of the time frame for results to be available.
- Educate the client about the importance of following up with provider if results are abnormal.

62.1 Pap and HPV screening guidelines

The American Cancer Society provides guidelines for the prevention and early detection of cervical cancer. See www.cancer.org. QEBP

Testing recommendations by age

21	All women begin screening for cervical cancer.
21 TO 29	Pap test every 3 years. HPV unnecessary unless needed following an abnormal Pap test.
30 TO 65	Pap and HPV every 5 years.
OLDER THAN 65	May discontinue testing if regular screenings have been negative. If diagnosed with cervical precancer, continue to screen.
	Screening is unnecessary for women who have had a hysterectomy with removal of the cervix and have a negative history of cervical cancer.
	Women who are at high risk for cervical cancer need to be screened more frequently based on the advice of her provider.

Colposcopy and cervical biopsy

A colposcopy is the examination of the tissues of the vagina and cervix using an electric microscope. Typically, the provider also performs a biopsy. Several options are available.

- The provider may perform an endocervical curettage if a lesion is visible.
- A cone biopsy is an extensive surgical biopsy. The provider excises a cone-shaped sample of tissue to remove potentially harmful cells. In some cases, anesthesia is used for the procedure. Margins of the excised tissue are examined to ensure removal of all harmful cells. The surgeon may destroy the cells using a scalpel, cryosurgery (extreme cold, which freezes the tissue), lasers, or a procedure known as loop electrosurgical excision (LEEP). LEEP uses an electric current, and the laser procedure uses a laser beam that vaporizes the abnormal tissue.
- The best time to perform the procedure is in the early phase of the menstrual cycle because the cervix is less vascular.

INDICATIONS

Pap tests that demonstrate atypical or abnormal cells must be followed up with a colposcopy and cervical biopsy.

CONSIDERATIONS

PREPROCEDURE

NURSING ACTIONS
- Provide psychological support.
- Explain the procedure to the client and inform her that when the specimen is obtained, she can expect to experience temporary discomfort and cramping.
- Preprocedure care is the same as that for a Pap test, except a sterile biopsy cup will be needed instead of the other equipment.

POSTPROCEDURE

NURSING ACTIONS
- Postprocedure care is the same as for a Pap test.
- Provide client with perineal pad and tissues.

CLIENT EDUCATION Qᴘᴄᴄ
- Instruct the client to rest for the first 24 hr after the procedure.
- Instruct the client to abstain from sexual intercourse and avoid using a douche, vaginal creams, or tampons until all discharge has stopped (usually about 2 weeks).
- Instruct the client to avoid lifting heavy objects for approximately 2 weeks to allow time for the cervix to heal.
- Instruct the client to use analgesics as directed by the provider, but to avoid the use of aspirin because it can cause bleeding. Qₛ
- Instruct the client to report excessive bleeding, fever, or foul-smelling drainage to the provider.

COMPLICATIONS

Bleeding

Heavy bleeding can result from the excision of tissue.

NURSING ACTIONS: Assess for heavy bleeding.

CLIENT EDUCATION: Instruct the client to notify the provider for heavy vaginal bleeding.

Infection

Infection can result from this invasive procedure.

NURSING ACTIONS: Assess the client for fever, chills, severe pain, foul odor, or purulent vaginal discharge.

CLIENT EDUCATION: Instruct the client to notify the provider regarding manifestations of infection.

Endometrial biopsy

A thin, hollow tube is inserted through the cervix, and a curette or suction equipment is used to obtain the endometrial tissue sample.

INDICATIONS

POTENTIAL DIAGNOSES: Endometrial biopsies are done to assess for uterine cancer as well as evaluate for menstrual irregularities and potential causes of infertility.

CLIENT PRESENTATION: Abnormal or postmenopausal bleeding

CONSIDERATIONS

PREPROCEDURE

NURSING ACTIONS
- Obtain the client's menstrual history.
- Administer an analgesic prior to the procedure.
- Prepare the client using same procedure as pelvic examination.
- Witness consent.

CLIENT EDUCATION Qᴘᴄᴄ
- Educate the client about the procedure.
  - Biopsies are done with the client awake.
  - The client will feel some discomfort and cramping.
  - Instruct the client on use of relaxation techniques.
- Have the client empty her bladder.

POSTPROCEDURE

NURSING ACTIONS
- Postprocedure care is the same as that for a Pap test.
- Encourage the client to rest on the examination table until cramping has diminished.

CLIENT EDUCATION
- Inform the client that spotting can be present for 1 to 2 days.
- Tell the client that results will be available in approximately 72 hr.
- Instruct the client to abstain from sexual intercourse and avoid using a douche, vaginal creams, or tampons until all discharge has stopped (usually about 1 to 2 days).
- Have the client notify the provider of heavy vaginal bleeding, fever, severe pain, or foul discharge.

COMPLICATIONS

Bleeding

Heavy vaginal bleeding is a potential complication of an endometrial biopsy.

NURSING ACTIONS: Assess for heavy bleeding.

CLIENT EDUCATION: Instruct the client to notify the provider of heavy vaginal bleeding.

Infection

Infection can result from this invasive procedure.

NURSING ACTIONS: Assess for fever, chills, severe pain, foul odor, and purulent vaginal discharge.

CLIENT EDUCATION: Instruct the client to notify the provider regarding manifestations of infection.

Screening for reproductive disorders

Syphilis

There are two serologic (blood) studies used to screen for syphilis. ⓠEBP
- Venereal disease research laboratory (VDRL): the oldest test for syphilis that is still performed
- Rapid plasma reagin (RPR): a newer test for syphilis and has replaced the VDRL test in many institutions

INTERPRETATION OF FINDINGS
- Both tests are done using a sample of blood and reported as nonreactive (negative for syphilis) or reactive (positive for syphilis).
- False positives can occur secondary to infection, pregnancy, malignancies, and autoimmune disorders.
- If either test is reactive, diagnosis should be confirmed using one of the following tests:
  - Fluorescent treponemal antibody absorbed (FTA-ABS)
  - Microhemagglutination assays for antibody to *T. pallidum*

Human immune deficiency virus (HIV)

The enzyme immunoassay (EIA) test and Western blot assay are used to detect the presence of HIV.

INTERPRETATION OF FINDINGS
- The EIA test, formerly the enzyme-linked immunosorbent assay (ELISA) is an antibody test used to measure the client's response to HIV. The test is typically positive 3 weeks to 3 months after the infection occurs, but it can be delayed for as long as 36 months. False positive results can occur, so further testing is needed.
- If the EIA is positive, the Western blot assay is used to confirm the diagnosis of HIV.

Genital herpes

Although a diagnosis of genital herpes can be based on the client's history and physical, it can be confirmed with laboratory testing, which include the following.
- **Herpes viral culture:** Fluid from a lesion is obtained using a swab and placed in a cup for culture.
- **Polymerase chain reaction (PRC) test:** Identifies genetic material of the virus. Cells from a lesion, blood, or other body fluids can be tested. Identifies type of virus (herpes simplex 1 [HSV 1] or herpes simplex 2 [HSV 2]).
- **Antibody test:** Blood is tested for antibodies to the virus. Some tests can identify the type of virus. The HerpeSelect Immunoblot, HerpeSelect ELISA, and Western Blot can be used to differentiate between HSV 1 and HSV 2.

Mammography

During a mammogram, a breast is mechanically compressed both vertically and horizontally by the x-ray machine while radiologic pictures are taken of each breast.

INDICATIONS

Screening mammograms detect breast cancer lesions in women who do not have manifestations. Screening mammograms decrease cancer death rates because the treatment options and outcomes are best when the cancer is detected early. Q EBP

> A number of organizations provide guidelines for screening mammograms, including the American Cancer Society and the U.S. Preventive Services Task Force. For current guidelines, see www.cancer.org and www.uspreventiveservicestaskforce.org.

Diagnostic mammograms are used when a screening mammogram reveals abnormal findings or when breast cancer manifestations are present. The diagnostic mammogram provides a more detailed picture and is more accurate than the screening mammogram.

There are two types of mammography screening tools. Traditional mammography images are stored on film. Digital mammography takes an electronic image, which can be stored electronically. Both types are effective diagnostic tools; however, the digital mammogram can be more useful in women who have dense breast tissue. It is also more costly.

A breast ultrasound can be used to determine whether a mass is fluid-filled (cyst) or a solid mass, which could be a cancerous lesion. A wire needle biopsy can be used if the abnormal area is too small to be palpated. Ultrasound is used to identify the area of concern. Then a small wire is placed into the area. Subsequently the surgeon performs a biopsy using the wire to locate the area.

CONSIDERATIONS

PREPROCEDURE Q PCC

CLIENT EDUCATION
- Instruct the client to avoid the use of deodorant, lotion, or powders in the axillary region or on the breasts prior to the exam.
- Tell the client she should not have a mammogram if she is pregnant.

INTRAPROCEDURE

Radiologic technicians are often the members of the health care team who perform mammograms.

NURSING ACTIONS: The client can feel slight, temporary discomfort when the breast is compressed.

POSTPROCEDURE

CLIENT EDUCATION
- Inform the client that she will be contacted about results of diagnostic examination.
- Reinforce education about self-breast examinations.
- Encourage the client to follow the advice of her provider regarding when to return for a follow-up mammogram.

Hysterosalpingography

- Visualization of the cervix, uterus, and fallopian tubes by x-ray with injection of contrast dye
- Performed 2 to 5 days following menstrual period to avoid harm to an existing pregnancy

INDICATIONS

- Evaluation of fibroids, tumors and fistulas
- Assessment of fertility

CONSIDERATIONS

PREPROCEDURE

NURSING ACTIONS Q S
- Confirm date of client's last menstrual cycle.
- Assess for allergy to iodine.
- Witness informed consent.
- Prepare client as for a pelvic exam.

INTRAPROCEDURE

NURSING ACTIONS
- Remain with the client and provide support.
- Have ready the necessary equipment for the provider during the procedure.

POSTPROCEDURE

NURSING ACTIONS: Provide the client with perineal pad and tissues.

CLIENT EDUCATION Q PCC
- Inform the client that minimal bleeding can occur from the cervix.
- Instruct the client to take analgesics as prescribed by the provider for pelvic cramping. Inform the client she can also experience referred pain to the shoulder.
- Inform the client of the time frame for results to be available.
- Instruct the client to notify the provider if bleeding continues for 4 or more days and to report any manifestations of infection, such as fever, severe pain, or foul discharge.

Hysterectomy

- A hysterectomy is the removal of the uterus.
- A bilateral salpingo oophorectomy is the removal of the ovaries and fallopian tubes.
- There are three methods of performing a hysterectomy.
  - Abdominal approach, also known as a total abdominal hysterectomy
  - Vaginal approach
  - Laparoscopy-assisted vaginal hysterectomy
- There are a number of options available for a woman who requires a hysterectomy or other reproductive procedure. In some cases, the decision regarding which procedure is based on the client's preference in conjunction with the surgeon's recommendation.
  - Total hysterectomy: Uterus and cervix are removed.
  - Subtotal hysterectomy: Uterus is removed; cervix is not.
  - Bilateral salpingo oophorectomy: Ovaries and fallopian tubes are removed.
  - Panhysterectomy: Uterus, cervix, ovaries, and fallopian tubes are removed.
  - Radical hysterectomy: Uterus, cervix, upper part of the vagina, and adjacent tissue (including lymph nodes) are removed.
- To treat leiomyomas (benign fibroid tumors), uterine-sparing procedures are available.

INDICATIONS

POTENTIAL DIAGNOSES
- Uterine cancer
- Noncancerous conditions: fibroids, endometriosis (inflammation of the endometrium), and genital prolapse: that cause pain, bleeding, or emotional stress

CLIENT PRESENTATION
- Painful intercourse
- Hypermenorrhea
- Pelvic pressure
- Urinary urgency or frequency
- Constipation

CONSIDERATIONS

PREPROCEDURE

NURSING ACTIONS Qs
- Ensure that clients who have been taking anticoagulant medications, aspirin, nonsteroidal anti-inflammatory drugs (NSAIDs), or vitamin E have discontinued their use.
- Rule out pregnancy.
- Administer preoperative antibiotics.
- Place antiembolism stockings.
- Complete psychological assessment.
- Maintain NPO status.
- Ensure that informed consent has been obtained.

CLIENT EDUCATION Qs
- Teach the client how to turn, cough, and deep breathe, and the importance of early ambulation.
- Instruct the client how to use an incentive spirometer.
- Teach the client about preoperative and postoperative medications.

POSTPROCEDURE QEBP

NURSING ACTIONS
- Postoperatively, the nurse must monitor the client for vaginal bleeding. Excess bleeding is more than one saturated pad in 4 hr.
- An indwelling urinary catheter is generally inserted intraoperatively and in place for the first 24 hr postoperatively.
- Priority assessments and interventions following a total abdominal hysterectomy:
  - Monitor vital signs (fever, hypotension).
  - Monitor breath sounds (risk of atelectasis; turn, cough, and deep breathe; use of incentive spirometry; ambulation).
  - Monitor bowel sounds (risk of paralytic ileus).
  - Monitor urine output. (Call the provider if less than 30 mL/hr.)
  - Provide IV fluid and electrolyte replacement until bowel sounds return.
  - Monitor the incision (infection, integrity, risk of dehiscence).
  - Monitor for indications of thrombophlebitis (warmth, tenderness, edema).
  - Take thromboembolism precautions (sequential compression devices, ambulation).
  - Monitor blood loss (Hgb and Hct, vital signs).

CLIENT EDUCATION
- Instruct the client about a well-balanced diet that is high in protein and vitamin C for wound healing, and high in iron if the client is anemic.
- If the client's ovaries have been removed, she can develop menopausal manifestations. Discuss issues related to hormone therapy with the client.
- Instruct the client to restrict activity (heavy lifting, strenuous activity, driving, stairs, sexual activity) for as long as 6 weeks depending on the procedure that was performed. Qs
- Remind the client to avoid the use of tampons.
- Tell the client to notify the surgeon of temperatures greater than 37.8° C (100° F), foul-smelling drainage from incision, pain, redness, swelling in calf, or burning on urination.

COMPLICATIONS

Complications for clients following a hysterectomy are similar to that of clients who are postoperative following other abdominal surgeries. Monitor the client for complications, including the following.

Hypovolemic shock

Hypovolemic shock due to blood loss is a potential complication following a hysterectomy.

NURSING ACTIONS
- Monitor vital signs, Hgb, and Hct.
- Check for excessive vaginal bleeding (more than one saturated perineal pad in 4 hr).
- Provide fluid replacement therapy and/or blood transfusions as indicated.

Infection

Can be indicated by foul-smelling vaginal drainage, temperatures greater than 37.8° C (100° F), and redness, swelling, or drainage at the site of the incision.

Psychological reactions

Psychological reactions can occur months to years after surgery.

NURSING ACTIONS
- Encourage the client to discuss the positive aspects of life.
- Understand that occasional sadness in the client is normal, but persistent sadness or depression indicates a need for counseling assistance.

CLIENT EDUCATION: Encourage the client to attend a support group. Qpcc

Application Exercises

1. A nurse in a clinic is reviewing the facility's testing process and procedures for human immune deficiency virus (HIV) with a new employee. Which of the following information should the nurse include in the review?

   A. In the presence of HIV, the enzyme immunoassay (EIA) test is typically reactive within 72 hr after the client is infected.

   B. The Western blot assay is used to confirm diagnosis of HIV.

   C. The polymerase chain reaction (PRC) test is used to confirm diagnosis of HIV.

   D. CD4+ cell counts will be elevated in a client who is infected with HIV.

2. A nurse is providing instructions to a client prior to her first mammogram. Which of the following information should the nurse provide prior to the procedure?

   A. "You should not take any aspirin products prior to the mammogram."

   B. "Do not use apply any deodorant the day of the exam."

   C. "You will need to avoid sexual intercourse the day before the mammogram."

   D. "You should avoid exercise prior to the exam."

3. A nurse is providing education to a client prior to her first Papanicolaou (Pap) test. Which of the following statements should the nurse make?

   A. "You should urinate immediately after the procedure is over."

   B. "You will not feel any discomfort."

   C. "You may experience some bleeding after the procedure."

   D. "You will need to hold your breath during the procedure."

4. A nurse in a provider's office is reviewing a client's laboratory results, which shows a positive rapid plasma regain (RPR). Which of the following tests will be administered to the client to confirm the diagnosis of syphilis?

   A. Venereal Disease Research Laboratory (VDRL)

   B. D-dimer

   C. Fluorescent treponemal antibody absorbed (FTA-ABS)

   D. Sickledex

5. A nurse is providing teaching for a client who is to undergo a cervical biopsy. Which of the following information should the nurse include in the instructions? (Select all that apply.)

   A. "The procedure is painless."

   B. "Avoid heavy lifting for approximately 2 weeks after the procedure."

   C. "Heavy bleeding is common during the first 12 hours after the procedure."

   D. "Plan to rest for the first 72 hours after the procedure."

   E. "Avoid the use of tampons for 2 weeks after the procedure."

PRACTICE Active Learning Scenario

A nurse is planning care for a client who will have a total abdominal hysterectomy. Use the ATI Active Learning Template: Therapeutic Procedure to complete this item.

NURSING ACTIONS (PRE, INTRA, POST): List at least two nursing actions the nurse should include preprocedure and at least four actions the nurse should include postprocedure.

Application Exercises Key

1. A. The EIA test is typically reactive 3 weeks to 3 months after the infection occurs, but it can be delayed for as long as 36 months.

   B. **CORRECT:** Confirming HIV is a two-step process. If the EIA is positive, a second test (the Western blot assay) is done.

   C. The PRC test is used to confirm the diagnosis of genital herpes.

   D. The EIA test is typically reactive 3 weeks to 3 months after the infection occurs, but it can be delayed for as long as 36 months.

   Ⓝ *NCLEX® Connection: Reduction of Risk Potential, Laboratory Values*

2. A. Taking aspirin products does not alter the accuracy of a mammogram.

   B. **CORRECT:** Applying deodorant or powder can alter the accuracy of a mammogram by causing a shadow to appear.

   C. Having sexual intercourse does not alter the accuracy of a mammogram.

   D. Exercising does not alter the accuracy of a mammogram.

   Ⓝ *NCLEX® Connection: Reduction of Risk Potential, Therapeutic Procedures*

3. A. The client is instructed to urinate immediately before the procedure.

   B. The client can experience discomfort when the provider obtains the cervical sample.

   C. **CORRECT:** The client can experience a small amount of vaginal bleeding due to scraping of the cervix.

   D. The client should use relaxation techniques, such as taking deep breaths during the procedure.

   Ⓝ *NCLEX® Connection: Reduction of Risk Potential, Therapeutic Procedures*

4. A. The VDRL is another screening test for syphilis.

   B. The D-dimer is a test used measure fibrin and is used to diagnose disseminated intravascular coagulation.

   C. **CORRECT:** The fluorescent treponemal antibody absorbed is used to confirm the diagnosis of syphilis.

   D. The sickledex is used to diagnose sickle cell anemia.

   Ⓝ *NCLEX® Connection: Reduction of Risk Potential, Laboratory Values*

5. A. Typically the client will experience temporary discomfort and cramping when the specimen is obtained.

   B. **CORRECT:** The client should avoid heavy lifting until the cervix has healed, which takes approximately 2 weeks.

   C. Some bleeding is common after a cervical biopsy, but excessive bleeding is a complication and should be reported to the provider.

   D. The client should plan to rest for the first 24 hr after the procedure.

   E. **CORRECT:** The client should not use tampons until the cervix has healed, which takes approximately 2 weeks.

   Ⓝ *NCLEX® Connection: Reduction of Risk Potential, Therapeutic Procedures*

PRACTICE Answer

Using the ATI Active Learning Template: Therapeutic Procedure

NURSING ACTIONS (PRE, INTRA, POST)

Preprocedure
- Maintain NPO status.
- Ensure that informed consent has been obtained.
- Teach the client to turn, cough, and deep breathe; to use the incentive spirometer; and the importance of early ambulation
- Teach the client about preoperative and postoperative medications.
- Rule out pregnancy.
- Ensure that clients who have been taking anticoagulant medications, aspirin, nonsterodial anti-inflammatory drugs (NSAIDs), or vitamin E have discontinued their use.
- Administer preoperative antibiotics.
- Place antiembolism stockings.
- Complete psychological assessment.

Postprocedure
- Monitor vaginal bleeding. The client should have no more than one saturated perineal pad in 4 hr.
- Maintain indwelling urinary catheter and monitor urine output. The client should have at least 30 mL/hr.
- Monitor vital signs.
- Monitor breath sounds and use of incentive spirometer.
- Assist with ambulation.
- Monitor bowel sounds.
- Provide IV fluid and electrolyte replacement.
- Monitor the client's incision.
- Monitor the Hgb and Hct.
- Monitor for indications of thrombosis and take thromboembolism precautions.
- Instruct the client about diets that promote wound healing (high protein and vitamin C).
- Instruct the client to restrict activity.
- If ovaries have been removed, discuss issues related to hormone therapy.
- Remind the client to avoid the use of tampons.
- Tell the client to notify the surgeon of temperature over 37.8° C (100° F), foul-smelling drainage from incision, pain, redness, swelling in calf, and burning on urination.
- Assess psychological status.

Ⓝ *NCLEX® Connection: Reduction of Risk Potential, Therapeutic Procedures*

CHAPTER 63 # Menstrual Disorders and Menopause

The average age of menarche (first menses) is 12.4 years but can occur from 9 to 17 years. Assessment is indicated if an adolescent has not begun menstruation by 16.5 years of age.

Menstrual cycles are typically 28 days long, with a range from 23 to 35 days. The first day of menstruation is day 1 of a menstrual cycle. Ovulation typically occurs around day 14. Menstruation begins 14 days after ovulation and typically lasts 4 to 6 days, but it can continue for up to 9 days.

Menstrual cycles continue until menopause or surgical removal of the uterus. Menopause is when ovulation ceases and menstrual cycles become irregular and eventually stop. The median age of onset of menopause is 51 years.

Menstrual disorders

Painful menstruation, or dysmenorrhea, is common in adolescents and young women. In many women, this pain is significantly decreased after the birth of a child or as the woman becomes older.

Dysfunctional uterine bleeding (DUB) is believed to be due to a hormonal imbalance of decreased estrogen and can include menorrhagia and metrorrhagia.
- **Menorrhagia** is excessive menstrual bleeding (in amount and duration), possibly with clots that saturates more than one tampon or pad per hour.
- **Metrorrhagia** is bleeding between menstrual periods. It is more common in women who are entering menopause and in adolescent females.

Amenorrhea is the absence of menses. In a woman who has had menstrual cycles, this can be an indication of pregnancy or a medical disorder, such as thyroid disorder or structural disorders of the reproductive system. A common cause is low percentage of body fat in women who are involved in sports or strenuous physical activity. Anorexia nervosa also can result in amenorrhea due to a decrease in body fat.

Premenstrual syndrome (PMS) is thought to be caused by an imbalance between estrogen and progesterone.
- Manifestations can vary among women and can vary for an individual woman from one cycle to the next. Common manifestations include irritability, impaired memory, depression, poor concentration, mood swings, binge eating, breast tenderness, bloating, weight gain, headache, and back pain.
- **Premenstrual dystrophic disorder (PMDD)** is a severe form of PMS seen in only a small number of women, and it interferes with a woman's ability to carry out her daily activities. With either condition, manifestations begin a few days before the menstrual period and end a few days after the onset of the menstrual period.

Endometriosis is characterized by an overgrowth of endometrial tissue that extends outside the uterus into the fallopian tubes, onto the ovaries, and into the pelvis. Blockage of the fallopian tubes by endometrial tissue is a common cause of infertility.

ASSESSMENT

When assessing a client who has a menstrual disorder the nurse should assess the client's:
- Menstrual history (age of first menses, monthly cycle)
- Sexual history
- Nutritional history

EXPECTED FINDINGS

- Report of premenstrual depression, irritability, changes in appetite, abdominal bloating, fatigue, emotional lability, or fluid retention
- Characteristics of flow
- Characteristics and location of pain during menstrual cycle
- Pelvic tenderness during palpation of the lower abdomen and the pelvic examination
- Metabolic disorders (thyroid disorders)

LABORATORY TESTS

Hemoglobin and hematocrit can be below the expected reference range due to excessive blood loss.

CA-125 is an immunodiagnostic test in which findings are elevated in ovarian cancer. Endometriosis and other conditions can also cause CA-125 to be elevated above the expected reference range.

DIAGNOSTIC PROCEDURES

Endometrial biopsy determines the relationship between menstrual flow and the hormone cycle, as well as possible pathologic reasons for bleeding, such as uterine cancer.

Transvaginal ultrasound can identify the presence of uterine fibroids, endometrial abnormalities, or leiomyomas.

PATIENT-CENTERED CARE

MEDICATIONS

Hormonal contraceptives

- Can be used to decrease manifestations of PMS, PMDD, dysmenorrhea, and DUB
- Might be the initial treatment for endometriosis

Diuretic

An aldosterone antagonist (spironolactone) can be used to treat bloating and weight gain associated with PMS and PMDD.

Leuprolide: synthetic luteinizing hormone

- Reduces the follicle-stimulating and luteinizing hormone levels in DUB
- Suppresses estrogen and testosterone production in the body, making it an effective treatment for endometriosis (promotes atrophy of ectopic tissue)
- Can cause birth defects, so the client should use a reliable form of contraception Qs
- Can cause decreased libido and increased risk of osteoporosis

NSAIDs: ibuprofen

- Prescribed for endometriosis to inhibit production of prostaglandins
- Aids in treatment of pain and discomfort related to PMS and PMDD

Oral iron supplements

Used to treat anemia associated with DUB

SSRIs: fluoxetine, sertraline

Used to treat the emotional and physical manifestations of PMS and PMDD

THERAPEUTIC PROCEDURES

DUB

Dilatation and curettage: Used to diagnose and treat DUB. The cervix is dilated, and the wall of the uterus is scraped with a curette. Endometrium scraped from the uterine wall is sent to the laboratory for examination.

Endometrial ablation: Used to remove endometrial tissue in the uterus. The tissue may be removed by laser, heat, electricity, or cryotherapy.

Hysterectomy: If other treatments are unsuccessful

Endometriosis

Laparoscopic removal of ectopic tissue and adhesions: A laser may be used to remove tissue.

Menopause

- Menopause is the cessation of menses. Menses will appear on an infrequent cycle for a period of time that does not exceed 2 years. Menopause is considered complete when no menses have occurred for 12 months.
- The client can have natural or surgically induced menopause.

ASSESSMENT

EXPECTED FINDINGS

Vasomotor manifestations: Hot flashes and irregular menses

Genitourinary: Atrophic vaginitis, shrinking of labia, decreased vaginal secretions, dyspareunia, increased vaginal pH, vaginal dryness, incontinence

Psychological: Mood swings, changes in sleep patterns, decreased REM sleep

Skeletal: Decreased bone density

Cardiovascular: Decreased HDL, increased LDL

Dermatological: Decreased skin elasticity, loss of hair on the head and pubic area

Reproductive: Breast tissue changes

LABORATORY TESTS

Follicle stimulating hormone (FSH): Increased during menopause

Blood, urine, and saliva hormone levels: Estrogens, progesterone, testosterone

DIAGNOSTIC PROCEDURES

Pelvic examination with Papanicolaou (Pap) test to rule out cancer in cases of abnormal bleeding

Breast examination with mammogram to rule out cancer in cases of a palpable change from predominantly glandular tissue to fatty tissue

Biopsy of uterine lining in cases of undiagnosed abnormal uterine bleeding in a woman older than 40 years of age, or in a woman whose menses has stopped for 1 year and bleeding has begun again

Bone mineral density measurement using dual-energy x-ray absorptiometry DXA) to determine the client's risk for osteoporosis

PATIENT-CENTERED CARE

MEDICATIONS

Menopausal hormone therapy (HT)

- Estrogen deficiency manifestations occur naturally as part of the aging process during menopause. Menopausal hormone therapy is prescribed to suppress hot flashes associated with menopause, to prevent atrophy of vaginal tissue, and to reduce the risk of fractures due to osteoporosis. For a woman who has a uterus, HT includes estrogen and progestin. For a woman who no longer has a uterus (following a hysterectomy), estrogen alone is prescribed.
- Many preparations of HT are available (oral, transdermal, intravaginal, intramuscular). The provider may prescribe HT as a continuous, combined estrogen-progesterone therapy or a variety of cyclic patterns.
- Based on their individual risk factors and health care needs, women should discuss the risks and benefits of using HT with their providers.
  - The risk associated with the use of HT depends on many factors (the age of the woman, her personal/family history, the regimen prescribed).
  - HT places women at risk for a number of adverse conditions, including coronary heart disease, myocardial infarction, deep-vein thrombosis, stroke, and breast cancer.
- If HT is required for management of menopausal manifestations, the best recommendation is to use HT on a short-term basis.

CLIENT EDUCATION
- Reinforce to the client the advantages and disadvantages of HT. HT can be beneficial in the prevention of age-related problems such as osteoporosis and fractures.
- Atrophic vaginitis, which is characterized by vaginal burning and bleeding, pruritus, and painful intercourse, can improve with HT. Vaginal instillations of estrogen can be the best option because systemic absorption is reduced.
- Instruct the client in self-administration of HT.
- Advise the client to quit smoking immediately if applicable.
- Teach the client how to prevent and assess the development of venous thrombosis. Qs
  - Avoid wearing knee-high stockings and clothing or socks that are restrictive.
  - Note and report manifestations of unilateral leg pain, edema, warmth, and redness.
  - Avoid sitting for long periods of time.
  - Take short walks throughout the day to promote circulation.
  - Perform frequent ankle pumps, and move and stretch legs.
- Women often experience atypical manifestations of myocardial infarction (MI) rather than the classic chest pain often reported by male clients. Instruct the client about atypical manifestations of an MI (dyspnea, jaw discomfort, indigestion, pain between the shoulders), and instruct the client to seek assistance immediately.

- If oral therapy causes nausea, taking medication with food can help.
- If the client is using vaginal creams or suppositories of estrogen compounds, be sure to refrain from inserting them prior to intercourse, or the client's partner can absorb some of the product.

Alternative therapies

- Ask the client about her use of complementary and alternative therapies such as black cohosh, ginseng, and red clover to relieve the effects of menopause. Research regarding their usefulness is inconsistent.
- Phytoestrogens interact with estrogen receptors in the body, which can result in a decrease in the manifestations of menopause. Vegetables such as dandelion greens, alfalfa sprouts, black beans, and soy beans contain phytoestrogens. QEBP
- Vitamins E and B_6 are reported to decrease hot flashes in some women.

CLIENT EDUCATION
- Older adult clients can decrease the risk of osteoporosis by performing regular weight-bearing exercises; increasing intake of high-protein and high-calcium foods; avoiding alcohol, caffeine, and tobacco; and taking calcium with vitamin D supplements. ⓖ

COMPLICATIONS

Embolic complications

Risk increased by concurrent smoking
- Myocardial infarction, especially during the first year of therapy
- Stroke
- Venous thrombosis: Thrombophlebitis, especially during the first year of therapy

Cancer

- In some studies, long-term use of HT has been found to increase the risk for breast cancer.
- Some studies indicate that long-term use of estrogen-only HT increases the risk for ovarian and endometrial cancer.

Application Exercises

1. A school nurse is providing an education session about menstruation with a group of adolescent female students. Which of the following statements should the nurse include? (Select all that apply.)

   A. "The average age of onset of menstruation is 10."

   B. "The range for a typical menstrual cycle is between 23 and 35 days."

   C. "The first day of the menstrual cycle begins with the last day of the menstrual period."

   D. "Ovulation typically occurs around the 14th day of the menstrual cycle."

   E. "A menstrual period can last as long as 9 days."

2. A nurse is reviewing the medical record of a client who has premenstrual syndrome (PMS). The nurse should identify that which of the following medications are used to treat PMS? (Select all that apply.)

   A. Fluoxetine

   B. Spironolactone

   C. Ethinyl estradiol/drospirenone

   D. Ferrous sulfate

   E. Methylergonovine

3. A nurse in a provider's office is providing information to a client who has dysfunctional uterine bleeding (DUB). Which of the following statements by the client indicate understanding of the information? (Select all that apply.)

   A. "My heavy bleeding can be due to a hormonal imbalance."

   B. "If I experience menstrual pain, I should take aspirin."

   C. "Oral contraceptives are contraindicated for women who heavy uterine bleeding like mine."

   D. "My doctor may perform a D&C to find out what's causing my abnormal bleeding."

   E. "My condition is more common in women who are in their 30s."

4. A nurse is providing support to a client who has a new diagnosis of endometriosis. The nurse should inform the client that which of the following conditions is a possible complication of endometriosis?

   A. Insulin resistance

   B. Infertility

   C. Vaginitis

   D. Pelvic inflammatory disease

5. A nurse is reviewing the medical record of a client who is menopausal. Which of the following findings should the nurse expect? (Select all that apply.)

   A. Increased vaginal secretions

   B. Decreased bone density

   C. Increased HDL level

   D. Decreased skin elasticity

   E. Increased pubic hair growth

   F. Decreased follicle stimulating hormone level

PRACTICE Active Learning Scenario

A nurse is instructing a client who is being evaluated for premenstrual syndrome (PMS) to journal her manifestations to aid in diagnosis. Use the ATI Active Learning Template: System Disorder to complete this item.

EXPECTED FINDINGS: Identify six manifestations of PMS.

Application Exercises Key

1. A. Although some females experience the onset of menstruation as early as age 9, the average age is 12.4 years of age.

   B. **CORRECT:** Although a typical menstrual cycle is 28 days, a range of 23 to 35 days is considered a regular menstrual cycle.

   C. The first day of the menstrual cycle begins with the first day of the menstrual period.

   D. **CORRECT:** The first half of the menstrual cycle is the follicular phase, and the second half is the luteal phase. Ovulation typically occurs around the middle of the cycle, or day 14 in a 28-day cycle.

   E. **CORRECT:** A menstrual period typically lasts from 4 to 6 days but can continue for up to 9 days.

   (N) *NCLEX® Connection: Physiological Adaptation, Pathophysiology*

2. A. **CORRECT:** Fluoxetine, an SSRI, is used to treat the emotional manifestations of PMS, such as irritability and mood swings, and has an added effect of treating physical manifestations.

   B. **CORRECT:** Spironolactone is a diuretic and can reduce bloating and weight gain associated with PMS.

   C. **CORRECT:** Oral contraceptives can be prescribed to reduce the manifestations of PMS.

   D. Oral iron supplements, such as ferrous sulfate, are used to treat anemia associated with dysfunctional uterine bleeding.

   E. Methylergonovine is used to treat postpartum hemorrhage.

   (N) *NCLEX® Connection: Pharmacological and Parenteral Therapies, Medication Administration*

3. A. **CORRECT:** The client should be aware that DUB can be caused by a progesterone deficiency.

   B. The client should avoid aspirin due to the increased risk for bleeding. NSAIDs can be recommended as needed for menstrual pain or discomfort.

   C. The client should be aware that contraceptives can be prescribed to treat DUB.

   D. **CORRECT:** The client should be aware that when the provider performs a dilatation and curettage, endometrium scraped from the uterine wall is sent to the laboratory for evaluation.

   E. The client should be aware that DUB is more common in adolescent girls and in women who are nearing menopause.

   (N) *NCLEX® Connection: Physiological Adaptation, Pathophysiology*

4. A. Insulin resistance is a complication of polycystic ovary syndrome.

   B. **CORRECT:** Infertility is a complication of endometriosis because endometrial tissue overgrowth can block the fallopian tubes.

   C. Vaginitis is typically caused by an infection.

   D. Pelvic inflammatory disease is caused by an infection of the pelvic organs.

   (N) *NCLEX® Connection: Reduction of Risk Potential, Potential for Complications from Surgical Procedures and Health Alterations*

5. A. Clients who are menopausal are expected to have decreased vaginal secretions.

   B. **CORRECT:** Clients who are menopausal are expected to have decreased bone density.

   C. Clients who are menopausal are expected to have a decreased HDL level and increased LDL level.

   D. **CORRECT:** Clients who are menopausal are expected to have decreased skin elasticity.

   E. Clients who are menopausal are expected to have a loss of hair on the head and in the pubic area.

   F. Clients who are menopausal are expected to have an increased follicle stimulating hormone (FSH) level.

   (N) *NCLEX® Connection: Basic Care and Comfort, Nutrition and Oral Hydration*

PRACTICE Answer

Using the ATI Active Learning Template: System Disorder

EXPECTED FINDINGS

- Irritability
- Impaired memory
- Depression
- Poor concentration
- Mood swings
- Binge eating
- Breast tenderness
- Bloating
- Weight gain
- Headache
- Back pain

(N) *NCLEX® Connection: Physiological Adaptation, Pathophysiology*

CHAPTER 64 *Disorders of Female Reproductive Tissue*

Pelvic organ prolapse occurs when the female client's pelvic floor muscles and ligaments become weakened or damaged, resulting in a cystocele or rectocele. A cystocele is a protrusion of the posterior bladder through the anterior vaginal wall. It is caused by weakened pelvic muscles and/or structures. A rectocele is a protrusion of the anterior rectal wall through the posterior vaginal wall. It is caused by a defect of the pelvic structures, a difficult delivery, or a forceps delivery. Uterine prolapse is another form of pelvic organ prolapse.

Medical treatment is possible for clients who have a cystocele or a rectocele causing mild manifestations. If treatment is unsuccessful, the provider may recommend surgical intervention.

Fibrocystic breast condition is a noncancerous breast condition. It is most common in younger women. It occurs less frequently in postmenopausal women. The condition is thought to occur due to cyclic hormonal changes. Fibrosis (of connective tissue) and cysts (fluid-filled sacs) develop.

Cystocele and rectocele

HEALTH PROMOTION AND DISEASE PREVENTION

- Advise clients who are at risk to lose weight if obese.
- Instruct clients to eat high-fiber diets and drink adequate fluids to prevent constipation.

ASSESSMENT

RISK FACTORS

- Cystocele and rectocele can develop in older adult females, usually following menopause.
- Older adult clients are more susceptible to constipation and chronic bearing down during elimination, which can displace weakened structures. Ⓒ

Cystocele

- Obesity
- Advanced age (loss of estrogen)
- Family history
- Multiparity
- Increased abdominal pressure during pregnancy
- Strain and injury during vaginal childbirth

Rectocele

- Pelvic structure defects
- Obesity
- Aging
- Constipation
- Family history
- Difficult vaginal childbirth necessitating repair of a tear

EXPECTED FINDINGS

Cystocele

- Urinary frequency and/or urgency
- Stress incontinence
- History of frequent urinary tract infections
- Sense of vaginal fullness
- Dyspareunia
- Fatigue
- Back and pelvic pain

Rectocele

- Constipation and/or the need to place fingers in the vagina to elevate the rectocele to complete evacuation of feces
- Sensation of a mass in the vagina
- Pelvic/rectal pressure or pain
- Dyspareunia
- Fecal incontinence
- Uncontrollable flatus
- Hemorrhoids

DIAGNOSTIC PROCEDURES

Cystocele

- A pelvic examination reveals a bulging of the anterior vaginal wall when the client is instructed to bear down.
- Bladder ultrasound measures residual urine.
- Urine culture and sensitivity is used to diagnose urinary tract infection associated with urinary stasis.
- A cystography is performed to identify the degree of bladder protrusion.
- An x-ray can help assess the degree of cystocele.

Rectocele

- A pelvic examination reveals a bulging of the posterior wall when the client is instructed to bear down.
- A rectal examination reveals the presence of a rectocele.

PATIENT-CENTERED CARE

THERAPEUTIC PROCEDURES

Intravaginal estrogen: Intravaginal estrogen is used to prevent atrophy of the pelvic muscles in women who are postmenopausal.

Bladder training: Contributes to urinary continence

Vaginal pessary (64.1)

- A removable rubber, plastic, or silicone device inserted into the vagina to provide support and block protrusion of other organs into the vagina. The provider selects the type of pessary and ensures that it fits correctly.
- NURSING ACTIONS
  - Teach the client how to insert, remove, and clean the device.
  - Inform the client that routine checks by the provider are necessary to ensure proper fit, and to monitor for complications.
  - Instruct the client to notify the provider if she experiences pain, discomfort, or vaginal discharge.
  - Ensure that the client does not have a latex allergy if a rubber pessary is prescribed. **Qs**

Kegel exercises

- Exercises the client performs to strengthen the pelvic floor muscles, which results in reduction or prevention of pelvic organ prolapse and stress urinary incontinence
- CLIENT EDUCATION
  - Teach the client how to perform the exercises.
  - Contract the circumvaginal and perirectal muscles.
  - Tightening pelvic muscles.
  - Gradually increase the contraction period to 10 seconds.
  - Follow each contraction period with a relaxation period of 10 seconds.
  - Perform while lying down, sitting, and standing.
  - Perform the exercises 30 to 80 times daily.
  - Keep abdominal muscles relaxed during contractions.

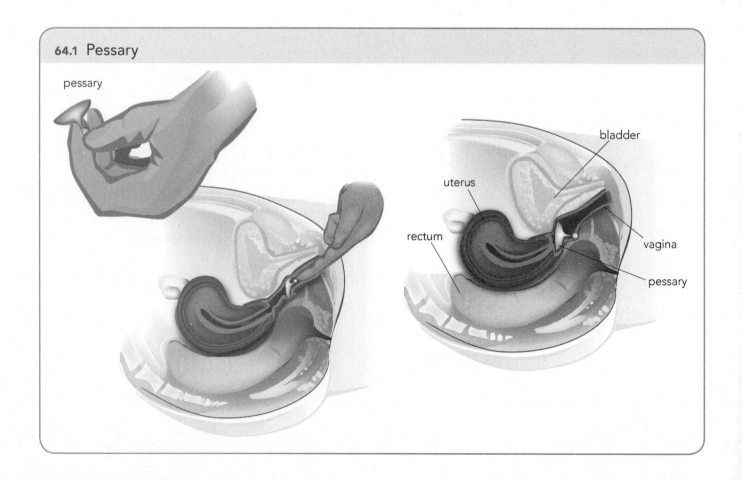

64.1 Pessary

pessary

bladder

uterus

rectum

vagina

pessary

Transvaginal repair: A transvaginal repair is performed to treat prolapse of pelvic organs. Vaginal mesh or tape is used to create a sling that supports the pelvic floor.

Anterior-posterior repair: Surgical repair of both a cystocele and a rectocele.

Hysterectomy: May be performed at the same time as cystocele or rectocele repair.

Cystocele

Anterior colporrhaphy: Using a vaginal or laparoscopic approach, the pelvic muscles are shortened and tightened, resulting in increased bladder support.

Rectocele

Posterior colporrhaphy: Using a vaginal/perineal approach, the pelvic muscles are shortened and tightened, resulting in a reduction of rectal protrusion into the vaginal canal.

POSTOPERATIVE NURSING ACTIONS

- Provide routine postoperative care to prevent complications.
- Administer analgesics, antimicrobials, and stool softeners/laxatives as prescribed.
- Apply a warm compress to the abdomen to decrease discomfort.
- Suggest that the client take frequent sitz baths to soothe the perineal area.
- Provide a low-residue diet until normal bowel function returns.

CLIENT EDUCATION Qs

- Instruct the client to notify the provider about indications of infection (elevated temperature, pulse, or respirations; foul-smelling or purulent vaginal discharge; or consistent pain).
- Caution the client to avoid straining at defecation; sneezing; coughing; lifting; and sitting, walking, or standing for prolonged periods following surgery.
- Instruct the client to tighten and support pelvic muscles when coughing or sneezing.
- Advise the client of postoperative restrictions, including avoidance of strenuous activity, lifting anything weighing greater than 5 lb, and sexual intercourse, for 6 weeks.
- Inform the client that the sutures are absorbable and do not require removal.

COMPLICATIONS

Complications are similar to those associated with a vaginal hysterectomy.

- Vaginal erosion and serious infection has led to the recall of some surgical mesh or tape used to repair pelvic organ prolapse. For more information, see www.fda.gov.
- Provide the client with written information from the manufacturer regarding the specific product used. Qs
- Dyspareunia (painful sexual intercourse) is a possible surgical complication due to surgical alteration of the vaginal orifice.

Fibrocystic breast condition

ASSESSMENT

RISK FACTORS

- Premenopausal status
- Postmenopausal hormone replacement therapy

EXPECTED FINDINGS

- Breast pain
- Tender lumps, commonly in upper, outer quadrant

PHYSICAL ASSESSMENT FINDINGS: Palpable rubberlike lumps, usually in the upper, outer quadrant

DIAGNOSTIC PROCEDURES

Breast ultrasound is used to confirm the diagnosis.

Fine-needle aspiration is used to confirm the diagnosis or to reduce pain due to fluid build-up.

PATIENT-CENTERED CARE

NURSING CARE

- Suggest that the client reduce the intake of salt before menses, wear a supportive bra, and apply either local heat or cold to temporarily reduce pain.
- Discuss the risks (liver disease, stroke) of hormonal medication therapy with clients considering this form of treatment.
- Encourage the client to follow the provider's recommendations and to journal the effectiveness of the treatment plan.
- Inform the client that having fibrocystic breast condition does not increase her risk of breast cancer.

MEDICATIONS

- Over-the-counter analgesics such as acetaminophen or ibuprofen
- Oral contraceptives or hormonal medication therapy if manifestations are severe to suppress estrogen/progesterone secretion
- Diuretics to decrease breast engorgement

Application Exercises

1. A nurse is instructing a client how to perform Kegel exercises. Which of the following instructions should the nurse include? (Select all that apply.)

   A. Perform exercises about 50 times each day.

   B. Contract the circumvaginal and/or perirectal muscles.

   C. Gradually increase the contraction period to 10 seconds.

   D. Follow each contraction with at least a 10-second relaxation period.

   E. Perform while sitting, lying, and standing.

   F. Tighten abdominal muscles during contractions.

2. A nurse is performing a preoperative assessment for a client who is scheduled for an anterior colporrhaphy. Which of the following client statements should the nurse expect?

   A. "I have to push the feces out of a pouch in my vagina with my fingers."

   B. "I have pain and bleeding when I have a bowel movement."

   C. "I have had frequent urinary tract infections."

   D. "I am embarrassed by uncontrollable flatus."

3. A nurse is reviewing the medical record of a client who has a cystocele. Which of the following findings should the nurse identify as a risk factor for the development of this disorder?

   A. BMI of 18

   B. Nulliparity

   C. Chronic constipation

   D. Postmenopausal

4. A nurse is preparing to discharge a client following an anterior and posterior colporrhaphy. Which of the following instructions should the nurse provide?

   A. "Do not bend over for at least 6 weeks."

   B. "You can lift objects as heavy as 10 pounds."

   C. "Do not engage in intercourse for at least 6 weeks."

   D. "You might have foul-smelling drainage for the first week after surgery."

5. A nurse in a provider's office is reviewing the medical record of a client who has fibrocystic breast condition. Which of the following findings should the nurse expect?

   A. Palpable rubberlike lump in the upper outer quadrant

   B. BRCA1 gene mutation

   C. Elevated CA-125

   D. *Peau d'orange* dimpling of the breast

PRACTICE Active Learning Scenario

A nurse is preparing an educational session for a group of women on medications used to treat fibrocystic breast condition. Use the ATI Active Learning Template: Medication to complete this item.

THERAPEUTIC USES: Identify three types of medications used to treat the condition, and provide a brief description of the purpose of the medications in treating fibrocystic breast condition.

Application Exercises Key

1. A. **CORRECT:** The client should perform Kegel exercises 30 to 80 times a day.

   B. **CORRECT:** The client should contract her circumvaginal and perirectal muscles as if trying to stop the flow of urine or passing flatus.

   C. **CORRECT:** The client should hold the contraction for 10 seconds. She might need to gradually increase the contraction period to reach this goal.

   D. **CORRECT:** The client should follow each contraction with a relaxation period of 10 seconds.

   E. **CORRECT:** The client can perform the exercises while lying, sitting, or standing.

   F. The client should relax her other muscles, such as those in her abdomen and her thighs.

   Ⓝ *NCLEX® Connection: Health Promotion and Maintenance, Health Promotion/Disease Prevention*

2. A. Pouching of feces is an expected finding associated with a rectocele. The surgical procedure for a rectocele is posterior colporrhaphy.

   B. Pain and bleeding with a bowel movement is an expected finding associated with a rectocele.

   C. **CORRECT:** Due to urinary stasis associated with a cystocele, this finding is an expected finding of a cystocele. The surgery for a cystocele is an anterior colporrhaphy.

   D. Uncontrollable flatus is an expected finding associated with a rectocele.

   Ⓝ *NCLEX® Connection: Physiological Adaptation, Alterations in Body Systems*

3. A. The nurse should identify obesity as a risk factor for the development of a cystocele. A BMI of 18 indicates the client is underweight.

   B. The nurse should identify multiparity as a risk factor for the development of a cystocele.

   C. The nurse should identify constipation as a risk factor for the development of a rectocele.

   D. **CORRECT:** The nurse should identify that the advancing age and loss of estrogen that correlate with postmenopausal status are risk factors for the development of a cystocele.

   Ⓝ *NCLEX® Connection: Health Promotion and Maintenance, Health Promotion/Disease Prevention*

4. A. The client does not have a restriction regarding bending over.

   B. The client should not lift an object that weighs more than 5 lb.

   C. **CORRECT:** The client should refrain from intercourse to allow time for the surgical site to heal, which is typically about 6 weeks.

   D. Foul-smelling drainage is an indication of infection, which should be reported to the provider.

   Ⓝ *NCLEX® Connection: Reduction of Risk Potential, Therapeutic Procedures*

5. A. **CORRECT:** Clients who have fibrocystic breast condition typically have breast pain and rubbery palpable lumps in the upper outer quadrant of the breasts.

   B. BRCA1 gene mutation is a risk factor for breast cancer.

   C. An elevated CA-125 is a finding associated with ovarian cancer.

   D. *Peau d'orange* dimpling of the breast is a finding associated with breast cancer.

   Ⓝ *NCLEX® Connection: Physiological Adaptation, Pathophysiology*

PRACTICE Answer

Using ATI Active Learning Template: Medication

THERAPEUTIC USES

- Analgesics, such as acetaminophen or ibuprofen, are used to relieve pain.
- Oral contraceptives or hormonal medication therapy suppress estrogen/progesterone secretion.
- Diuretics decrease breast engorgement.

Ⓝ *NCLEX® Connection: Physiological Adaptation, Pathophysiology*

CHAPTER 65

Diagnostic Procedures for Male Reproductive Disorders

Changes to the prostate gland are common as men age, and routine diagnostic procedures are recommended to evaluate these changes. Enlargement of the prostate gland is usually benign and is called benign prostatic hyperplasia (BPH). Prostate cancer is one of the most common forms of cancer in men. Q̲EBP

Diagnostic procedures for male reproductive disorders include prostate-specific antigen (PSA), early prostate cancer antigen (EPCA-2), digital rectal exam (DRE), and transrectal ultrasound (TRUS).

Prostate-specific antigen, early prostate cancer antigen, and digital rectal exam

PSA measures the amount of a protein produced by the prostate gland in the bloodstream. It is performed prior to the DRE because a rise in PSA can occur due to the irritation that occurs upon palpation of the gland. A sample of blood is used to determine the PSA level.

EPCA-2 measures the amount of protein in the blood that is only produced by abnormal prostate cells.

DRE is done in an office or clinic.
- With the client leaning over the examination table, the provider places a gloved, lubricated finger in the client's anus and palpates the posterior portion of the prostate gland through the rectal wall. The client also can be placed on his side or in the lithotomy position for the exam. Q̲PCC
- If the DRE reveals an abnormality, the location of the potentially cancerous prostate lesion is determined by ultrasonography and confirmed by a biopsy.

INDICATIONS

- Many providers recommend an annual PSA and DRE for men older than 50 years to help ensure early detection of prostate cancer. African American men and men who have a family history of prostate cancer should begin screening at an earlier age.
- Because the EPCA-2 is highly sensitive in detecting prostate cancer some providers are using this test in place of a biopsy. The EPCA-2 is also used to monitor the client's response to treatment for prostate cancer.
- For additional information regarding screening for and treatment of prostate cancer, see www.cdc.gov.

CLIENT PRESENTATION: As the prostate gland enlarges, it encroaches on the urethra and causes diminished flow and retention of urine. Blood can also be found in the urine. These findings can indicate BPH or prostate cancer.

INTERPRETATION OF FINDINGS

PSA: An increase can indicate that a client has prostatic cancer.
- PSA levels increase with age. For a man younger than 50 years of age, a PSA level of 2.5 ng/mL is within the expected range.
- The client can have an elevated PSA level for up to 6 weeks following a urinary tract infection.
- A PSA value greater than 4 ng/mL requires further evaluation. An elevated PSA is an indication of a number of conditions, including prostate cancer, BPH, and acute prostatitis.

EPCA-2: A value of 30 ng/mL or greater is highly suggestive of prostate cancer.

DRE: Abnormal findings during the DRE include an abnormally large and hard prostate with an irregular shape or lumps.

Transrectal ultrasound

- With the client in a left, side-lying position, a probe is inserted into the client's rectum, and sound waves are bounced off the surface of the prostate gland to provide an image.
- The provider may prescribe an enema prior to the procedure.
- The procedure is contraindicated for clients who have a latex allergy. The rectal ultrasound probe is covered by a latex sac. Therefore, it is important to check the client for a latex allergy prior to the procedure. Q̲s

INDICATIONS

A TRUS is done if a client's PSA is elevated or the DRE reveals a possible abnormality.

INTERPRETATION OF FINDINGS

If an irregularity is found, the image is used to guide a needle biopsy.

Application Exercises

1. A nurse at a provider's office is caring for an older adult client who is having an annual physical exam. Which of the following findings indicates additional follow-up is needed in regard to the prostate gland? (Select all that apply.)

   A. Prostate-specific antigen (PSA) is 7.1 ng/mL.

   B. A digital rectal exam (DRE) reveals an enlarged and nodular prostate.

   C. The client reports a weak urine stream.

   D. The client reports urinating once during the night.

   E. Smegma is present below the glans of the penis.

2. A nurse is providing information to a client who is scheduled for a transrectal ultrasound (TRUS). Which of the following information should the nurse include?

   A. "This procedure will determine whether you have prostate cancer."

   B. "The procedure is contraindicated if you have an allergy to eggs."

   C. "Sound waves will be used to create a picture of your prostate."

   D. "You should avoid having a bowel movement for 1 hr prior to the procedure."

Application Exercises Key

1. A. **CORRECT:** Although the PSA level is typically elevated in an older adult male, a PSA level greater than 4 ng/mL warrants additional follow-up.

   B. **CORRECT:** An enlarged and nodular prostate is a possible indication of prostate cancer and requires further evaluation.

   C. **CORRECT:** A weak urine stream is a manifestation of benign prostatic hyperplasia and warrants follow-up

   D. Urinating once during the night is an expected finding for an older adult male.

   E. Smegma is a normal secretion that can accumulate beneath the glans penis.

   Ⓝ *NCLEX® Connection: Health Promotion and Maintenance, Health Screening*

2. A. A biopsy or EPCA-2 is used to make the diagnosis of prostate cancer.

   B. A TRUS is contraindicated if the client has an allergy to latex.

   C. **CORRECT:** A transrectal ultrasound creates an image of the prostate using sound waves.

   D. The provider may prescribe an enema prior to the procedure to decrease the interference of feces with obtaining accurate test results.

   Ⓝ *NCLEX® Connection: Reduction of Risk Potential, Diagnostic Tests*

PRACTICE Answer

Using ATI Active Learning Template: Diagnostic Procedure

DESCRIPTION OF PROCEDURE

PSA: A blood sample is taken to measure a specific protein produced by the prostate gland that is present in the bloodstream. The PSA is performed first because examination of the prostate irritates the prostate and can cause the PSA to rise.

DRE: With the client leaning over the exam table, or placed on his side, or in the lithotomy position, the examiner uses a gloved, lubricated finger to palpate the prostate through the rectal wall to identify any abnormalities in size, shape, and consistency.

INDICATIONS

- Age greater than 50 years old
- African American descent
- Family history of prostate cancer

Ⓝ *NCLEX® Connection: Reduction of Risk Potential, Diagnostic Tests*

CHAPTER 66 *Benign Prostatic Hyperplasia*

As an adult male ages, the prostate gland enlarges. When the enlargement of the gland begins to cause urinary dysfunction, it is called benign prostatic hyperplasia (BPH). BPH is a very common condition of the older adult male.

BPH can significantly impair the outflow of urine from the bladder, making a client susceptible to infection and retention. Excessive amounts of urine retained can cause reflux of urine into the kidney, dilating the ureter and causing kidney infections.

ASSESSMENT

RISK FACTORS

- Increased age
- Smoking, chronic alcohol use
- Sedentary lifestyle, obesity
- Western diet (high fat, protein, carbohydrate; low fiber)
- Diabetes mellitus, heart disease

EXPECTED FINDINGS

- The International Prostate Symptom Score (I-PSS) is an assessment tool used to determine the severity of manifestations and their effect on the client's quality of life. The client rates the severity of lower urinary tract manifestations using a 0 to 5 scale and also rates his quality of life as affected by urinary tract manifestations.
- Clients who have BPH typically report urinary frequency, urgency, hesitancy, or incontinence; incomplete emptying of the bladder; dribbling post-voiding; nocturia; diminished force of urinary stream; straining with urination; and hematuria.
- Urinary stasis and persistent urinary retention leads to frequent urinary tract infections.
- If BPH persists, back flow of urine into the ureters and kidney can lead to kidney damage.

LABORATORY TESTS

Urinalysis and culture: WBCs elevated and bacteria present with urinary tract infection

CBC: WBCs elevated if systemic infection present, RBCs possibly decreased due to hematuria

BUN and creatinine: Elevated, indicating kidney damage

Prostate-specific antigen: To rule out prostate cancer

Culture and sensitivity of prostatic fluid: Can be performed if fluid is expressed during digital rectal examination

DIAGNOSTIC PROCEDURES

Digital rectal exam will reveal an enlarged, smooth prostate.

Transrectal ultrasound with needle aspiration biopsy is performed to rule out prostate cancer in the presence of an enlarged prostate.

Early prostate cancer antigen serum blood test may be prescribed instead of a biopsy to rule out prostate cancer.

PATIENT-CENTERED CARE

NURSING CARE

CLIENT EDUCATION
- Frequent ejaculation releases retained prostatic fluids, thereby decreasing the size of the prostate.
- Tell the client to avoid drinking large amounts of fluids at one time, and to urinate when the urge is initially felt.
- Tell the client to avoid bladder stimulants, such as alcohol and caffeine.
- Tell the client to avoid medications that cause decreased bladder tone, such as anticholinergics, decongestants, and antihistamines.
- Medication is used for conservative treatment of BPH.

MEDICATIONS

The goal of medication for BPH is to re-establish uninhibited urine flow out of the bladder.

Dihydrotestosterone (DHT)-lowering medications

5-alpha reductase inhibitor (5-ARI), such as finasteride
- DHT-lowering medications decrease the production of testosterone in the prostate gland.
- Decreasing DHT often causes a decrease in the size of the prostate.

CLIENT EDUCATION
- Reinforce that it can take 6 months to 1 year before effects of the medication are evident.
- Inform the client that impotence and a decrease in libido are possible adverse effects.
- Advise the client to report breast enlargement to the provider.
- Finasteride is teratogenic to a male fetus. The medication is potentially absorbed through the skin. Women who are pregnant or who could become pregnant should avoid contact with tablets that are crushed or broken and with the semen of a client currently taking this medication. Qs

Alpha-blocking agents: tamsulosin

- Alpha-adrenergic receptor antagonists cause relaxation of the bladder outlet and prostate gland.
- These agents decrease pressure on the urethra, thereby re-establishing a stronger urine flow.

CLIENT EDUCATION
- Warn the client that postural hypotension can occur, and to slowly make changes in position.
- Warn the client that concurrent use with cimetidine can potentiate the hypotensive effect.

THERAPEUTIC PROCEDURES

Transurethral needle ablation

Low-level radiation is used to shrink the prostate.

Transurethral microwave therapy

Heat is applied to the prostate to decease its size.

Prostatic stent

Placed to keep the urethra patent, especially if client is a poor candidate for surgery

Interstitial laser coagulation

- Also called contact laser prostatectomy
- Laser energy is used to coagulate excess prostatic tissue.

Electrovaporization of the prostate

High-frequency electrical current is used to cut and vaporize excess tissue.

Surgical resection

An option for clients who do not receive adequate relief from conservative measures

Transurethral incision of the prostate

Involves incisions into the prostate to relieve constriction of the urethra
- Tissue is not removed with this procedure.
- It is minimally invasive and typically performed in an outpatient setting.

Holmium laser enucleation of the prostate

Uses a laser to remove excess prostatic tissue that is obstructing the client's urethra
- The tissue is then moved to the bladder where the client eliminates it in the urine.
- The client often has an indwelling urinary catheter that is left in place overnight.

Transurethral resection of the prostate (TURP)

The most common surgical procedure for BPH
- TURP is performed using a resectoscope (similar to a cystoscope) that is inserted through the urethra and trims away excess prostatic tissue, enlarging the passageway of the urethra through the prostate gland.
- Typically, epidural and spinal anesthesia are used.

PREOPERATIVE NURSING ACTIONS
- Carefully assess cardiovascular, respiratory, and renal systems.
- Ensure that the client fully understands the procedure and what to expect postoperatively.

POSTOPERATIVE NURSING ACTIONS
- Postoperative treatment for a TURP usually includes placement of an indwelling three-way catheter.
  - The urinary catheter drains urine and allows for instillation of a continuous bladder irrigation (CBI) of normal saline (isotonic) or another prescribed irrigating solution to keep the catheter free from obstruction.
  - The rate of the CBI is adjusted to keep the irrigation return pink or lighter. For example, if bright-red or ketchup-appearing (arterial) bleeding with clots is observed, the nurse should increase the CBI rate.
  - If the catheter becomes obstructed (bladder spasms, reduced irrigation outflow), turn off the CBI and irrigate with 50 mL irrigation solution using a large piston syringe or per facility or surgeon protocol. Contact the surgeon if unable to dislodge the clot.
  - Record the amount of irrigating solution instilled (generally very large volumes) and the amount of return. The difference equals urine output.
  - The catheter has a large balloon (30 to 45 mL). The catheter is taped tightly to the leg, creating traction so that the balloon will apply firm pressure to the prostatic fossa to prevent bleeding. This makes the client feel a continuous need to urinate. Instruct the client to not void around the catheter as this causes bladder spasms. Avoid kinks in the tubing.
- Monitor vital signs and urinary output.
- Administer/provide increased fluids.
- Monitor for bleeding (persistent bright-red bleeding unresponsive to increase in CBI and traction on the catheter or reduced Hgb levels) and report to the provider.
- Assist the client to ambulate as soon as possible to reduce the risk of deep-vein thrombosis and other complications that occur due to immobility.
- Administer medications.
  - Analgesics (surgical manipulation or incisional discomfort)
  - Antispasmodics (bladder spasms)
  - Antibiotics (prophylaxis)
  - Stool softeners (avoid straining)
- When the catheter is removed, monitor urinary output. The initial voiding following removal can be uncomfortable, red in color, and contain clots. The color of the urine should progress toward amber in 2 to 3 days. Instruct the client that expected output is 150 to 200 mL every 3 to 4 hr. The client should contact the provider if unable to void.

CLIENT EDUCATION

- Tell the client to avoid heavy lifting, strenuous exercise, straining, and sexual intercourse for the prescribed length of time (usually 2 to 6 weeks).
- Tell the client to drink 12 or more 8-oz glasses of water each day unless contraindicated.
- Tell the client to avoid nonsteroidal anti-inflammatory medications due to increased risk for bleeding.
- Tell the client to avoid bladder stimulants, such as caffeine and alcohol.
- Tell the client that if urine becomes bloody, to stop activity, rest, and increase fluid intake.
- Tell the client to contact the surgeon for persistent bleeding or obstruction (less than expected output or distention).

COMPLICATIONS

Complications of procedures to treat BPH include regrowth of prostate tissue and reoccurrence of bladder neck obstruction.

TURP complications

- Urethral trauma, urinary retention, bleeding, and infection are complications associated with TURP.

NURSING ACTIONS
- Monitor the client and intervene for bleeding.
- Provide antibiotic prophylaxis to the client.

Application Exercises

1. A nurse in a provider's office is obtaining a history from a client who is undergoing an evaluation for benign prostatic hyperplasia (BPH). The nurse should identify that which of the following findings are indicative of this condition? (Select all that apply.)
   - A. Backache
   - B. Frequent urinary tract infections
   - C. Weight loss
   - D. Hematuria
   - E. Urinary incontinence

2. A nurse is caring for a client who has a new diagnosis of benign prostatic hyperplasia (BPH). The nurse should anticipate a prescription for which of the following medications?
   - A. Oxybutynin
   - B. Diphenhydramine
   - C. Ipratropium
   - D. Tamsulosin

3. A nurse is instructing a client who is scheduled for a transurethral resection of the prostate (TURP) about his postoperative care. Which of the following information should the nurse include in the teaching?
   - A. "You may have a continuous sensation of needing to void even though you have a catheter."
   - B. "You will be on bed rest for the first 2 days after the procedure."
   - C. "You will be instructed to limit your fluid intake after the procedure."
   - D. "Your urine should be clear yellow the evening after the surgery."

4. A nurse is providing discharge instructions to a client who is postoperative following a TURP. Which of the following instructions should the nurse include? (Select all that apply.)
   - A. Avoid sexual intercourse for 3 months after the surgery.
   - B. If urine appears bloody, stop activity and rest.
   - C. Avoid drinking caffeinated beverages.
   - D. Take a stool softener once a day.
   - E. Treat pain with ibuprofen.

PRACTICE Active Learning Scenario

A nurse is teaching a client who has a new prescription for finasteride about the medication. Use the ATI Active Learning Template: Medication to complete this item.

THERAPEUTIC USES: Identify the therapeutic use of this medication for this client.

CLIENT EDUCATION: Identify four instructions the nurse should include.

Application Exercises Key

1. A. Backache occurs in the presence of prostate cancer that has spread to other areas of the body.

   B. **CORRECT:** In the presence of BPH, pressure on urinary structures leads to urinary stasis, which in turn promotes the occurrence of urinary tract infections.

   C. Weight loss occurs in the presence of prostate cancer.

   D. **CORRECT:** Hematuria occurs in the presence of BPH.

   E. **CORRECT:** Overflow incontinence occurs in the presence of BPH due to an increased volume of residual urine.

   Ⓝ NCLEX® Connection: Physiological Adaptation, Pathophysiology

2. A. Oxybutynin is an anticholinergic medication that is used to treat overactive bladder. Anticholinergic medications are contraindicated for a client who has BPH. Oxybutynin causes urinary retention.

   B. Diphenhydramine is an antihistamine and is contraindicated for a client who has BPH. Diphenhydramine causes urinary retention.

   C. Ipratropium is an anticholinergic medication used to treat asthma and other respiratory conditions. Ipratropium causes urinary retention.

   D. **CORRECT:** Tamsulosin is an alpha-adrenergic receptor antagonist that relaxes the bladder outlet and the prostate gland, which improves urinary flow.

   Ⓝ NCLEX® Connection: Pharmacological and Parenteral Therapies, Medication Administration

3. A. **CORRECT:** To reduce the risk of postoperative bleeding, the client will have a catheter with a large balloon that places pressure on the internal sphincter of the bladder. Pressure on the sphincter causes a continuous sensation of needing to void.

   B. The client is ambulated early in the postoperative period to reduce the risk of deep-vein thrombosis and other complications that occur due to immobility.

   C. The client is encouraged to increase his fluid intake unless contraindicated by another condition. A liberal fluid intake reduces the risks of urinary tract infection and dysuria.

   D. The client's urine is expected to be pink the first 24 hr after surgery.

   Ⓝ NCLEX® Connection: Reduction of Risk Potential, Therapeutic Procedures

4. A. The client should follow the provider's instructions, which typically includes avoidance of sexual intercourse for 2 to 6 weeks after the surgery.

   B. **CORRECT:** Excessive activity can cause recurrence of bleeding. The client should rest to promote reclotting at the incisional site.

   C. **CORRECT:** The client should avoid caffeine and other bladder stimulants.

   D. **CORRECT:** The client should take a stool softener to keep the stool soft and thus prevent the complication of bleeding at the time of a bowel movement.

   E. The client should avoid taking nonsteroidal anti-inflammatory drugs because they can cause bleeding.

   Ⓝ NCLEX® Connection: Reduction of Risk Potential, Therapeutic Procedures

PRACTICE Answer

Using the ATI Active Learning Template: Medication

THERAPEUTIC USES: Finasteride inhibits 5-alpha reductase and enzyme, which converts testosterone to dihydrotesterone. Production of testosterone in the prostate gland is reduced, which in turn reduces the size of prostate tissue.

CLIENT EDUCATION
- The medication is prescribed on a long-term basis. It may take as long as 1 year before the effects of the medication are evident.
- Impotence and a decreased libido are possible adverse effects.
- Report breast enlargement to the provider.
- Finasteride is teratogenic to the male fetus. The medication can be absorbed through the skin. Women who are pregnant or who could become pregnant should avoid contact with tablets that are crushed or broken and with the semen of a client currently taking this medication.

Ⓝ NCLEX® Connection: Pharmacological and Parenteral Therapies, Medication Administration

NCLEX® Connections

When reviewing the following chapters, keep in mind the relevant topics and tasks of the NCLEX outline, in particular:

Client Needs: Basic Care and Comfort

MOBILITY/IMMOBILITY
Assess the client for mobility, gait, strength and motor skills.

Maintain/correct the adjustment of client's traction device.

Implement measures to promote circulation.

Client Needs: Reduction of Risk Potential

POTENTIAL FOR ALTERATIONS IN BODY SYSTEMS: Identify client with increased risk for insufficient vascular perfusion.

POTENTIAL FOR COMPLICATIONS OF DIAGNOSTIC TESTS/TREATMENTS/PROCEDURES
Position the client to prevent complications following tests/treatments/procedures.

Use precautions to prevent injury and/or complications associated with a procedure or diagnosis.

SYSTEM SPECIFIC ASSESSMENTS: Assess the client for peripheral edema.

Client Needs: Physiological Adaptation

ALTERATIONS IN BODY SYSTEMS: Provide wound care or assist with dressing change.

ILLNESS MANAGEMENT
Promote and provide continuity of care in illness management activities.

Provide postoperative care.

MEDICAL EMERGENCIES: Notify primary health care provider about client unexpected response/emergency situation.

CHAPTER 67 *Musculoskeletal Diagnostic Procedures*

Imaging studies are the primary diagnostic procedures for musculoskeletal disorders. Muscle weakness is an indication for evaluating the conduction of electrical impulses. Arthroscopy assesses the condition of a joint and allows the repair of tears and other joint defects.

Musculoskeletal diagnostic procedures that nurses should be knowledgeable about include arthroscopy, nuclear scans (bone scan, gallium scan, thallium scan), dual-energy x-ray absorptiometry scans (DXA), electromyography (EMG), and nerve conduction studies. Other diagnostic procedures that help detect joint problems and identify musculoskeletal structures are x-ray studies, ultrasound, computed tomography (CT) scans, and magnetic resonance imaging (MRI).

Arthroscopy

- Arthroscopy allows visualization of the internal structures of a joint, most commonly the knee or shoulder joints. It is a sterile procedure.
- Number and placement of incisions depend on the area of the joint undergoing visualization and the extent of the repair.
- Infection in the joint and a lack of joint mobility are contraindications for arthroscopy.

INDICATIONS

POTENTIAL DIAGNOSES: A client who has a joint injury can undergo arthroscopy to ascertain the extent of damage, during which the provider can use the arthroscope to repair a torn ligament or meniscus or perform a synovial biopsy.

CLIENT PRESENTATION
- Joint swelling, pain, and crepitus
- Joint instability

CONSIDERATIONS

PREPROCEDURE

NURSING ACTIONS
- Teach the client postprocedure exercises or refer him to a physical therapist (straight-leg raising, quadriceps setting isometrics).
- Ensure that the client signed the informed consent form.

CLIENT EDUCATION
- Provide postoperative joint exercises.
- Reinforce explanation of the procedure.

POSTPROCEDURE

NURSING ACTIONS
- Postprocedure care is on an outpatient basis.
- Assess neurovascular status and dressings on the client's limb every hour or per the facility's protocol. Qs

CLIENT EDUCATION
- Apply ice for the first 24 hr.
- Elevate the extremity for 12 to 24 hr.
- Instruct the client to take an analgesic for pain.
- Apply a splint or sling.
- Maintain activity restrictions.
- Have the client use crutches if the provider allows limited weight bearing.
- Monitor the color and temperature of the extremity, as well as pain and sensation.
- Notify the provider of any changes, such as swelling, increased joint pain, thrombophlebitis, or infection (redness, swelling, purulent drainage).

COMPLICATIONS

Infection

Complications are uncommon after this procedure, but infection can occur as with any procedure that disrupts the integrity of the skin.

CLIENT EDUCATION: Notify the provider immediately of swelling, redness, or fever.

Nuclear scans

Bone scans

Bone scans evaluate the entire skeletal system.
- A radionuclide test involves a radioactive isotope via injection 2 to 3 hr before scanning.
- Bone scans can detect hairline bone fractures, tumors, fractures, and diseases of the bone (osteomyelitis, osteoporosis, vertebral compression fractures).
- Bone scans are becoming less common due to the increased availability of MRI equipment.

Gallium and thallium scans

Gallium and thallium scans are more sensitive for detecting bone problems than a bone scan.
- The radioisotope migrates to tissues of the brain, liver, and breast, and helps detect disease of these organs.
- The client receives the radionuclide injection 4 to 6 hr before scanning.
- The scan takes 30 to 60 min and can require sedation to help the client lie still during that time. Repeat scanning occurs at 24, 48, and 72 hr.

INDICATIONS

Gallium and thallium scans

POTENTIAL DIAGNOSES
- Arthritis
- Osteomyelitis
- Fractures
- Osteoporosis
- Primary or metastatic bone cancer
- Bone pain of unknown origin

CLIENT PRESENTATION: Bone pain

CONSIDERATIONS

PREPROCEDURE

NURSING ACTIONS
- Inform the client about the procedure.
- Assess for allergy to radioisotope or conditions that would prevent performing the procedure (pregnancy, kidney disease).

CLIENT EDUCATION
- Explain the need to lie still during the entire procedure.
- Instruct the client to empty the bladder before the procedure to promote visualization of pelvic bones. QEBP

POSTPROCEDURE

CLIENT EDUCATION
- Following the procedure, the client does not need to take any radioactive precautions.
- Encourage the client to drink fluids to increase excretion of radioisotope in the urine and feces.

Dual-energy x-ray absorptiometry

- DXA scans estimate the density of bone mass—usually in the hip or spine—and the presence/extent of osteoporosis.
- A DXA scan uses two beams of radiation. A computer analyzes the findings and a radiologist interprets them. Clients do not receive contrast material. Clients receive a score that relates their amount of bone density to that of other people with demographic similarities.
- Clients lie on an x-ray table during scanning of the hip or spine.

Note: These scores are not gender-specific.

INDICATIONS

POTENTIAL DIAGNOSES
- Osteoporosis
- Postmenopausal state (baseline: at age 40)

CLIENT PRESENTATION
- Loss of height
- Bone pain
- Fractures

CONSIDERATIONS

PREPROCEDURE CLIENT EDUCATION
- Inform the client about the procedure.
- Instruct the client to stay dressed but remove metallic objects.

POSTPROCEDURE CLIENT EDUCATION: Follow up with the provider to discuss possible supplements and medications if bone loss is present.

Electromyography and nerve conduction studies

EMG and nerve conduction studies determine the presence and cause of muscle weakness.

EMG

- Clients undergo EMG at the bedside or in an EMG laboratory.
- The technician places thin needles in the muscle under study. Electrodes attach the needles to an oscilloscope, which records activity during a muscle contraction.

Nerve conduction study

- The technician attaches surface or needle electrodes to the skin.
- Low electrical currents go through the electrodes, producing a recording of the muscle response to the stimulus.

INDICATIONS

POTENTIAL DIAGNOSES
- Neuromuscular disorders
- Motor neuron disease
- Peripheral nerve disorders (carpal tunnel)

CONSIDERATIONS

PREPROCEDURE

NURSING ACTIONS
- Inform the client about what to expect.
- Instruct the client to avoid the application of cream or lotion to the area on the day of the procedure.
- Determine whether the client takes an anticoagulant, because anticoagulation is a contraindication for this procedure due to the risk for bleeding within the muscle with needle insertion.
- Check for any skin infections in the area of assessment. Infection is a contraindication for this procedure due to the risk for transmission of the infection to the muscle. Qs
- Ask whether the client takes any muscle relaxants. The provider might discontinue these prior to the procedure to ensure accurate test results.
- Make sure the client signed the consent form.

CLIENT EDUCATION
- Teach the client that discomfort is possible during needle insertion and when the electrical current goes through the electrodes.
- Tell the client she might have to flex her muscle during needle insertion.

POSTPROCEDURE

CLIENT EDUCATION
- Inform the client that some bruising can occur at needle insertion sites.
- Tell the client to report swelling or tenderness at any of the sites to the provider.
- Instruct the client to apply ice to prevent hematoma formation at the needle insertion sites and to reduce swelling or warm compresses to relieve residual discomfort.

Application Exercises

1. A nurse is completing preoperative teaching for a client who is to undergo an arthroscopy to repair a shoulder injury. Which of the following statements should the nurse include? (Select all that apply.)

   A. "Avoid damage or moisture to the cast on your arm."

   B. "Inspect your incision daily for indications of infection."

   C. "Apply ice packs to the area for the first 24 hours."

   D. "Keep your arm in a dependent position."

   E. "Perform isometric exercises."

2. A nurse is planning care for a client who is postoperative following an arthroscopy of the knee. Which of the following actions should the nurse take? (Select all that apply.)

   A. Assess color and temperature of the extremity.

   B. Apply warm compresses to incision sites.

   C. Place pillows under the extremity.

   D. Administer analgesic medication.

   E. Assess pulse and sensation in the foot.

3. A nurse is teaching a client who is going to have a bone scan. Which of the following statements should the nurse include?

   A. "You will receive an injection of a radioactive isotope when the scanning procedure begins."

   B. "You will be inside a tube-like structure during the procedure."

   C. "You will need to take radioactive precautions with your urine for 24 hours after the procedure."

   D. "You will have to urinate just before the procedure."

4. A nurse is educating clients at a health fair about dual-energy x-ray absorptiometry (DXA) scans. Which of the following information should the nurse include in the teaching? (Select all that apply.)

   A. The test requires the use of contrast material.

   B. The hip and spine are the usual areas the device scans.

   C. The scan detects osteoarthritis.

   D. Bone pain can indicate a need for a scan.

   E. At age 40 years, you should have a baseline scan.

5. A nurse is planning care for a client who will undergo an electromyography (EMG). Which of the following actions should the nurse include in the plan of care? (Select all that apply.)

   A. Assess for bruising.

   B. Apply ice to insertion sites.

   C. Determine whether the client takes a muscle relaxant.

   D. Instruct the client to flex her muscles during needle insertion.

   E. Expect swelling, redness, and tenderness at the insertion sites.

Application Exercises Key

1. A. The client should wear a sling to immobilize the arm of the affected shoulder to limit activity and promote healing.

   B. **CORRECT:** The client should inspect the incision for evidence of infection, such as redness, swelling, or purulent drainage.

   C. **CORRECT:** The client should apply ice packs to the affected area for the first 24 hr to reduce swelling and discomfort.

   D. The client should elevate the affected extremity for 12 to 24 hr to reduce swelling.

   E. **CORRECT:** The client should perform the isometric exercises as the provider prescribed and as physical therapist directed.

   Ⓝ *NCLEX® Connection: Reduction of Risk Potential, Therapeutic Procedures*

2. A. **CORRECT:** Assessing color and temperature of the affected extremity helps the nurse identify alterations in circulation.

   B. Cold compresses on the incisional site for the first 24 hr help decrease swelling and pain.

   C. **CORRECT:** Elevating the leg will help decrease swelling and pain in the affected extremity.

   D. **CORRECT:** Administering analgesic medication helps relieve joint pain in the affected extremity.

   E. **CORRECT:** Assessing pulse and sensation of the affected extremity helps the nurse identify alterations in circulation.

   Ⓝ *NCLEX® Connection: Physiological Adaptation, Alterations in Body Systems*

3. A. The nurse should inform the client that the radioactive isotope is injected through an IV 2 to 3 hr before the scanning.

   B. The nurse should inform the client that the procedure does not use a tube-like structure as for an MRI.

   C. The nurse should inform the client that radioactive precautions for his urine are not necessary following the procedure.

   D. **CORRECT:** The nurse should inform the client that he will need to urinate prior to the procedure. An empty bladder promotes visualization of the pelvic bones.

   Ⓝ *NCLEX® Connection: Reduction of Risk Potential, Therapeutic Procedures*

4. A. The nurse should inform the client that a DXA scan does not require contrast material.

   B. **CORRECT:** The nurse should inform the client that the most common areas for a DXA scan are the hip and spine for more clear visualization of a large area of bone.

   C. The nurse should inform the client that a DXA scan detects osteoporosis, not osteoarthritis.

   D. **CORRECT:** The nurse should inform the client that bone pain, loss of height, and fractures are findings that can indicate the need for a DXA scan.

   E. **CORRECT:** The nurse should inform the client that a baseline scan at age 40 is helpful for comparison with a scan during the postmenopausal period.

   Ⓝ *NCLEX® Connection: Reduction of Risk Potential, Therapeutic Procedures*

5. A. **CORRECT:** Some bruising can occur at the needle insertion sites.

   B. **CORRECT:** The nurse should apply ice to the insertion sites to prevent hematoma development.

   C. **CORRECT:** The nurse should assess the client's medications to determine whether she takes a muscle relaxant, which can decrease the accuracy of the test results.

   D. **CORRECT:** The nurse should ask the client to flex her muscles for an easier insertion of the needle into the muscle.

   E. The nurse should instruct the client to report swelling, redness, and tenderness at the insertion sites to the provider because this can indicate an infection.

   Ⓝ *NCLEX® Connection: Reduction of Risk Potential, Diagnostic Tests*

PRACTICE Active Learning Scenario

A nurse is teaching a client who is having a gallium scan. What information should the nurse include in the teaching? Use the ATI Active Learning Template: Diagnostic Procedure to complete this item.

DESCRIPTION OF PROCEDURE

INDICATIONS: List three.

NURSING INTERVENTIONS (PRE, INTRA, POST): List two preprocedure and one postprocedure.

PRACTICE Answer

Using ATI Active Learning Template: Diagnostic Procedure

DESCRIPTION OF PROCEDURE: A gallium scan involves a radioisotope called radionuclide that is injected into the client 4 to 6 hr before the scan to view the client's bones. The radionuclide also migrates to the tissues of the brain, liver, and breast and is used to detect disease of these organs.

INDICATIONS: Detect fractures, osteoporosis, bone lesions, osteomyelitis, and arthritis.

NURSING INTERVENTIONS (PRE, INTRA, POST)
Preprocedure
- Assess for allergy to radioisotopes.
- Assess for existing conditions, such as pregnancy or kidney disease, that are contraindications for the procedure.
- Have the client empty his bladder before the procedure.
Postprocedure: Inform the client to increase fluid intake to promote the excretion of the radioisotope in the urine and feces.

Ⓝ *NCLEX® Connection: Reduction of Risk Potential, Therapeutic Procedures*

UNIT 10   NURSING CARE OF CLIENTS WHO HAVE
MUSCULOSKELETAL DISORDERS
SECTION: DIAGNOSTIC AND THERAPEUTIC PROCEDURES

CHAPTER 68 *Arthroplasty*

Most musculoskeletal surgical procedures are performed to repair damaged joints, particularly the knees and the hips.

Arthroplasty refers to the surgical removal of a diseased joint due to osteoarthritis, osteonecrosis, rheumatoid arthritis, trauma, or congenital anomalies, and replacing it with prosthetics or artificial components made of metal and/or plastic.

Total joint arthroplasty, also called total joint replacement, involves replacement of all components of an articulating joint.

Total knee arthroplasty involves the replacement of the distal femoral component, the tibia plate, and the patellar button. Total knee arthroplasty is a surgical option when conservative measures fail. **(68.1)**

Unicondylar knee replacement is done when a client's joint is diseased in one compartment of the joint.

Total hip arthroplasty involves the replacement of the acetabular cup, femoral head, and femoral stem. **(68.2)**

Hemiarthroplasty refers to half of a joint replacement. Fractures of the femoral neck can be treated only with the replacement of the femoral component.

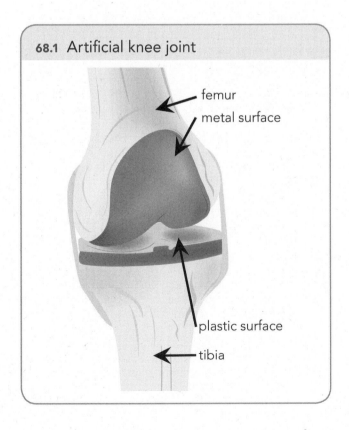

68.1 Artificial knee joint

femur
metal surface
plastic surface
tibia

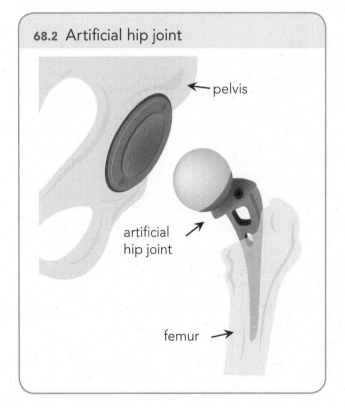

68.2 Artificial hip joint

pelvis
artificial hip joint
femur

INDICATIONS

The goal of both hip and knee arthroplasty is to eliminate pain, restore joint motions, and improve a client's functional status and quality of life.

POTENTIAL DIAGNOSES
- Knee and hip arthroplasty treats degenerative disease (osteoarthritis, rheumatoid arthritis).
- Osteonecrosis is a necrosis of the bone secondary to lack of blood flow with trauma or chronic steroid therapy as the cause.

CLIENT PRESENTATION
- Pain when bearing weight on the joint (walking, running)
- Joint crepitus and stiffness
- Joint swelling (primarily occurs in the knees)

CONSIDERATIONS

CONTRAINDICATIONS

- Recent or active infection (urinary tract infection), which can cause micro-organisms to migrate to the surgical area and cause the prosthesis to fail
- Arterial impairment to the affected extremity
- Client inability to follow the postsurgical regimen
- A comorbid condition (uncontrolled diabetes mellitus or hypertension, advanced osteoporosis, progressive inflammatory condition, unstable cardiac or respiratory conditions)

PREPROCEDURE

NURSING ACTIONS: Review diagnostic test results.
- **CBC, urinalysis, electrolytes, BUN, creatinine:** Assess surgical readiness, and rule out anemia, infection, or organ failure. Epoetin alfa may be prescribed several weeks preoperatively to increase Hgb for a client who has mild anemia.
- **Chest x-ray:** Rule out pulmonary surgical contraindications (infection, tumor).
- **ECG:** Gather baseline rhythm to identify cardiovascular surgical contraindications (dysrhythmia).

CLIENT EDUCATION
- Teach the client that postoperative care includes incentive spirometry, transfusion, surgical drains, dressing, pain control, transfer, exercises, and activity limits.
- Teach the client about autologous blood donation. The client donates blood prior to procedure to be used during or after the procedure.
- Remind the client to scrub the surgical site with a prescribed antiseptic soap the night before and the morning of surgery to decrease bacterial count on skin, which helps lower the chance of infection.
- Instruct the client to wear clean clothes and sleep on clean linens the night before surgery.
- Tell the client to take antihypertensive and other medications the surgeon allows with a sip of water the morning of surgery.

INTRAPROCEDURE

- General or spinal anesthesia can be used.
- Joint components are removed and replaced with artificial components.
- Components can be cemented in place. Components that do not use cement allow the bone to grow into the prosthesis to stabilize it. Weight bearing is delayed several weeks until the femoral shaft has grown into the prosthesis.

POSTPROCEDURE

CLIENT EDUCATION
- The client requires extensive physical therapy to regain mobility. The client can be discharged home or to an acute rehabilitation facility. If discharged home, outpatient or in-home therapy must be provided. Home care should be available for 4 to 6 weeks.
- Monitor for evidence of incisional infection (fever, increased redness, swelling, purulent drainage).
- Care for the incision (clean daily with soap and water).
- Monitor for deep vein thrombosis (swelling, redness, pain in calf), pulmonary embolism (shortness of breath, chest pain), and bleeding if the client is taking an anticoagulant.

Knee arthroplasty

NURSING ACTIONS
- Provide postoperative care, and prevent postoperative complications (venous thromboembolism developing into deep vein thrombosis [DVT], which can lead to a pulmonary embolism, anemia, infection, neurovascular compromise).
- Older adult clients are at a higher risk for medical complications related to chronic conditions, including hypertension, diabetes mellitus, coronary artery disease, and obstructive pulmonary disease. Ⓖ
- A continuous passive motion (CPM) machine may be prescribed to promote motion in the knee, promote circulation, and prevent scar tissue formation. CPM is usually placed and initiated immediately after surgery. CPM provides passive range of motion from full extension to the prescribed amount of flexion. Follow the prescribed duration of use, but turn it off during meals.
- Positions of flexion of the knee are limited to avoid flexion contractures.
  - Avoid knee gatch and pillows placed behind the knee.
  - Place one pillow under the lower calf and foot to cause a slight extension of the knee joint and to prevent flexion contractures. The knee can also rest flat on the bed.
- To prevent pressure ulcers from developing on the heels, place a small blanket or pillow slightly above the ankle area to keep heels off the bed.

- Provide medications as prescribed. Focus needs to be about pain medications. This promotes client participation in early ambulation.
  - **Analgesics:** Opioids (epidural, PCA, IV, oral), NSAIDs
  - **Peripheral nerve blockade:** Inject the femoral or sciatic nerve with a local anesthetic, or the client can receive a continuous infusion of local anesthetic directly into sciatic or femoral nerve.
    - A continuous peripheral nerve block provides localized pain relief.
    - Monitor for systemic effects of local anesthetic, such as metallic taste in the mouth, tinnitus, slurred speech, decreased respiratory rate, hypotension, bradycardia, restlessness, or seizure.
  - **Antibiotics:** Prophylaxis is generally administered 30 min before the surgical incision is made and postoperatively to prevent infection.
  - **Anticoagulant:** Warfarin, fondaparinux, rivaroxaban, or low-molecular-weight heparin, such as enoxaparin. The client can have a prescription for sequential compression devices, foot pumps, and/or antiembolism stockings to prevent venous thromboembolism formation that can develop into DVT.
- Apply ice or cold therapy to the incisional area to reduce postoperative swelling.
- Monitor neurovascular status of the surgical extremity (movement, sensation, color, pulse, capillary refill) every 2 to 4 hr, and compare with the contralateral extremity.
- Assess frequently for overt bleeding and manifestations of hypovolemia, such as hypotension and tachycardia.
- Monitor the compression bandage and wound suction drain for excessive drainage.
- Monitor the autotransfusion drainage system, if used, and re-infuse blood as prescribed.

CLIENT EDUCATION: Dislocation is not common following total knee arthroplasty. However, kneeling and deep-knee bends are limited indefinitely.

Hip arthroplasty

NURSING ACTIONS
- Provide postoperative care, and prevent complications.
- Check the dressing site frequently, noting any evidence of bleeding. Monitor and record drainage from surgical drains.
- Monitor daily laboratory values, including Hgb and Hct levels. Hgb and Hct can continue to drop for 48 hr after surgery. Autologous blood from presurgery donation or blood salvaged intraoperatively or postoperatively using collection devices may be used for postoperative blood replacement. Blood transfusions are relatively common for Hgb levels less than 9 g/dL.
- Monitor the neurovascular status of the surgical extremity (movement, sensation, color, pulse, capillary refill, and compare with contralateral extremity) every 2 to 4 hr.

- Provide medications as prescribed.
  - **Analgesics:** Opioids (epidural, PCA, IV, oral), NSAIDs
  - **Antibiotics:** Generally administered 30 min before the surgical incision is made as a prophylaxis, and postoperatively to prevent infection
  - **Anticoagulant:** Warfarin, dalteparin, fondaparinux, rivaroxaban, or low-molecular-weight heparin, such as enoxaparin
- Provide early ambulation.
  - Transfer the client out of bed from his unaffected side into a chair or wheelchair.
  - Weight-bearing status is determined by the orthopedic surgeon and by choice of cemented (usually partial/full weight-bearing as tolerated) vs. non-cemented prostheses (usually only partial or minimal weight-bearing [toe touch] until after a few weeks of bone growth).
  - Use assistive (walker) and adaptive (raised toilet seat, grab bars, and shower chairs) devices when caring for the client. Qs
  - Apply ice to the surgical site following ambulation as a nonpharmacological measure to decrease pain and discomfort.
- Place the client supine with the head slightly elevated and the affected leg in a neutral position. Place a pillow or abduction device between the legs when turning to the unaffected side. The client should not be turned to the operative side, which could cause hip dislocation.
- Use total hip precautions to prevent dislocation of the new joint.
- Monitor for new joint dislocation: acute onset of pain, reports hearing "a pop," internal rotation of the affected extremity, and shortened affected extremity.

CLIENT EDUCATION
- Arrange for and instruct the client about the use of raised toilet seats, and care items (long-handled shoehorn, dressing sticks).
- Teach the client to follow position restrictions to avoid dislocation.
  - Use elevated seating and a raised toilet seat.
  - Use straight chairs with arms.
  - Use an abduction pillow or regular pillow, if prescribed, between the legs while in bed (and with turning, if restless, or in an altered mental state).
  - Externally rotate the toes.
  - Use extended handles on shoehorns and dressing sticks to prevent flexion greater than 90°.
  - Avoid flexion of hip greater than 90°.
  - Avoid low chairs.
  - Do not cross the legs.
  - Do not internally rotate the toes.
  - Avoid turning to the operative side, unless prescribed.

COMPLICATIONS

HIP ARTHROPLASTY

Venous thromboembolism

Can develop into a DVT resulting in a pulmonary embolism, a life-threatening complication after total hip arthroplasty

NURSING CONSIDERATIONS
- Monitor for manifestations of pulmonary embolism, including acute dyspnea, tachycardia, and pleuritic chest pain.
- Follow venous thromboembolism prophylaxis to include pharmacological management, antiembolic stockings, and sequential compression devices or foot pumps while in bed.
- Encourage plantar flexion, dorsiflexion, and circumduction exercises to prevent clot formation.
- Encourage early ambulation with physical and occupational therapy.

Hip dislocation, infection, anemia, neurovascular compromise

NURSING CONSIDERATIONS
- Older adult clients are at an increased risk for medical complications related to chronic conditions, including hypertension, diabetes mellitus, coronary artery disease, and obstructive pulmonary disease. Ⓖ
- Older adult clients are at the greatest risk for a potentially life-threatening complication (venous thromboembolism formation that develops into DVT, pulmonary emboli) due to age and compromised circulation before surgery.
- Clients who are obese or who have a history of venous thromboembolism formation are also at increased risk for developing DVT or pulmonary emboli.
- Monitor for bleeding.

Application Exercises

1. A nurse is reviewing the health record of a client who is to undergo total joint arthroplasty. The nurse should recognize which of the following findings as a contraindication to this procedure?

   A. Age 78 years

   B. History of cancer

   C. Previous joint replacement

   D. Bronchitis 2 weeks ago

2. A nurse is admitting a client to the orthopedic unit following a total knee arthroplasty. Which of the following actions by the nurse are appropriate? (Select all that apply.)

   A. Check continuous passive motion device settings.

   B. Palpate dorsal pedal pulses.

   C. Place a pillow behind the knee.

   D. Elevate heels off bed.

   E. Apply heat therapy to incision.

3. A nurse is planning discharge teaching for a client who had a total hip arthroplasty. Which of the following should the nurse include in the teaching? (Select all that apply.)

   A. Clean the incision daily with soap and water.

   B. Turn the toes inward when sitting or lying.

   C. Sit in a straight-backed armchair.

   D. Bend at the waist when putting on socks.

   E. Use a raised toilet seat.

4. A nurse is assessing a client who is scheduled to undergo a right knee arthroplasty. The nurse should expect which of the following findings? (Select all that apply.)

   A. Skin reddened over the joint

   B. Pain when bearing weight

   C. Joint crepitus

   D. Swelling of the affected joint

   E. Limited joint motion

5. A nurse is completing a preoperative teaching plan for a client who is scheduled to have a total hip arthroplasty. Which of the following should the nurse include in the teaching plan? (Select all that apply.)

   A. Encourage complete autologous blood donation.

   B. Sit in a low reclining chair.

   C. Instruct the client to roll onto the operative hip.

   D. Use an abductor pillow when turning the client.

   E. Perform isometric exercises.

PRACTICE Active Learning Scenario

A nurse is preparing to administer enoxaparin to a client who had a total knee arthroplasty. What should the nurse consider before administering the medication? Use the ATI Active Learning Template: Medication and the Pharmacology Review Module to complete this item.

EXPECTED PHARMACOLOGICAL ACTION: Define.

NURSING INTERVENTIONS: List two nursing interventions.

CLIENT EDUCATION: List three client teaching points.

Application Exercises Key

1. A. Age greater than 70 is not a contraindication for a total joint arthroplasty unless there are comorbidity factors.

   B. History of cancer is not a contraindication for a total joint arthroplasty unless there are comorbidity factors.

   C. Previous joint arthroplasty surgery is a contraindication for total joint arthroplasty unless there are comorbidity factors.

   D. **CORRECT:** The client who recently had bronchitis or a recent infection can cause micro-organisms to migrate to the surgical area and cause the prosthesis to fail.

   Ⓝ *NCLEX® Connection: Physiological Adaptation, Pathophysiology*

2. A. **CORRECT:** The nurse should check the continuous passive motion device settings to determine if the settings are as prescribed.

   B. **CORRECT:** The nurse should assess the strength of the pulses of both lower extremities to help determine adequate circulation.

   C. The nurse should place one pillow under the lower calf and foot to cause a slight extension of the knee joint and to prevent flexion contractures. The knee can also rest flat on the bed.

   D. **CORRECT:** The nurse should prevent pressure ulcers on the client's heels by elevating the heels off the bed with a pillow.

   E. The nurse should apply cold therapy to reduce postoperative swelling.

   Ⓝ *NCLEX® Connection: Reduction of Risk Potential, Therapeutic Procedures*

3. A. **CORRECT:** The client should wash the surgical incision daily with soap and water to decrease the risk of infection.

   B. The client should externally rotate toes to prevent dislocation of the hip prosthesis.

   C. **CORRECT:** Using a straight-backed armchair decreases the chance of bending at a greater than 90° angle, which can cause dislocation of the hip prosthesis.

   D. Bending at the waist places the hip in a position greater than a 90° angle, which can cause dislocation of the hip prosthesis.

   E. **CORRECT:** Using a toilet riser decreases the chance of bending greater than 90°, which can cause dislocation of the hip prosthesis.

   Ⓝ *NCLEX® Connection: Reduction of Risk Potential, Potential for Complications of Diagnostic Tests/Treatments/Procedures*

4. A. Skin over the knee that is red can indicate infection and is not an expected finding.

   B. **CORRECT:** Pain when bearing weight is an expected finding due to degeneration of the joint.

   C. **CORRECT:** Joint crepitus due to degeneration of the joint tissue is an expected finding.

   D. **CORRECT:** Swelling of the affected joint due to degeneration of the joint tissue is an expected finding.

   E. **CORRECT:** Limited joint motion is due to degeneration of the joint tissue and is an expected finding.

   Ⓝ *NCLEX® Connection: Physiological Adaptation, Alterations in Body Systems*

5. A. **CORRECT:** The nurse should encourage the client to donate blood that can be used postoperatively.

   B. The nurse should have the client sit in a hard back chair to keep the hip at a 90° angle. This prevents dislocation.

   C. The nurse should avoid turning the client to the operative side to prevent dislocation of the prosthesis.

   D. **CORRECT:** The nurse should place an abductor device or pillow between the client's legs when turning to prevent dislocation of the affected hip.

   E. **CORRECT:** The nurse should instruct the client to perform isometric exercises to prevent blood clots and maintain muscle tone.

   Ⓝ *NCLEX® Connection: Reduction of Risk Potential, Therapeutic Procedures*

PRACTICE Answer

Using ATI Active Learning Template: Medication

EXPECTED PHARMACOLOGICAL ACTION: Enoxaparin is an anticoagulant. Use low molecular-weight heparin after abdominal and orthopedic surgery to prevent deep vein thrombosis that may lead to pulmonary embolism.

NURSING INTERVENTIONS
- Do not expel the air bubble from the syringe before injection. It's nitrous oxide and allows the client to receive all the medication during the injection.
- Rotate injection sites.
- Monitor for manifestations of unexplained bleeding.

CLIENT EDUCATION
- Encourage the use of a soft toothbrush and shaving with an electric razor to prevent bleeding.
- Avoid over-the-counter medication unless prescribed by a provider.
- Don't take enoxaparin with garlic, ginger, ginkgo, or feverfew. These supplements may increase the risk of bleeding.

Ⓝ *NCLEX® Connection: Pharmacological and Parenteral Therapies, Expected Actions/Outcomes*

UNIT 10   NURSING CARE OF CLIENTS WHO HAVE
MUSCULOSKELETAL DISORDERS
SECTION: DIAGNOSTIC AND THERAPEUTIC PROCEDURES

CHAPTER 69 *Amputations*

Amputation is the removal of a body part, most commonly an extremity. Amputations can be elective due to complications of peripheral vascular disease and arteriosclerosis, congenital deformities, chronic osteomyelitis, or malignant tumor; or traumatic due to an accident.

Amputations are described in regard to the extremity and whether they are located above or below the designated joint. The term disarticulation describes an amputation performed through a joint.

The higher the level of amputation, the greater the amount of effort that will be required to use a prosthesis. The level of the amputation is determined by the presence of adequate blood flow needed for healing.

Older adult clients are poor candidates for prosthetic training due to the amount of energy required for ambulation. Ⓖ

Significant changes to body image occur after an amputation and should be addressed during the perioperative and rehabilitative phases.

UPPER EXTREMITY AMPUTATIONS

- Upper extremity amputations include above- and below-the-elbow amputations, wrist and shoulder disarticulations, and finger amputations.
- Traumatic amputation caused by accidents, war, or injury is the primary cause of upper extremity amputations.

LOWER EXTREMITY AMPUTATIONS

- Lower extremity amputations include above- and below-the-knee amputations, hip and knee disarticulations, Syme's amputation (removal of foot with ankle saved), and mid-foot and toe amputations.
- Lower extremity amputations are usually done due to peripheral vascular disease as a result of arteriosclerosis.
- Every effort is made to save as much of the extremity as possible. Even loss of the big toe can significantly affect balance, gait, and push-off ability during ambulation. Salvage of the knee with a below-the-knee amputation also improves function vs. an above-the-knee amputation.

HEALTH PROMOTION AND DISEASE PREVENTION

- Clients who have diabetes mellitus should monitor blood glucose and maintain it within the expected reference range.
- Use safety measures when working with heavy machinery or in areas where there is a risk of electrocution or burns.
- Encourage clients to quit or not start smoking, maintain a healthy weight, and exercise regularly.
- Tell clients to maintain good foot care and to seek early medical attention for non-healing wounds.

ASSESSMENT

RISK FACTORS

- Traumatic injury: motor vehicle crashes, industrial equipment, and war-related injuries
- Thermal injury: frostbite, electrocution, burns
- Peripheral vascular disease
- Malignancy
- Older adult clients have a higher risk of peripheral vascular disease and diabetes mellitus resulting in decreased tissue perfusion and peripheral neuropathy. Both conditions place older adult clients at risk for lower extremity amputation. Ⓖ

CHRONIC DISEASE PROCESSES
- Peripheral vascular disease resulting in ischemia/gangrene
- Diabetes mellitus resulting in peripheral neuropathy and peripheral vascular disease
- Infection (osteomyelitis)

EXPECTED FINDINGS

Decreased tissue perfusion
- Clients might report pain.
- History of injury or disease process precipitating amputation
- Altered peripheral pulses (can need to use Doppler)
- Differences in temperature of extremities (level of leg at which temperature becomes cool)
- Altered color of extremities (black indicates gangrene; cyanosis indicates vascular compromise)
- Presence of infection and open wounds
- Lack of sensation in the affected extremity

NURSING ACTIONS
- Monitor capillary refill by comparing the extremities. In older adult clients, capillary refill can be difficult to monitor due to thickened and opaque nails.
- Observe for edema, necrosis, and lack of hair distribution of the extremity due to inadequate peripheral circulation.

DIAGNOSTIC PROCEDURES

To determine blood flow at various levels of an extremity

Angiography: Allows visualization of peripheral vasculature and areas of impaired circulation

Doppler laser and ultrasonography studies: Measures speed of blood flow in an extremity

Transcutaneous oxygen pressure (TcPO₂): Measures oxygen pressures in an extremity to indicate blood flow in the extremity, which is a reliable indicator for healing

Ankle–brachial index: Measures difference between ankle and brachial systolic pressures

PATIENT-CENTERED CARE

NURSING CARE

- Prevent postoperative complications (hypovolemia, pain, infection).
- Assess surgical site for bleeding. Monitor vital signs frequently.
- Monitor tissue perfusion of end of residual limb.
  ○ Palpate residual limb for warmth. Heat can indicate infection.
  ○ Compare pulse most proximal to incision with pulse in other extremity.
- Monitor for manifestations of infection and non-healing of incision. Infection can lead to osteomyelitis.
  ○ Amputation might not heal if performed below the level of adequate tissue perfusion.
  ○ Position the affected extremity in dependent position to promote blood flow/oxygenation.
  ○ Administer antibiotics and change dressings as prescribed if open amputation was performed.
  ○ Record characteristics of drainage, such as amount, color, and odor.

Management of traumatic amputation

- Implement a medical emergency system (EMS).
- Apply direct pressure using gauze, if available, or clean cloth to prevent life-threatening hemorrhage.
- Elevate the extremity above the heart to decrease blood loss.
- Wrap the severed extremity in dry sterile gauze (if available) or in a clean cloth, and place in a sealed plastic bag. Submerge the bag in ice water (one part ice and three parts water), and send with the client.

Pain

- Monitor and treat pain.
- Differentiate between phantom limb and incisional pain.

Incisional pain is treated with analgesics.

Phantom limb pain
- The sensation of pain in the location of the extremity following the amputation
- Related to severed nerve pathways and is a frequent complication in clients who experienced chronic limb pain before the amputation

- Can be experienced immediately after surgery, up to several weeks, or indefinitely
- Occurs less frequently following traumatic amputation
- Often described as deep and burning, cramping, shooting, or aching
- Treated much differently from incisional pain
  ○ Administration of calcitonin during the first week of after having an amputation can decrease phantom limb pain.
  ○ Administering beta blockers, such as propranolol, can relieve the continual dull, burning sensation associated with the amputated limb.
  ○ Administering antiepileptics, such as gabapentin or pregabalin, can relieve sharp, stabbing, and burning phantom limb pain.
  ○ Some clients can have relief from antispasmodics, such as baclofen, and antidepressant medication.
  ○ The nurse should recognize the pain is real and manage it accordingly.
  ○ Alternative treatment for phantom limb pain can include nonpharmacological methods, such as massage, heat, transcutaneous electrical nerve stimulation (TENS), ultrasound therapy, biofeedback, or relaxation therapy.
  ○ Teach the client how to push the residual limb down toward the bed while supported on a soft pillow. This helps reduce phantom limb pain and prepare the limb for a prosthesis.

Client perception and feelings regarding amputation

- Allow for the client and family to grieve for the loss of the body part and change in body image.
- Feelings can include depression, anger, withdrawal, and grief.
- The nurse should assess the psychosocial well-being of the client. Assess for feelings of altered self-concept and self-esteem, and willingness and motivation for rehabilitation.
- The nurse should facilitate a supportive environment for the client and family so grief can be processed. Refer the client to religious/spiritual adviser, social worker, or counselor.
- Rehabilitation should include adaptation to a new body image and integration of prosthetic and adaptive devices into self-image.

Residual limb preparation and prosthesis fitting

Residual limb must be shaped and shrunk in preparation for prosthetic training.

SHRINKAGE INTERVENTIONS
- Wrap the stump, using elastic bandages (figure-eight wrap) to prevent restriction of blood flow and decrease edema.
- Use a stump shrinker sock (easier for the client to apply).
- Use an air splint (plastic inflatable device) inflated to protect and shape the residual limb and for easy access to inspect the wound.

CLIENT EDUCATION

- Explain to the client how to care for and wrap the residual limb, and how to perform limb-strengthening exercises.
- Reinforce the proper application and care of the prosthesis.
- Explain how to safely transfer and use mobility devices and adaptive aids. Qs
- Explain how to manage phantom limb pain.

THERAPEUTIC PROCEDURES

Closed amputation: This is the most common technique used. A skin flap is sutured over the end of the residual limb, closing the site.

Open amputation: This technique is used when an active infection is present. A skin flap is not sutured over the end of the residual limb, allowing for drainage of infection. The skin flap is closed at a later date.

INTERPROFESSIONAL CARE

Intensive efforts by the interprofessional team are necessary to facilitate successful rehabilitation.
- A certified prosthetic orthotist will fit client with prosthesis after the wound is healed and the stump has shrunk.
- A physical therapist will train the client in the application and care of the prosthesis and mobility aids.

- A psychologist can be needed to help with adjustment to loss of the extremity.
- A social worker will assist the client who has financial issues and can refer the client to resources and a support group or organization for people who have had amputations.

COMPLICATIONS

Flexion contractures

Flexion contractures are more likely with the hip or knee joint following amputation due to improper positioning.

NURSING ACTIONS
- Prevention includes range-of-motion (ROM) exercises and proper positioning immediately after surgery.
- To prevent hip or knee flexion contracture, some providers do not advocate elevating the stump on a pillow. However, other providers allow elevation for the first 24 to 48 to reduce swelling and discomfort.
- Have the client lie prone for 20 to 30 min several times a day to help prevent hip flexion contractures.
- Discourage prolonged sitting.

CLIENT EDUCATION
- Have a physical therapist teach the client some exercises that will prevent contractures.
- Teach the client to stand using good posture with residual limb in extension. This also will aid in balance.

Application Exercises

1. A nurse is presenting information to a group of clients at a health fair about measures to reduce the risk of amputation. Which of the follow information should the nurse provide? (Select all that apply.)

   A. Encourage clients who smoke to consider smoking cessation programs.

   B. Encourage clients who have diabetes mellitus to maintain blood glucose within the expected reference range.

   C. Instruct clients to unplug electrical equipment when performing repairs.

   D. Encourage clients who have vascular disease to maintain good foot care.

   E. Advise clients to wait 2 hr after taking pain medication before driving.

2. A nurse is assessing an older adult client who has arteriosclerosis and is scheduled for a possible right lower extremity amputation. Which of the following are expected findings in the affected extremity? (Select all that apply.)

   A. Skin cool to touch from mid-calf to the toes

   B. Lower leg appearing dusky when client is sitting

   C. Palpable pounding pedal pulse

   D. Lack of hair on lower leg

   E. Blackened areas on several toes

3. A nurse is caring for a client following a below-the-elbow amputation. Which of the following actions should the nurse take? (Select all that apply.)

   A. Encourage dependent positioning of the residual limb.

   B. Inspect for presence and amount of drainage.

   C. Implement shrinkage intervention of the residual limb.

   D. Wrap the residual limb in a circular manner using gauze.

   E. Assess for feelings of body image changes.

4. A nurse is caring for a client who had an above-the-knee amputation. The client reports a sharp, stabbing type of phantom pain. Which of the following actions should the nurse take?

   A. Facilitate counseling services.

   B. Encourage use of cold therapy.

   C. Question whether the pain is real.

   D. Administer an antiepileptic medication.

5. A nurse is preparing a plan of care to prevent a client from developing flexion contractions following a below-the-knee amputation 24 hr ago. Which of the following actions should the nurse include in the plan of care?

   A. Limit any type of exercise to the residual limb for the first 48 hr after surgery.

   B. Position the client prone several times each day.

   C. Wrap the stump in a figure-eight pattern.

   D. Encourage sitting in a chair during the day.

Application Exercises Key

1. A. **CORRECT:** The nurse should provide information about smoking cessation, which can decrease the development of arteriosclerosis and possible amputation of a lower extremity.

   B. **CORRECT:** The nurse should provide information about regulating blood glucose levels within a normal reference range to prevent the development of arteriosclerosis and possible amputation of a lower extremity.

   C. **CORRECT:** The nurse should provide information about unplugging electrical equipment when performing repairs to prevent electrocution and injury to an extremity, which can lead to amputation.

   D. **CORRECT:** The nurse should provide information about maintaining good foot care to prevent infection, which can result in amputation.

   E. Driving under the influence of pain medication can lead the client to an accident or injury to an extremity requiring amputation.

   Ⓝ *NCLEX® Connection: Health Promotion and Maintenance, Health Promotion/Disease Prevention*

2. A. **CORRECT:** The client can have coolness of the affected extremity where decreased vascularization starts.

   B. **CORRECT:** The affected extremity can become dusky when sitting due to decreased vascularization of the extremity.

   C. The client will have a lack of or diminished pedal pulse of the affected extremity due to decreased vascularization.

   D. **CORRECT:** The client can have decreased hair growth on areas of the affected extremity due to decreased vascularization.

   E. **CORRECT:** The client can have blackened areas on several toes suggestive of gangrene due to decreased vascularization to the affected extremity.

   Ⓝ *NCLEX® Connection: Physiological Adaptation, Pathophysiology*

3. A. **CORRECT:** The nurse should place the residual limb in a dependent position to improve circulation to the end of the stump and promote healing.

   B. **CORRECT:** The nurse should inspect the residual limb for the presence and amount of drainage to determine early manifestations of infection.

   C. **CORRECT:** The nurse should prepare the residual limb to include shrinkage interventions before fitting of the prosthesis.

   D. The nurse should wrap the residual limb with an elastic bandage in a figure-eight manner to prevent restriction of blood flow before fitting for the prosthesis.

   E. **CORRECT:** The nurse should assess for feelings of depression, anger, withdrawal, and grief due to body image changes.

   Ⓝ *NCLEX® Connection: Physiological Adaptation, Alterations in Body Systems*

4. A. Counseling services can assist the client to cope with body image changes and is not prescribed for treatment of phantom pain.

   B. Heat therapy, not cold therapy, to the residual limb is an alternative therapy that the nurse can implement to relieve phantom pain.

   C. Phantom pain is related to the severed nerve pathways following the amputation. The nurse should not question whether the pain is real.

   D. **CORRECT:** An antiepileptic medication can relieve a sharp, stabbing type of phantom pain.

   Ⓝ *NCLEX® Connection: Pharmacological and Parenteral Therapies, Pharmacological Pain Management*

5. A. To avoid flexion contractures, the nurse should encourage the client to perform range-of-motion exercise to the residual limb to prevent flexion contractures.

   B. **CORRECT:** The nurse should have the client lie prone several times each day for 20 to 30 min to prevent flexion contractures.

   C. The client can have the residual limb wrapped in a figure eight to prepare for the prosthesis, but this action does not prevent flexion contractures.

   D. The client can develop flexion contractures by allowing the residual stump to hang in a bent position when sitting for an extended period following the amputation.

   Ⓝ *NCLEX® Connection: Reduction of Risk Potential, Potential for Complications of Diagnostic Tests/Treatments/Procedures*

PRACTICE Active Learning Scenario

A nurse is completing discharge planning for a client who had an amputation. What members of an interprofessional team should the nurse include in the discharge planning process? Use the ATI Active Learning Template: Basic Concept to complete this item.

RELATED CONTENT: List three members of the interprofessional team and describe the principal purpose of each member.

PRACTICE Answer

Using the ATI Active Learning Template: Basic Concept

RELATED CONTENT
- Certified prosthetic orthotist fits the client with the prosthesis following healing and shrinking of the stump.
- Physical therapist provides training for applying the prosthesis, assists in mobility training, and reviews mobility aids.
- Psychologist assists the client and family in adjusting to the loss of an extremity.
- Social worker provides referral information for financial assistance, resources and support groups, or organizations to help adjust to life-changing physical conditions.

Ⓝ *NCLEX® Connection: Health Promotion and Maintenance, Aging Process*

UNIT 10   **NURSING CARE OF CLIENTS WHO HAVE MUSCULOSKELETAL DISORDERS**
SECTION: MUSCULOSKELETAL DISORDERS

CHAPTER 70   *Osteoporosis*

Osteoporosis is a common chronic metabolic bone disorder resulting in low bone density. Osteoporosis occurs when the rate of bone resorption (osteoclast cells) exceeds the rate of bone formation (osteoblast cells) resulting in fragile bone tissue and can lead to fractures. Common sites of osteoporotic fractures include the wrists, hips, and the spine, although any bone can sustain a fracture.

Osteopenia, the precursor to osteoporosis, refers to low bone mineral density relative to the client's age and gender. Bone mineral density peaks between the ages of 18 to 30. After peak years, bone density decreases, with a significant increase in the rate of loss in postmenopausal women due to estrogen loss.

HEALTH PROMOTION AND DISEASE PREVENTION

- Ensure the client's diet includes adequate amounts of calcium and vitamin D, especially before age 35.
  - Foods rich in vitamin D are most fish, egg yolks, fortified milk, and cereal.
  - Foods rich in calcium are milk products, green vegetables, fortified orange juice and cereals, red and white beans, and figs.
- Encourage the client to take a calcium supplement with vitamin D if dietary intake is inadequate (lactose intolerance).
- Encourage the client to limit the amount of carbonated beverages, which contain phosphates and can cause calcium loss.
- Encourage the client to expose areas of skin to sun 5 to 30 min twice a week. Exposure to the sun for any length of time should include wearing sunscreen to avoid getting a sunburn.
- Encourage female clients to discuss the pros and cons of hormone replacement therapy postmenopausally with her provider.
- Encourage the client to engage in weight-bearing exercises (e.g., walking, lifting weights).

ASSESSMENT

RISK FACTORS

- Female gender, family history, and thin, lean body build are precursors to low bone density.
- Increased bone loss can occur with the following.
  - Age older than 60
  - Female who has postmenopausal estrogen deficiency or low levels of calcitonin
  - Male who has low testosterone
- History of low calcium intake with suboptimal levels of vitamin D decreases bone formation.
- A diet deficient or excessive in protein can contribute to the development of osteoporosis. Clients who limit protein have a reduced ability to use calcium because up to 50% of calcium is bound to protein. Clients who follow a high-protein, low-carbohydrate diet can eliminate important nutrients, such as calcium-rich foods.
- History of smoking and high alcohol intake (three or more drinks per day) causes decreased bone formation and increased bone absorption.
- Excess caffeine consumption causes excretion of calcium in the urine.
- Inadequate intake of calcium and vitamin D stimulates the parathyroid hormone to be released and triggers calcium to be pulled from the bone.
- History of gastric bypass surgery (bypassing of the duodenum where the majority of calcium is absorbed) limits the amount of calcium available.
- Lack of physical activity or prolonged immobility places the client at risk for osteoporosis because bones need the stress of weight-bearing activity for bone rebuilding and maintenance.
- Secondary osteoporosis results from medical conditions.
  - Co-morbidities including hyperparathyroidism, hyperthyroidism, diabetes mellitus, Cushing's syndrome, rheumatoid arthritis, malabsorption syndrome, kidney impairment, anorexia nervosa, and chronic airway disorders (COPD, asthma) that affect calcium absorption and bone development.
  - Medication use over a prolonged period—including loop diuretics, corticosteroids, thyroid medications, and anticonvulsants—affects calcium absorption and bone metabolism.
  - Long-term lack of weight-bearing (spinal cord injury, sedentary life-style)
- Older adult clients have an increased risk of falls related to impaired balance, generalized weakness, gait changes, and impaired vision and hearing. Medication side effects can cause orthostatic hypotension, urinary frequency, or confusion, which can also raise the risk for falls. The body also does not absorb and use calcium as efficiently, but it does excrete calcium more readily than occurs in the younger adult. Ⓖ

EXPECTED FINDINGS

- Reduced height (postmenopausal)
- Acute back pain after lifting or bending (worse with activity, relieved by rest)
- Restriction in movement and spinal deformity
- History of fractures (wrist, femur, thoracic spine)
- Thoracic (kyphosis) of the dorsal spine **(70.1)**
- Pain upon palpation over affected area

LABORATORY TESTS

- Serum calcium, vitamin D, phosphorus, and alkaline phosphatase levels are drawn to rule out other metabolic bone diseases (Paget's disease or osteomalacia).
- 24-hr urine can evaluate the rate of calcium excretion.

DIAGNOSTIC PROCEDURES

Radiographs

Radiographs of the spine and long bones reveal low bone density and fractures.

Dual-energy x-ray absorptiometry (DXA)

- A DXA scan is used to screen for early changes in bone density and is usually done on the hip or spine.
- A peripheral DXA scan is used to assess the bone density of the heel, forearm, or finger.
- DXA uses two beams of radiation. Findings are analyzed by a computer and interpreted by a radiologist. Clients receive a score that relates their amount of bone density that of young, healthy adults (T score). Another reading, a Z score, compares the client's readings with those of a group of age-matched clients who serve as a control.
- The client will lie on an x-ray table while a scan of a selected area is done. Although clothing is not removed for the test, metallic objects that might interfere with the scanning procedure should be removed.

Peripheral quantitative ultrasound (pQUS)

- An ultrasound, usually of the heel, tibia, and patella, is performed.
- pQUS is an inexpensive, portable, and low-risk method to determine osteoporosis and assessing for risk of fracture, especially in men over age 70 years.

Quantitative computed tomography

Quantitative computer tomography is used to measure bone density, especially in the vertebral column.

PATIENT-CENTERED CARE

NURSING CARE

- Administer medications as prescribed.
- Instruct the client and family regarding dietary calcium food sources.
- Instruct the client to limit excess caffeine, alcohol, and carbonated beverages, which increase bone loss.
- Provide information regarding calcium and vitamin D supplementation. (Take with food.)
- Instruct the client on the need for adequate amounts of protein, magnesium, vitamin K, and other trace minerals needed for bone formation.
- Reinforce the need for exposure to vitamin D (moderate sun exposure using sunscreen, fortified milk).
- Encourage weight-bearing exercises (at least 30 min, three to five times a week) to improve strength and reduce bone loss.
- Assess the home environment for safety (remove throw rugs, provide adequate lighting, clear walkways) to prevent falls, which can result in fractures. **Qs**
  - Reinforce the use of safety equipment and assistive devices.
  - Instruct the client to avoid inclement weather (ice, slippery surfaces).
  - Clearly mark thresholds, doorways, and steps.

MEDICATIONS

Medications such as calcium and vitamin D can slow or prevent osteoporosis. A combination of several of these medications may be used in place of just one.

Thyroid hormone

Calcitonin human, calcitonin salmon

THERAPEUTIC USES: Decreases bone resorption by inhibiting osteoclast activity for treatment of osteoporosis, hypercalcemia, and Paget's disease of the bone

NURSING CONSIDERATIONS
- Calcitonin human can only be administered subcutaneously.
- Calcitonin salmon can be administered subcutaneously, intramuscularly, and intranasally.

Teriparatide

THERAPEUTIC USES
- A parathyroid hormone that stimulates osteoblasts to increase new bone formation to increase bone mass
- Stimulates calcium absorption
- Limited use in clients who are at high risk for fractures and those who have prolonged corticosteroid use

NURSING CONSIDERATIONS
- Administered only subcutaneously
- Contraindicated for hypercalcemia, history of bone cancer, radiation, or Paget's disease
- Report leg cramps or bone pain to the provider.
- Orthostatic hypotension can occur up to 4 hr after receiving the medication.

Estrogen hormone supplements

Estrogen, estrogen, medroxyprogesterone

THERAPEUTIC USES: Replaces estrogen lost due to menopause or surgical removal of ovaries

NURSING CONSIDERATIONS
- Instruct client on potential complications, including breast and endometrial cancers and deep-vein thrombosis (DVT).
- Reinforce monthly breast self-examinations. Estrogen should be given along with progesterone in women who still have their uterus.

Selective estrogen receptor modulators

Raloxifene

THERAPEUTIC USES
- Decreases osteoclast activity, subsequently decreasing bone resorption and increasing bone mineral density
- Prevents and treats postmenopausal osteoporosis and breast cancer

NURSING CONSIDERATIONS
- Avoid for clients who have a history of DVT.
- Monitor liver function tests.
- Instruct client on need for calcium and vitamin D supplements.
- Monitor and instruct clients to report unusual calf pain or tenderness, acute migraine, insomnia, urinary tract infection, or vaginal burning/itching to the provider.
- Discontinue use 72 hr before prolonged bed rest.

Calcium supplement

Calcium carbonate, calcium citrate

THERAPEUTIC USES: Supplements calcium consumed in food products to promote healthy bones (not to slow osteoporosis)

NURSING CONSIDERATIONS
- Give with food in divided doses with 6 to 8 oz of water.
- Calcium supplements can cause GI upset.
- Monitor for constipation and development of hypercalcemia.

Vitamin D supplement

THERAPEUTIC USES
- Increases absorption of calcium from the intestinal tract and availability of calcium in the serum needed for remineralization of bone
- Needed by individuals who are not exposed to adequate amounts of sunlight or who do not meet its daily requirements

NURSING CONSIDERATIONS: Vitamin D is a fat-soluble vitamin, so toxicity can occur. Symptoms of toxicity include weakness, fatigue, nausea, constipation, and kidney stones.

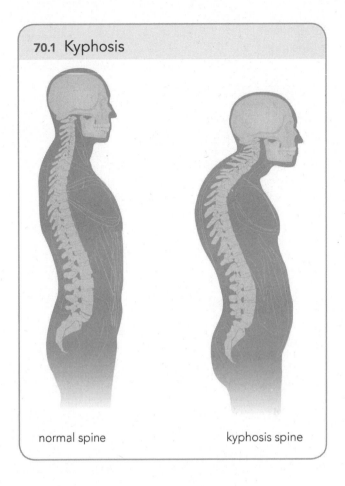

70.1 Kyphosis

normal spine   kyphosis spine

Bisphosphonates

Alendronate, ibandronate, risedronate, zoledronic acid, pamidronate

THERAPEUTIC USES
- Decreases number and actions of osteoclasts, subsequently inhibiting bone resorption for prevention and treatment of osteoporosis, hypercalcemia, and Paget's disease of the bone
- Ibandronate, zoledronic acid and pamidronate are available as IV preparations.
- Alendronate, ibandronate, and risedronate are available as oral medications.

NURSING CONSIDERATIONS
- Risk for esophagitis and esophageal ulcers with oral preparations. Report early signs of indigestion, chest pain, difficulty swallowing, or bloody emesis to the provider immediately.
- Take with 8 oz water in the early morning before eating.
- Remain upright for 30 min after taking oral medication.
- Monitor calcium levels in clients receiving IV preparations.
- Clients using IV preparations should have dental examinations and preventative treatment prior to starting therapy to minimize the risk of osteonecrosis of the jaw.

Monoclonal antibody

Denosumab

THERAPEUTIC USES
- Decreases formation and function of osteoclasts, reducing bone resorption and increases bone density
- Limited use in clients who are at high risk for fractures

NURSING CONSIDERATIONS
- Contraindicated for clients who have hypocalcemia.
- Monitor calcium levels.
- Clients should have dental examinations and preventative treatment prior to starting therapy to minimize the risk of osteonecrosis of the jaw.
- Instruct client to notify the provider if manifestations of infection develop.
- Administer subcutaneously into the upper arm, upper thigh, or abdomen.

THERAPEUTIC PROCEDURES

Orthotic devices

Orthotic devices are available for immobilization of the spine immediately after a compression fracture of the spine.
- The device provides support and decreases pain.
- A physical therapist fits the device for the client and teaches him how to apply it.

NURSING ACTIONS
- Teach the client how to check for skin breakdown under the orthotic device.
- Instruct the client on the importance of good posture and body mechanics.
- Teach the client to log roll when getting out of bed.
- Instruct the client to use heat and back rubs to promote muscle relaxation.

Joint repair or joint arthroplasty

Can be necessary to repair or replace a joint weakened by osteoporosis. This is most often the hip joint.

Vertebroplasty or kyphoplasty

Minimally invasive procedures performed by a surgeon or radiologist
- Bone cement is injected into the fractured space of the vertebral column with or without balloon inflation.
- Balloon inflation of the fracture is to contain the cement and add height to the fractured vertebra.
- Mild sedation is used.
- Client lies in a supine position for 1 to 2 hr following procedure.

NURSING ACTIONS
- Monitor vital signs for shortness of breath and the puncture site for bleeding.
- Complete a neurological assessment.
- Apply cold therapy to the injection site.

CLIENT EDUCATION
- Avoid driving for 24 hr following the procedure
- Keep the dressing dry. Remove it the day following the procedure.
- Monitor the site for signs of infection.
- Resume activities such as walking the day following the procedure and gradually increase activity level as tolerated.

INTERPROFESSIONAL CARE

- Physical therapy may be used to establish an exercise regimen: 20 to 30 min of aerobic exercise (e.g., walking) at least three times per week in addition to weightlifting.
- Clients can need rehabilitation if fractures cause immobilization or disability.
- Most hip fractures are due to osteoporosis. Joint repair or joint arthroplasty requires physical therapy for a full recovery.

COMPLICATIONS

Fractures

Fractures are the leading complication of osteoporosis. Early recognition and treatment is essential.

NURSING ACTIONS
- Review risk factors for osteoporosis and falls.
- Assess dietary intake of calcium.
- Reinforce daily exercise including weight-bearing activities.
- Ensure proper screening with a DXA scan.

Application Exercises

1. A nurse is admitting an older adult client who has suspected osteoporosis. Which of following is an expected finding? (Select all that apply.)

   A. History of consuming one glass of wine daily

   B. Loss in height of 2 in (5.1 cm)

   C. Body mass index (BMI) of 21

   D. Kyphotic curve at upper thoracic spine

   E. History of lactose intolerance

2. A nurse is providing care for a client who had a vertebroplasty of the thoracic spine. Which of the following is an appropriate action by the nurse?

   A. Apply heat to the puncture site.

   B. Place the client in a supine position.

   C. Turn the client every 1 hr.

   D. Ambulate the client within the first hour postprocedure.

3. A nurse is providing dietary teaching about calcium-rich foods to a client who has osteoporosis. Which of the following foods should the nurse include in the instructions?

   A. White bread

   B. White beans

   C. White meat of chicken

   D. White rice

4. A nurse is performing health screenings at a health fair. Which of the following clients are at risk for osteoporosis? (Select all that apply.)

   A. A 40-year-old client who takes prednisone for asthma

   B. A 30-year-old client who jogs 3 miles daily

   C. A 45-year-old client who takes phenytoin for seizures

   D. A 65-year-old client who has a sedentary lifestyle

   E. A 70-year-old client who has smoked for 50 years

5. A nurse is planning discharge teaching on home safety for an older adult client who has osteoporosis. Which of the following information should the nurse include in the teaching? (Select all that apply.)

   A. Remove throw rugs in walkways.

   B. Use prescribed assistive devices.

   C. Remove clutter from the environment.

   D. Walk with caution on icy surfaces.

   E. Maintain lighting of doorway areas.

PRACTICE Active Learning Scenario

A nurse is administering raloxifene to a client who has osteoporosis. What should the nurse consider before administering the medication? Use the ATI Active Learning Template: Medication to complete this item.

THERAPEUTIC USES: List two.

NURSING INTERVENTIONS: Describe two.

EVALUATION OF MEDICATION EFFECTIVENESS: Describe one.

Application Exercises Key

1. A. A client who consumes more than three glasses of alcohol each day is at risk for developing osteoporosis because alcohol can increase bone loss.

   B. **CORRECT:** The loss of 2 inches of height is suggestive of osteoporosis due to fractures of the vertebral column.

   C. **CORRECT:** A client who has a BMI of 21 is at risk of developing osteoporosis due to low body weight and thin body build, suggesting decreased bone mass.

   D. **CORRECT:** Kyphosis curve is highly suggestive of osteoporosis due to fractures of the vertebrae causing the curve.

   E. **CORRECT:** Lactose intolerance is highly suggestive of osteoporosis due to possible lack of calcium intake.

   Ⓝ *NCLEX® Connection: Physiological Adaptation, Pathophysiology*

2. A. The client should have cold therapy applied to the puncture site to decrease bleeding and swelling following the procedure.

   B. **CORRECT:** The client should remain in a supine position with bed flat for the first 1 to 2 hr following the procedure to allow for hardening of the cement.

   C. The client should remain in a supine position with bed flat for 1 to 2 hr following the procedure.

   D. The client should remain in a supine position with bed flat for 1 to 2 hr following the procedure.

   Ⓝ *NCLEX® Connection: Reduction of Risk Potential, Therapeutic Procedures*

3. A. White bread is not a calcium-rich food, but it is a good source of carbohydrates.

   B. **CORRECT:** White beans should be included in the teaching because they are a good source of calcium.

   C. White meat of chicken is not a calcium-rich food, but it is a good source of protein.

   D. White rice is not a calcium-rich food, but it is a good source of carbohydrates.

   Ⓝ *NCLEX® Connection: Basic Care and Comfort, Nutrition and Oral Hydration*

4. A. **CORRECT:** Prednisone affects the absorption and metabolism of calcium and places the client at risk for osteoporosis.

   B. Weight-bearing activities decrease the risk for osteoporosis due to placing stress on bones, which promotes bone rebuilding and maintenance.

   C. **CORRECT:** Phenytoin affects the absorption and metabolism of calcium and places the client at risk for osteoporosis.

   D. **CORRECT:** A sedentary lifestyle places the client at risk for osteoporosis because bones need the stress of weight bearing activity for bone rebuilding and maintenance.

   E. **CORRECT:** Smoking increases the risk for osteoporosis because it decreases osteogenesis.

   Ⓝ *NCLEX® Connection: Health Promotion and Maintenance, Health Promotion/Disease Prevention*

5. A. **CORRECT:** Removing throw rugs in walkways can help to prevent a fall and bone fracture.

   B. **CORRECT:** Using prescribed assistive devices can help to prevent a fall and bone fracture.

   C. **CORRECT:** Removing clutter from the environment can help to prevent tripping, falling, and a bone fracture.

   D. The client should avoid walking on icy surfaces during inclement weather to help prevent a fall and bone fracture.

   E. **CORRECT:** Good lighting in doorway areas can prevent a fall and bone fracture.

   Ⓝ *NCLEX® Connection: Safety and Infection Control, Home Safety*

PRACTICE Answer

Using the ATI Active Learning Template: Medication

THERAPEUTIC USES
Selective estrogen receptor modulator
- Decreases bone resorption and increases bone density
- Treatment of postmenopausal osteoporosis
- Treatment of breast cancer by reducing the risk of cancer metastasis

NURSING INTERVENTIONS
- Avoid administering to a client who has a history of deep vein thrombosis (DVT).
- Instruct the client to report unusual calf pain or tenderness, a sign of DVT.
- Assess liver function tests periodically.
- Review need for calcium and vitamin D supplements when taking the medication.

EVALUATION OF MEDICATION EFFECTIVENESS
- Improved bone mineral density
- No further loss in height
- No metastasis of the cancer

Ⓝ *NCLEX® Connection: Pharmacological and Parenteral Therapies, Medication Administration*

CHAPTER 71 *Musculoskeletal Trauma*

A fracture is a break in a bone secondary to trauma or a pathological condition. Fractures caused by trauma are the most common type of bone fracture. Pathological fractures can be caused by metastatic cancer, osteoporosis, or Paget's disease.

Bone is continually going through a process of remodeling as osteoclasts release calcium from the bone and osteoblasts build up the bone. Remodeling of bone occurs at equal rates until an individual reaches their thirties. From this age on, the activity of the osteoclasts outpace the osteoblasts, increasing an individual's risk of osteoporosis. In women, this process significantly increases following menopause. Subsequently, women experience fractures secondary to osteoporosis about decade earlier than men.

Fractures

- A **closed (simple) fracture** does not break through the skin surface.
- An **open (compound) fracture** disrupts the skin integrity, causing an open wound and tissue injury with a risk of infection.
- Open fractures are graded based upon the extent of tissue injury.
  - **Grade I:** minimal skin damage
  - **Grade II:** damage includes skin and muscle contusions but without extensive soft tissue injury
  - **Grade III:** damage is excessive to skin, muscles, nerves, and blood vessels
- A **complete fracture** goes through the entire bone, dividing it into two distinct parts. An **incomplete fracture** goes through part of the bone.
- A **simple fracture** has one fracture line, while a **comminuted fracture** has multiple fracture lines splitting the bone into multiple pieces.
- A **displaced fracture** has bone fragments that are not in alignment, and a **non-displaced fracture** has bone fragments that remain in alignment.
- A **fatigue (stress) fracture** results when excess strain occurs from recreational and athletic activities.

- A **pathological (spontaneous) fracture** occurs to bone that is weak from a disease process, such as bone cancer or osteoporosis.
- **Compression fracture** occurs from a loading force pressing on callus bone. This condition is common older adult clients who have osteoporosis.

COMMON TYPES OF FRACTURES

Comminuted: Bone is fragmented.

Oblique: Fracture occurs at oblique angle and across bone.

Spiral: Fracture occurs from twisting motion (common with physical abuse).

Impacted: Fractured bone is wedged inside opposite fractured fragment.

Greenstick: Fracture occurs on one side (cortex) but does not extend completely through the bone (most often in children).

Hip fractures are the most common injury in older adults and are usually associated with falls.

HEALTH PROMOTION AND DISEASE PREVENTION

- Ensure recommended intake of calcium for developmental stage in life.
- Ensure adequate intake of vitamin D and/or exposure to sunlight.
- Monitor for development of osteoporosis, especially in postmenopausal clients and clients who have a thyroid disorder.
- Engage in weight-bearing exercise on a regular basis.
- Take a bisphosphonate if prescribed to slow bone resorption and treat osteoporosis.
- Use caution to prevent falls or accidents.
- Prevent injury with the use of seat belts and helmets.

71.1 X-ray of leg fracture

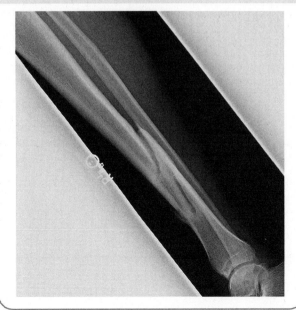

ASSESSMENT

RISK FACTORS

- Osteoporosis
  - Excessive exercising and weight loss from dieting and malnutrition can lead to osteoporosis.
  - Women who do not use estrogen replacement therapy after menopause lose estrogen and are unable to form strong new bone.
  - Clients on long-term corticosteroid therapy lose calcium from their bones due to direct inhibition of osteoblast function, inhibition of gastrointestinal calcium absorption, and enhancement of bone resorption.
- Falls
- Motor vehicle crashes
- Substance use disorder
- Diseases (bone cancer, Paget's disease)
- Contact sports and hazardous recreational activities (football, skiing)
- Physical abuse
- Lactose intolerance
- Age, as bone becomes less dense with advancing age ©

EXPECTED FINDINGS

- History of trauma, metabolic bone disorders, chronic conditions, and possible use of corticosteroid therapy
- Pain and reduced movement manifest at the area of fracture or the area distal to the fracture.

PHYSICAL ASSESSMENT FINDINGS

- Crepitus: A grating sound created by the rubbing of bone fragments
- Deformity: Internal rotation of extremity, shortened extremity, visible bone with open fracture
- Muscle spasms: Due to the pulling forces of the bone when not aligned
- Edema: Swelling from trauma
- Ecchymosis: Bleeding into underlying soft tissues from trauma

DIAGNOSTIC PROCEDURES

- Standard radiographs, computed tomography (CT) imaging scan used to detect fractures of the hip and pelvis, and/or magnetic resonance imagery (MRI)
  - Identify the type of fracture and location.
  - Indicate pathological fracture resulting from tumor or mass.
  - Determine soft tissue damage around fracture (MRI).
- Bone scan using radioactive material determines hairline fractures and complications/delayed healing.

PATIENT-CENTERED CARE

NURSING CARE

- Provide emergency care at time of injury.
- Maintain ABCs.
- Monitor vital signs and neurological status because injury to vital organs can occur due to bone fragments (fractures of pelvis, ribs).
- Stabilize the injured area, including the joints above and below the fracture, by using a splint and avoiding unnecessary movement.
- Maintain proper alignment of the affected extremity.
- Elevate the limb above the heart and apply ice.
- Assess for bleeding and apply pressure, if needed.
- Cover open wounds with a sterile dressing.
- Remove clothing and jewelry near the injury or on the affected extremity.
- Keep the client warm.
- Assess pain frequently and follow pain management protocols, both pharmacological and nonpharmacological.
- Initiate and continue neurovascular checks at least every hour. Immediately report any change in status to the provider.
- Prepare the client for any immobilization procedure appropriate for the fracture.

Immobilizing interventions: Casts, splints, and traction

Immobilization secures the injured extremity in order to
- Prevent further injury.
- Promote healing/circulation.
- Reduce pain.
- Correct a deformity.

TYPES OF IMMOBILIZATION DEVICES
- Casts
- Splints/immobilizers
- Traction
- External fixation
- Internal fixation

Closed reduction: When a pulling force (traction) is applied manually to realign the displaced fractured bone fragments. Once the fracture is reduced, immobilization is used to allow the bone to heal.

Open reduction: When a surgical incision is made and the bone is manually aligned and kept in place with plates and screws. This is known as an open reduction and internal fixation procedure.

PATIENT-CENTERED CARE

NURSING CARE

Neurovascular assessment

Neurovascular assessment is essential throughout immobilization. Assessments are performed every hour for the first 24 hr and every 1 to 4 hr thereafter following initial trauma to monitor neurovascular compromise related to edema and/or the immobilization device. Neurovascular assessment includes the following.

Pain: Assess pain level, location, and frequency. Assess pain using a 0 to 10 pain rating scale, and have the client describe the pain. Immobilization, ice, and elevation of the extremity with the use of analgesics should relieve most of the pain.

Sensation: Assess for numbness or tingling of the extremity. Loss of sensation can indicate nerve damage.

Skin temperature: Check the temperature of the affected extremity. The extremity should be warm, not cool, to touch. Cool skin can indicate decreased arterial perfusion.

Capillary refill: Press nail beds of affected extremity until blanching occurs. Blood return should be within 3 seconds. Prolonged refill indicates decreased arterial perfusion. Nail beds that are cyanotic can indicate venous congestion.

Pulses: Pulses should be palpable and strong. Pulses should be equal to the unaffected extremity. Edema can make it difficult to palpate pulses, so Doppler ultrasonography might be required.

Movement: Client should be able to move affected extremity in active motion.

Casts

Casts are more effective than splints or immobilizers because the client is unable to remove.
- Casts, as circumferential immobilizers, are applied once the swelling has subsided (to avoid compartment syndrome). If the swelling continues after cast application and causes unrelieved pain, the cast can be split on one side (univalve) or on both sides (bivalved).
- A window can be placed in an area of the cast to allow for skin inspection (e.g., if the client has a wound under the cast).
- Moleskin is used over any rough area of the cast that can rub against the client's skin.
- A fitted stockinette is placed under the plaster cast.

TYPES OF CASTS
- Short and long arm and leg casts
- Walking cast (a rubber walking pad on the sole of the cast assists the client in ambulating when weight bearing is allowed)
- Spica casts (a portion of the trunk and one or two extremities; typically used on children who have congenital hip dysplasia)
- Body casts (encircle the trunk of the body)

CASTING MATERIALS
- Plaster of Paris casts are heavy, not water-resistant, and can take 24 to 72 hr to dry.
- Synthetic fiberglass casts are light, stronger, water-resistant, and dry very quickly (in 30 min).

NURSING ACTIONS
- Monitor neurovascular status every hour for first 24 hr and assess pain. Qs
- Apply ice for 24 to 48 hr.
- Handle a plaster cast with the palms, not fingertips, until the cast is dry to prevent denting the cast.
- Avoid setting the cast on hard surfaces or sharp edges.
- Prior to casting, the area is cleaned and dried. Tubular cotton web roll is placed over the affected area to maintain skin integrity. The casting material is then applied.
- After cast application, position the client so that warm, dry air circulates around and under the cast (support the casted area without pressure under or directly on the cast) for faster drying and to prevent pressure from changing the shape of the cast. Use gloves to touch the cast until it is completely dry.
- Elevate the cast above the level of the heart during the first 24 to 48 hr to prevent edema of the affected extremity. Use a cloth-covered pillow instead of plastic while cast is drying.
- Ensure that cast is not too tight; there should be room for one finger between the skin and cast.
- Document presence of drainage and report sudden increase in drainage. Circling drainage on cast is an unreliable indicator of drainage amount and can increase client anxiety.
- Older adult clients have an increased risk for impaired skin integrity due to the loss of elasticity of the skin and decreased sensation (comorbidities).

CLIENT EDUCATION
- Instruct clients not to place any foreign objects inside the cast to avoid trauma to the skin. Itching under the cast is relieved by blowing cool air from a hair dryer into the cast.
- Cover the cast with plastic if needed to avoid soiling from urine or feces.
- Demonstrate how plastic bags can cover the cast during baths and showers to keep the cast dry.
- Report any areas under the cast that are painful, have a "hot spot," have increased drainage, are warm to the touch, or have an odor, which can indicate infection.
- Instruct the client to report change in mobility and complications such as shortness of breath, skin breakdown, and constipation.

Traction

- Traction uses a pulling force to promote and maintain alignment of the injured area.
- Traction prescriptions should include the type of traction, amount of weight, and whether traction can be removed for nursing care.

GOALS OF TRACTION

- Prevent soft tissue injury.
- Realign of bone fragments.
- Decrease muscle spasms and pain.
- Correct or prevent further deformities.

TYPES OF TRACTION

- **Manual:** A pulling force is applied by the hands of the provider for temporary immobilization, usually with sedation or anesthesia, in conjunction with the application of an immobilizing device.
- **Straight or running:** The counter traction is provided by the client's body by applying a pulling force in a straight line. Movement of the client's body can alter the traction provided.
  - **Skin:** Primary purpose is to decrease muscle spasms and immobilize the extremity prior to surgery. The pulling force is applied by weights that are attached by rope to the client's skin with tape, straps, boots, or cuffs. Examples include Bryant's traction (used for congenital hip dislocation in children) and Buck's traction (used preoperatively for hip fractures for immobilization in adult clients). **(71.2)**
- **Balanced suspension:** The counter traction is produced by devices such as slings or splints to support the fractured extremity off the bed while pulling with ropes and weights. The client's body can move without altering the traction. **(71.3)**
  - **Skeletal:** Screws are inserted into the bone (e.g., Halo traction). Can use heavier weights (15 to 30 lb) and longer traction time to realign the bone. Provide frequent pin site care to prevent infection. **(71.4)** Qs

NURSING ACTIONS

- Assess neurovascular status of the affected body part every hour for 24 hr and every 4 hr after that.
- Maintain body alignment and realign if the client seems uncomfortable or reports pain.
- Avoid lifting or removing weights.
- Ensure that weights hang freely and are not resting on the floor.
- If the weights are accidentally displaced, replace the weights. If the problem is not corrected, notify the provider.
- Ensure that pulley ropes are free of knots, fraying, loosening, and improper positioning at least every 8 to 12 hr.
- Notify the provider if the client experiences severe pain from muscle spasms unrelieved with medications or repositioning. Move the client in halo traction as a unit, without applying pressure to the rods. This will prevent loosening of the pins and pain.
- Routinely monitor skin integrity and document.
- Use heat/massage as prescribed to treat muscle spasms.
- Use therapeutic touch and relaxation techniques.

PIN SITE CARE

- Pin care is done frequently throughout immobilization (skeletal traction and external fixation methods) to prevent and to monitor for manifestations of infection.
  - Drainage and redness (color, amount, odor)
  - Loosening of pins
  - Tenting of skin at pin site (skin rising up pin)
- Pin care protocols (chlorhexidine) are based on provider preference and facility policy. A primary concept of pin care is that one cotton swab is designated for each pin to avoid cross-contamination.
- Pin care is provided usually once a shift, 1 to 2 times a day, or per facility protocol.

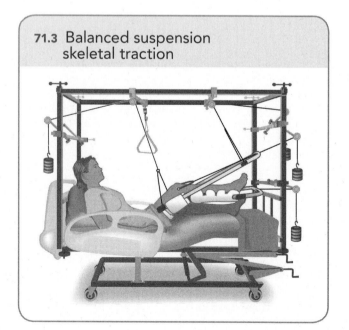

71.3 Balanced suspension skeletal traction

71.2 Buck's traction

MEDICATIONS

Analgesics
- Opioid and nonopioid analgesics as needed to control pain.
- NSAIDs decrease associated tissue inflammation.

Muscle relaxants: Relieve muscle spasms.

Stool softener: To prevent constipation

Antibiotic: Prophylactic antibiotics to decrease the risk of infection for open fractures.

THERAPEUTIC PROCEDURES

Splints and immobilizers

Splints and immobilizers provide support, control movement, and prevent additional injury.
- Splints are removable and allow for monitoring of skin swelling or integrity.
- Splints can support fractured/injured areas until casting occurs and swelling is decreased. Casting is then used for post-paralysis injuries to avoid joint contracture.
- Immobilizers are prefabricated and typically fasten with hook-and-loop fastener straps.

CLIENT EDUCATION
- Ensure the client is aware of application protocol regarding full-time or part-time use.
- Instruct the client to observe for skin breakdown at pressure points.

External fixation

External fixation involves fracture immobilization using percutaneous pins and wires that are attached to a rigid external frame.

USED TO TREAT
- Comminuted fracture or nonunion fractures with extensive soft tissue damage
- Leg length discrepancies from congenital defects
- Bone loss related to tumors or osteomyelitis

ADVANTAGES
- Immediate fracture stabilization
- Minimal blood loss occurring in comparison with internal fixation
- Allowing for early mobilization and ambulation
- Maintaining alignment of closed fractures that could not be maintained in cast or splint
- Permitting wound care with open fractures

71.4 Halo fixation device

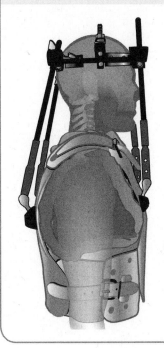
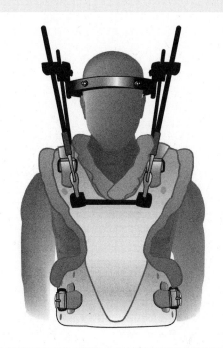

DISADVANTAGES
- Risk of pin site infection leading to osteomyelitis
- Potential overwhelming appearance to client
- Noncompliance issues

NURSING ACTIONS
- Elevate extremity.
- Monitor neurovascular status and skin integrity.
- Assess body image.
- Perform pin care every 8 to 12 hr. Monitor site for drainage, color, odor, redness.
- Observe for manifestations of fat and pulmonary embolism.
- Provide antiembolism stockings and sequential compression device to prevent deep-vein thrombosis (DVT).

CLIENT EDUCATION
- Teach the client pin care.
- Discuss clothing and other materials that can be used to cover the device.
- If activity is restricted, advise the client to perform deep breathing and leg exercises and other techniques to prevent complications to immobilization, such as pneumonia or thrombus formation.

Open reduction and internal fixation

- Open reduction refers to visualization of a fracture through an incision in the skin, and internal fixation with plates, screws, pins, rods, and prosthetics as needed.
- After the bone heals, the hardware might be removed, depending on the location and type of hardware.
- Circular external fixation: Technique to promote new bone growth for malunion and nonunion fracture. Device is turned four times per day to pull apart the cortex of the bone and stimulate growth.

NURSING ACTIONS
- Prevent dislocation, especially of hip. Qᴘᴄᴄ
- Monitor skin integrity.
- Ensure heels are off bed at all times and inspect bony prominence every shift.
- Perform a neurovascular assessment.
- Observe the cast or dressing for postoperative drainage. The cast can have a window cut in it through which the incision can be viewed. An elastic wrap is used to keep the window block cover in place to decrease localized edema.
- Monitor for manifestations of fat and pulmonary embolism.
- Provide antiembolism stockings and a sequential compression device to prevent DVT and administer prescribed anticoagulants.
- Monitor the client's pain level.
  - Administer analgesics, antispasmodics, and/or anti-inflammatory medication (NSAIDs) and assess relief.
  - Position for comfort and with ice on the surgical site.
- Monitor for manifestations of infection.
  - Monitor vital signs, observing for fever, tachycardia, incisional drainage, redness, and odor.
  - Monitor laboratory values (WBC, ESR).
  - Provide surgical aseptic wound care.
- Increase physical mobility as appropriate.
  - Consult physical and occupational therapy for ambulation and activities of daily living.
  - Monitor orthostatic blood pressure when the client gets out of bed for the first time.
  - Turn and reposition the client every 2 hr.
  - Have the client get out of bed from the unaffected side.
  - Position the client for comfort (within restrictions).
- Support nutrition.
  - Encourage increased calorie intake.
  - Ensure use of calcium supplements.
  - Encourage small, frequent meals with snacks.
  - Monitor for constipation.

COMPLICATIONS

Compartment syndrome

- Compartment syndrome usually affects extremities and occurs when pressure within one or more of the muscle compartments (an area covered with an elastic tissue called fascia) of the extremity compromises circulation, resulting in an ischemia-edema cycle.
- Capillaries dilate in an attempt to pull oxygen into the tissue. Increased capillary permeability from the release of histamine leads to edema from plasma proteins leaking into the interstitial fluid space.
- Increased edema causes pressure on the nerve endings, resulting in pain. Blood flow is further reduced and ischemia persists, resulting in compromised neurovascular status.
- Pressure can result from external sources, such as a tight cast or a constrictive bulky dressing.
- Internal sources, such as an accumulation of blood or fluid within the muscle compartment, can cause pressure as well.

MANIFESTATIONS
- Compartment syndrome is assessed by using the five P's (pain, paralysis, paresthesia, pallor, and pulselessness).
  - Increased pain unrelieved with elevation or by pain medication. Intense pain when passively moved.
  - Paresthesia or numbness, burning, and tingling are early manifestations.
  - Paralysis, motor weakness, or inability to move the extremity indicate major nerve damage and are late manifestations.
  - Color of tissue is pale (pallor), and nail beds are cyanotic.
  - Pulselessness is a late manifestation of compartment syndrome.
  - Palpated muscles are hard and swollen from edema.
- If untreated, tissue necrosis can result. Neuromuscular damage occurs within 4 to 6 hr.
- Surgical treatment is a fasciotomy.
- A surgical incision is made through the subcutaneous tissue and fascia of the affected compartment to relieve the pressure and restore circulation.
- After the fasciotomy, the open wounds require sterile packings and dressings until secondary closure occurs. Skin grafts might be necessary. Negative pressure wound therapy can be used to reduce edema.

NURSING ACTIONS
Prevention includes the following.
- Assess neurovascular status frequently.
- Notify the provider when compartment syndrome is suspected.
- The provider will cut the cast on one side (univalve) or both sides (bivalve).
- Loosen the constrictive dressing or cut the bandage or tape.

CLIENT EDUCATION
- Instruct the client to report pain not relieved by analgesics or pain that continues to increase in intensity.
- Remind the client to report numbness, tingling, or a change in color of the extremity.

Fat embolism

- Adults older than age 70 are at a high risk of developing a fat embolism. Hip and pelvis fractures are common causes. Ⓖ
- Fat embolism can occur after the injury, usually within 12 to 48 hr following long bone fractures or with total joint arthroplasty.
- Fat globules from the bone marrow are released into the vasculature and travel to the small blood vessels, including those in the lungs, resulting in acute respiratory insufficiency and impaired organ perfusion. Careful diagnosis should differentiate between fat embolism and pulmonary embolism.

MANIFESTATIONS

- Early manifestations
  - Dyspnea, increased respiratory rate, decreased oxygen saturation
  - Headache
  - Decreased mental acuity related to low arterial oxygen level
  - Respiratory distress
  - Tachycardia
  - Confusion
  - Chest pain
- Late manifestation: Cutaneous petechiae: pinpoint-sized subdermal hemorrhages that occur on the neck, chest, upper arms, and abdomen (from the blockage of the capillaries by the fat globules). This is a discriminating finding from pulmonary embolism.

NURSING ACTIONS

- Maintain the client on bed rest.
- Prevention includes immobilization of fractures of the long bones and minimal manipulation during turning if immobilization procedure has not yet been performed.
- Treatment includes oxygen for respiratory compromise, corticosteroids for cerebral edema, vasopressors, and fluid replacement for shock, as well as pain and antianxiety medications as needed.

Venous thromboembolism

Deep-vein thrombosis and pulmonary embolism:
Deep-vein thrombosis is a common complication following trauma, surgery, or disability related to immobility.

NURSING ACTIONS

- Encourage early ambulation.
- Apply antiembolism stockings, sequential compression device.
- Administer anticoagulants as prescribed.
- Encourage intake of fluids to prevent hemoconcentration.
- Instruct the client to rotate feet at the ankles and perform other lower extremity exercises as permitted by the particular immobilization device.
- Monitor for manifestations (swollen, reddened calf).

Osteomyelitis

Osteomyelitis is an infection of the bone that begins as an inflammation within the bone secondary to penetration by infectious organisms (virus, bacteria, or fungi) following trauma or surgical repair of a fracture.

MANIFESTATIONS

- Bone pain that is constant, pulsating, localized, and worse with movement
- Erythema and edema at the site of the infection
- Fever: Older adults might not have an elevated temperature. Ⓖ
- Leukocytosis and possible elevated sedimentation rate
- Many of these manifestations will disappear if the infection becomes chronic.

DIAGNOSTIC PROCEDURES

- Bone scan using radioactive material to diagnose osteomyelitis and MRI can also facilitate a diagnosis.
- Cultures are performed for detection of possible aerobic and anaerobic organisms.
- If septicemia develops, blood cultures will be positive for offending microbes.

TREATMENT

- Long course (3 months) of IV and oral antibiotic therapy.
- Surgical debridement can be indicated. If a significant amount of the bone requires removal, a bone graft can be necessary.
- Hyperbaric oxygen treatments can promote healing in chronic cases of osteomyelitis.
- Surgically implanted antibiotic beads in bone cement are packed into the wound as a form of antibiotic therapy.
- Unsuccessful treatment can result in amputation.

NURSING ACTIONS

- Administer antibiotics as prescribed to maintain a constant blood level.
- Administer analgesics as needed.
- Conduct neurovascular assessments if debridement is done.
- If the wound is left open to heal, standard precautions are adequate, and clean technique can be used during dressing changes.

Avascular necrosis

- Avascular necrosis results from the circulatory compromise that occurs after a fracture. Blood flow is disrupted to the fracture site and the resulting ischemia leads to tissue (bone) necrosis.
- Commonly found in hip fractures or in fractures with displacement of a bone.
- Clients receiving long-term corticosteroid therapy are at greater risk for developing avascular necrosis.
- Replacement of damaged bone with a bone graft or prosthetic replacement can be necessary.

Failure of fracture to heal

A fracture that has not healed within 6 months of injury is considered to be experiencing delayed union.
- **Malunion:** Fracture heals incorrectly
- **Nonunion:** Fracture that never heals
  - Electrical bone stimulation and bone grafting can treat nonunion.
  - Low intensity pulse ultrasound can promote healing to treat nonunion.
  - Can occur more frequently in older adult clients due to impaired healing process. Ⓖ
- Malunion or nonunion can cause immobilizing deformity of the bone involved.

Carpal tunnel syndrome

Compression of the median nerve in the wrist from swollen or thickened synovium, causing pain and numbness.

ASSESSMENT

RISK FACTORS

- Some metabolic and connective tissue diseases such as rheumatoid arthritis (synovitis) and diabetes mellitus (reduced circulation)
- Occupational injury from repetitive stress of hand activities such as pinching or grasping during wrist flexion (computer users)
- Repetitive sports injury (tennis)
- Children and adolescents due to use of computers and handheld devices
- Growth of a space occupying lesion, such as a ganglia or lipoma

EXPECTED FINDINGS

- Diagnosis is made based on history and report of pain and numbness in affected hand.
- Pain is often worse at night and can radiate to the arm, shoulder, and neck or chest.
- Paresthesia (painful tingling): Sensory changes occur weeks or months before motor.
- Phalen's maneuver (positive in most clients who have carpal tunnel syndrome)
  - Ask the client to place the back of his hands together and flex both wrists at the same time.
  - Tinel's sign: Tap lightly over the median nerve area of the wrist
  - A positive result is paresthesia in the median nerve distribution (palmer side of thumb, index, middle and half of ring finger)

PATIENT-CENTERED CARE

NURSING CARE

- Medication therapy
  - NSAIDs for relief of pain and inflammation
  - Corticosteroid injections directly into the carpal tunnel
- Splint or hand brace to immobilize the wrist: can use during the day, during the night, or both
- Laser or ultrasound therapy
- Yoga and exercise
- Surgery can relieve the pressure by decompressing the pressure on the nerve.
  - Endoscopic carpal tunnel release: less invasive but a longer recovery period of postoperative pain and numbness
  - Open carpal tunnel release

POSTOPERATIVE CARE

- Monitor vital signs and check dressing for drainage and tightness.
- Elevate hand above the heart to reduce swelling.
- Check neurovascular status of fingers every hour and encourage the client to move them frequently.
- Offer pain medications.

CLIENT EDUCATION

- Hand movements and heavy lifting might be restricted 4 to 6 weeks.
- The client can expect weakness and discomfort for weeks or months.
- Remind the client to report any changes in neurovascular status including increase in pain to surgeon immediately.

Sprains and strains

Strain

- Excessive stretching or pulling of a muscle or tendon that is weak or unstable
- Often caused by falls, lifting a heavy item, and exercise

CLASSIFICATIONS OF STRAINS

- **First-degree (mild) strain** causes mild inflammation and little bleeding. There can be swelling, ecchymosis, and tenderness.
- **Second-degree (moderate) strain** involves partial tearing of the muscle or tendon fibers. Involves impaired muscle function.
- **Third-degree (severe) strain** involves a ruptured muscle or tendon with separation of muscle from muscle, tendon from muscle, or tendon from bone. Causes severe pain and immobility.

Sprain

- Excessive stretching of a ligament. Twisting motions from a fall or sports activity can be the cause of the injury.
- Classification of sprains are according to severity.

PATIENT-CENTERED CARE

Management of strain

- Cold and heat application, exercise, and activity limitations.
- Anti-inflammatory medications to decrease inflammation and pain.
- Surgical repair if needed for third-degree strains to repair ruptured muscle or tendon.

Management of sprain

- RICE (rest, ice, compression, elevation) for mild sprains.
- Second-degree require immobilization and partial weight bearing while the tear heals.
- Immobilization for 4 to 6 weeks is necessary for third-degree sprains. Arthroscopic surgery if needed.

> **PRACTICE** Active Learning Scenario
>
> A nurse is performing a neurovascular assessment on a client who has a cast applied following a right arm fracture. What interventions should the nurse take? Use the ATI Active Learning Template: Basic Concept to complete this item:
>
> **RELATED CONTENT:** Identify the purpose of neurovascular assessment.
>
> **UNDERLYING PRINCIPLES:** Identify the six components of a neurovascular assessment.
>
> **NURSING INTERVENTIONS:** Describe a nursing intervention related to each of the six components.

Application Exercises

1. A nurse is teaching a client how to manage an external fixation device upon discharge. Which of the following statements by the client indicates an understanding of the teaching? (Select all that apply.)
   - A. "I will clean the pins twice a day."
   - B. "I will use a separate cotton swab for each pin."
   - C. "I will report loosening of the pins to my doctor."
   - D. "I will move my leg by lifting the device in the middle."
   - E. "I will report increased redness at the pin sites."

2. A nurse is assessing a client who has a casted compound fracture of the femur. Which of the following findings is a manifestation of a fat emboli?
   - A. Altered mental status
   - B. Reduced bowel sounds
   - C. Swelling of the toes distal to the injury
   - D. Pain with passive movement of the foot distal to the injury

3. A nurse is assessing a client who had an external fixation device applied 2 hr ago for a fracture of the left tibia and fibula. Which of the following findings is a manifestation of compartment syndrome? (Select all that apply.)
   - A. Intense pain when the client's left foot is passively moved
   - B. Capillary refill of 3 sec on the client's left toes
   - C. Hard, swollen muscle in the client's left leg
   - D. Burning and tingling of the client's left foot
   - E. Client report of minimal pain relief following a second dose of opioid medication

4. A nurse is completing discharge teaching to a client who had a wound debridement for osteomyelitis. Which of the following information should the nurse include in the teaching?
   - A. Antibiotic therapy should continue for 3 months.
   - B. Relief of pain indicates the infection is eradicated.
   - C. Airborne precautions are used during wound care.
   - D. Expect paresthesia distal to the wound.

5. A nurse in the emergency department is planning care for a client who has a right hip fracture. Which of the following immobilization devices should the nurse anticipate in the plan of care?
   - A. Skeletal traction
   - B. Buck's traction
   - C. Halo traction
   - D. Bryant's traction

1. A. **CORRECT:** Clean the external fixation pins one to two times each day to remove exudate that can harbor bacteria.

   B. **CORRECT:** Using a separate cotton swab on each pin will decrease the risk of cross-contamination, which could cause pin site infection.

   C. **CORRECT:** Notify the provider if a pin is loose because the provider will know how much to tighten the pin and prevent damage to the tissue and bone.

   D. The external fixation device should never be used to lift or move the affected leg, due to the risk of injuring and dislocating the fractured bone.

   E. **CORRECT:** The client should report redness, heat, and drainage at the pin sites, which can indicate an infection that can lead to osteomyelitis.

   Ⓝ *NCLEX® Connection: Basic Care and Comfort, Mobility/Immobility*

2. A. **CORRECT:** Altered mental status is an early manifestation of fat emboli. Other manifestations include dyspnea, chest pain, and hypoxemia.

   B. Reduced bowel sounds is an adverse effect of opioid narcotics and can result in constipation.

   C. Swelling of the toes distal to the injury is a manifestation of reduced circulation and can be the result of a tight cast. The nurse should elevate the extremity and apply ice.

   D. Pain with passive movement of the foot distal to the injury is an expected finding. Severe pain or pain unrelieved by narcotics is a manifestation of compartment syndrome.

   Ⓝ *NCLEX® Connection: Basic Care and Comfort, Mobility/Immobility*

3. A. **CORRECT:** Intense pain of the left foot when passively moved can indicate pressure from edema on nerve endings and is a manifestation of compartment syndrome.

   B. Capillary refill of 3 seconds is within the expected reference range. Pallor is a manifestation of compartment syndrome.

   C. **CORRECT:** A hard, swollen muscle on the affected extremity indicates edema build-up in the area of injury and is a manifestation of compartment syndrome.

   D. **CORRECT:** Burning and tingling of the left foot indicates pressure from edema on nerve endings and is an early manifestation of compartment syndrome.

   E. **CORRECT:** Minimal pain relief after receiving opioid medication can indicate pressure from edema on nerve endings and is an early manifestation of compartment syndrome.

   Ⓝ *NCLEX® Connection: Reduction of Risk Potential, Potential for Complications from Surgical Procedures and Health Alterations*

4. A. **CORRECT:** Treatment of osteomyelitis includes continuing antibiotic therapy for 3 months.

   B. Relief of pain does not indicate that osteomyelitis is resolved, and the client should continue antibiotic therapy as prescribed.

   C. When performing wound care contact precautions are implemented to prevent spread of the organism.

   D. The client should monitor and report manifestations of neurovascular compromise, such as paresthesia.

   Ⓝ *NCLEX® Connection: Reduction of Risk Potential, Potential for Complications from Surgical Procedures and Health Alterations*

5. A. Skeletal traction is an immobilization device applied surgically to a long bone (femur, or tibia), and cervical spine. It is not used for a hip fracture.

   B. **CORRECT:** Buck's traction is a temporary immobilization device applied to a client who has a femur or hip fracture to diminish muscle spasms and immobilize the affected extremity until surgery is performed.

   C. Halo traction immobilizes the cervical spine when a cervical fracture occurs.

   D. Bryant's traction is used for congenital hip dislocation in children.

   Ⓝ *NCLEX® Connection: Reduction of Risk Potential, Therapeutic Procedures*

PRACTICE Answer

Using the ATI Active Learning Template: Basic Concept

RELATED CONTENT:
Neurovascular assessment is performed to monitor for any compromise in the affected extremity caused by edema and or immobilization device.

UNDERLYING PRINCIPLES
- Assess for pain level, location, and type and frequency.
- Assess sensation of the distal extremity.
- Assess skin temperature for warmth.
- Assess capillary refill.
- Assess the pulses distal to the fracture.
- Assess finger movement.

NURSING INTERVENTIONS
- Pain: Administer pain medication, elevate the extremity, and apply ice.
- Sensation: Notify the provider of numbness, tingling, or loss of sensation.
- Skin temperature: Notify the provider if the affected extremity is cool compared to the unaffected extremity.
- Capillary refill: Notify the provider if nail beds are cyanotic.
- Pulses: Notify the provider if pulse is absent.
- Finger movement: Notify the provider if the client is unable to perform passive or active movement of the fingers.

Ⓝ *NCLEX® Connection: Reduction of Risk Potential, Therapeutic Procedures*

UNIT 10   NURSING CARE OF CLIENTS WHO HAVE
MUSCULOSKELETAL DISORDERS
SECTION: MUSCULOSKELETAL DISORDERS

CHAPTER 72 *Osteoarthritis and*
Low-Back Pain

Osteoarthritis (OA), or degenerative joint disease (DJD), is a disorder characterized by progressive deterioration of the articular cartilage. It is a noninflammatory (unless localized), nonsystemic disease.

It is no longer thought to be only a wear-and-tear disease associated with aging, but rather a process in which new tissue is produced as a result of cartilage destruction within the joint. The destruction outweighs the production. The cartilage and bone beneath the cartilage erode and osteophytes (bone spurs) form, resulting in narrowed joint spaces. The changes within the joint lead to pain, immobility, muscle spasms, and potential inflammation.

Early in the disease process of OA, it can be difficult to distinguish from rheumatoid arthritis (RA). (72.1)

Low-back pain (LBP) occurs along the lumbosacral area of the vertebral column. LBP can be acute (self-limiting) or chronic (longer than 3 months or repeated episodes of pain).

In addition to back pain, the client can experience foot, ankle, and leg weakness or burning/stabbing pain radiating to the leg or foot. LBP can be related to an injury, fall, or heavy lifting. LBP is the leading cause of work disability. It is most prevalent between ages 30 and 60. Smoking and obesity contribute to LBP.

HEALTH PROMOTION AND DISEASE PREVENTION

Osteoarthritis

- Encourage the client to use joint-saving measures (good body mechanics, labor-saving devices).
- Encourage the client to maintain a healthy weight to decrease joint degeneration of the hips and knees.
- Recommend that the client stop smoking to reduce cartilage loss, especially if there is a family history of OA.
- Encourage the client to avoid or limit repetitive strain on joints (jogging, contact sports, risk-taking activities).
- Recommend wearing well-fitted shoes with supports to prevent falls.

Low-back pain

- Exercise to keep back healthy and strong.
- Use body mechanics and proper lifting techniques (ergonomics).
- Maintain correct posture.
- Wear low-heeled shoes.
- Maintain a healthy weight.
- Smoking cessation, as smoking is linked to disk degeneration. Q EBP
- Avoid prolonged sitting/standing.
- Healthy diet including adequate calcium and vitamin D.

72.1 Characteristics of osteoarthritis and rheumatoid arthritis

	Osteoarthritis	Rheumatoid arthritis
DISEASE PROCESS	Cartilage destruction with bone spur growth at joint ends; degenerative	Synovial membrane inflammation resulting in cartilage destruction and bone erosion; inflammatory
FINDINGS	Pain with activity that improves at rest	Swelling, redness, warmth, pain at rest or after immobility (morning stiffness)
EFFUSIONS	Localized inflammatory response	All joints
BODY SIZE	Usually overweight	Usually underweight
NODES	Heberden's and Bouchard's nodes	Swan neck and boutonnière deformities of hands
SYSTEMIC INVOLVEMENT	No: articular	Yes: lungs, heart, skin, and extra-articular
SYMMETRICAL	No	Yes
DIAGNOSTIC TESTS	X-rays	X-rays and positive rheumatoid factor

ASSESSMENT

RISK FACTORS

Osteoarthritis

- Aging: majority of adults over age 60 have joint changes on x-ray).
- Genetic factors
- Joint injury due to acute or repetitive stress on joints predisposes to later OA.
- Obesity: OA affects weight-bearing joints such as knees, hips in overweight clients.
- Metabolic disorders, such as diabetes, and blood disorders, such as sickle cell disease predisposes to joint degeneration.

Low-back pain

- Can occur at any time but most prevalent from ages 30 to 60
- Family history of back pain or history of a back injury
- Being pregnant (changes in posture and weight distribution)
- History of spine problems, back surgery, or compression fracture
- Job or occupation that requires heavy lifting, twisting, or repetitive motion
- Smoking (linked to disk degeneration)
- Overweight
- Having poor posture

72.2 Heberden's and Bouchard's nodes

CAUSES OF LOW-BACK PAIN

- Muscle strain/spasm
- Ligament sprain
- Osteoarthritis
- Osteoporosis
- Scoliosis
- Compression fracture
- A defect of a vertebrae (spondylolysis)
- A vertebra that slips forward on the one below it (spondylolisthesis)
- Narrowing of the spinal canal (spinal stenosis)
- Herniated disk (herniated nucleus pulposus), which can cause sciatic nerve involvement with burning or stabbing pain into one leg or foot

EXPECTED FINDINGS

Osteoarthritis

- Joint pain and stiffness
- Pain with joint palpation or range of motion (observe for muscle atrophy, loss of function, limp when walking, and restricted activity due to pain)
- Crepitus in one or more of the affected joints
- Enlarged joint related to bone hypertrophy
- Heberden's nodes enlarged at the distal interphalangeal joints
- Bouchard's nodes located at the proximal interphalangeal joints (OA is not a symmetrical disease, but these nodes can occur bilaterally). These nodes can be inflamed and painful.
- Inflammation resulting from secondary synovitis, indicating advanced disease
- Joint effusion (excess joint fluid) that is easily moved from one area of the joint to another area
- Vertebral radiating pain affected by cervical or lumbar compression of nerve roots
- Limping gait due to hip or knee pain
- Back pain due to OA of the spine

Low-back pain

- Dull or sharp low back pain
- Pain aggravated by coughing, sneezing, or straining
- Muscle spasms, cramping, and stiffness
- Pain in the buttock
- Sciatic nerve compression causes severe pain when leg is straightened and held up.
- Numbness/tingling of the leg (paresthesia); burning or stabbing pain in the leg or foot
- Report chills/fever, bowel or bladder incontinence, progression of decreased ability to move, and paresthesias to the provider promptly (can indicate a more serious condition). **Qs**

LABORATORY TESTS

OA: Laboratory tests are usually normal with OA. Erythrocyte sedimentation rate and high-sensitivity C-reactive protein can be increased slightly related to secondary synovitis.

LBP: CBC, erythrocyte sedimentation rate and urinalysis may be ordered with LBP to rule out cancer or infection. Serum electrophoresis can help to rule out multiple myeloma.

DIAGNOSTIC PROCEDURES

X-rays: to rule out fracture, spondylosis (spinal degeneration), or neoplasm

Magnetic resonance imaging with or without contrast: shows soft tissue structures of the back, including intervertebral disks, the spinal cord and spinal nerves

Computed tomography (CT) scans
- Shows injuries or pathology that involves bone
- Can be done with or without contrast

Nuclear bone scan
- Provides ability to scan entire skeleton
- Detects tumors, arthritis, osteomyelitis, osteoporosis, vertebral compression fractures, and unexplained bone pain

CT myelogram
- Uses x-ray and contrast which is put into the subarachnoid space with a thin needle (lumbar puncture)
- The contrast moves through the space so the nerve roots and spinal cord can be visualized

Electromyogram (EMG) and nerve conduction
- Measures electrical impulses produced by nerves and muscle response.
- Looks for bone, nerve or muscle problems that might be causing pain

Arthrogram
- X-ray study of a joint after contrast medium (air or contrast, or both) has been injected to enhance visualization
- Bone chips, torn ligaments, or other loose bodies within a joint can be visualized

PATIENT-CENTERED CARE

NURSING CARE

PAIN ASSESSMENT/MONITORING
- Location, characteristics, quality, severity, precipitating or relieving factors
- Sciatic nerve pain becomes worse when the leg is held straight and lifted upward

MUSCULOSKELETAL ASSESSMENT/MUSCLE TONE AND STRENGTH
- Inspect back for vertebral alignment and tenderness
- Degree of functional limitation; ability to perform ADLs
- Gait ability and characteristics
- Proper functional/joint alignment (OA)/vertebral alignment (low back pain)
- Levels of fatigue and pain after activity
- Range of motion

NEUROLOGICAL ASSESSMENT/SENSORY PERCEPTION
- Genitourinary: bowel or bladder problems
- Home barriers

PSYCHOSOCIAL ASSESSMENT Qpcc
- Pain interference with sexuality
- Depression related to pain
- Anxiety related to pain
- Alteration in self-esteem and body image due to joint deformities and nodules in OA

CLIENT EDUCATION
- Acute LBP often resolves spontaneously.
- Positioning (e.g., William's position: semi-Fowler's position with a pillow under flexed knees) can alleviate pain associated with LBP from a herniated disk. Qebp
- Instruct the client about the use of analgesics and NSAIDs prior to activity and around the clock as needed.
- Balance rest with activity.
- Instruct the client on proper body mechanics.
- Encourage the use of thermal applications: heat (dry or moist) to alleviate pain and ice for acute inflammation.
- Encourage the use of complementary and alternative therapies, including acupuncture, tai chi, hypnosis, magnets, and music therapy.
- Encourage the use of splinting for joint protection, and the use of larger joints.
- Encourage the use of assistive devices to promote safety and independence, including an elevated toilet seat, shower bench, long-handled reacher, and shoe horn.
- Encourage the use of a daily schedule of activities that will promote independence (high-energy activities in the morning).
- Encourage a well-balanced diet and ideal body weight. Consult a dietitian to provide meal planning for balanced nutrition.

MEDICATIONS

Analgesic therapy

Acetaminophen does not provide anti-inflammatory benefits, which might not be needed if synovitis is not present

NURSING ACTIONS
- Limit administration of acetaminophen to a maximum of 4,000 mg/24 hr. Some experts recommend a maximum daily dose of 2,500 to 3,000 mg/day when used long-term to prevent liver toxicity. Qs
- Make sure clients are aware of opioids that contain acetaminophen, such as hydrocodone bitartrate 5 mg/acetaminophen 500 mg, which contains various amounts of hydrocodone and acetaminophen.
- Monitor liver function tests.

Nonsteroidal anti-inflammatory drugs (NSAIDs)

- Analgesics and anti-inflammatories (celecoxib, naproxen, ibuprofen) are used to relieve pain and synovitis if present.
- Baseline liver and kidney function tests and CBC are needed if NSAIDs are to be given.
- May replace acetaminophen with an NSAID if adequate relief is not obtained.
- Topical NSAID (diclofenac epolamine patch) may be used and is non-systemic.

NURSING ACTIONS
- Monitor kidney function (BUN and creatinine).
- Educate the client that NSAIDs are nephrotoxic and should be taken as prescribed. Qs
- Teach the client to report evidence of black tarry stool, indigestion, and shortness of breath.

Muscle relaxants

- Cyclobenzaprine hydrochloride may be given for muscles spasms due to LBP.
- Can cause acute confusion in older adults. Ⓖ
- Do not drive or operate dangerous equipment.

Opioids

Opioid analgesics, such as hydrocodone and oxycodone, are appropriate for treating moderate to severe pain.

- Tramadol is considered a weak opioid that can be used for OA.
- Monitor and intervene for adverse effects of opioid use, especially for older adults.
- If used, opioids should be taken on a short-term basis by most clients. Some clients who have chronic back pain may receive prescriptions for opioids for long-term use. ⓆEBP

Topical analgesics

Trolamine salicylate: Can provide varying amounts of temporary pain relief, depending on client response.

- Apply topically over the area of involvement.
- Contains salicylate.

Lidocaine 5% patch: Can be helpful for nerve pain and OA of knees for short-term use.

- Apply to clean, dry, intact skin for 12 hr each day.
- Can cause skin irritation.
- Contraindicated with class I antidysrhythmic medications.

Capsaicin: Can provide varying amounts of temporary pain relief depending on client response.

- Apply topically over an area of involvement.
- Use gloves for application; wash hands thoroughly to prevent burning of eyes.
- Made from alkaloid that is derived from hot peppers.
- It is thought to prevent transmission of pain sensations from peripheral neural transmitters.

CLIENT EDUCATION FOR CAPSAICIN

- Instruct the client to wear gloves during application of capsaicin. ⓆPCC
- Advise the client to wear nitrile gloves when applying capsaicin patch.
- Instruct the client to avoid applying tight dressings to area where capsaicin cream was applied to prevent skin irritation.
- Tell the client to wash hands immediately after applying capsaicin and avoid touching eyes or applying over broken skin areas, which can cause painful burning.
- Explain to the client that a burning sensation of the skin after application is normal and should subside.
- Instruct the client to apply frequently (up to four times a day) for maximum benefit.

COMPLEMENTARY AND ALTERNATIVE THERAPIES FOR SHORT-TERM PAIN RELIEF

- Chiropractic or spinal manipulation
- Imagery, acupuncture, acupressure, music therapy, massage, biofeedback, and herbal medicines

Glucosamine supplements

- Glucosamine is a naturally occurring chemical involved in the makeup of cartilage. Glucosamine sulfate is believed to aid in the synthesis of synovial fluid and rebuild cartilage.
- Glucosamine can decrease the cells that cause joint inflammation and degradation of cartilage.
- Glucosamine is often taken in combination with chondroitin and might not have a pain reduction effect.

CLIENT EDUCATION

- Consult the provider regarding use and dosage. ⒼS
- Contraindicated for clients who have hypertension or are pregnant or breastfeeding.
- Chondroitin can cause bleeding, especially for clients taking anticoagulants.
- Can cause mild GI upset (nausea, heartburn).
- Use with caution with shellfish allergy.
- Question clients about concurrent use of chondroitin, NSAIDs, heparin, and warfarin.

Intra-articular injections

- Glucocorticoids are used to treat localized inflammation. One joint may be injected no more than 4 times a year.
- Hyaluronic acid is used to replace the body's natural hyaluronic acid, which is destroyed by joint inflammation. It is currently only approved for treatment of hip and knee joints.

CLIENT EDUCATION: For hyaluronic acid, instruct clients to notify the provider of allergy to birds, feathers, or eggs because this medication is made from combs of chickens.

INTERPROFESSIONAL CARE

Physical therapy: Services can teach muscle strengthening exercises, application of heat, diathermy (treatment with electrical currents), ultrasonography (treatment with sound waves), or stretching and strengthening exercises. ⓆTC

- Phonophoresis: application of a topical medication, such as lidocaine, followed by ultrasound or iontophoresis (using heat and dexamethasone) may be used by a physical therapist to force medication into subcutaneous tissue and increase relief of pain.
- A transcutaneous electrical nerve stimulation (TENS) unit may be prescribed by the provider and applied by the physical therapist with client instruction on how to use it.

A nutritionist: may assist the client in diet for weight loss or control in relation to reduced activity level, providing teaching regarding foods high in calcium and vitamin D.

Occupational therapy: to increase independent function such as personal care or home skills.

THERAPEUTIC PROCEDURES

Conservative therapy includes balancing rest with activity, exercising with water therapy, joint positioning, using bracing or splints, cane, proper posture, wearing supportive shoes, and applying thermal therapies (heat or cold).

Osteoarthritis

Total joint arthroplasty or total joint replacement: When all other conservative measures fail, the client may choose to undergo total joint arthroplasty to relieve the pain and improve mobility and quality of life.

- Joint replacement is contraindicated with any type of infection.
- A dental exam and/or dental procedures should be done before surgery to decrease risk of infection.
- Uncontrolled diabetes or hypertension can cause major postoperative complications.

Low-back pain

MINIMALLY INVASIVE SURGERY

- **Microscopic endoscopic diskectomy or percutaneous endoscopy diskectomy:** Fluoroscopy is used to guide a tubular device through which the herniated disk is removed by cutting it out, or suctioning out the center of the disk.
- **Laser-assisted laparoscopic lumbar diskectomy:** Laparoscope and laser are used to treat the herniated disks.
- **Kyphoplasty:** A needle is inserted into the back to inflate a balloon to help the vertebra regain its shape. Then a cement substance is injected into the space. Vertebroplasty is very similar, but a balloon is not used.

OPEN SURGICAL PROCEDURES

- **Open diskectomy:** removal of the herniated disk
- **Laminectomy:** removal of part of the laminae and facet joints
- **Surgery for tumors or infection**
- **Arthrodesis/spinal fusion:** surgery to join or fuse two or more vertebrae
  - A bone graft from the pelvic bone or bone bank is used to make a bridge between vertebrae that are next to each other.
  - Metal implants can also be used.

Application Exercises

1. A nurse is assessing a client who has osteoarthritis of the knees and fingers. Which of the following manifestations should the nurse expect to find? (Select all that apply.)

   A. Heberden's nodes

   B. Swelling of all joints

   C. Small body frame

   D. Enlarged joint size

   E. Limp when walking

2. A nurse is providing information to a client who has osteoarthritis of the hip and knee. Which of the following information should the nurse include in the information? (Select all that apply.)

   A. Apply heat to joints to alleviate pain.

   B. Ice inflamed joints following activity.

   C. Install an elevated toilet seat.

   D. Take tub baths.

   E. Complete high-energy activities in the morning.

3. A nurse is providing information about capsaicin cream to a client who reports continuous knee pain from osteoarthritis. Which of the following information should the nurse include in the discussion?

   A. Continuous pain relief is provided.

   B. Inspect for skin irritation and cuts prior to application.

   C. Cover the area with tight bandages after application.

   D. Apply the medication every 2 hr during the day.

4. A nurse is caring for a client who injured her lower back during a fall and describes sharp pain in her back and down her left leg. In which of the following positions should the nurse plan to place the client to attempt to decrease her pain?

   A. Prone without use of pillows

   B. Semi-Fowler's with a pillow under the knees

   C. High-Fowler's with the knees flat on the bed

   D. Supine with the head flat

5. A nurse is providing teaching for a client who has a history of low back injury. Which of the following instructions should the nurse give the client to prevent future problems with low back pain? (Select all that apply)

   A. Engage in regular exercise including walking.

   B. Sit for up to 10 hr each day to rest the back.

   C. Maintain weight within 25% of ideal body weight.

   D. Create a smoking cessation plan.

   E. Wear low-heeled shoes.

Application Exercises Key

1. A. **CORRECT:** Heberden's nodes are enlarged nodules on the distal interphalangeal joints of the hands and feet of a client who has osteoarthritis.

   B. Swelling and pain of all joints is a manifestation of rheumatoid arthritis. A local inflammation of a joint is related to osteoarthritis.

   C. A small body frame is a risk factor for rheumatoid arthritis. Obesity is a risk factor for osteoarthritis.

   D. **CORRECT:** A client can manifest enlarged joints due to bone hypertrophy.

   E. **CORRECT:** A client can manifest a limp when walking due to pain from inflammation in the localized joint.

   Ⓝ *NCLEX® Connection: Physiological Adaptation, Pathophysiology*

2. A. **CORRECT:** Applying heat to joints can provide temporary relief of pain.

   B. **CORRECT:** Applying ice to inflamed joints following activity can decrease edema.

   C. **CORRECT:** Installing an elevated toilet seat can help decrease strain and pain of the affected joints.

   D. Taking a tub bath places the client at risk for increased strain and pain on the affected joints when getting in and out of the tub and increases the risk for falls.

   E. **CORRECT:** Encouraging high-energy activity in the morning is recommended as part of a daily routine to promote independence.

   Ⓝ *NCLEX® Connection: Physiological Adaptation, Alterations in Body Systems*

3. A. Capsaicin cream provides temporary relief of pain rather than continuous relief when applied several times daily.

   B. **CORRECT:** Inspect the skin for irritation and cuts before applying capsaicin cream, because hot peppers in the cream can cause a painful burning sensation in areas of skin breakdown.

   C. After capsaicin cream is applied, avoid covering the area with a tight bandage, which can cause increased skin irritation.

   D. For maximum pain relief benefit, apply capsaicin cream up to four times a day.

   Ⓝ *NCLEX® Connection: Pharmacological and Parenteral Therapies, Medication Administration*

4. A. Prone position without use of pillows has not been found to decrease acute low back pain.

   B. **CORRECT:** Williams position, with the client in semi-Fowler's position with the knees flexed by pillows, has been found to relieve low-back pain caused by a bulging disk and nerve root involvement.

   C. High-Fowler's position with the knees flat has not been found to decrease acute low back pain.

   D. Supine position with the head flat has not been found to decrease acute low back pain.

   Ⓝ *NCLEX® Connection: Basic Care and Comfort, Non–Pharmacological Comfort Interventions*

5. A. **CORRECT:** Regular exercise, including walking or swimming, is a strategy that can prevent low back pain

   B. Long periods of sitting or standing can cause low-back pain. Advise the client to use footstools or ergonomic chairs when sitting is necessary.

   C. The client should maintain weight within 10% of ideal body weight, as obesity can cause low-back pain.

   D. **CORRECT:** Stopping or cutting down on smoking is a strategy that can decrease problems with low-back pain, as smoking can cause disk degeneration.

   E. **CORRECT:** Wearing low-heeled, well-fitting shoes can prevent low back pain. The nurse should instruct the client to avoid high-heeled shoes.

   Ⓝ *NCLEX Connection: Physiological Integrity, Mobility/Immobility*

PRACTICE Active Learning Scenario

A nurse is providing information on collaborative and nonpharmacologic therapies for a client who is having continual joint pain from osteoarthritis. What information should the nurse include? Use the ATI Active Learning Template: Basic Concept to complete this item.

RELATED CONTENT: Describe two activities each for collaborative care involving physical therapy and nutrition therapy.

NURSING INTERVENTIONS: Describe three actions the nurse could add to a teaching plan for this client.

PRACTICE Answer

Using the ATI Active Learning Template: Basic Concept

RELATED CONTENT
Physical therapy
- Apply heat, diathermy, and ultrasound.
- Perform stretching and strengthening exercises.
- Use transcutaneous electrical nerve stimulation (TENS).
Nutritional therapy
- Provide nutritional information on weight loss.
- Provide nutritional information on a balanced diet.
- Provide information on use of vitamin D and calcium.

NURSING INTERVENTIONS
- Balance rest with activity.
- Use braces, splints, and cane.
- Apply thermal therapies (heat or cold).
- Use assistive devices such as a long-handled reacher and an elevated toilet seat.
- Plan high-energy activities in the morning when feeling most rested.

Ⓝ *NCLEX® Connection: Health Promotion and Maintenance, Health Promotion/Disease Prevention*

When reviewing the following chapters, keep in mind the relevant topics and tasks of the NCLEX outline, in particular:

Client Needs: Basic Care and Comfort

MOBILITY/IMMOBILITY: Implement measures to promote circulation.

NUTRITION AND ORAL HYDRATION: Evaluate the impact of disease/illness on the nutritional status of client.

Client Needs: Reduction of Risk Potential

LABORATORY VALUES: Obtain specimens other than blood for diagnostic testing.

POTENTIAL FOR ALTERATIONS IN BODY SYSTEMS: Identify the client's potential for skin breakdown.

SYSTEM SPECIFIC ASSESSMENTS: Identify client with increased risk for insufficient vascular perfusion.

Client Needs: Physiological Adaptation

ALTERATIONS IN BODY SYSTEMS
Apply knowledge of nursing procedures, pathophysiology and psychomotor skills when caring for a client with an alteration in body systems.

Monitor wounds for signs and symptoms of infection.

Perform wound care or dressing change.

FLUID AND ELECTROLYTE IMBALANCES: Identify signs and symptoms of client fluid and/or electrolyte imbalance.

MEDICAL EMERGENCIES: Apply knowledge of pathophysiology when caring for a client experiencing a medical emergency.

UNIT 11   NURSING CARE OF CLIENTS WHO HAVE
INTEGUMENTARY DISORDERS

SECTION: DIAGNOSTIC AND THERAPEUTIC PROCEDURES

CHAPTER 73 *Integumentary Diagnostic Procedures*

Integumentary diagnostic procedures involve identification of pathogenic micro-organisms. The most accurate and definitive way to identify micro-organisms and cell characteristics is by examining blood, body fluids, and tissue samples under a microscope.

Skin lesions or changes in the skin can need confirmation by microscope to determine if the cause is viral, fungal, or bacterial.

Skin diagnostic studies

Wood's light examination

- Ultraviolet light is used to produce specific colors to reveal a skin infection.
- Examination is performed in a dark room to evaluate pigment changes in a light-skinned client.

Diascopy

A glass slide or lens is pressed down over the area to be examined to test for blanchability. It is used to determine whether the lesion is vascular (inflammatory) or nonvascular (nevus) or hemorrhagic (petechiae or purpura). Hemorrhagic and nonvascular lesions do not blanch, but inflammatory lesions do.

Skin culture and sensitivity

- **Culture** refers to isolation of the pathogen on culture media. Q EBP
- **Sensitivity** refers to the effect that antimicrobial agents have on the micro-organism.
  - If the micro-organism is killed by the antimicrobial, the microbe is considered to be sensitive to that medication.
  - If tolerable levels of the medication are unable to kill the microbe, the microbe is considered to be resistant to that medication.
- A culture and sensitivity can be done on a sample of purulent drainage from a skin lesion.
- Cultures should be done prior to initiating antimicrobial therapy.
- Results of a culture and sensitivity test usually are available preliminarily within 24 to 48 hr, and final results in 72 hr.

INDICATIONS

CLIENT PRESENTATION

- Skin lesions, which can be infectious, can appear raised, reddened, edematous, and/or warm.
- There can be purulent drainage and/or fever.

CONSIDERATIONS

PREPROCEDURE

NURSING ACTIONS
- Use standard precautions when collecting and handling specimens. Q s
- Most specimens will be collected by the nurse or provider.

INTRAPROCEDURE

Bacterial or viral specimens

NURSING ACTIONS
- Express material from the lesion by lifting or puncturing the crusted or scabbed area over the lesion using a small-gauge sterile needle or 0.9% sodium chloride and a sterile cotton swab.
- Culturette tubes are specific for specimen collection and contain a sterile cotton-tipped applicator and a fixative that is released after the infectious exudate is applied to the applicator and inserted in the tube.
- A specimen obtained for a viral culture is immediately placed on ice and sent to the laboratory.

Fungal specimen

NURSING ACTIONS
- Requires a sufficient quantity of scales collected using a wooden tongue depressor and placing the specimen in a clean container to be sent to the laboratory.
- If a fungal culture is needed because of inconclusive results due to a deeper fungal infection, a punch biopsy is performed.
- Specimens must be properly labeled and delivered to the laboratory promptly for appropriate storage and analysis.

POSTPROCEDURE

NURSING ACTIONS: Teach the client about measures to prevent the spread of an infectious skin disorder.

- **Bacterial infection:** Bathe daily using an antibacterial soap.
  - Do not squeeze bacterial lesions but remove the crusted exudate so the antibacterial topical medication can penetrate into the lesion.
  - Apply warm compresses twice daily for comfort to furuncles or areas where cellulitis is present. Qpcc
- **Viral lesion:** Apply compress of Burow's solution (aluminum acetate in water) for 20 min, three times a day to promote the formation of a crust and healing.
  - Avoid tight, restrictive clothing that can irritate a lesion.
  - Allow a lesion to dry between treatments, and avoid lying on the lesion to promote circulation and comfort.
  - Use good hand hygiene to prevent cross-contamination of the infection.
  - Avoid sharing personal items (combs, brushes, clothing, footwear).

Medication therapy for bacterial infections

- Superficial skin infections are treated with topical antibacterial cream or ointment.
- Extensive bacterial skin infections involving the lymphatic system, or if cellulitis is present, are treated with systemic antibiotic therapy (cephalosporins or penicillins).
- If allergic to cephalosporins and penicillins, the provider can prescribe tetracycline, erythromycin, azithromycin, or tobramycin.
- If the skin lesion is cultured as having methicillin-resistant *Staphylococcus aureus*, IV vancomycin or oral linezolid or clindamycin is prescribed.

Medication for viral infections

Topical treatment with acyclovir, valacyclovir, or famciclovir decreases the number of active viruses on the surface of the skin and reduces the discomfort associated with a herpetic infection or lesion.

Medication for fungal infections

- Yeast infections or dermatophyte infections are treated with topical cream or powder. For example, clotrimazole cream is applied to the infected skin twice a day and for 1 to 2 weeks after the lesions are no longer present, or as prescribed by the provider.
- Skin must be clean and dry before applying topical ointments or creams.

INTERPRETATION OF FINDINGS

BACTERIAL INFECTION
- The microbe responsible for the infection is identified in the culture, and the antimicrobials that are sensitive to that microbe are listed.
- Heavy growth of greater than 100,000 colonies definitively diagnoses an infection.
- Indeterminate results are 10,000 to 100,000 colonies.
- Negative results are less than 10,000 colonies.
- Appropriate medications are those with three to four degrees of sensitivity.

VIRAL INFECTION: Herpes virus: A cotton-tipped applicator is used to obtain vesicle fluid from intact lesions for culture.

Tzanck smear

A microscopic cytology examination is completed after extracting cells from the base of a lesion. Microscopic examination reveals multinucleated giant cells to confirm the lesion is viral.

Potassium hydroxide (KOH) test

- The test confirms a fungal skin lesion.
- A microscopic examination of the scales scraped off a lesion is mixed with KOH. Specimen is positive for fungus if there is the presence of fungal hyphae (threadlike filaments).

Biopsy

- Biopsy is the removal of a sample of tissue by excision or needle aspiration for cytological (histological) examination.
- Biopsy confirms or rules out malignancy.
- Skin biopsies are performed under local anesthesia.
- Biopsy for skin lesions can be a punch biopsy, shave biopsy, or excisional biopsy.

Punch biopsy: A small plug of tissue approximately 2 to 6 mm is removed with a specific cutting instrument, with or without sutures to close the site.

Shave biopsy: Removal of only the part of the lesion that is raised above the surrounding tissue using a scalpel or razor blade with no suturing.

Excisional biopsy: A larger and deeper specimen is obtained, and suturing is required.

INDICATIONS

POTENTIAL DIAGNOSES: A biopsy is commonly performed to establish an exact diagnosis or to rule out diseases such as cancer.

CLIENT PRESENTATION: Evidence of skin lesion can include an area of discoloration that is thickened, thinned, raised, flat, rough, painful, open, dry, and/or itchy.

CONSIDERATIONS

PREPROCEDURE

NURSING ACTIONS
- Ensure that the client has signed the informed consent form.
- Explain the procedure to the client.

CLIENT EDUCATION
- Inform the client about what to expect in regard to the formation of a scar.
- Teach the client about what to expect about the test or procedure.

INTRAPROCEDURE

NURSING ACTIONS
- Explain to the client what to expect according to the type of biopsy.
- Assist the provider with the test or procedure as needed, and assist with local anesthesia.
- Establish a sterile field. Qs
- Place the tissue sample in a container containing appropriate solution, label, and send to the laboratory.
- Apply pressure to the biopsy site to control bleeding as appropriate.
- Place a sterile dressing over the biopsy site as appropriate.

POSTPROCEDURE

Postbiopsy discomfort usually is relieved by mild analgesics.

NURSING ACTIONS: Monitor the biopsy site as appropriate.

CLIENT EDUCATION
- Teach the client to report excessive bleeding or evidence of infection (redness, warmth, drainage, fever) to the provider. Qs
- Teach the client to check the incision daily. The incision should be clean, dry, and intact.
- The client may remove dressings after 8 hr, and may use tap water or 0.9% sterile sodium chloride to clean the biopsy site of dried blood or crusts.
- If prescribed, the client may apply an antibacterial topical medication to prevent infection.
- If sutures are used, the client should return to the provider for removal in 7 to 10 days.

INTERPRETATION OF FINDINGS

After a biopsy is completed, the tissue sample is sent to pathology for interpretation.

Application Exercises

1. A nurse is caring for a client who has a suspected viral skin lesion. Which of the following laboratory findings should the nurse anticipate reviewing to confirm this diagnosis?

   A. Potassium hydroxide (KOH)

   B. Diascopy

   C. Tzanck smear report

   D. Biopsy

2. A nurse in a clinic is preparing to obtain a skin specimen from a client who has a suspected herpes infection. Which of the following actions should the nurse take? (Select all that apply.)

   A. Scrape the site with a wooden tongue depressor.

   B. Puncture the crusted area with a sterile needle.

   C. Swab the crusted area with a sterile cotton-tipped applicator.

   D. Place cotton-tipped applicator in culturette tube.

   E. Place culturette tube in ice.

3. A nurse is instructing a client on home care after a culture for a bacterial infection and cellulitis. Which of the following information should the nurse include in the teaching?

   A. Bathe daily with moisturizing soap.

   B. Apply antibacterial topical medication to the crusted exudate.

   C. Apply warm compresses to the affected area.

   D. Cover affected area with snug-fitting clothing.

4. A nurse is providing discharge instructions to a client who had a skin biopsy with sutures. The nurse should identify that which of the following client statements indicates that the teaching has been effective?

   A. "I can expect redness around the site for 5 to 7 days."

   B. "I will most likely have a fever for the first few days."

   C. "I should apply an antibiotic ointment to the area."

   D. "I will make a return appointment in 3 days for removal of my sutures."

5. A nurse is providing teaching to a client about a new prescription for clotrimazole topical cream. Which of the following statements should the nurse include in the teaching?

   A. "It reduces the discomfort of a herpetic infection but does not cure the infection."

   B. "This is a cream to treat a bacterial infection."

   C. "Apply the topical medication for up to 2 weeks after the fungal lesions are gone."

   D. "Apply the cream to lesions while they are moist."

Application Exercises Key

1. A. Findings of a potassium hydroxide (KOH) test reveal if skin lesions are fungal in origin.

   B. Diascopy provides increased visibility of a skin lesion by blanching the skin over the lesion, thus eliminating erythema which can obscure findings.

   C. **CORRECT:** A Tzanck smear report confirms whether a skin lesion is viral in origin.

   D. Findings of a biopsy report confirm or rule out if a lesion is malignant.

   Ⓝ *NCLEX® Connection: Reduction of Risk Potential, Diagnostic Tests*

2. A. A wooden tongue depressor is used to scrape cells of a skin lesion to test for a fungus.

   B. **CORRECT:** Exudate under the crusted area should be collected. The crust or scab should be punctured or lifted to obtain a reliable specimen.

   C. Swab the moist lesion bed under the crust with a sterile cotton-tipped applicator to obtain a reliable specimen.

   D. **CORRECT:** The cotton-tipped applicator is placed in liquid fixative within the culturette tube.

   E. **CORRECT:** The culturette tube is immediately placed in ice when obtaining a viral specimen.

   Ⓝ *NCLEX® Connection: Reduction of Risk Potential, Diagnostic Tests*

3. A. The client should use antibacterial soap to reduce the bacteria count on the skin.

   B. The client should apply topical medication directly to the moist lesion bed. The medication will not penetrate the crusted exudate.

   C. **CORRECT:** The client should apply warm compresses to the affected area to promote comfort.

   D. The client should wear loose-fitting clothes to avoid irritating the lesion.

   Ⓝ *NCLEX® Connection: Reduction of Risk Potential, Therapeutic Procedures*

4. A. The client should report redness, pain, drainage, or warmth at the biopsy site to the provider.

   B. A fever is an indication of an infection, and the provider should be notified.

   C. **CORRECT:** Antibiotic ointment is applied as prescribed by the provider to prevent infection.

   D. Removal of the sutures following a biopsy is done 7 to 10 days postprocedure.

   Ⓝ *NCLEX® Connection: Reduction of Risk Potential, Therapeutic Procedures*

5. A. Clotrimazole is not an antiviral medication to treat a herpetic infection.

   B. Clotrimazole is not an antibacterial medication.

   C. **CORRECT:** Clotrimazole is a medication used to treat a fungal infection and is applied for 1 to 2 weeks after the infection is resolved.

   D. Clotrimazole should be applied to clean, dry skin. Wash the skin gently and pat dry before applying.

   Ⓝ *NCLEX® Connection: Pharmacological and Parenteral Therapies, Medication Administration*

PRACTICE Active Learning Scenario

A nurse is caring for a client who will have a biopsy of a skin lesion. What should the nurse consider in planning for the procedure? Use the ATI Active Learning Template: Basic Concept to complete this item.

UNDERLYING PRINCIPLES: List and describe the three types of integumentary biopsies.

NURSING INTERVENTIONS: Describe two intraprocedure nursing actions.

PRACTICE Answer

Using the ATI Active Learning Template: Basic Concept

UNDERLYING PRINCIPLES

- Punch biopsy: A 2 to 6 mm plug of tissue is removed from the skin lesion, followed with or without suturing.
- Shave biopsy: A scalpel or razor blade removes only the raised area of the lesion, with no suturing.
- Excisional biopsy: A large, deep specimen of tissue is obtained, followed with suturing.

NURSING INTERVENTIONS

- Assist with setting up materials for placement of a local anesthetic.
- Apply pressure to the biopsy site to control bleeding.
- Place a sterile dressing over the biopsy site if needed.

Ⓝ *NCLEX® Connection: Reduction of Risk Potential, Therapeutic Procedures*

CHAPTER 74 *Skin Disorders*

Psoriasis is a skin disorder characterized by scaly, dermal patches and caused by overproduction of keratin. This overproduction can occur at a rate up to seven times the rate of normal cells. It is thought to be an autoimmune disorder and has periods of exacerbations and remissions. Although lesions can appear anywhere, they are commonly present on the elbows, knees, trunk, scalp, sacrum, and the lateral aspects of extremities. Psoriasis can be classified as psoriasis vulgaris, exfoliative, or palmoplantar pustulosis. In some clients, psoriasis affects the joints, causing arthritis-type changes and pain.

Dermatitis is an inflammation of the skin resulting from exposure to allergens (internal or external) that causes changes in the skin structure or tissue destruction. Manifestations of dermatitis can be nonspecific and include itching, lesions without distinct borders, and different distribution patterns. Rashes can evolve from acute to chronic, and place the client at increased risk for bacterial infection resulting from breaks in the skin caused by scratching. Dermatitis can be classified as eczematous, contact, or atopic.

Psoriasis

ASSESSMENT

RISK FACTORS

- Infections (severe streptococcal throat infection, Candida infection, upper respiratory infection)
- Skin trauma (recent surgery, sunburn)
- Genetics
- Stress (related to overstimulation of the immune system)
- Seasons (warm weather improves symptoms)
- Hormones (puberty or menopause)
- Medications (lithium, beta-blocker, indomethacin)
- Obesity
- Female gender

EXPECTED FINDINGS

- **Psoriasis vulgaris** presents as reddened, thickened skin with silvery white scales with bilateral distribution.
- **Exfoliative psoriasis** displays as erythema and scaling from a severe inflammatory reaction with no obvious lesions. The reaction can cause dehydration and hypothermia or hyperthermia.
- **Palmoplantar pustulosis** manifests as reddened hyperkeratotic areas (accelerated maturation of epidermal cells) due to an inflammatory disorder. Plaques form and pustules turn brown, peel, and form a crust on the palms of the hands and soles of the feet. The course of the disease is cyclic.
- Exacerbation and remission of pruritic lesions

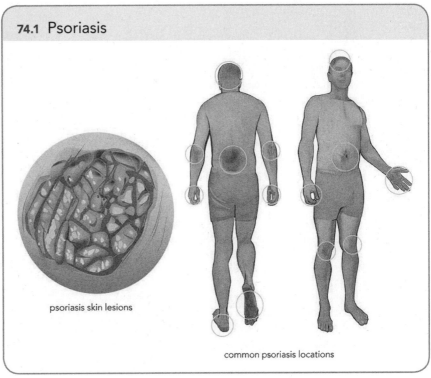

74.1 Psoriasis

psoriasis skin lesions

common psoriasis locations

PHYSICAL ASSESSMENT FINDINGS
- Scaly patches
- Bleeding stimulated by removal of scales
- Skin lesions primarily on the scalp, elbows and knees, sacrum, and lateral areas of the extremities (psoriasis vulgaris)
- Pitting, crumbling nails

PATIENT-CENTERED CARE

MEDICATIONS

Topical therapies

Corticosteroids (triamcinolone, betamethasone): reduce secondary inflammatory response of lesions and suppresses cellular division/proliferation.
- NURSING ACTIONS
  - Observe skin for thinning, striae, or hypopigmentation with high-potency corticosteroids.
  - Instruct client on proper application
- CLIENT EDUCATION
  - Instruct the client to apply high-potency corticosteroids as prescribed to prevent adverse effects and take periodic medication vacations.
  - The provider may instruct the client to use warm, moist, occlusive dressings of plastic wrap (gloves, plastic garments, booties) after applying the topical medication. These can be left in place up to 8 hr each day.
  - Instruct the client to avoid application of medication on face or into skin folds. May apply medication to scalp.

Tar preparations: coal tar and tars made from trees (juniper, birch, and pine) that suppress cellular division/proliferation and reduces inflammation.
- NURSING ACTIONS
  - Monitor skin for irritation.
  - Instruct the client on proper application
- CLIENT EDUCATION
  - Advise the client that tar applications can cause stinging and burning.
  - Advise the client that tar applications can cause staining of the skin and hair.
  - Due to odor and staining, the client should apply this product at night and cover areas of body with old pajamas, gloves, and socks.

Vitamin D analogs (calcipotriene, calcitriol): prevents cellular proliferation
- NURSING ACTIONS
  - Monitor for itching, irritation, and erythema.
  - Monitor for hypercalcemia (elevated serum calcium, muscle weakness, fatigue, anorexia).
- CLIENT EDUCATION
  - Instruct client to limit sun exposure due to increased risk of developing skin cancer.
  - Instruct client on proper application.
  - Instruct client on recognition of cancerous lesions.

Vitamin A (tazarotene): slows cellular division and reduces inflammation
- NURSING ACTIONS
  - Contraindicated during pregnancy. Qpcc
  - Monitor for localized reactions, inflammation, and desquamation of the skin.
- CLIENT EDUCATION
  - Instruct clients on proper application.
  - Instruct clients to avoid exposure to sun or artificial UV light.
  - Instruct clients to use reliable forms of birth control
  - Discontinue use and notify provider if pregnancy occurs.

Systemic medications

Cytotoxic medications (methotrexate, acitretin): reduce turnover of epidermal cells; used for severe, intractable cases
- NURSING ACTIONS
  - Monitor liver function tests for liver toxicity if methotrexate or acitretin therapy is being used.
  - Methotrexate can cause bone marrow suppression (leukopenia, thrombocytopenia, anemia).
  - Contraindicated during pregnancy and can cause fetal death or congenital anomalies.
- CLIENT EDUCATION
  - Instruct the client to avoid alcohol while taking these medications.
  - Advise the client to monitor for fever, sore throat, increased bleeding or bruising, and fatigue.
  - Inform the client these medications can decrease the effectiveness of contraceptives.

Biologic agents: first-line treatment for moderate to severe plaque psoriasis that suppress immune function (adalimumab, etanercept, ustekinumab, alefacept, and infliximab)
- NURSING ACTIONS
  - Evaluate for latent tuberculosis and hepatitis B virus.
  - Inspect prefilled syringe for particles or discoloration.
  - Rotate injection sites, and do not rub after administration.
  - Protect medication from light.
- CLIENT EDUCATION
  - Inform the client not to take if pregnant or breastfeeding.
  - Teach the client how to administer subcutaneous medication.
  - Instruct the client to report signs of infection.
  - Educate the client about need for lifelong treatment and the increased risk of cancer.
  - Instruct the client to not receive any live vaccines while taking the medication.

Cyclosporine and azathioprine
- Immunosuppressant medications are administered when lesions do not respond to other therapies.
- Nephrotoxicity occurs and increases the risk of infections.

THERAPEUTIC PROCEDURES

Photochemotherapy and ultraviolet light (PUVA therapy)
- A psoralen photosensitizing medication (methoxsalen) is administered followed by long-wave ultraviolet A (UVA) to decrease proliferation of epidermal cells.
- Methoxsalen is given orally 2 hr before UV treatments.
- Treatments are given two to three times per week, avoiding consecutive days.
- NURSING ACTIONS
  - Monitor the skin's response to light (redness, tenderness, tanning).
  - Ensure that the client wears eye protection during treatment and for 24 hr following a treatment (indoors and outside). Qs
- CLIENT EDUCATION
  - Instruct the client to notify the provider of extreme redness, swelling, and discomfort.
  - Inform the client of the long-term effects of premature skin aging, cataracts, and skin cancer.

Narrow-band ultraviolet B light therapy can be implemented without medication application, and requires fewer treatments.

Dermatitis

HEALTH PROMOTION AND DISEASE PREVENTION

- If the cause is identified, avoidance therapy is used.
- Do not scratch affected areas because it can cause secondary skin infections.
- Use products (soap, laundry detergent, cosmetics) that do not contain fragrance.
- Avoid the use of fabric softener dryer sheets.
- Wash skin thoroughly after exposure to irritants.
- Apply cool, damp compresses to rash to decrease inflammation.
- Use colloidal oatmeal baths to relieve itching.

ASSESSMENT

RISK FACTORS

- External skin exposure to allergens
- Internal exposure to allergens and irritants
- Stress (eczematous dermatitis)
- Genetic predisposition (eczematous dermatitis)
- Specific cause not always known

EXPECTED FINDINGS

Eczematous dermatitis

- Development of thickened areas of skin
- Can appear dry or moist and crusted
- Pruritus
- Symmetrical involvement usually of face, neck, arms, legs, and feet

Contact dermatitis

- Caused by exposure to allergen, chemical, or mechanical irritation.
- Rash is well-demarcated.
- Distribution varies depending upon the cause and the exposure to the allergen.

Atopic dermatitis

- Chronic rash.
- Can be caused by allergens or chronic skin disease.
- Development of thickened areas of skin along with scaling and desquamation.
- Pruritus can be intense.
- Distribution includes face, neck, and upper torso along with skin folds (antecubital, popliteal).

PATIENT-CENTERED CARE

Avoidance therapy if cause identified

MEDICATIONS

Steroid therapy: topical, intralesional, systemic (hydrocortisone, betamethasone, triamcinolone, prednisone)
- Reduce secondary inflammatory response of lesions.
- NURSING ACTIONS
  - Instruct clients using steroids for long periods to taper doses when discontinuing medication.
  - Monitor for adrenal suppression.
  - Advise clients to avoid using topical steroids on lesions that are infected.
  - Instruct client about proper application.
- CLIENT EDUCATION Qpcc
  - Warm, moist dressings may be used over topical application to increase absorption of medication.
  - Advise the client to avoid the use of occlusive dressings over rash after applying topical steroid medications.

Antihistamines: topical, systemic (diphenhydramine, cetirizine, fexofenadine)
- Relief of redness, pruritus, and edema
- NURSING ACTIONS: Monitor for urinary retention with the use of systemic medications.
- CLIENT EDUCATION
  - Advise client that product can cause photosensitivity.
  - Caution the client to avoid operating machinery and driving while taking systemic antihistamine.
  - Advise client to take systemic form at bedtime, as product can cause drowsiness.

Topical immunosuppressants: tacrolimus, pimecrolimus
- For use in treatment of eczematous dermatitis that has been resistant to glucocorticoid treatment
- Relieves inflammation
- NURSING ACTIONS
  - Instruct client on application of medication.
  - Monitor for erythema, burning sensation.
  - Avoid the use of occlusive dressings.
- CLIENT EDUCATION
  - Avoid use if infection is present.
  - Discontinue use when rash clears.
  - Avoid direct sunlight and the use of tanning beds.

Application Exercises

1. A nurse is providing information about a new prescription for corticosteroid cream to a client who has mild psoriasis. Which of the following instructions should the nurse include? (Select all that apply.)

   A. Apply an occlusive dressing after application.

   B. Apply three to four times per day.

   C. Wear gloves after application to lesions on the hands.

   D. Avoid applying in skin folds.

   E. Use medication continuously over a period of several months.

2. A nurse is teaching a client who has a history of psoriasis about photochemotherapy and ultraviolet light (PUVA) treatments. Which of the following instructions should the nurse include in the teaching?

   A. Apply vitamin A cream before each treatment.

   B. Administer a psoralen medication before the treatment.

   C. Use this treatment every evening.

   D. Remove the scales gently following each treatment.

3. A nurse is educating a female client on the use of calcipotriene topical medication for the treatment of psoriasis. Which of the following information should the nurse include? (Select all that apply.)

   A. Recommended for facial lesions.

   B. Expect a stinging sensation upon application.

   C. Apply to the scalp.

   D. Obtain a pregnancy test.

   E. Limit application to skin folds.

4. A nurse is providing teaching to the parent of a child who has contact dermatitis. Which of the following information should the nurse include?

   A. Use fabric softener dryer sheets when drying the child's clothing.

   B. Apply a warm, dry compress to the rash area.

   C. Place the child in a bath with colloidal oatmeal.

   D. Leave the child's hands uncovered during the night.

5. A nurse caring for a client who has contact dermatitis and has a new prescription for diphenhydramine. For which of the following adverse effects should the nurse monitor?

   A. Elevated blood glucose levels

   B. Urinary retention

   C. Hyperpigmentation of the skin

   D. Insomnia

PRACTICE Active Learning Scenario

A nurse is providing information to a client who has a prescription for pimecrolimus to treat severe eczematous dermatitis. What information should the nurse include? Use the ATI Active Learning Template: Medication to complete this item.

THERAPEUTIC USES

NURSING INTERVENTIONS: Describe two.

CLIENT EDUCATION: Describe two teaching points.

Application Exercises Key

1. A. **CORRECT:** An occlusive dressing can enhance the efficacy of the topical corticosteroid on the exposed lesions.

   B. Corticosteroid cream is applied twice daily to prevent development of local and systemic adverse effects.

   C. **CORRECT:** Gloves worn after the medication can enhance the efficacy of the topical corticosteroid on the exposed lesions of the hands.

   D. **CORRECT:** Corticosteroid cream applied to lesions in skin folds increases the risk of yeast infections.

   E. The client should take periodic medication "vacations" to minimize the risk for development of local and systemic adverse effects.

   Ⓝ *NCLEX® Connection: Pharmacological and Parenteral Therapies, Medication Administration*

2. A. PUVA treatment does not involve the use of vitamin A cream.

   B. **CORRECT:** PUVA treatment involves the administration of a medication, such as a psoralen, to enhance photosensitivity.

   C. PUVA treatments are completed two to three times each week and not on consecutive days.

   D. Removal of scales can cause bleeding and is not recommended when treating psoriasis.

   Ⓝ *NCLEX® Connection: Reduction of Risk Potential, Therapeutic Procedures*

3. A. Applying calcipotriene to the face is not recommended because it can cause facial dermatitis.

   B. **CORRECT:** Calcipotriene causes stinging and burning sensations when applied to the lesions.

   C. **CORRECT:** Calcipotriene solution is applied to scalp lesions.

   D. **CORRECT:** Calcipotriene can cause birth defects. Female clients should obtain a pregnancy test before using the medication.

   E. **CORRECT:** Applying calcipotriene to skin folds can cause a possible local reaction of itching, irritation, and erythema.

   Ⓝ *NCLEX® Connection: Pharmacological and Parenteral Therapies, Medication Administration*

4. A. The parent should avoid the use of fabric softener dryer sheets when cleaning the child's clothing. Liquid fabric softener may be used.

   B. The parent should apply a cool, moist compress to the child's rash area to decrease inflammation.

   C. **CORRECT:** The use of a colloidal oatmeal bath will relieve the child's itching.

   D. The parent should apply mittens on the child's hands at night to decrease unconscious scratching of the rash, which can lead to a secondary infection.

   Ⓝ *NCLEX® Connection: Health Promotion and Maintenance, Health Promotion/Disease Prevention*

5. A. Glucocorticoids such as prednisone can increase blood glucose levels. However, this is not an adverse effect of diphenhydramine.

   B. **CORRECT:** The nurse should monitor the client's urinary output, as retention is a possible adverse effect of diphenhydramine.

   C. Hyperpigmentation of the skin can be seen in clients who have adrenal insufficiency, but is not associated with the use of diphenhydramine.

   D. Diphenhydramine is a first-generation antihistamine and can cause excessive drowsiness rather than insomnia.

   Ⓝ *NCLEX® Connection: Pharmacological and Parenteral Therapies, Medication Administration*

PRACTICE Answer

Using the ATI Active Learning Template: Medication

THERAPEUTIC USES: Relieve itching

NURSING INTERVENTIONS
- Instruct client on application of medication.
- Monitor for erythema, burning sensation.
- Avoid the use of occlusive dressings.

CLIENT EDUCATION
- Avoid use if infection is present.
- Discontinue use when rash clears.
- Avoid direct sunlight and the use of tanning beds.

Ⓝ *NCLEX® Connection: Pharmacological and Parenteral Therapies, Medication Administration*

UNIT 11   NURSING CARE OF CLIENTS WHO HAVE
            INTEGUMENTARY DISORDERS
            SECTION: INTEGUMENTARY DISORDERS

CHAPTER 75 *Burns*

Dry heat, moist heat, direct contact with hot surfaces, chemicals, electricity, and ionizing radiation can cause burns, which result in cellular destruction of the skin layers and underlying tissue. The type and severity of the burn affect the treatment plan.

In addition to destruction of body tissue, a burn injury results in the loss of temperature regulation, sweat and sebaceous gland function, and sensory function. Metabolism increases to maintain body heat as a result of burn injury and tissue damage.

TYPES OF BURNS

Dry heat injuries result from open flames and explosions.

Moist heat injuries result from contact with hot liquid or steam. Scald injuries are more common in older adults and younger children.

Contact burns occur when hot metal, tar, or grease contacts the skin.

Chemical burns result from exposure to a caustic agent. Cleaning agents in the home (drain cleaner, oven cleaner, bleach) and agents in the industrial setting (caustic soda, sulfuric acid) can cause chemical burns.

Electrical burns result when an electrical current passes through the body and can cause severe damage, including loss of organ function, tissue destruction with subsequent need for amputation of a limb, and cardiac or respiratory arrest.

Thermal burns result when clothes ignite from heat or flames that electrical sparks produce.

Flash (arc) burns result from contact with electrical current that travels through the air from one conductor to another.

Conductive electrical injury results when a person touches electrical wiring or equipment.

Radiation burns most often result from therapeutic treatment for cancer or from sunburn.

SEVERITY OF THE BURNS

Percentage of total body surface area (TBSA): Use standardized charts for age groups to identify the extent of the injury and calculate medication doses, fluid replacement volumes, and caloric needs. QEBP

Depth of the burn: Classify burns according to the layers of skin and tissue involved: superficial, partial, full, and deep full thickness.

Body location of the burn: In areas where the skin is thinner, there is more damage to underlying tissue (any part of the face, hand, perineum, feet).

Age: Young clients and older adult clients have less reserve capacity to deal with a burn injury. Skin thins with aging, so more damage to underlying tissue can occur. ©

Causative agent: Thermal, chemical, electrical, or radioactive.

Presence of other injuries: Fractures or other injuries increase the risk of complications.

Involvement of the respiratory system: Inhalation of deadly fumes, smoke, steam, and heated air can cause respiratory failure or airway edema. Carbon monoxide poisoning also can occur, especially if the injury took place in an enclosed area.

Overall health of the client: A client who has a chronic illness has a greater risk of complications and a worse prognosis.

METHODS TO ASSESS BURNS

Rule of Nines: Quick method to approximate the extent of burns by dividing the body into multiples of nine. The sum equals the TBSA.

Lund and Browder Method: A more exact method estimating the extent of burn by the percentage of surface area of specific anatomic parts, particularly the head and legs.

Palmar Method: Quick method to approximate scattered burns using the palm of the client's hand. The palm of the hand (including the fingers) is equal to 1% TBSA.

Other more accurate evaluation methods include indocyanine green video angiography and laser Doppler imaging. Both show areas of high and low tissue perfusion.

THREE PHASES OF BURN CARE

Emergent (resuscitative phase)

- Begins with the injury and continues for 24 to 48 hr.
- Priorities include securing the airway, supporting circulation and organ perfusion by fluid replacement, managing pain, preventing infection through wound care, maintaining body temperature, and providing emotional support.

Acute

- Begins 36 to 48 hr after injury when the fluid shift resolves.
- Ends with closure of the wound.
- Priorities include assessment and maintenance of the cardiovascular, respiratory, and gastrointestinal systems (including nutrition); wound care; pain control; and psychosocial interventions.

Rehabilitative

- Begins when most of the burn area has healed.
- Ends when the client achieves the highest level of functioning possible.
- Priorities include psychosocial support; prevention of scars and contractures; and resumption of activities, including work, family, and social roles.
- This phase can last for years.

HEALTH PROMOTION AND DISEASE PREVENTION

- Ensure that the number and placement of fire extinguishers and smoke alarms in the home is adequate and operable. Family members should know how to use the extinguishers.
- Keep emergency numbers near the phone. Qs
- Have a family exit and meeting plan for fires. Reinforce that no one should ever re-enter a burning building.
- Review with clients of all ages that in the event that clothing or skin is on fire, they should "stop, drop, and roll" to extinguish the fire.
- Store matches and lighters out of reach and out of sight of children and adults who lack the ability to protect themselves.
- Reduce the setting on water heaters to 48.9° C (120° F).
- Have an annual professional inspection and cleaning of the chimney and fireplace.
- Turn handles of pots and pans to the side, or use back burners.
- Don't leave hot cups on the edge of the counter.
- Cover electrical outlets.
- Keep flammable objects away from space heaters.
- Wear gloves when handling chemicals.
- Teach clients to wear protective clothing during sun exposure and to use sunscreen.
- Instruct clients to avoid using tanning beds.
- Avoid smoking in bed and when under the influence of alcohol or sedating medications.
- Do not smoke or have open flames in a room where oxygen is in use.
- Never add flammable substances (gasoline, lighter fluid, kerosene) to an open flame.

75.1 Depth of injury

	Superficial thickness	Superficial partial thickness	Deep partial thickness	Full thickness	Deep full thickness
AREA INVOLVED	Damage to epidermis	Damage to the entire epidermis and some parts of the dermis	Damage to entire epidermis and deep into the dermis	Damage to the entire epidermis and dermis Can extend into the subcutaneous tissue Nerve damage	Damage to all layers of skin Extends to muscle, tendons, and bones
APPEARANCE	Pink to red No blisters Mild edema No eschar	Pink to red Blisters Mild to moderate edema No eschar	Red to white No blisters Moderate edema Eschar soft and dry	Red, black, brown, yellow, or white No blisters Severe edema Eschar hard and inelastic	Black No blisters No edema Eschar hard and inelastic
SENSATION/ HEALING	Painful/ Tender Sensitive to heat Heals within 3 to 6 days No scarring	Painful Heals within 3 weeks No scarring, but minor pigment changes	Painful and sensitive to touch Heals in 2 to 6 weeks Scarring likely Possible grafting	Sensation minimal or absent Heals within weeks to months Scarring Grafting	Heals within weeks to months Scarring Grafting
EXAMPLE	Sunburn Flash burn (sudden intense heat)	Flash flame and scalds Brief contact with hot object	Flame and scalds Grease, tar, or chemical burns Prolonged exposure to hot objects	Scalds Grease, tar, chemical, or electrical burns Prolonged exposure to hot objects	Electrical burns Flames

ASSESSMENT

RISK FACTORS

- Inhalation injury
- OLDER ADULTS Ⓖ
  - Higher risk for damage to subcutaneous tissue, muscle, connective tissue, and bone because of thinner skin
  - Higher risk for complications from burns because of chronic illnesses (e.g., diabetes mellitus, cardiovascular disease)

EXPECTED FINDINGS

- Report of burn agent (dry heat, moist heat, chemical, electrical, ionizing radiation)
- Duration of contact
- Body area of the burn
- Demographic data: age, weight, height
- Health history, including pre-existing illnesses

PHYSICAL ASSESSMENT FINDINGS (75.2)

Levels of care

Inhalation damage findings include singed nasal hair, eyebrows, and eyelashes; sooty sputum; hoarseness; wheezing; edema of the nasal septum; and smoky smelling breath. Indications of the impending loss of the airway include hoarseness, brassy cough, drooling or difficulty swallowing, and audible wheezing, crowing, and stridor. Ⓠs

Carbon monoxide inhalation (from burns in an enclosed area) findings include headache, weakness, dizziness, confusion, erythema (pink or cherry red skin) and upper airway edema, followed by sloughing of the respiratory tract mucosa.

Hypovolemia and shock can result from fluid shifts from the intercellular and intravascular space to the interstitial space. Additional findings include hypotension, tachycardia, and decreased cardiac output.

LABORATORY TESTS

Resuscitation phase: Initial fluid shift (occurs in the first 12 hr and continues for 24 to 36 hr)
- **CBC** with differential
- **Glucose:** elevated due to stress
- **BUN:** elevated due to fluid loss
- **Hct and Hgb:** elevated (hemoconcentration) due to the loss of fluid volume and the fluid shift into the interstitial space (third spacing)
- Electrolytes
  - **Sodium:** decreased due to third spacing (hyponatremia)
  - **Potassium:** increased due to cell destruction (hyperkalemia)
- **Carboxyhemoglobin:** more than 10% strongly indicates smoke inhalation
- Other: total protein, albumin, ABGs, liver enzymes, urinalysis, and clotting studies

Fluid remobilization (starts at about 24 hr; diuretic stage begins at 48 to 72 hr after injury)
- **Hgb and Hct:** decreased (hemodilution) due to the fluid shift from the interstitial space back into vascular fluid
- **Sodium:** remains decreased due to renal and wound loss
- **Potassium:** decreased due to renal loss and movement back into cells (hypokalemia)
- **WBC count:** initial increase then decrease with left shift
- **Blood glucose:** elevated due to the stress response
- **ABGs:** slight hypoxemia and metabolic acidosis
- **Total protein and albumin:** low due to fluid loss

75.2 Burn staging

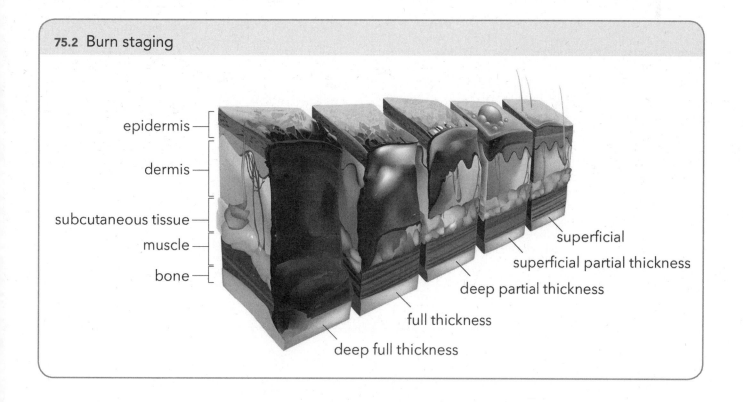

epidermis
dermis
subcutaneous tissue
muscle
bone

superficial
superficial partial thickness
deep partial thickness
full thickness
deep full thickness

DIAGNOSTIC PROCEDURES

Diagnostic studies can include renal scans, computed tomography, ultrasonography, bronchoscopy, and magnetic resonance imaging to determine extent of the burn injury.

PATIENT-CENTERED CARE

NURSING CARE

Minor burns

- Stop the burning process. Q_EBP
  ○ Remove clothing or jewelry that might conduct heat.
  ○ Apply cool water soaks or run cool water over injury; do not use ice.
  ○ Flush chemical burns with a large volume of water.
  ○ Cover the burn with a clean cloth to prevent contamination and hypothermia.
  ○ Provide warmth.
- Provide analgesics.
- Cleanse with mild soap and tepid water. (Avoid excess friction.)
- Use antimicrobial ointment.
- Apply a dressing (nonadherent, hydrocolloid) if clothing is irritating the burn.
- Educate the family to avoid using greasy lotions or butter on the burn.
- Teach the family to observe for evidence of infection.
- Determine the need for a tetanus immunization.

Moderate and major burns

During the initial (resuscitation) phase (from the time of injury to 12 to 48 hr later) following a major burn, sympathetic nervous system manifestations such as tachycardia, increased respiratory rate, decreased gastrointestinal motility, and increased blood glucose are expected findings.

Cardiovascular system: Presence of edema, central and peripheral pulses, capillary refill, pulse oximetry, invasive or noninvasive blood pressure, and electrocardiographic changes

Respiratory system
- Assess respiratory rate and depth.
- Upper airway edema becomes pronounced 8 to 12 hr after the beginning of fluid resuscitation. Crowing, stridor, or dyspnea requires nasal or oral intubation.
- Provide humidified supplemental oxygen.
- Support the airway and ventilation. Mechanical ventilation and paralytic medications (atracurium or vecuronium) can become necessary.
- Provide care for tracheotomy when long-term intubation is expected.
- Monitor and maintain chest tubes.
- Instruct the client to cough, breathe deeply, and use incentive spirometry every hour.
- Suction (endotracheal or nasotracheal) every hour or as needed. Consider the need for additional analgesics.

Gastrointestinal system
- Clients at risk for aspiration might need NG tube insertion. Some clients experience gastroparesis and vomiting.
- Monitor stool, vomitus, and gastric secretions for blood.
- Keep the head of the bed elevated at all times.

Urinary system
- Insert an indwelling urinary catheter.
- Monitor I&O.
- Monitor urine characteristics, specific gravity, BUN, creatinine, and sodium.

Fluid replacement: To maintain cardiac output.
- Hypovolemic shock is a common cause of death in the resuscitation phase.
- Initiate IV access using a large-bore needle. If burns cover a large area of the body, the client requires insertion of a central venous catheter or intraosseous catheter.
- Fluid replacement is important during the first 24 hr.
- Third spacing (capillary leak syndrome) is a continuous leak of plasma from the vascular space into the interstitial space, which results in electrolyte imbalance and hypotension.
- Rapid fluid replacement during the emergent phase maintains tissue perfusion and prevents hypovolemic (burn) shock.
- Fluid resuscitation meets individual clients' needs (TBSA of burn, burn depth, inhalation injury, associated injuries, age, urine output, cardiac output, blood pressure, status of electrolytes).
- Administer half of the total 24-hr IV fluid volume within the first 8 hr and the remaining volume over the next 16 hr. Q_EBP
- Infuse isotonic crystalloid solutions, such as 0.9% sodium chloride or lactated Ringer's.
- Infuse colloid solutions, such as albumin or synthetic plasma expanders, after the first 24 hr of burn recovery.
- Monitor vital signs.
- Assess for fluid overload: edema, engorged neck veins, rapid and thready pulse, lung crackles, wheezes.
- Weigh the client daily.
- Maintain urine output of 30 mL/hr (0.5 mL/kg/hr).
- Prepare to administer blood products.
- Monitor for manifestations of shock.
  ○ Alterations in sensorium (confusion)
  ○ Increased capillary refill time
  ○ Urine output less than 30 mL/hr
  ○ Rapid elevations of temperature
  ○ Decreased bowel sounds
  ○ Blood pressure average or low.
- Maintain thermoregulation.

Hypothermia
- The skin helps control the body's temperature. With skin injury, the body loses heat.
- Use warm, inspired air, a warm room, warming blankets, and warmers for infusing fluids.

Hyperthermia
- Hypermetabolic conditions increase core body temperature.
- Low-grade temperature develops as a compensatory mechanism.

Pain management

- Monitor pain and the effectiveness of pain treatment.
- Avoid routes other than IV during the resuscitation phase due to decreased absorption from other routes.
- Use IV opioid analgesics, such as morphine, hydromorphone, and fentanyl or anesthetics, such as ketamine, and nitrous oxide. Q**EBP**
- Monitor for respiratory depression when administering opioid analgesics. Q**S**
- The use of patient-controlled analgesia (PCA) is appropriate for some clients. PCA helps manage pain, and the client benefits from having a sense of control.
- Administer pain medication prior to dressing changes and procedures.
- Use nonpharmacologic methods for pain control, such as guided imagery, music therapy, and therapeutic touch, to enhance the effects of analgesic medications and manage pain more effectively.

Infection prevention

- Maintain a protective environment.
- Restrict plants and flowers due to the risk of contact with *Pseudomonas aeruginosa*.
- Restrict consumption of fresh fruits and vegetables.
- Limit visitors.
- Monitor for manifestations of infection and report them to the provider.
- Use client-dictated equipment, such as blood pressure cuffs and thermometers.
- Administer tetanus toxoid.
- Administer antibiotics to treat infection. Monitor peak and trough levels.
- Use strict asepsis with wound care.

Nutritional support

- Large burn areas create a hypermetabolic and hypercatabolic state, requiring 5,000 calories/day. Caloric needs double or triple 4 to 12 days after the burn.
- Increase caloric intake to meet increased metabolic demands and prevent hypoglycemia.
- Increase protein intake to prevent tissue breakdown and promote healing.
- Decreased gastrointestinal motility and increased caloric needs require enteral therapy or total parenteral nutrition.

Restoration of mobility

- Maintain correct body alignment, splint extremities, and facilitate position changes to prevent contractures.
- Maintain active and passive range of motion.
- Assist with ambulation as soon as the client is stable.
- Apply pressure dressings to prevent contractures and scarring.
- Monitor areas at high risk for pressure sores (heels, sacrum, back of the head).

Psychological support of client and family

- Provide emotional support. Q**PCC**
- Assist with coping.

MEDICATIONS

Apply topical agents (antimicrobial creams, ointments, solutions).

Silver nitrate 0.5%

Apply with a gauze dressing.

ADVANTAGES
- Reduces fluid evaporation
- Bacteriostatic
- Inexpensive

DISADVANTAGES
- Does not penetrate eschar
- Stains clothing and linen
- Depletes sodium and potassium

Silver sulfadiazine 1%

Apply a thin layer with a clean glove.

ADVANTAGES
- Usually pain-free
- Effective against gram-negative bacteria, gram-positive bacteria, and yeast

DISADVANTAGES
- Can cause transient neutropenia
- Sulfa allergy is a contraindication
- Penetrates eschar minimally
- Can cause a gray or blue-green discoloration
- Decreases granulocyte formation

Mafenide acetate

Apply twice daily.

ADVANTAGES
- Penetrates eschar and goes into underlying tissues
- Bacteriostatic against gram-negative and gram-positive bacteria

DISADVANTAGES
- Painful to apply and remove
- Can cause metabolic acidosis

Polymyxin B-bacitracin

Apply every 2 to 8 hr to keep the burn moist.

ADVANTAGES
- Bacteriostatic against gram-positive organisms
- Painless and easy to apply

DISADVANTAGES: Hypersensitivity can develop.

Gentamicin topical

Aminoglycoside anti-infective agent

ADVANTAGES: Bactericidal aminoglycoside

DISADVANTAGES
- Nephrotoxic: Monitor kidney function.
- Ototoxic: Monitor for hearing loss weekly.

THERAPEUTIC PROCEDURES

Escharotomy

Incision through the eschar relieves pressure from the constricting force of fluid buildup under circumferential burns on the extremity or chest and improves circulation.

Fasciotomy

Incision through eschar and fascia relieves tissue pressure when escharotomy alone does not.

Wound care

Nonsurgical management, such as hyperbaric oxygen therapy

NURSING ACTIONS Qpcc
- Premedicate the client with an analgesic.
- Remove all previous dressings.
- Assess for odors, drainage, and discharge. Assess for sloughing, eschar, bleeding, and new skin-cell regeneration.
- Cleanse the wound thoroughly, removing all previous ointments.
- Assist with debridement.
  - **Mechanical:** Use scissors and forceps to cut away the dead tissue during the hydrotherapy treatment.
  - **Hydrotherapy:** Assist the client into a warm tub of water or use warm running water, as if to shower, to cleanse the wound.
    - Use mild soap or detergent to wash burns gently, and then rinse with room-temperature water.
    - Encourage the client to exercise his joints during the hydrotherapy treatment.
  - **Enzymatic:** Apply a topical enzyme to break down and remove dead tissue.
  - Apply topical enzyme agents such as collagenase to the wound during a daily dressing change.
- Ensure that the client does not become hypothermic during the treatment.
- Use surgical asepsis while applying a thin layer of topical antibiotic ointment and cover it with a dressing.

Skin coverings

Biologic skin coverings temporarily promote healing of large burns. Additionally, biologic skin coverings promote the retention of water and protein and provide coverage of nerve endings, thus reducing pain. The provider stipulates whether to leave skin coverings open or protect them with a dressing.
- Allograft (homograft): Skin donations from human cadavers for partial- and full-thickness burn wounds
- Xenograft (heterograft): Skin from animals, such as pigs, for partial-thickness burn wounds
- Amnion: From human placenta; requires frequent changes
- Cultured skin: Grows from a small specimen of epidermal cells from an unburned area
- Artificial skin: Two layers of skin made beef collagen and shark cartilage
- Synthetic skin coverings: For partial-thickness burn wounds

Permanent skin coverings can be the treatment of choice for burns covering large areas of the body.
- Autografts: Skin from another area of the client's body
  - Sheet graft: Sheet of skin for covering the wound
  - Mesh graft: Sheet of skin in which a mesher has created small slits, so the graft can stretch over large areas of the burn
- Artificial skin: Synthetic product for faster healing of partial- and full-thickness burns
- Cultured epithelium: Epithelial cells to use for clients who have few grafting sites

NURSING ACTIONS
- Maintain immobilization of graft sites.
- Elevate extremities.
- Provide wound care to the donor site.
- Administer analgesics.
- Monitor for infection before and after applying skin coverings or grafts. QEBP
  - Discoloration of unburned skin surrounding burn wound
  - Green subcutaneous fat
  - Degeneration of granulation tissue
  - Development of subeschar hemorrhage
  - Hyperventilation indicating systemic involvement of infection
  - Unstable body temperature

CLIENT EDUCATION
- Instruct the client to keep the extremity elevated.
- Instruct the client to report symptoms of infection.
- Determine the client's level of pain, and provide additional measures to control donor site pain.
- Instruct the client to continue to perform range-of-motion exercises and to work with a physical therapist to prevent contractures.
- Show the client how to observe the wound for infection and how to perform wound care.

INTERPROFESSIONAL CARE

- Initiate referrals to a dietitian, social worker (for community support services), psychological counselor, and physical therapist.
- Respiratory therapy can help improve pulmonary function.
- Consult a case manager to coordinate the client's post-discharge care.
- Initiate a referral for home health nursing care. QTC
- Initiate a referral to occupational therapy for evaluation of the home environment and assistance to relearn how to perform ADLs.

COMPLICATIONS

Airway injury

- Thermal injuries to the airway can result from steam or chemical inhalation, aspiration of scalding liquid, and external explosion while breathing. If the injury took place in an enclosed space, suspect carbon monoxide poisoning.
- Effects might not manifest for 24 to 48 hr. They include progressive hoarseness, brassy cough, difficulty swallowing, drooling, copious secretions, adventitious breath sounds, and expiratory sounds that include audible wheezes, crowing, and stridor.

NURSING ACTIONS: Support the airway and ventilation, and administer supplemental oxygen.

CLIENT EDUCATION: Educate the client and family about airway management, such as deep breathing, coughing, and elevating the head of the bed.

Fluid and electrolyte imbalances

NURSING ACTIONS
- Assess fluid volume status. Weigh the client daily, and document I&O.
- Monitor laboratory results and compare them to previous data.
- Administer IV fluids and electrolytes.

CLIENT EDUCATION: Educate the client and family about signs and symptoms of electrolyte imbalances and the need to alert the provider immediately.

Wound infections

Burns can leave skin vulnerable to bacterial infection and increase risk of infection and sepsis.

NURSING ACTIONS
- Assess for discoloration, edema, odor, and drainage.
- Assess for fluctuations in temperature and heart rate.
- Obtain specimens for wound culture.
- Administer antibiotics.
- Monitor laboratory results, observing for anemia and infection.
- Use surgical aseptic technique with dressing changes.

CLIENT EDUCATION: Educate the client and family about the importance of infection control.

Muscle and joint mobility

Scarring and contractures: Deep burns can limit movement of bones and joints. Scar tissue can form and cause shortening and tightening of skin, muscles, and tendons (contractures).

NURSING ACTIONS
- Assist with active or passive range–of–motion exercises at least three times daily.
- Encourage neutral positions with limited flexion. Encourage the use of splints.
- Encourage ambulation as soon as possible.
- Use compression dressings for up to 24 months to increase mobility and reduce scarring.

Application Exercises

1. A nurse in a provider's office is assessing a client who has a severe sunburn. Which of the following classifications should the nurse use to document this burn?

   A. Superficial thickness
   B. Superficial partial thickness
   C. Deep partial thickness
   D. Full thickness

2. A nurse is caring for a client who has sustained burns over 35% of his total body surface area. Of this total, 20% are full-thickness burns on the arms, face, neck, and shoulders. The client's voice has become hoarse. He has a brassy cough and is drooling. The nurse should identify these findings as indications that the client has which of the following?

   A. Pulmonary edema
   B. Bacterial pneumonia
   C. Inhalation injury
   D. Carbon monoxide poisoning

3. A nurse is assessing a client who sustained deep partial-thickness and full-thickness burns over 40% of his body 24 hr ago. Which of the following are findings should the nurse expect? (Select all that apply.)

   A. Dyspnea
   B. Bradycardia
   C. Hyperkalemia
   D. Hyponatremia
   E. Decreased hematocrit

4. A nurse is preparing to administer fentanyl to a client who sustained deep partial-thickness and full-thickness burns over 60% of his body 24 hr ago. The nurse should plan to use which of the following routes to administer the medication?

   A. Subcutaneous
   B. Oral
   C. Intravenous
   D. Transdermal

5. A nurse is planning care for an adult client who sustained severe burn injuries. Which of the following interventions should the nurse include in the plan of care? (Select all that apply.)

   A. Limit visitors in the client's room.
   B. Encourage fresh vegetables in the diet.
   C. Increase protein intake.
   D. Instruct the client to consume 2,000 calories/day.
   E. Restrict fresh flowers in the room.

Application Exercises Key

1. A. **CORRECT:** A sunburn is a superficial thickness burn. Superficial burns damage the top layer of the skin.

   B. A superficial partial-thickness burn results from flames or scalds. This damages the entire epidermis layer of the skin.

   C. A deep partial-thickness burn can result from contact with hot grease. This affects the deep layers of the skin.

   D. A full-thickness burn can result from contact with hot tar. This affects the dermis and sometimes the subcutaneous fat layer.

   Ⓝ *NCLEX® Connection: Physiological Adaptation, Pathophysiology*

2. A. Difficulty breathing and production of pink frothy sputum indicate pulmonary edema.

   B. Productive cough and a fever are indicative of a bacterial infection.

   C. **CORRECT:** Wheezing and hoarseness indicate inhalation injury with impending loss of the airway. These require immediate reporting to the provider.

   D. Confusion and headaches indicate carbon monoxide poisoning.

   Ⓝ *NCLEX® Connection: Physiological Adaptation, Pathophysiology*

3. A. **CORRECT:** Dyspnea can occur during the initial phase following a burn due to airway injury and fluid shifts.

   B. Tachycardia occurs during the initial phase following a burn due to sympathetic nervous system compensation.

   C. **CORRECT:** Hyperkalemia occurs during the initial phase following a burn as a result of leakage of fluid from the intracellular space.

   D. **CORRECT:** Hyponatremia occurs during the initial phase of a burn as a result in sodium retention in the interstitial space.

   E. Hct increases during the initial phase of a burn due to hemoconcentration.

   Ⓝ *NCLEX® Connection: Physiological Adaptation, Pathophysiology*

4. A. The nurse should not give subcutaneous injections due to the difficulty of absorption from tissue during the resuscitation phase.

   B. The nurse should not give oral (including buccal, sublingual) medications due to decreased motility in the gastrointestinal tract during the resuscitation phase.

   C. **CORRECT:** The nurse should use the IV route to administer pain medication for rapid absorption and fast pain relief during the resuscitation phase.

   D. The nurse should not use the transdermal route of administration due to delays in absorption during the resuscitation phase.

   Ⓝ *NCLEX® Connection: Pharmacological and Parenteral Therapies, Pharmacological Pain Management*

5. A. **CORRECT:** The nurse should limit the number of visitors and limit the amount of time they can visit to decrease the risk of infection.

   B. The client should restrict consumption of fresh vegetables due to the presence of bacteria on the surface and the increased risk for infection.

   C. **CORRECT:** The client should increase protein consumption, which promotes wound healing and prevents tissue breakdown.

   D. The client should consume up to 5,000 calories/day because caloric needs double or triple beginning 4 to 12 days following the burn.

   E. **CORRECT:** Flowers should not be in the client's room due to the bacteria they carry, which increase the risk for infection.

   Ⓝ *NCLEX® Connection: Physiological Adaptation, Illness Management*

PRACTICE Active Learning Scenario

A nurse is reviewing the care of a client who has an autograft skin covering over a burn injury with a nurse who will assume care of the client at the end of the day. What should the nurse include in the review? Use the ATI Active Learning Template: Therapeutic Procedure to complete this item.

DESCRIPTION OF PROCEDURE

NURSING INTERVENTIONS: Describe at least four.

PRACTICE Answer

Using the ATI Active Learning Template: Therapeutic Procedure

DESCRIPTION OF PROCEDURE: An autograft is donor skin from another area of the client's body. This is a permanent skin covering and used for burns on larger areas of the body.

NURSING INTERVENTIONS
- Maintain immobilization of the graft site.
- Elevate the extremity.
- Provide wound care to the donor site.
- Administer analgesics.
- Monitor for evidence of infection before and after skin coverings or grafts are applied.
  - Discoloration of unburned skin surrounding burn wound
  - Green color to subcutaneous fat
  - Degeneration of granulation tissue
  - Development of subeschar hemorrhage
  - Hyperventilation indicating systemic involvement of infection
  - Unstable body temperature

Ⓝ *NCLEX® Connection: Physiological Adaptation, Illness Management*

NCLEX® Connections

When reviewing the following chapters, keep in mind the relevant topics and tasks of the NCLEX outline, in particular:

Client Needs: Pharmacological and Parenteral Therapies

ADVERSE EFFECTS/CONTRAINDICATIONS/SIDE EFFECTS/INTERACTIONS: Assess the client for actual or potential side effects and adverse effects of medications.

DOSAGE CALCULATION: Use clinical decision making/critical thinking when calculating dosages.

MEDICATION ADMINISTRATION: Educate client on medication self-administration procedures.

Client Needs: Reduction of Risk Potential

DIAGNOSTIC TESTS: Apply knowledge of related nursing procedures and psychomotor skills when caring for clients undergoing diagnostic testing.

LABORATORY VALUES: Notify primary health care provider about laboratory test results.

THERAPEUTIC PROCEDURES: Educate client about treatments and procedures.

Client Needs: Physiological Adaptation

FLUID AND ELECTROLYTE IMBALANCES: Apply knowledge of pathophysiology when caring for the client with fluid and electrolyte imbalances.

ILLNESS MANAGEMENT: Educate client about managing illness.

PATHOPHYSIOLOGY: Identify pathophysiology related to an acute or chronic condition.

CHAPTER 76 *Endocrine Diagnostic Procedures*

Disorders of the endocrine system relate to either the excess or deficiency of a hormone or to a defect in a receptor site for a hormone. Laboratory tests for evaluating endocrine function vary according to the organ or system under analysis.

Many of these tests are blood, urine, or saliva tests that determine an excess or lack of a particular hormone in the body. Some of these tests stimulate a reaction in the body that will facilitate diagnosis of a particular disorder.

Stimulation testing involves giving hormones to stimulate the target gland to determine if the gland is capable of normal hormone production. Suppression testing involves giving medications or substances to evaluate the body's ability to suppress excessive hormone production.

Posterior pituitary gland

The posterior pituitary gland secretes the hormone vasopressin (antidiuretic hormone [ADH]). ADH increases permeability of the renal distal tubules, causing the kidneys to reabsorb water.

- A deficiency of ADH causes diabetes insipidus, which is the excretion of a large quantity of dilute urine.
- Excessive secretion of ADH causes the syndrome of inappropriate antidiuretic hormone (SIADH). With SIADH, the kidneys retain water, urine becomes concentrated, urinary output decreases, and extracellular fluid volume increases.
- Diagnostic tests for the posterior pituitary gland include the water deprivation test, ADH, serum and urine electrolytes and osmolality, and urine specific gravity.

INDICATIONS

Water deprivation test

The water deprivation test measures the kidneys' ability to concentrate urine in light of an increased plasma osmolality and a low plasma vasopressin level. It requires a controlled setting with careful observation of the client for complications of dehydration.

- This test helps identify causes and types of diabetes insipidus (DI).
  - Nephrogenic DI: failure of the kidneys to respond to ADH for a variety of reasons, such as hypokalemia and hypocalcemia
  - Central (neurogenic) DI: head injury, tumor, irradiation of the pituitary gland, or serious infection
  - Medication-induced DI: lithium, demeclocycline
- This test requires that the client have a baseline sodium level within the expected reference range and a urine osmolality less than 300 mOsm/kg H_2O.
- The expected reference range for osmolality is 285 to 295 mOsm/kg H_2O.
- Osmolality increases with dehydration and decreases with overhydration, so it provides important information about fluid and electrolyte balance.
- Contraindications for this test include renal insufficiency, uncontrolled diabetes mellitus, hypovolemia, and adrenal or thyroid hormone deficiency.

Tests that diagnose SIADH

ADH, serum and urine electrolytes and osmolality, and urine-specific gravity tests identify SIADH.

CONSIDERATIONS

Water deprivation test

PREPROCEDURE

- Begin the test by withholding fluids for a specific number of hours, or until the client loses a specific amount of body weight.
- The osmolality must be greater than 288 mOsm/kg before administering the ADH hormone.
- Monitor closely to identify and intervene for severe dehydration.
- Establish IV access.

INTRAPROCEDURE

- Place the client in a recumbent position for 30 min. The client may sit or stand during urination and weight determination.
  - Ask the client to empty his bladder. Record the amount, and send the specimen to the laboratory for immediate processing to determine osmolality.
  - Weigh the client to nearest tenth of a kilogram (0.1 kg). Record the weight. Measure and record blood pressure and pulse.
- Initiate complete fluid restriction. Have the client maintain a semi-recumbent position except to urinate.
  - Repeat the three steps: weigh and measure urine osmolality hourly until a specific number of hourly tests (two to three) show a urine osmolality increase of less than 30 mOsm/kg H_2O.
  - Obtain serum osmolality and record any findings.
  - Administer a dose of vasopressin or desmopressin at a predetermined point during the test and obtain urine osmolality again after 30 to 60 min.

ADH

- The client should fast and avoid stress for 12 hr prior to the test.
- Some medications (including acetaminophen, antidepressants, diuretics, opioids, phenytoin) can interfere with the test. Review medications with the provider.
- Collect a blood sample and transport it to the laboratory within 10 min.

Electrolytes

- No pre- or postprocedure care is necessary.
- The laboratory analyzes samples of blood for electrolyte components.

Urine electrolytes and osmolality

- No pre- or postprocedure care is necessary.
- The laboratory analyzes samples of urine for electrolyte components.

Urine specific gravity

The laboratory usually performs this test but nurses can use a calibrated hydrometer or a temperature-compensated refractometer to perform it on a clinical unit.

INTERPRETATION OF FINDINGS

Water deprivation test

- Clients who have nephrogenic DI have up to a 9% decrease in urine osmolality during the test due to the kidneys' inability to concentrate urine.
- Clients who have central (neurogenic) DI have a rise in osmolality of more than 9% following administration of vasopressin.
- Clients who have medication-induced DI have an osmolality less than 9% and take longer to become dehydrated during the test than are clients who have central DI.

ADH

Increased ADH indicates SIADH.

EXPECTED REFERENCE RANGE: 1 to 5 pg/mL (1 to 5 ng/L)

Electrolytes

- Low sodium is expected with SIADH.
- Decreased osmolality and increased urine osmolality indicate SIADH.

EXPECTED REFERENCE RANGE
- **Sodium:** 136 to 145 mEq/L
- **Potassium:** 3.5 to 5.0 mEq/L
- **Chloride:** 98 to 106 mEq/L
- **Magnesium:** 1.3 to 2.1 mEq/L

Urine electrolytes and osmolality

- High urine sodium content is expected with SIADH.
- Increased urine osmolality indicates SIADH.

EXPECTED REFERENCE RANGE
- **Urine sodium:** 40 to 220 mEq/24 hr in a 24-hr collection or greater than 20 mEq/L in a random urine collection
- **Urine potassium:** 25 to 100 mEq/L/24 hr, depending on potassium intake
- **Urine chloride:** 110 to 250 mEq/24 hr
- **Urine osmolality:** 50 to 1,200 mOsm/kg H_2O, depending on fluid intake

Urine-specific gravity

A decrease in urine output and an increase in urine specific gravity occur as a result of excess production of ADH.

EXPECTED REFERENCE RANGE: 1.010 to 1.025

COMPLICATIONS

Water deprivation test

Dehydration can occur due to a decrease in vascular volume.

NURSING ACTIONS: Monitor closely for early indications of dehydration, including postural hypotension, tachycardia, and dizziness. Discontinue the test if the client loses more than 2 kg (or a specific amount) of body weight.

Adrenal cortex

- A hyperfunctioning adrenal cortex and an excess production of cortisol characterize Cushing's disease and Cushing's syndrome (hypercortisolism).
- Hypofunctioning of the adrenal cortex and a consequent lack of adequate amounts of serum cortisol characterize Addison's disease.
- Diagnostic tests for the adrenal cortex include the dexamethasone suppression test, plasma and salivary cortisol, 24-hr urine for cortisol, adrenocorticotropic hormone (ACTH), and ACTH stimulation tests.
- A CT scan and an MRI identify atrophy of the adrenal glands causing hypofunction.

INDICATIONS

Dexamethasone suppression test

This test determines whether dexamethasone, a synthetic steroid similar to cortisol, has an effect on cortisol levels.

CONSIDERATIONS

Dexamethasone suppression test

- Typically, the client takes a dose of dexamethasone by mouth, and a blood sample the next morning determines whether cortisol is present.
- A low dose of dexamethasone screens a client for Cushing's disease; high doses help determine the cause of the disease.
- The client should stop taking some medications (diuretics, antibiotics, oral contraceptives) and try to reduce stress prior to and during testing, as these can affect the test results.

Plasma cortisol

The provider determines the best time for testing, usually with blood sampling at 8 a.m. and again at 4 p.m.

Salivary cortisol

- Midnight is the usual time for salivary collection.
- A salivary cushion pad inside the client's cheek, directly over the salivary gland, collects the sample.

Urinary cortisol

- The laboratory measures cortisol in a 24-hr urine collection.
- Physical exercise and emotional stress elevate cortisol levels.
- The client empties his bladder and then collects all urine he excretes during the next 24-hr period.
- The client keeps the urine in a container with boric acid in it and keeps it on ice or in a refrigerator.
- Some medications, such as diuretics, interfere with the test results, so the client should stop taking them, with the provider's approval, for several days prior to urine collection.

ACTH

ACTH is most accurate with morning blood samples.

ACTH stimulation test

Administer cosyntropin IV, and obtain specimens for plasma cortisol levels at 30 min and 1 hr.

INTERPRETATION OF FINDINGS

Dexamethasone suppression test

- When the pituitary gland produces decreased amounts of ACTH, the adrenal glands release decreased amounts of cortisol.
- When clients who have Cushing's disease receive dexamethasone, there is no decrease in the production of ACTH and cortisol.

Plasma cortisol

Higher levels can indicate hypercortisolism (Cushing's disease). Low levels can indicate hypocortisolism (Addison's disease).

EXPECTED REFERENCE RANGE: Cortisol varies according to the time of day. Because it has a diurnal (daily) pattern, higher levels are present in the early morning, and the lowest levels occur around midnight, or 3 to 5 hr after the onset of sleep.

Salivary cortisol

High levels indicate hypercortisolism.

EXPECTED REFERENCE RANGE: Salivary cortisol is at its lowest point around midnight and at its highest point between 7 and 9 a.m.

Urinary cortisol

Higher levels can indicate hypercortisolism (Cushing's disease). Low levels can indicate hypocortisolism (Addison's disease).

EXPECTED REFERENCE RANGE: Less than 100 mcg/day in a 24-hr urine collection

ACTH

ACTH increases with Addison's disease and either increases or decreases with Cushing's disease (depending on the cause of the syndrome).

ACTH stimulation test

- An increase in cortisol after administration of ACTH is expected.
- If cortisol does not increase after administration of cosyntropin (an ACTH-like medication), the test is positive for Addison's disease or hypocortisolism.
- The ACTH stimulation test determines the functioning of the pituitary gland in relation to stimulating the secretion of adrenal hormones of cortisol.
- A 24-hr test or a 3-day test is an option with IV infusions of cosyntropin over several hours.

Adrenal medulla

- Disorders of the adrenal medulla, such as a tumor, can cause hypersecretion of catecholamines, resulting in stimulation of a sympathetic response, such as tachycardia, hypertension, and diaphoresis. These tests determine whether the cause of a client's unrelieved hypertension is a pheochromocytoma.
- Diagnostic tests for the adrenal medulla include plasma-free metanephrine testing and the clonidine suppression test.

INDICATIONS

Plasma-free metanephrine test

- Identification of a pheochromocytoma
- The laboratory tests blood samples for both metanephrine and normetanephrine.

Clonidine suppression test

- Identification of a pheochromocytoma
- The laboratory measures plasma catecholamines levels prior to and 3 hr after administration of clonidine.

CONSIDERATIONS

Plasma-free metanephrine test

PREPROCEDURE
- Caffeine, alcohol, and several medications interfere with the test results. Review the client's medications, including acetaminophen, with the provider. The client should stop taking a acetaminophen for 48 hr prior to test.
- Physical exercise and increased stress can interfere with test results.
- Assess the client's stress level. Having the client lie down and rest for 30 min prior to the test can reduce stress.
- Notify the provider about any interfering factors before obtaining a blood sample for the test.

CLIENT EDUCATION
- Instruct the client to maintain a moderate level of activity.
- Instruct the client about caffeine and alcohol restrictions.

Clonidine suppression test

PRE/INTRAPROCEDURE: Monitor for hypotension.

POSTPROCEDURE CLIENT EDUCATION
- Inform the client that fatigue can occur after the test.
- Continue monitoring blood pressure for at least 1 hr following the procedure.

INTERPRETATION OF FINDINGS

Plasma-free metanephrine test

- Elevation of both metanephrine and normetanephrine above the expected reference range indicates a pheochromocytoma.
- If only one of these catecholamines is elevated, a pheochromocytoma is probable.

Clonidine suppression test

- If a client does not have a pheochromocytoma, clonidine suppresses catecholamine release and decreases the level of catecholamines (decreases blood pressure).
- If the client has a pheochromocytoma, the clonidine has no effect (no decreased blood pressure).
- Hypovolemia is a contraindication due to the risk for severe hypotension.

Carbohydrate metabolism

- Insulin deficiency (as in type 1 diabetes mellitus) and insulin resistance (as in type 2 diabetes mellitus) can alter carbohydrate metabolism, resulting in hyperglycemia.
- Diagnostic tests to evaluate carbohydrate metabolism include fasting (no caloric intake for 8 hr) blood glucose, oral glucose tolerance testing, and glycosylated hemoglobin (HbA1c).

CONSIDERATIONS

Fasting blood glucose

- Ensure that the client has fasted (no food or beverages other than water) for the 8 hr prior to blood sampling.
- The client should postpone taking antidiabetes medications until after the blood sampling.

Random (casual) blood glucose

- Refers to any time of day without regard to mealtime.
- No pre- or postprocedure care is necessary. The test requires obtaining a random blood sample.

Oral glucose tolerance test

- Instruct the client to consume a balanced diet for 3 days prior to the test and fast for 10 to 12 hr prior to the test.
- The technician will obtain a blood specimen for a fasting blood glucose level at start of the test.
- The client then consumes a specific amount of glucose.
- The technician obtains blood samples at 30 min, 1 hr, 2 hr, 3 hr, and sometimes 4 hr after the client consumes glucose. Assess clients for hypoglycemia throughout the procedure.

Glycosylated hemoglobin (HbA1c)

- No pre- or postprocedure care is necessary. The test requires obtaining a random blood sample.
- Fasting is not necessary.

INTERPRETATION OF FINDINGS

Fasting blood glucose

- Determines blood glucose when the client has consumed no foods or fluids (other than water) for the past 8 hr.
- Fasting blood glucose greater than 126 mg/dL on two different occasions can indicate diabetes mellitus.
- Fasting blood glucose levels 100 to 125 mg/dL can indicate prediabetes.

EXPECTED REFERENCE RANGE
- Less than 100 mg/dL for adults and children older than 2 years
- Slightly increased for adults older than 50 years

Random (casual) blood glucose

EXPECTED REFERENCE RANGE: Less than 200 mg/dL

Oral glucose tolerance test

- Blood glucose greater than 200 mg/dL at 2 hr following glucose ingestion can indicate diabetes. The test may be repeated on another day to check results.
- Determines the ability to metabolize a standard amount of glucose.

EXPECTED REFERENCE RANGE
- Less than 200 mg/dL 1 hr following glucose ingestion
- Less than 140 mg/dL 2 hr following glucose ingestion
- 70 to 115 mg/dL 3 or 4 hr following glucose ingestion

Glycosylated hemoglobin (HbA1c)

- HbA1c is the best indicator of an average blood glucose level for the past 120 days.
- Assists in evaluating treatment effectiveness and adherence to the diet plan, medication regimen, and exercise schedule.

EXPECTED REFERENCE RANGE
- HbA1c 5.7% or less indicates no diabetes mellitus.
- HbA1c less than 7% indicates good diabetes control.
- HbA1c 8% to 9% indicates fair diabetes control.
- HbA1c 9% or greater indicates poor diabetes control.

Thyroid and anterior pituitary gland

Hyperthyroidism and hypothyroidism are disorders in which there are inappropriate amounts of the thyroid hormones triiodothyronine (T_3) and thyroxine (T_4) circulating. These inappropriate amounts of T_3 and T_4 cause an increase or decrease in metabolic rate that affects all body systems.

- The anterior pituitary gland secretes thyroid stimulating hormone (TSH). Hyposecretion of TSH can lead to secondary hypothyroidism, and hypersecretion of TSH can cause secondary hyperthyroidism.
- Diagnostic tests to evaluate the function of the thyroid and anterior pituitary glands include T_3 (triiodothyronine), T_4 (thyroxine), TSH, thyrotropin-releasing hormone (TRH) stimulation test, and radioactive iodine uptake.
- Ultrasounds and CT scans determine the size, shape, and presence of nodules and masses on these glands.

INDICATIONS

TSH

Results help monitor thyroid replacement therapy and differentiate types of thyroid disorders.

Thyroid scan

- A noninvasive gamma probe over the thyroid measures the amount of ^{123}I the gland absorbed.
- Evaluates size, shape, position and ability of the thyroid gland to function following an oral dose of ^{123}I

CONSIDERATIONS

T_3 and T_4

- No pre- or postprocedure care is necessary for either test.
- The laboratory requires a random blood sample.

TSH

- No pre- or postprocedure care is necessary.
- The laboratory requires a random blood sample.
- It stimulates the release of thyroid hormone by the anterior pituitary gland.

TRH

The TRH requires giving a bolus of thyrotropin-releasing hormone, and then assessing serum concentrations of TSH at intervals.

Thyroid scan

- The client receives an oral radioactive dose of ^{123}I, and a scintillation counter measures the amount the thyroid absorbed.
- Pregnancy and recent exposure to iodine-containing dye are contraindications.
- Explain to the client that ^{123}I has a very short half life, thus radiation precautions are not necessary for this test.

INTERPRETATION OF FINDINGS

T_3 and T_4

- Low and high levels of each indicate hypothyroidism and hyperthyroidism, respectively.
- A high level of T_3 is a better indicator hyperthyroidism than is T_4.

EXPECTED REFERENCE RANGE
- **T_3:** 70 to 205 ng/dL
- **T_4 (total):** 4.0 to 12.0 mcg/dL

TSH

- TSH can increase or decrease, depending on the cause.
- An increased value indicates primary hypothyroidism due to thyroid dysfunction or thyroiditis.
- A decreased value indicates hyperthyroidism (Graves' disease) or secondary hypothyroidism (due to pituitary or hypothalamus dysfunction).

TRH

- The expected reference range is relative to baseline.
- The TSH should double the baseline value shortly after administration of thyrotropin-releasing hormone.
- If the TSH increases twofold or more above baseline, this finding indicates hypothyroidism.

Thyroid scan

Clients who have hyperthyroidism absorb high amounts (greater than 35%) of ^{123}I.

Application Exercises

1. A nurse is caring for a client who asks why the provider bases his medication regimen on his HbA1c instead of his log of morning fasting blood glucose results. Which of the following responses should the nurse make?

   A. "HbA1c measures how well insulin is regulating your blood glucose between meals."

   B. "HbA1c indicates how well your have regulated your blood glucose over the past 120 days."

   C. "HbA1c is the first test your doctor prescribed to determine that you have diabetes."

   D. "HbA1c determines if the your doctor should adjust your insulin dosage."

2. A nurse is reviewing the laboratory findings for a client who might have hyperthyroidism. The nurse should identify an elevation which of the following substances as an indication that the client has this disorder

   A. Triiodothyronine

   B. Plasma-free metanephrine

   C. Urine cortisol

   D. Urine osmolality

3. A nurse is reviewing the health record of a client who has syndrome of inappropriate antidiuretic hormone (SIADH). Which of the following laboratory findings should the nurse expect? (Select all that apply.)

   A. Low sodium

   B. High potassium

   C. Increased urine osmolality

   D. High urine sodium

   E. Increased urine specific gravity

4. A nurse is caring for a client who has primary adrenal insufficiency and is preparing to undergo an ACTH stimulation test. Which of the following findings should the nurse expect after an IV injection of cosyntropin?

   A. No change in plasma cortisol

   B. Elevated fasting blood glucose

   C. Decrease in sodium

   D. Increase in urinary output

5. A nurse is assessing a client during a water deprivation test. For which of the following complications should the nurse monitor the client?

   A. Bradycardia

   B. Orthostatic hypotension

   C. Neck vein distention

   D. Crackles in lungs

PRACTICE Active Learning Scenario

A nurse is planning care for a client who will undergo a clonidine suppression test. What should the nurse include in the plan of care?

Use the ATI Active Learning Template: Diagnostic Procedure to complete this item to include the following.

INDICATIONS

INTERPRETATION OF FINDINGS

NURSING ACTIONS: Describe one intraprocedure.

Application Exercises Key

1. A. Capillary glucose monitoring evaluates how well insulin is regulating blood glucose between meals.

   B. CORRECT: HbA1c measures blood glucose control over the past 120 days

   C. A fasting blood glucose is the first test providers prescribe to diagnose diabetes mellitus. HbA1c is not a screening test.

   D. Capillary glucose monitoring evaluates how well insulin regulates blood glucose.

   Ⓝ *NCLEX® Connection: Reduction of Risk Potential, Laboratory Values*

2. A. CORRECT: Increased triiodothyronine (T3) indicates hyperthyroidism.

   B. A n increase in plasma-free metanephrine indicates the presence of a pheochromocytoma (tumor of the cells of the adrenal medulla).

   C. A high cortisol level indicates hyperfunction of the adrenal cortex and can indicate that the client has Cushing's disease.

   D. Increased urine osmolality indicates SIADH.

   Ⓝ *NCLEX® Connection: Reduction of Risk Potential, Laboratory Values*

3. A. CORRECT: SIADH results in water retention, causing a low sodium level.

   B. SIADH does not affect potassium levels.

   C. CORRECT: SIADH results in an increase in urine osmolality due to the decreased urine volume.

   D. CORRECT: SIADH results in water retention, causing a high urine sodium level.

   E. CORRECT: SIADH results in water retention, causing an increase in urine specific gravity.

   Ⓝ *NCLEX® Connection: Reduction of Risk Potential, Laboratory Values*

4. A. CORRECT: No change in plasma cortisol indicates primary adrenal insufficiency (Addison's disease or hypocortisolism) after an IV injection of cosyntropin during an ACTH stimulation test due to an inadequate production of cortisol.

   B. An elevated fasting blood glucose helps identify diabetes mellitus.

   C. An increase in sodium indicates primary adrenal insufficiency (Addison's disease or hypocortisolism).

   D. A decrease in urinary output indicates primary adrenal insufficiency (Addison's disease or hypocortisolism).

   Ⓝ *NCLEX® Connection: Pharmacological and Parenteral Therapies, Expected Actions/Outcomes*

5. A. Tachycardia is a complication the nurse should monitor for during a water deprivation test due to dehydration.

   B. CORRECT: The nurse should monitor for orthostatic hypotension resulting from dehydration during a water deprivation test.

   C. Flat neck veins are likely during a water deprivation test due to dehydration.

   D. T he nurse should monitor the client for dizziness rather than lung crackles during a water deprivation test.

   Ⓝ *NCLEX® Connection: Reduction of Risk Potential, Diagnostic Tests*

PRACTICE Answer

Using the ATI Active Learning Template: Diagnostic Procedure

INDICATIONS: Confirms a pheochromocytoma

INTERPRETATION OF FINDINGS
- If client does not have a pheochromocytoma, clonidine suppresses catecholamine release and decreases the serum level of catecholamines (decreases blood pressure).
- If client has a pheochromocytoma, clonidine has no effect (no decrease in blood pressure).

NURSING ACTIONS: Monitor the client for hypotension.

Ⓝ *NCLEX® Connection: Reduction of Risk Potential, Diagnostic Tests*

CHAPTER 77 *Pituitary Disorders*

The pituitary gland (hypophysis) is known as the "master gland" due to its regulation of many bodily functions. Located underneath the hypothalamus, at the base of the skull, the pituitary gland is regulated by the hypothalamus. It is divided into two lobes; anterior (adenohypophysis) and posterior (neurohypophysis), which secrete regulatory hormones. The anterior pituitary gland secretes six hormones while the posterior pituitary secretes two hormones.

The hormones associated with the posterior pituitary are produced in the hypothalamus and stored in the posterior pituitary, where they are released into the circulation as needed.

HORMONES

Anterior pituitary

Thyroid-stimulating hormone: Stimulation of the thyroid gland

Adrenocorticotropic hormone (ACTH): Stimulation of the adrenal glands to secrete glucocorticoids

Luteinizing hormone
• WOMEN: stimulates maturation of ova and ovulation
• MEN: stimulates production of testosterone

Follicle-stimulating hormone
• WOMEN: stimulates growth of ovarian follicles and estrogen secretion
• MEN: stimulates sperm production

Prolactin: Stimulates breast milk production during lactation

Growth hormone (GH): Stimulates protein synthesis and growth of muscle and bone

Posterior pituitary

Antidiuretic hormone (ADH) (vasopressin): Increases resorption of water in the kidneys

Oxytocin (OT)
• Stimulates contraction of uterus following delivery
• Stimulates ejection of breast milk during lactation

DISORDERS

Altered function of the pituitary gland can be caused by disease of the pituitary gland or the hypothalamus, trauma, tumor, or vascular lesion. Hyperfunction or hypofunction of the anterior and posterior pituitary gland can occur independently of one another.
• Oversecretion of ACTH from the anterior pituitary gland results in Cushing's disease
• Over secretion of GH results in gigantism in children and acromegaly in the adult client. In the adult client, acromegaly manifests as enlargement of body parts without affecting the client's height.
• Undersecretion of GH in children results in dwarfism.
• Insufficient secretion of hormones in the anterior pituitary typically affects all the hormones, termed panhypopituitarism. It affects the target organs of the hormones produced in the anterior pituitary, including the thyroid, adrenal cortex, and gonads.
• A deficiency of ADH causes diabetes insipidus (DI). DI is characterized by the excretion of a large quantity of diluted urine.
• Excessive secretion of ADH causes the syndrome of inappropriate antidiuretic hormone (SIADH). In SIADH, the kidneys retain water, urine output decreases, and extracellular fluid volume is increased.
• Posterior pituitary disorders result in fluid and electrolyte imbalances.

Acromegaly

- Characterized by excess growth hormone in adults, which causes an increase in size of body parts but not height.
- Manifestations are widespread, including overgrowth of the skin; bones of the forehead, jaw, feet and hands; and enlargement of organs including the liver and the heart.
- If left untreated can cause hypertension, diabetes mellitus, and heart problems.
- Onset is gradual and can progress for years before becoming noticeable.

ASSESSMENT

RISK FACTORS

- Age (adulthood)
- Benign tumors (pituitary adenoma)

EXPECTED FINDINGS

- Severe headaches
- Visual disturbances (diplopia, decreased visual acuity)
- Thick lips with coarse facial structures
- Joint pain
- Decreased libido
- Enlarged hands and feet
- Hyperglycemia
- Barrel-shaped chest
- Lower jaw protrusion
- Increasing head size
- Change in voice characteristics
- Change in menstrual pattern
- Sleep apnea
- Increases in intracranial pressure (decreased LOC, pupillary changes, severe hypertension, widened pulse pressure, bradycardia, seizures) **Qs**

LABORATORY TESTS

Growth hormone suppression test

Growth hormone level is measured as a baseline and following administration of glucose, typically 0.5 g/kg or 100 g. Elevated glucose levels are expected to suppress GH; however, clients who have acromegaly will show only a slight decrease or no decrease at all in GH levels.

NURSING ACTIONS
- Obtain baseline GH and glucose levels.
- Administer prescribed glucose.
- Obtain GH and blood glucose levels at 10, 60, and 120 min after glucose administration

CLIENT EDUCATION: Client should receive nothing but water for 6 to 8 hr preceding the test

DIAGNOSTIC PROCEDURES

X-rays of the skull: Identify abnormalities of the sella tircica, the location of the pituitary gland within the skull.

CT or MRI of the head: Identify soft tissue lesions.

Cerebral angiography: Evaluation for the presence of vascular malformation or aneurysms.

PATIENT-CENTERED CARE

NURSING CARE

PREOPERATIVE
- Instruct client not to brush his teeth, blow his nose, or bend at the waist postoperatively. These actions can increase intracranial pressure. **Qs**
- Assess self-concept related to physical manifestations of disorder.

POSTOPERATIVE
- Monitor neurological status.
- Monitor drainage to mustache dressing (drip pad).
- Notify provider of the presence of glucose in the drainage (indication of leakage of cerebrospinal fluid).
- Maintain the client in a high-Fowler's position.
- Monitor fluid balance, especially greater output than intake (DI).
- Encourage deep breathing exercises, but limit coughing as this increases intracranial pressure and can cause a leak of cerebrospinal fluid (CSF).
- Assess for manifestations of meningitis.
- Administer replacement hormones.

MEDICATIONS

Dopamine agonists (bromocriptine mesylate, cabergoline) inhibit the release of GH.
CLIENT EDUCATION: Instruct the client to notify the provider immediately if chest pain, dizziness, or watery nasal discharge occurs while taking bromocriptine. This can indicate cardiac dysrhythmia, coronary artery spasms, or leakage of CSF. **Qs**

Somatostatin analogs (octreotide, lanreotide) inhibit GH release.

Growth hormone receptor blocker (pegvisomant) prevents GH receptor activity and blocks production of insulin-like growth factor.

THERAPEUTIC PROCEDURES

Hypophysectomy: Removal of the pituitary gland through an endoscopic transnasal (most common) or oronasal (transsphenoidal) approach. If these approaches do not provide access to the tumor, a craniotomy is indicated.

Radiation therapy: Shrinks pituitary tumor over a period of time.

CLIENT EDUCATION

- Hormone replacement therapy will be lifelong.
- Avoid activities that increase intracranial pressure.
- Report postnasal drip or increased swallowing.
- Rinse mouth frequently to minimize effects of mouth breathing.
- Use oral rinses and flossing to clean teeth. Avoid brushing teeth due to risk of trauma to the operative site.
- Consume a diet high in fiber to minimize straining to defecate.

Diabetes insipidus

- Diabetes insipidus results from a deficiency of ADH, which is secreted by the posterior lobe of the pituitary gland (neurohypophysis).
- Decreased ADH reduces the ability of the distal renal tubules in the kidneys to collect and concentrate urine, resulting in excessive diluted urination, excessive thirst, electrolyte imbalance, and excessive fluid intake.

TYPES OF DIABETES INSIPIDUS

Primary: A lack of ADH production or release; caused by defects in the hypothalamus or pituitary gland.

Secondary: A lack of ADH production or release; caused by infection, tumors in or near the hypothalamus or pituitary gland, head trauma, or brain surgery.

Nephrogenic: Inherited; renal tubules do not react to ADH

Drug-induced: Lithium carbonate or demeclocycline can alter the way the kidneys respond to ADH.

ASSESSMENT

RISK FACTORS

- Clients who have a head injury, tumor or lesion, surgery or irradiation near or around the pituitary gland, or infection (meningitis, encephalitis)
- Clients who are taking lithium carbonate or demeclocycline
- Older adult clients are at higher risk for dehydration due to lower water content of the body, decreased thirst response, decreased ability of the kidneys to concentrate urine, increased use of diuretics, swallowing difficulties, or inadequate food intake. ©

EXPECTED FINDINGS

- Polyuria (abrupt onset of excessive urination, urinary output of 4 to 30 L/day of dilute urine): failure of the renal tubules to collect and reabsorb water
- Polydipsia (excessive thirst, consumption of 2 to 20 L/day)
- Nocturia
- Fatigue
- Dehydration, as evidenced by extreme thirst, weight loss, muscle weakness, headache, constipation, and dizziness

PHYSICAL ASSESSMENT FINDINGS

- Sunken eyes
- Tachycardia
- Hypotension
- Loss or absence of skin turgor
- Dry mucous membranes
- Weak, poor peripheral pulses
- Decreased cognition

LABORATORY TESTS

Electrolyte imbalances: such as increased sodium

Urine chemistry: Think DILUTE.
- Decreased urine specific gravity (less than 1.005)
- Decreased urine osmolality (less than 200 mOsm/L)
- Decreased urine pH
- Decreased urine sodium
- Decreased urine potassium
- As urine volume increases, urine osmolality decreases.

Serum chemistry: Think CONCENTRATED.
- Increased serum osmolality (greater than 300 mOsm/L)
- Increased serum sodium
- Increased serum potassium
- As serum volume decreases, the serum osmolality increases.

DIAGNOSTIC PROCEDURES

Water deprivation test (ADH stimulation test)

- This is an easy and reliable diagnostic test. Dehydration is induced by withholding fluids.
- A subcutaneous injection of vasopressin produces urine output with an increased specific gravity and osmolality.
- The test is positive for DI if the kidneys are unable to concentrate urine despite increased plasma osmolarity.

NURSING ACTIONS

- Obtain baseline weight, vital signs, serum electrolytes and osmolarity, and urine specific gravity and osmolarity.
- Monitor hourly vital signs, urine specific gravity, osmolarity, and body weight.
  - Discontinue the test and rehydrate the client for a loss of more than 2 kg in body weight. Q EBP
- Monitor for severe dehydration.
  - Early indications of dehydration can be postural hypotension, tachycardia, and dizziness. Be prepared to discontinue the test if these indicators develop.

CLIENT EDUCATION

- Explain the test procedure to the client.
- Advise the client to report any dizziness, headache, or nausea.

Vasopressin test

A subcutaneous injection of vasopressin produces urine output with an increased specific gravity if the client has central diabetes insipidus. This differentiates central from nephrogenic diabetes insipidus.

NURSING ACTIONS: Administer vasopressin subcutaneously and obtain a urine sample for osmolality 30 to 60 min after administration.

CLIENT EDUCATION: Explain the test procedure to the client. Advise the client to notify the nurse of any dizziness, headache, or nausea.

PATIENT-CENTERED CARE

NURSING CARE

- Monitor vital signs, urinary output, central venous pressure, I&O, specific gravity, and laboratory studies (potassium, sodium, BUN, creatinine, specific gravity, osmolarity).
- Weigh the client daily.
- Promote the prescribed diet (regular diet with restriction of foods that exert a diuretic effect, such as caffeine).
- IV therapy: Hydration (I&O must be matched to prevent dehydration) and electrolyte replacement.
- Promote safety: Keep bedside rails up while client is in bed, and provide assistance with ambulation due to dizziness or muscle weakness. Ensure easy access to a bathroom or bedpan. Qs
- Add bulk foods and fruit juices to the diet if constipation develops. A laxative might be needed.
- Assess skin turgor and mucous membranes.
- Provide skin and mouth care, and apply a lubricant to cracked or sore lips. Use a soft toothbrush and mild mouthwash to avoid trauma to the oral mucosa. Use alcohol-free skin care products, and apply emollient lotion after baths.
- Encourage the client to drink fluids in response to thirst.

MEDICATIONS

ADH replacement agents

- Desmopressin, which is a synthetic ADH, or aqueous vasopressin administered intranasally, orally, or parenterally
- Results in increased water absorption from kidneys and decreased urine output

NURSING CONSIDERATIONS

- Monitor vital signs, urinary output, central venous pressure, I&O, specific gravity, and laboratory studies (potassium, sodium, BUN, creatinine, specific gravity, osmolarity).
- Dose can be adjusted depending on urine output.
- Give vasopressin cautiously to clients who have coronary artery disease because the medication can cause vasoconstriction.
- Monitor for headache, confusion, or other indications of water intoxication.

CLIENT EDUCATION

- Educate the client regarding lifelong self-administration of vasopressin therapy. Qpcc
- For an intranasal dose, teach the client to clear nasal passage and sit upright prior to inhalation.
- Instruct the client to monitor weight daily and notify the provider of a gain greater than 0.9 kg (2 lb) in 24 hr.
- Instruct the client to restrict fluids if directed and notify the provider of headache or confusion.

INTERPROFESSIONAL CARE

Home assistance for fluid, medication, and dietary management might be required.

CLIENT EDUCATION

- Instruct client on medications for home use.
- Instruct the client to weigh daily, eat a high-fiber diet, wear a medical alert wristband, and monitor fluid I&O.
- Teach the client to monitor for indications of dehydration (weight loss; dry, cracked lips; confusion; weakness).
- Advise the client to restrict fluids as prescribed to prevent water intoxication, and avoid consumption of alcohol.

COMPLICATIONS

Untreated DI can cause hypovolemia, hyperosmolarity, hypernatremia, circulatory collapse, unconsciousness, central nervous system damage, and seizures. Excessive urine output causing severe dehydration can lead to these complications.

NURSING ACTIONS: Monitor fluid balance and prevent dehydration by providing proper fluid intake.

CLIENT EDUCATION: Advise the client to seek early medical attention for any indications of DI and follow care instructions.

Syndrome of inappropriate antidiuretic hormone

SIADH, or Schwartz-Bartter syndrome, is an excessive release of ADH, also known as vasopressin, secreted by the posterior lobe of the pituitary gland (neurohypophysis).

Excess ADH leads to renal reabsorption of water and suppression of renin-angiotensin mechanism, causing renal excretion of sodium leading to water intoxication, cellular edema, and dilutional hyponatremia. Fluid shifts within compartments causes decreased serum osmolarity.

ASSESSMENT

RISK FACTORS

Conditions that stimulate the hypothalamus to hypersecrete ADH include malignant tumors, increased intrathoracic pressure (such as with positive pressure ventilation), head injury, meningitis, stroke, tuberculosis, and medications (chemotherapy agents, TCAs, SSRIs, opioids, fluoroquinolone antibiotics).

EXPECTED FINDINGS

- Early manifestations include headache, weakness, anorexia, muscle cramps, and weight gain (without edema because water, not sodium, is retained).
- As the serum sodium level decreases, the client experiences personality changes, hostility, sluggish deep tendon reflexes, nausea, vomiting, diarrhea, and oliguria with dark yellow concentrated appearance.

PHYSICAL ASSESSMENT FINDINGS
- Confusion, lethargy, and Cheyne–Stokes respirations herald impending crisis. When the serum sodium level drops further, seizures, coma, and death can occur.
- Manifestations of fluid volume excess include tachycardia, bounding pulses, possible hypertension, crackles in lungs, distended neck veins, taut skin, and weight gain without edema. Intake is greater than output.

LABORATORY TESTS

Urine chemistry: Think CONCENTRATED.
- Increased urine sodium
- Increased urine osmolarity
- As urine volume decreases, urine osmolarity increases.

Blood chemistry: Think DILUTE.
- Decreased serum sodium (dilutional hyponatremia)
- Decreased serum osmolarity (less than 270 mEq/L)
- As serum volume increases, serum osmolarity decreases.

PATIENT-CENTERED CARE

NURSING CARE

- Restrict oral fluids to 500 to 1,000 mL/day to prevent further hemodilution (first priority). During fluid restriction, provide comfort measures for thirst, such as mouth care, ice chips, lozenges, and staggered water intake.
- Flush all enteral and gastric tubes with 0.9% sodium chloride, instead of water, to replace sodium and prevent further hemodilution. Q**EBP**
- Monitor I&O. Report decreased urine output.
- Monitor vital signs for increased blood pressure, tachycardia, and hypothermia.
- Auscultate lung sounds to monitor for pulmonary edema (can develop rapidly and is a medical emergency).
- Monitor for decreased serum sodium/osmolarity and elevated urine sodium/osmolarity.
- Weigh the client daily. A weight gain of 1 kg (2.2 lb) indicates a gain of 1 L of fluid. Report this to the provider.
- Report altered mental status (headache, confusion, lethargy, seizures, coma).
- Reduce environmental stimuli and position the client as needed.
- Provide a safe environment for clients who have altered levels of consciousness. Maintain seizure precautions. Q**s**
- Monitor for indications of heart failure, which can occur from fluid overload. Use of a loop diuretic can be indicated.

MEDICATIONS

Tetracycline derivative (demeclocycline)

- Unlabeled use to correct fluid and electrolyte imbalances by stimulating urine flow.
- Contraindicated in clients who have impaired kidney function.

NURSING CONSIDERATIONS: Monitor for effective treatment, such as increased serum sodium/osmolarity and decreased urine sodium osmolarity.

CLIENT EDUCATION
- Instruct the client to avoid taking demeclocycline at the same time as calcium, iron, magnesium supplements, antacids containing aluminum, or milk products.
- Advise the client to monitor for indications of a yeast infection, such as a white, cheese-like film inside the mouth.
- Advise the client to avoid prolonged exposure to sunlight. Protective clothing and sunscreen should be used.
- Instruct the client to notify the provider if diarrhea develops.

Vasopressin antagonists (tolvaptan, conivaptan)

Promote water excretion without causing sodium losses.

NURSING CONSIDERATIONS Qᴘᴄᴄ
- Administration initiated in the acute care setting.
- Monitor blood glucose levels.
- Monitor serum sodium levels.
- Monitor intake and output.
- Monitor bowel patterns.

CLIENT EDUCATION
- Advise client to perform frequent oral care.
- Instruct client to monitor for indications of dehydration, such as weakness.

Loop diuretic (furosemide)

Used to increase water excretion from the kidneys

NURSING CONSIDERATIONS: Use with caution because loop diuretics cause sodium excretion and can worsen hyponatremia.

CLIENT EDUCATION
- Advise the client to change positions slowly in case of postural hypotension.
- Advise the client to notify the provider of findings of hyponatremia, such as nausea, decreased appetite, and vomiting.

THERAPEUTIC PROCEDURES

Hypertonic sodium chloride IV fluid

The goal is to elevate the sodium level enough to alleviate neurologic compromise.

NURSING ACTIONS
- In severe hyponatremia/water intoxication, administration of 200 to 300 mL hypertonic IV fluid (3% to 5% sodium chloride).
- Monitor for fluid overload and heart failure (distended neck veins, crackles in lungs).

CLIENT EDUCATION
- Explain the procedure to the client.
- Advise the client to report difficulty breathing or shortness of breath, which can indicate heart failure.
- Include information about medications with discharge instructions.
- Instruct the client to obtain daily weights, wear a medical alert wristband, and restrict fluid intake.
- Advise the client to monitor for indications of hypervolemia (weight gain, difficulty breathing) and any neurological changes (tremors, disorientation), which can lead to seizures. Qₛ
- Advise the client to notify the provider of indications of hyponatremia, such as nausea, decreased appetite, and vomiting.
- Advise the client to avoid consumption of alcohol.

INTERPROFESSIONAL CARE

Home care can be required for fluid, medication, and dietary management.

COMPLICATIONS

Water intoxication, cerebral/pulmonary edema, and severe hyponatremia

Without prompt treatment, SIADH can lead to these complications, which can result in coma and death.

NURSING ACTIONS
- Monitor for early manifestations of water intoxication, such as lung crackles, distended neck veins, changes in neurological state (confusion, headaches, twitching, disorientation), edema, and decreased urinary output.
- Monitor neurologic status frequently.
- Maintain seizure precautions.
- Administer medications as prescribed.
- Monitor serum sodium level.

CLIENT EDUCATION
- Instruct the client and family about fluid restrictions and offer information about the condition and treatment.
- Provide support to ease the client's fears.

Central pontine myelinolysis

Treatment for SIADH can result in this condition characterized by nerve damage that is caused by the destruction of the myelin sheath in the brainstem (pons). The most common cause is a rapid change in sodium levels in the body. This most commonly occurs when a client is being treated for hyponatremia and the sodium levels rise too fast.

NURSING ACTIONS: During treatment with a vasopressin antagonist, hypertonic saline, or loop diuretics, plasma osmolarity and serum sodium should be monitored every 2 to 4 hr. Report any deterioration in neurologic status immediately. Qₛ

CLIENT EDUCATION
- Inform the client and family about the condition.
- Explain all procedures and information about medication and treatment.

Application Exercises

1. A nurse is caring for a client who has syndrome of inappropriate antidiuretic hormone (SIADH). Which of the following findings should the nurse expect? (Select all that apply.)

   A. Decreased serum sodium

   B. Urine specific gravity 1.001

   C. Serum osmolarity 230 mOsm/L

   D. Polyuria

   E. Increased thirst

2. A nurse is caring for a client who has diabetes insipidus. Which of the following urinalysis laboratory findings should the nurse anticipate?

   A. Presence of glucose

   B. Decreased specific gravity

   C. Presence of ketones

   D. Presence of red blood cells

3. A nurse is providing teaching to a client who has a new diagnosis of diabetes insipidus. Which of the following client statements indicates an understanding of the teaching?

   A. "I can drink up to 2 quarts of fluid a day."

   B. "I will need to use insulin to control my blood glucose levels."

   C. "I should expect to gain weight during this illness."

   D. "Muscle weakness is a symptom of diabetes insipidus."

4. A nurse is planning care for client who has acromegaly and is postoperative following a transsphenoidal hypophysectomy. Which of the following interventions should the nurse include in the plan?

   A. Maintain the client in a low-Fowler's position.

   B. Encourage deep breathing and coughing.

   C. Encourage the client to brush his teeth when awake and alert.

   D. Observe dressing drainage for the presence of glucose.

PRACTICE Active Learning Scenario

A nurse is planning care for a client who has SIADH and a new prescription for demeclocycline. What should the nurse include in the plan of care?

Use the ATI Active Learning Template: Medication to complete this item.

THERAPEUTIC USES

NURSING INTERVENTIONS: Describe one.

CLIENT EDUCATION: Describe two.

Application Exercises Key

1. A. **CORRECT:** A decrease in serum sodium is caused by an increase in the secretion of ADH.

   B. A urine specific gravity greater than 1.030 is caused by an increase in the secretion of ADH.

   C. **CORRECT:** A decrease in serum osmolarity is caused by an increase in the secretion of ADH.

   D. Reduced urine output is caused by the increase in the secretion of ADH.

   E. Increased thirst is an expected finding in a client who has diabetes insipidus.

   Ⓝ *NCLEX® Connection: Physiological Adaptation, Pathophysiology*

2. A. Glucose in the urine is indicative of diabetes mellitus.

   B. **CORRECT:** The urine of a client who has diabetes insipidus will be dilute with a urine specific gravity of less than 1.005.

   C. Ketones in the urine is indicative of diabetes mellitus.

   D. Red blood cells in the urine is indicative of diabetes mellitus.

   Ⓝ *NCLEX® Connection: Reduction of Risk Potential, Laboratory Values*

3. A. Excessive thirst is a manifestation of diabetes insipidus. Consumption of 4 to 30 L/day can be expected, and fluid intake should not be limited.

   B. Elevated blood glucose levels are a manifestation of diabetes mellitus.

   C. Weight loss is a manifestation of diabetes insipidus.

   D. **CORRECT:** Muscle weakness, weight loss, extreme thirst, headache, constipation, and dizziness are manifestations of dehydration that occurs with diabetes insipidus.

   Ⓝ *NCLEX® Connection: Physiological Adaptation, Illness Management*

4. A. The client should be placed into a high-Fowler's position.

   B. Coughing should be limited in the client who is postoperative, as this increases intracranial pressure and can cause a leak of CSF.

   C. Oral care for the client who is postoperative following a transsphenoidal hypophysectomy includes oral rinses and flossing. Brushing teeth can cause a leak of CSF and is contraindicated.

   D. **CORRECT:** The nurse should monitor the drainage to the mustache dressing and observe for the presence of glucose, which would indicate the presence of CSF. Notify the provider if this occurs.

   Ⓝ *NCLEX Connection: Reduction of Risk Potential, Therapeutic Procedures*

PRACTICE Answer

Using the ATI Active Learning Template: Medication

THERAPEUTIC USES: Demeclocycline is a derivative of tetracycline and is used to treat SIADH.

NURSING INTERVENTIONS: Monitor effectiveness of treatment, such as increased serum sodium/osmolarity and decreased urine sodium osmolarity.

CLIENT EDUCATION

- Instruct the client to avoid taking demeclocycline at the same time as calcium, iron, magnesium supplements, antacids containing aluminum, or milk products.
- Advise the client to monitor for indications of a yeast infection, such as a white, cheese-like film inside the mouth.
- Advise the client to avoid prolonged exposure to sunlight. Protective clothing and sunscreen should be used.
- Instruct the client to notify the provider if diarrhea develops.

Ⓝ *NCLEX® Connection: Pharmacological and Parenteral Therapies, Medication Administration*

UNIT 12   NURSING CARE OF CLIENTS WHO
           HAVE ENDOCRINE DISORDERS
           SECTION: THYROID DISORDERS

CHAPTER 78 *Hyperthyroidism*

The thyroid gland produces three hormones: thyroxine (T_4), triiodothyronine (T_3), and thyrocalcitonin (calcitonin). Secretion of T_3 and T_4 is regulated by the anterior pituitary gland through a negative feedback mechanism.

When serum T_3 and T_4 levels decrease, thyroid-stimulating hormone (TSH) is released by the anterior pituitary. This stimulates the thyroid gland to secrete more hormones until normal levels are reached. T_3 and T_4 affect all body systems by regulating overall body metabolism, energy production, and controlling tissue use of fats, proteins, and carbohydrates.

Calcitonin inhibits mobilization of calcium from bone and reduces blood calcium levels. Dietary intake of protein and iodine is necessary for the production of thyroid hormones.

Hyperthyroidism is a clinical syndrome caused by excessive circulating thyroid hormones. Because thyroid activity affects all body systems, excessive thyroid hormone exaggerates normal body functions and produces a hypermetabolic state.

HEALTH PROMOTION AND DISEASE PREVENTION

CLIENT EDUCATION
- Advise the client to do the following.
  - Take all medications as directed.
  - Check with the provider prior to taking over-the-counter medications.
  - Keep all follow-up appointments.
  - Adjust diet to increased metabolism when needed.
  - Seek measures to reduce stress, and get rest as needed.
  - Notify the provider of fever, increased restlessness, palpitations, or chest pain.

ASSESSMENT

RISK FACTORS

CAUSES OF HYPERTHYROIDISM
- Graves' disease is the most common cause. Autoimmune antibodies result in hypersecretion of thyroid hormones. Autosomal recessive trait passed to females.
- Toxic nodular goiter, a less common form of hyperthyroidism, is caused by overproduction of thyroid hormone due to the presence of thyroid nodules.
- Exogenous hyperthyroidism is caused by excessive dosages of thyroid hormone.

EXPECTED FINDINGS
- Nervousness, irritability, hyperactivity, emotional lability, decreased attention span, cries or laughs without cause, change in mental or emotional status
- Weakness, easy fatigability, exercise intolerance
- Muscle weakness
- Heat intolerance
- Weight change (usually loss) and increased appetite
- Insomnia and interrupted sleep
- Frequent stools and diarrhea
- Menstrual irregularities (amenorrhea or decreased menstrual flow) and decreased fertility
- Libido initially increased in both men and women, followed by a decrease as the condition progresses
- Warm, sweaty, flushed skin with velvety-smooth texture
- Hair thins, and develops a fine, soft, silky texture
- Tremor, hyperkinesia, hyperreflexia

- Exophthalmos (Graves' disease only) due to edema in the extraocular muscles and increased fatty tissue behind the eye
- Blurred or double vision and tiring of eyes due to pressure on the optic nerve
- Photophobia (sensitivity to light)
- Excessive tearing and bloodshot appearance of eyes
- Pretibial myxedema: dry waxy swelling of the front surfaces of the lower legs that resembles benign tumors (Graves' disease only)
- Vision changes
  - Eyelid retraction (lag): movement of the eyelid is delayed when the eye moves downward
  - Globe (eyeball) lag: upper eyelid pulls back faster than the eyeball when the client gazes upward
- Hair thinning or loss
- Goiter
- Bruit over the thyroid gland
- Elevated systolic blood pressure and widened pulse pressure
- Tachycardia, palpitations, and dysrhythmias
- Dyspnea
- Findings in older adult clients are often more subtle than those in younger clients. Ⓖ
  - Occasionally, an older adult client who has hyperthyroidism will demonstrate apathy or withdrawal instead of the more typical hypermetabolic state.
  - Older adult clients who have hyperthyroidism often present with heart failure, angina, and atrial fibrillation.

LABORATORY TESTS

Serum TSH test: Decreased in the presence of Graves' disease (can be elevated in secondary or tertiary hyperthyroidism)

Free T$_4$ index, T$_4$ (total) T$_3$: Elevated in the presence of disease

Thyroid-stimulating immunoglobulins: Elevated in Graves' disease, normal in other types of hyperthyroidism

Thyrotropin receptor antibodies: elevation most indicative of Graves' disease

DIAGNOSTIC PROCEDURES

Ultrasound: Used to produce images of the thyroid gland and surrounding tissue

Electrocardiogram: Used to evaluate the effects of excessive thyroid hormone on the heart (tachycardia, dysrhythmias). ECG changes include atrial fibrillation, and changes in the P and T waveforms.

Radioactive iodine uptake: Nuclear medicine test
- Clarifies size and function of the gland.
- Contraindicated in pregnant women.
- An assessment for an allergy to iodine or shellfish should be completed prior to this test.
- The uptake of radioactive iodine, administered orally 24 hr prior to the test, is measured.
- An elevated uptake is indicative of hyperthyroidism.

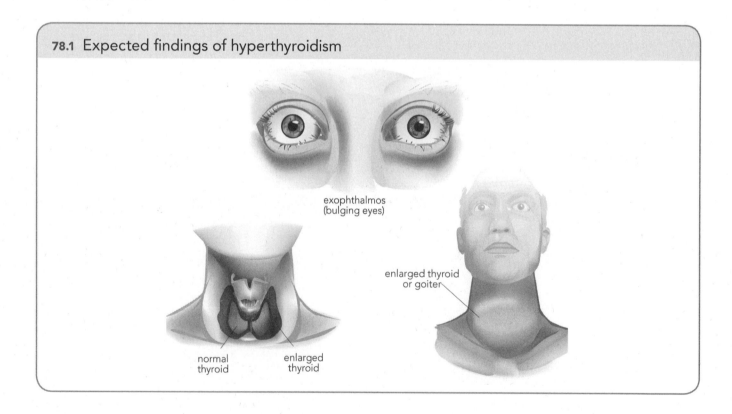

78.1 Expected findings of hyperthyroidism

exophthalmos (bulging eyes)

normal thyroid   enlarged thyroid

enlarged thyroid or goiter

NURSING CONSIDERATIONS

- Confirm that the client is not pregnant prior to the scan.
- Take a medication history to determine the use of iodides.
- Recent use of contrast media and oral contraceptives can cause falsely elevated serum thyroid hormone levels.
- Severe illness; malnutrition; and the use of aspirin, corticosteroids, and phenytoin sodium can cause a false decrease in serum thyroid hormone levels.
- Inform the provider if the client received any iodine contrast recently.

CLIENT EDUCATION

- Advise the client to avoid foods high in iodine for 1 week prior to the test.
- Suggest that the client use noniodized salt, and avoid fish, shellfish, and medications that contain iodine.

PATIENT-CENTERED CARE

NURSING CARE

- Minimize the client's energy expenditure by assisting with activities as necessary and by encouraging the client to alternate periods of activity with rest.
- Promote a calm environment.
- Assess mental status and decision-making ability. Intervene as needed to ensure safety.
- Monitor nutritional status. Provide increased calories, protein, and other nutritional support as necessary.
- Monitor I&O and the client's weight.
- Provide eye protection (patches, eye lubricant, tape to close eyelids) for a client who has exophthalmos.
- Monitor vital signs and hemodynamic parameters.
- Reduce room temperature.
- Provide cool shower/sponge bath to promote comfort.
- Provide linen changes as necessary.
- Report a temperature increase of 1° F or more to the provider immediately, because this is indicative of an impending thyroid crisis.
- Monitor ECG for dysrhythmias.
- Assure the family that any abrupt changes in the client's behavior are likely disease related and should subside with antithyroid therapy.
- Avoid excessive palpation of the thyroid gland.
- Administer antithyroid medications.
- Prepare the client for a total/subtotal thyroidectomy if the client is unresponsive to antithyroid medications or has an airway-obstructing goiter.

MEDICATIONS

Thionamides

- Methimazole and propylthiouracil inhibit the production of thyroid hormone.
- Thionamides are used to treat Graves' disease, as an adjunct to radioactive iodine therapy, to decrease hormone levels in preparation for surgery, and to treat thyrotoxicosis.

NURSING CONSIDERATIONS

- Monitor for manifestations of hypothyroidism, such as intolerance to cold, edema, bradycardia, increase in weight, or depression.
- Monitor CBC for leukopenia or thrombocytopenia.
- Monitor for indications of hepatotoxicity.

CLIENT EDUCATION

- Instruct the client to take the medication with meals.
- Advise the client to take the medication in divided doses at regular intervals to maintain an even therapeutic medication level.
- Advise the client to report fever, sore throat, or bruising to the provider.
- Advise the client to report any evidence of jaundice (yellowing of skin or eyes, darkening of urine).
- Advise the client to follow the provider's instructions about dietary intake of iodine.
- Remind women to advise the provider if they become pregnant.

Beta-adrenergic blockers

Propranolol, atenolol, and metoprolol treat sympathetic nervous system effects (tachycardia, palpitations). These medications counteract the effects of increased thyroid hormones but do not alter the levels of the hormones.

NURSING CONSIDERATIONS

- Monitor blood pressure, heart rate, and ECG.
- Monitor for hypoglycemia in clients who have diabetes mellitus.

CLIENT EDUCATION

- Advise the client that the medication can cause dizziness and to sit on the side of the bed for a few minutes before standing.
- Teach the client to check pulse prior to each dose and to notify the provider if heart rate falls below 60/min.
- Advise the client to discontinue the medication only on the advice of the provider.

Iodine solutions

Lugol's solution is a nonradioactive 5% elemental iodine in 10% potassium iodine that inhibits the release of thyroid hormone.

CLIENT EDUCATION

- These medications are for short-term use only (taken for 10 days followed by surgery).
- Administer 1 hr after an antithyroid medication.
- Use of these medications is contraindicated in pregnancy.
- Medication is available as a solution. Mix with juice or other liquid to mask the taste. Use a straw to avoid staining teeth. Take with food.
- These medications pass into breast milk and can have undesirable effects on a nursing infant.
- Instruct the client to notify the provider of fever, sore throat, and mouth ulcers.

THERAPEUTIC PROCEDURES

Radioactive iodine therapy

Radioactive iodine is taken up by the thyroid and destroys some of the hormone-producing cells (^{131}I).

- One dose can be sufficient, but a second or third dose might be needed.
- The degree of thyroid destruction varies and can require lifelong thyroid replacement.

NURSING CONSIDERATIONS

- Radioactive iodine therapy is contraindicated in women who are pregnant
- Monitor for manifestations of hypothyroidism, such as edema, intolerance to cold, bradycardia, increase in weight, and depression.

CLIENT EDUCATION Qs

- Advise the client that the effects of therapy might not be evident for 6 to 8 weeks.
- Advise the client to continue to take the medication as directed.
- Advise the client to stay away from pregnant women, infants, or small children for the first week following treatment. Avoid contact closer than 3 feet (1 meter) and limit contact to no more than 1 hr daily.
- Although a low dose of radiation is used, provide the client with precautions to prevent radiation exposure to others. Remind the client to follow directions from provider, which can include the following.
  - Do not use same toilet as others for 2 weeks.
  - Male clients should sit down to urinate.
  - Flush the toilet three times.
  - Take a laxative 2 to 3 days after treatment to help rid the body of stool contaminated with radiation.
  - Wear clothing that is washable, wash clothing separate from clothing of others, and run the washing machine for a full cycle after washing contaminated clothing.
  - Avoid contamination from saliva, do not share a toothbrush, and use disposable food service items (paper plates).

Thyroidectomy

The surgical removal of part or all of the thyroid gland

- **Subtotal thyroidectomy** can be performed for the treatment of hyperthyroidism when medication therapy fails or radiation therapy is contraindicated. It can also be used to correct diffuse goiter and thyroid cancer. After a subtotal thyroidectomy, the remaining thyroid tissue usually supplies enough thyroid hormone for normal function.
- If a **total thyroidectomy** is performed, the client will need thyroid hormone replacement therapy.

PREPROCEDURE NURSING CONSIDERATIONS

- Explain the purpose of the thyroidectomy to the client. Tell the client that there will be an incision in the neck, a dressing, and possibly a drain in place. Tell the client that some hoarseness and a sore throat from intubation and anesthesia can be experienced.
- The client usually receives propylthiouracil or methimazole 4 to 6 weeks before surgery.
- The client should receive iodine for 10 to 14 days before surgery. This reduces the gland's size and prevents excess bleeding.
- Beta blockers can be given to control hypertension, dysrhythmias, or tachycardia.
- The client can need to follow a high-protein, high-carbohydrate diet prior to surgery
- Instruct the client to support the neck when performing deep breathing and coughing exercises postoperatively.
- Notify the provider immediately if the client does not follow the medication regimen.

POSTPROCEDURE NURSING CONSIDERATIONS

- Keep the client in a semi-Fowler's position. Support head and neck with pillows. Avoid neck extension. Qs
- Following protocols, monitor vital signs typically every 15 min until stable then every 30 min.
- Assist with deep breathing exercises every 30 to 60 min.
- Provide oral and tracheal suction as needed.
- Check the surgical dressing and back of the neck for excessive bleeding. Respiratory distress can occur from compression of trachea due to hemorrhage, which is most likely to occur in the first 24 hr.
- Respiratory distress also can occur due to edema. Ensure that tracheostomy supplies are immediately available. Humidify air, assist to cough and deep breathe, and provide oral and tracheal suction if needed.
- Check for laryngeal nerve damage by asking the client to speak as soon as awake from anesthesia and every 2 hr thereafter.
- Administer medication to manage pain. Reassure the client that discomfort will resolve within a few days.
- Hypocalcemia and tetany can occur if parathyroid glands are damaged or removed. Indications are tingling of toes or around mouth, and muscle twitching. Check for positive Chvostek's and Trousseau's signs. Ensure that IV calcium gluconate or calcium chloride are immediately available.
  - Keep emergency equipment near the bedside. Qs
  - Monitor the client for evidence of hypocalcemia, such as tingling, muscle twitching, and numbness of mouth or distal extremities.
  - Advise the client to notify the nurse of any muscle twitching or tingling sensation of the mouth or distal extremities.

CLIENT EDUCATION

- Instruct the client to cough and breathe deeply while stabilizing the neck.
- Show the client how to change positions while supporting the back of the neck.
- Remind the client to be careful of the incisional drain if applicable.
- Advise the client that the voice will become hoarse, and to expect pain.
- Advise the client to notify the nurse of any tingling sensation of the mouth, tingling of the distal extremities, or muscle twitching.
- Remind the client that talking at intervals will be expected to check for nerve damage.
- Instruct the client to notify the surgeon of incisional drainage, swelling, or redness that can indicate infection.
- Advise the client and family to monitor for manifestations of hypothyroidism, such as hypothermia, lethargy, and weight gain.
- Instruct the client to take all medications as directed.
- Instruct clients who have had a total thyroidectomy that lifelong thyroid replacement medications will be required.
- Advise the client to check with the provider prior to taking over-the-counter medications.
- Instruct the client to keep all follow-up appointments.
- Advise the client to notify the surgeon of fever, increased restlessness, palpitations, or chest pain.

INTERPROFESSIONAL CARE

An endocrinologist, radiologist, pharmacist, and dietitian can collaborate in providing care for the client.

COMPLICATIONS

Hemorrhage at the incision site

Due to a loosened surgical tie, excessive coughing, or movement

NURSING CONSIDERATIONS

- Inspect the surgical incision and dressing for drainage and bleeding, especially at the back of the neck, and change the dressing as directed.
- Expect only scant drainage after 24 hr.
- Support the client's head and neck with pillows or sandbags. If the client is to be transferred from a stretcher to the bed, support the client's head and neck in good body alignment.

CLIENT EDUCATION

- To avoid pressure on the suture line, encourage the client to avoid neck flexion or extension.
- Instruct the client to cough and deep breathe while supporting the neck.
- Show the client how to change positions while supporting the back of the neck.

Thyroid storm/crisis

Thyroid storm/crisis results from a sudden surge of large amounts of thyroid hormones into the bloodstream, causing an even greater increase in body metabolism. This is a medical emergency with a high mortality rate.

- Precipitating factors include uncontrolled hyperthyroidism occurring most often with Graves' disease, infection, trauma, emotional stress, diabetic ketoacidosis, and digitalis toxicity, all of which increase demands on body metabolism. It also can occur following a surgical procedure or a thyroidectomy as a result of manipulation of the gland during surgery.
- Findings are hyperthermia, hypertension, delirium, vomiting, abdominal pain, tachydysrhythmias, chest pain, dyspnea, and palpitations.

NURSING CONSIDERATIONS

- Maintain a patent airway.
- Provide continuous cardiac monitoring for dysrhythmias.
- Administer acetaminophen to decrease temperature.

> ! Salicylate antipyretics (aspirin) are contraindicated because they release thyroxine from protein-binding sites and increase free thyroxine levels.

- Provide cool sponge baths, or apply ice packs to decrease fever. If fever continues, obtain a prescription for a cooling blanket for hyperthermia.
- Administer thionamides (methimazole or propylthiouracil) to prevent further synthesis and release of thyroid hormones.
- Administer sodium iodide as prescribed, 1 hr after administering thionamide medication.
- Administer beta-adrenergic blocking agents, such as propranolol, to block sympathetic nervous system effects.
- Administer glucocorticoids if adrenal insufficiency is suspected or to treat shock.
- Administer IV fluids to provide adequate hydration and prevent vascular collapse. Fluid volume deficit can occur due to increased fluid excretion by the kidneys or excessive diaphoresis. Monitor intake and output hourly to prevent fluid overload or inadequate replacement.
- Administer supplemental O_2 to meet increased oxygen demands.

CLIENT EDUCATION

- Provide support and information to the client and family about the condition and all procedures.
- Advise the client to notify the provider of fever, increased restlessness, palpitations, and chest pain.

Airway obstruction

Hemorrhage, tracheal collapse, tracheal mucus accumulation, laryngeal edema, and vocal cord paralysis can cause respiratory obstruction, with sudden stridor and restlessness.

NURSING CONSIDERATIONS
- A tracheostomy tray should be kept near the client at all times during the immediate recovery period. Qs
- Maintain the bed in a high-Fowler's position to decrease edema and swelling of the neck.
- If the client reports that the dressing feels tight, alert the provider immediately.
- Listen for respiratory stridor.
- Provide humidified air.
- Have suction equipment at the bedside.
- Medicate as prescribed to reduce swelling.

CLIENT EDUCATION: Instruct the client to notify the nurse of tightness or difficulty breathing.

Hypocalcemia and tetany

Damage to parathyroid gland causes hypocalcemia and tetany.

NURSING CONSIDERATIONS
- Monitor for indications of hypocalcemia (tingling of the fingers and toes, carpopedal spasms, convulsions).
- Assess for Chvostek's and Trousseau's signs, which are indicators of neuromuscular irritability from hypocalcemia.
- Have IV calcium gluconate available for emergency administration. Qs
- Maintain seizure precautions.

CLIENT EDUCATION: Advise the client to notify the nurse of any tingling sensation of the mouth, tingling of distal extremities, or muscle twitching.

Nerve damage

- Nerve damage can lead to vocal cord paralysis and vocal disturbances.
- Incisional damage or swelling can cause nerve damage.

NURSING CONSIDERATIONS
- Teach the client that he will be hoarse, be able to speak only rarely, and need to rest his voice for several days.
- After the procedure, monitor the client's ability to speak every 2 hr and document any changes.
- Assess the client's voice tone and quality, and compare it with the preoperative voice.

CLIENT EDUCATION: Remind the client that he will be asked to try to talk at intervals to check for nerve damage. Advise the client that a hoarse voice is not typically permanent.

Application Exercises

1. A nurse in a provider's office is reviewing the health record of a client who is being evaluated for Graves' disease. The nurse should identify that which of the following laboratory results is an expected finding?

   A. Decreased thyrotropin receptor antibodies
   B. Decreased thyroid-stimulating hormone (TSH)
   C. Decreased free thyroxine index
   D. Decreased triiodothyronine

2. A nurse is reviewing the manifestations of hyperthyroidism with a client. Which of the following findings should the nurse include? (Select all that apply.)

   A. Anorexia
   B. Heat intolerance
   C. Constipation
   D. Palpitations
   E. Weight loss
   F. Bradycardia

3. A nurse is providing instructions to a client who has Graves' disease and has a new prescription for propranolol. Which of the following information should the nurse include?

   A. "An adverse effect of this medication is jaundice."
   B. "Take your pulse before each dose."
   C. "The purpose of this medication is to decrease production of thyroid hormone."
   D. "You should stop taking this medication if you have a sore throat."

4. A nurse is preparing to receive a client from the PACU who is postoperative following a thyroidectomy. The nurse should ensure that which of the following equipment is available? (Select all that apply.)

   A. Suction equipment
   B. Humidified oxygen
   C. Flashlight
   D. Tracheostomy tray
   E. Chest tube tray

5. A nurse in a provider's office is planning care for a client who has a new diagnosis of Graves' disease and a new prescription for methimazole. Which of the following interventions should the nurse include in the plan of care? (Select all that apply.)

   A. Monitor CBC.
   B. Monitor triiodothyronine (T_3).
   C. Instruct the client to increase consumption of shellfish.
   D. Advise the client to take the medication at the same time every day.
   E. Inform the client that an adverse effect of this medication is iodine toxicity.

6. A nurse is assessing a client who is 12 hr postoperative following a thyroidectomy. The nurse should identify which of the following findings as indicative of thyroid crisis? (Select all that apply.)

   A. Bradycardia
   B. Hypothermia
   C. Dyspnea
   D. Abdominal pain
   E. Mental confusion

PRACTICE Active Learning Scenario

A nurse is reinforcing teaching with a client who will have radioactive iodine therapy. What should the nurse include in the teaching? Use the ATI Active Learning Template: Therapeutic Procedure to complete this item.

DESCRIPTION OF PROCEDURE: Provide a brief description of the procedure.

CLIENT EDUCATION: Identify five client instructions the nurse should include.

Application Exercises Key

1. A. In the presence of Graves' disease, elevated thyrotropin receptor antibodies is an expected finding.

   B. **CORRECT:** In the presence of Graves' disease, low TSH is an expected finding. The pituitary gland decreases the production of TSH when thyroid hormone levels are elevated.

   C. In the presence of Graves' disease, elevated free thyroxine index is an expected finding.

   D. In the presence of Graves' disease, elevated triiodothyronine is an expected finding.

   Ⓝ *NCLEX® Connection: Reduction of Risk Potential, Laboratory Values*

2. A. The client who has hyperthyroidism has an increased metabolic rate, resulting in increased hunger.

   B. **CORRECT:** Hyperthyroidism increases the client's metabolism, causing heat intolerance.

   C. Diarrhea is an expected finding for the client who has hyperthyroidism.

   D. **CORRECT:** Hyperthyroidism increases the client's metabolism, causing palpitations.

   E. **CORRECT:** Hyperthyroidism increases the client's metabolism, causing weight loss.

   F. Hyperthyroidism increases the client's metabolism, causing tachycardia.

   Ⓝ *NCLEX® Connection: Physiological Adaptation, Pathophysiology*

3. A. Yellowing of the skin is an adverse effect of methimazole.

   B. **CORRECT:** Propranolol can cause bradycardia. The client should take his pulse before each dose. If there is a significant change, he should withhold the dose and consult the provider.

   C. The purpose of propranolol is to suppress tachycardia, diaphoresis, and other effects of Graves' disease.

   D. Sore throat is not an adverse effect of this medication. The client should not discontinue taking this medication because this action can result in tachycardia and dysrhythmias.

   Ⓝ *NCLEX® Connection: Pharmacological and Parenteral Therapies, Medication Administration*

4. A. **CORRECT:** The client can require oral or tracheal suctioning. The nurse should ensure that suctioning equipment is available.

   B. **CORRECT:** The client can require supplemental oxygen due to respiratory complications. Humidified oxygen thins secretions and promotes respiratory exchange. This equipment should be available.

   C. A flashlight is used to measure the reaction of the pupils to light for a client who has an intracranial disorder. Checking pupil reaction with a flashlight is not indicated for this client.

   D. **CORRECT:** The client can experience respiratory obstruction. A tracheostomy tray should be available at the bedside.

   E. A chest tube tray would be used for a client who develops a hemothorax or pneumothorax. This is not an expected complication of a thyroidectomy. This equipment is not indicated for this client.

   Ⓝ *NCLEX® Connection: Physiological Adaptation, Illness Management*

5. A. **CORRECT:** Methimazole can cause a number of hematologic effects, including leukopenia and thrombocytopenia. The nurse should monitor CBC.

   B. **CORRECT:** Methimazole reduces thyroid hormone production. The nurse should monitor T_3.

   C. Methimazole reduces thyroid hormone production by blocking iodine. The nurse should instruct the client to limit iodine containing foods such as shellfish.

   D. **CORRECT:** Methimazole should be taken at the same time every day to maintain blood levels.

   E. Iodine toxicity is an adverse effect of potassium iodide solution.

   Ⓝ *NCLEX® Connection: Pharmacological and Parenteral Therapies, Medication Administration*

6. A. When thyroid crisis occurs, the client experiences an extreme rise in metabolic rate, which results in tachycardia.

   B. When thyroid crisis occurs, the client experiences an extreme rise in metabolic rate, which results in a high fever.

   C. **CORRECT:** Excessive levels of thyroid hormone can cause the client to experience dyspnea.

   D. **CORRECT:** When thyroid crisis occurs, the client can experience gastrointestinal conditions, such as vomiting, diarrhea, and abdominal pain.

   E. **CORRECT:** Excessive thyroid hormone levels can cause the client to experience mental confusion.

   Ⓝ *NCLEX® Connection: Reduction of Risk Potential, Potential for Complications from Surgical Procedures and Health Alterations*

PRACTICE Answer

Using the ATI Active Learning Template: Therapeutic Procedure

DESCRIPTION OF PROCEDURE: Radioactive iodine (^{131}I) is administered orally 24 hr prior to a thyroid scan. The thyroid absorbs the radiation, which results in destruction of cells that produce thyroid hormone.

CLIENT EDUCATION

- Advise the client that the effects of the therapy might not be evident for 6 to 8 weeks.
- Advise the client to take medication as directed.
- Provide the client with precautions to prevent radiation exposure to others.

- Remind the client to follow directions from provider, which can include the following.
  ○ Do not use same toilet as others for 2 weeks.
  ○ Sit down to urinate.
  ○ Flush the toilet three times.
  ○ Take a laxative 2 to 3 days after treatment to rid the body of stool contaminated with radiation.
  ○ Wear clothing that is washable, wash clothing separate from clothing of others, and run the washing machine for a full cycle after washing contaminated clothing.
  ○ Avoid infants or small children for 2 to 4 days after the procedure.
  ○ Avoid contamination from saliva, do not share a toothbrush, and use disposable food service items (paper plates).

Ⓝ *NCLEX® Connection: Reduction of Risk Potential, Therapeutic Procedures*

CHAPTER 79 *Hypothyroidism*

Hypothyroidism is a condition in which there is an inadequate amount of circulating thyroid hormones triiodothyronine (T_3) and thyroxine (T_4), causing a decrease in metabolic rate that affects all body systems.

Because hypothyroidism can have manifestations that mimic the aging process, hypothyroidism is often undiagnosed in older adult clients. This can lead to potentially serious adverse effects from medications (sedatives, opiates, anesthetics). ©

CLASSIFICATIONS BY ETIOLOGY

Primary hypothyroidism stems from dysfunction of the thyroid gland. This is the most common type of hypothyroidism and is caused by the following.
- Disease: autoimmune thyroiditis
- Use of medications that decrease the synthesis of thyroid hormone
- Loss of the thyroid gland: iodine deficiency, radioactive iodine treatment, surgical removal of the gland

Secondary hypothyroidism is caused by failure of the anterior pituitary gland to stimulate the thyroid gland or failure of the target tissues to respond to the thyroid hormones (pituitary tumors).

Tertiary hypothyroidism is caused by failure of the hypothalamus to produce thyroid-releasing hormone.

ASSESSMENT

RISK FACTORS

- Women 30 to 60 years old are affected 7 to 10 times more often than men.
- Many individuals who have mild hypothyroidism are frequently undiagnosed, but the hormone disturbance can contribute to an acceleration of atherosclerosis or complications of medical treatment (intraoperative hypotension, cardiac complications following surgery).
- Use of certain medications (lithium, amiodarone)
- Inadequate intake of iodine
- Radiation therapy to the head and neck

EXPECTED FINDINGS

Hypothyroidism is often characterized by vague and varied findings that develop slowly over time. Manifestations can vary and are related to the severity of the condition.
- Fatigue, lethargy
- Irritability
- Intolerance to cold
- Constipation
- Weight gain without an increase in caloric intake
- Pale skin
- Thick, brittle fingernails
- Depression and apathy
- Periorbital edema
- Joint or muscle pain
- Bradycardia, hypotension, dysrhythmias
- Slow thought processes and speech
- Hypoventilation, pleural effusion
- Thickening of the skin
- Thinning of hair on the eyebrows
- Dry, flaky skin
- Swelling in face, hands, and feet (myxedema [non-pitting, mucinous edema])
- Decreased acuity of taste and smell
- Hoarse, raspy speech
- Abnormal menstrual periods (menorrhagia/amenorrhea)
- Decreased libido

LABORATORY TESTS

T_3 expected reference range
- 70 to 205 ng/dL in adults ages 20 to 50
- 40 to 180 ng/dL in clients older than 50

T_4 expected reference range
- 4 to 12 mcg/dL in men
- 5 to 12 mcg/dL in women

EXPECTED RESULTS WITH HYPOTHYROIDISM
- **T_3:** Decreased
- **Serum thyroid-stimulating hormone (TSH)**
  - Increased with primary hypothyroidism
  - Decreased or within the expected reference range in secondary hypothyroidism
- **Free thyroxine index and T_4 levels:** Decreased
- **T_3 resin uptake:** Decreased
- **Thyrotropin receptor antibodies:** No response
- **Serum cholesterol:** Increased

DIAGNOSTIC PROCEDURES

Radioisotope (^{123}I) scan and uptake: Clients who have hypothyroidism have a low uptake of the iodine preparation.

ECG: Sinus bradycardia, dysrhythmias

PATIENT-CENTERED CARE

NURSING CARE

- Monitor for cardiovascular changes (low blood pressure, bradycardia, dysrhythmias).
- Monitor the client's weight. Assess for peripheral edema.
- If mental status is compromised, orient the client periodically, and provide safety measures. Qs
- Increase the client's activity level gradually, and provide frequent rest periods to avoid fatigue and decrease myocardial oxygen demands.
- Apply antiembolism stockings, and elevate the client's legs to assist venous return.
- Monitor respiratory status including rate, depth, pattern, oximetry, and arterial blood gases. Encourage the client to cough and breathe deeply to prevent pulmonary complications.
- Consult with a dietitian. Provide a low-calorie, high-bulk diet, and encourage fluids and activity to prevent constipation and promote weight loss. Administer cathartics and stool softeners as needed. Avoid fiber laxatives, which interfere with absorption of levothyroxine. Qᴛᴄ
- Provide meticulous skin care. Turn and reposition the client every 2 hr if the client is on extended bed rest. Use alcohol-free skin care products and an emollient lotion after bathing.
- Provide extra clothing and blankets for clients who have decreased cold tolerance. Dress the client in layers, adjust room temperature, and encourage intake of warm liquids if possible.
- Caution the client against using electric blankets or other electric heating devices because the combination of vasodilation, decreased sensation, and decreased alertness can result in unrecognized burns. Qs
- Encourage the client to verbalize feelings and fears about changes in body image. Return to the euthyroid (normal thyroid gland function) state takes time. The client might need frequent reassurance that most physical manifestations are reversible.
- Use caution with medications due to alteration in metabolism. Qs
  - CNS depressants (barbiturates or sedatives) are used with caution due to the risk of respiratory depression.
  - If CNS depressants are prescribed, the dose should be significantly less than for a client who does not have hypothyroidism.
  - Hypothyroidism alters metabolism and excretion of medications. The provider uses caution in prescribing medications to clients who have this condition.

MEDICATIONS

Thyroid hormone replacement therapy

Levothyroxine
- Thyroid hormone replacement therapy is the treatment of choice.
- Levothyroxine increases the effects of warfarin and can increase the need for insulin and digoxin.
- Medications that decrease the absorption of levothyroxine include cimetidine, lansoprazole, sucralfate, and colestipol. Administration of these medications should be separated from levothyroxine by at least 4 hr.
- Medications that can accelerate the metabolism of levothyroxine include phenytoin, carbamazepine, rifampin, sertraline, and phenobarbital, thus requiring an increase in dosage of levothyroxine to achieve therapeutic levels.
- Use caution when starting thyroid hormone replacement with older adult clients and those who have coronary artery disease to avoid coronary ischemia because of increased oxygen demands of the heart. It is preferable to start with much lower doses and increase gradually, taking 1 to 2 months to reach full replacement doses. Ⓒ

NURSING CONSIDERATIONS
- Administer thyroid hormone replacement therapy.
- Monitor for cardiovascular compromise (e.g., chest pain, palpitations, rapid heart rate, shortness of breath).

CLIENT EDUCATION
- Instruct the client that treatment begins slowly and that the dosage is increased every 2 to 3 weeks until the desired response is obtained. Serum TSH is monitored at scheduled times to ensure correct dosage.
- Remind the client to take the dose prescribed. Do not stop taking the medication or change the dose.
- Tell the client to take the medication on an empty stomach, typically 30 to 60 min before breakfast.
- Inform the client that fiber supplements, calcium, iron, and antacids interfere with absorption. Before taking any over-the-counter medications, the client must consult with the provider.
- Instruct the client to monitor for and report manifestations of hyperthyroidism (irritability, tremors, tachycardia, palpitations, heat intolerance, rapid weight loss).
- Inform the client that the treatment is considered to be lifelong, requiring ongoing medical assessment of thyroid function.

INTERPROFESSIONAL CARE

A home health nurse might need to visit the client and assess for adverse effects during the first few weeks of therapy.

COMPLICATIONS

Myxedema

Myxedema coma is a life-threatening condition that occurs when hypothyroidism is untreated or when a stressor (e.g., acute illness, surgery, chemotherapy, discontinuing thyroid replacement therapy, or use of sedatives/opioids) affects a client who has hypothyroidism.

MANIFESTATIONS

- Respiratory failure
- Hypotension
- Hypothermia
- Bradycardia, dysrhythmia
- Hyponatremia
- Hypoglycemia
- Coma

NURSING CONSIDERATIONS

- Maintain airway patency with ventilatory support if necessary.
- Provide continuous ECG monitoring.
- Monitor ABGs to detect hypoxia, hypercapnia, respiratory acidosis.
- Monitor mental status.
- Cover the client with warm blankets.
- Monitor body temperature hourly until stable.
- Replace fluid with 0.9% sodium chloride IV.
- Replace thyroid hormone by administering large doses of levothyroxine IV bolus. Monitor vital signs because rapid correction of hypothyroidism can cause adverse cardiac effects.
- Monitor I&O and daily weights. With treatment, urine output should increase, and body weight should decrease. Failure to do so should be reported to the provider.
- Treat hypoglycemia with glucose.
- Administer corticosteroids.
- Initiate aspiration precautions
- Check for possible sources of infection (blood, sputum, urine) that might have precipitated the coma. Treat any underlying illness.

PRACTICE Active Learning Scenario

A nurse is reviewing information about hypothyroidism with a client. What information should the nurse include in the discussion? Use the ATI Active Learning Template: System Disorder to complete this item.

ALTERATION IN HEALTH (DIAGNOSIS):
Provide a brief description of the disorder.

RISK FACTORS: Identify two risk factors.

DIAGNOSTIC PROCEDURES: Identify two laboratory tests that are used to diagnose hypothyroidism.

Application Exercises

1. A nurse in a provider's office is reviewing laboratory results of a client who is being evaluated for secondary hypothyroidism. Which of the following laboratory findings is expected for a client who has this condition?

   A. Elevated serum T_4

   B. Decreased serum T_3

   C. Elevated serum thyroid stimulating hormone

   D. Decreased serum cholesterol

2. A nurse is collecting an admission history from a female client who has hypothyroidism. Which of the following findings should the nurse expect? (Select all that apply.)

   A. Diarrhea

   B. Menorrhagia

   C. Dry skin

   D. Increased libido

   E. Hoarseness

3. A nurse is reinforcing teaching with a client who has a new prescription for levothyroxine to treat hypothyroidism. Which of the following information should the nurse include in the teaching? (Select all that apply.)

   A. Weight gain is expected while taking this medication.

   B. Medication should not be discontinued without the advice of the provider.

   C. Follow-up serum TSH levels should be obtained.

   D. Take the medication on an empty stomach.

   E. Use fiber laxatives for constipation.

4. A nurse in an intensive care unit is planning care for a client who has myxedema coma. Which of the following actions should the nurse include? (Select all that apply.)

   A. Observe cardiac monitor for dysrhythmias.

   B. Observe for evidence of urinary tract infection.

   C. Initiate IV fluids using 0.9% sodium chloride.

   D. Administer a levothyroxine IV bolus.

   E. Provide warmth using a heating pad.

5. A nurse in a provider's office is assessing a client who has hypothyroidism and recently began treatment with thyroid hormone replacement therapy. Which of the following findings should indicate to the nurse that the client might need a decrease in the dosage of the medication?

   A. Hand tremors

   B. Bradycardia

   C. Pallor

   D. Slow speech

Application Exercises Key

1. A. Decreased serum T₄ is an expected finding for a client who has hypothyroidism.

   B. **CORRECT:** Decreased serum T₃ is an expected finding for a client who has hypothyroidism.

   C. Decreased thyroid stimulating hormone level is an expected finding in a client who has secondary hypothyroidism.

   D. Elevated serum cholesterol is an expected finding for a client who has hypothyroidism.

   Ⓝ *NCLEX® Connection: Reduction of Risk Potential, Laboratory Values*

2. A. Constipation is a manifestation of hypothyroidism.

   B. **CORRECT:** Abnormal menstrual periods, including menorrhagia and amenorrhea, are manifestations of hypothyroidism.

   C. **CORRECT:** Dry skin is a manifestation of hypothyroidism.

   D. Decreased libido is a manifestation of hypothyroidism.

   E. **CORRECT:** Hoarseness is a manifestation of hypothyroidism.

   Ⓝ *NCLEX® Connection: Physiological Adaptation, Pathophysiology*

3. A. Levothyroxine speeds up metabolism. Weight loss is an expected effect.

   B. **CORRECT:** The provider carefully titrates the dosage of this medication. It should be increased slowly until the client reaches a euthyroid state. The client should not discontinue the medication unless directed to do so by the provider.

   C. **CORRECT:** Serum TSH levels are used to monitor the effectiveness of the medication.

   D. **CORRECT:** The medication should be taken on an empty stomach to promote absorption.

   E. Fiber laxatives reduce absorption of the medication and should be avoided.

   Ⓝ *NCLEX® Connection: Pharmacological and Parenteral Therapies, Medication Administration*

4. A. **CORRECT:** A client who has myxedema can have a flat or inverted T wave as well as ST deviations.

   B. **CORRECT:** An infection, such as in the urinary tract, can precipitate myxedema coma. The nurse should observe the client for manifestations of infection so that the underlying illness can be treated.

   C. **CORRECT:** Hyponatremia is an expected finding in the presence of myxedema coma. IV therapy is administered using 0.9% sodium chloride.

   D. **CORRECT:** Myxedema coma is a severe complication of hypothyroidism that if left untreated can lead to coma or death. Levothyroxine is administered IV bolus to treat the condition.

   E. The nurse should provide warmth with extra clothing and blankets. Electric heating devices should be avoided because the combination of vasodilation, decreased sensation, and decreased alertness places the client at risk for burns.

   Ⓝ *NCLEX® Connection: Physiological Adaptation, Medical Emergencies*

5. A. **CORRECT:** The nurse should identify hand tremors as a manifestation of hyperthyroidism that can result from thyroid hormone replacement therapy. The nurse should report this finding to the provider due to the possible need for a decrease in the dosage of medication.

   B. Bradycardia is an expected finding for hypothyroidism. This finding indicates the need for continued thyroid hormone replacement therapy with a possible increase in dosage.

   C. Pallor is an expected finding for hypothyroidism. This finding indicates the need for continued thyroid hormone replacement therapy with a possible increase in dosage.

   D. Slow thought processes and speech are expected findings for hypothyroidism. This finding indicates the need for continued thyroid hormone replacement therapy with a possible increase in dosage.

   Ⓝ *NCLEX® Connection: Physiological Adaptation, Medical Emergencies*

PRACTICE Answer

Using the ATI Active Learning Template: System Disorder

ALTERATION IN HEALTH (DIAGNOSIS): Hypothyroidism is a condition in which there is an inadequate amount of circulating thyroid hormones triiodothyronine (T₃) and thyroxine (T₄), causing a decrease in metabolic rate that affects all body systems.

RISK FACTORS
- Female clients age 30 to 60 years
- Use of lithium or amiodarone

LABORATORY TESTS
- Serum T₃
- Serum T₄
- Free T₄ index
- T₃ resin uptake
- Thyroid antibodies
- THR stimulation test
- TSH
- Serum cholesterol

Ⓝ *NCLEX® Connection: Physiological Adaptation, Illness Management*

CHAPTER 80 *Cushing's
Disease/Syndrome*

Cushing's disease (hypercortisolism) and Cushing's syndrome are caused by an oversecretion of the hormones the adrenal cortex produces.

Cushing's disease can be the result of a tumor in the pituitary gland resulting in release of the hormone ACTH. The ACTH then stimulates the adrenal cortex to increase the secretion of the glucocorticoid hormone cortisol. It can also be the result of hyperplasia of the adrenal cortex.

Cushing's syndrome results from long-term use of glucocorticoids to treat other conditions, such as asthma or rheumatoid arthritis.

ADRENAL CORTEX HORMONES

Mineralocorticoids: Aldosterone increases sodium absorption, and causes potassium excretion in the kidney.

Glucocorticoids: Cortisol affects glucose, protein, and fat metabolism; the body's response to stress; and the body's immune function.

Sex hormones: Androgens and estrogens

HEALTH PROMOTION AND DISEASE PREVENTION

- Advise the client to take medications and watch for adverse reactions. Advise the client that the need for medication therapy can be lifelong.
- Advise the client to eat foods high in calcium and vitamin D. The client should not ingest alcohol or caffeine. Advise the client to monitor for indications of gastric bleeding, such as coffee-ground emesis or black, tarry stools.
- Advise the client to avoid infection by using good hygiene and avoiding crowds or individuals who have infections. Qs
- Advise the client that he might need assistance at home due to residual muscle weakness.
- Instruct the client to monitor weigh himself every day and report weight gain.

ASSESSMENT

RISK FACTORS

Women between the ages of 20 and 40 years

Cushing's disease

ENDOGENOUS CAUSES OF INCREASED CORTISOL
- Adrenal hyperplasia
- Adrenocortical carcinoma
- Pituitary carcinoma that secretes adrenocorticotropic hormone (ACTH)
- Carcinomas of the lung, gastrointestinal (GI) tract, or pancreas (these tumors can secrete ACTH)

Cushing's syndrome

EXOGENOUS CAUSES OF INCREASED CORTISOL:
Therapeutic use of glucocorticoids for the following.
- Organ transplant
- Chemotherapy
- Autoimmune diseases
- Asthma
- Allergies
- Chronic inflammatory diseases

EXPECTED FINDINGS

- Weakness, fatigue, sleep disturbances
- Back and joint pain
- Altered emotional state (irritability, depression)
- Decreased libido

PHYSICAL ASSESSMENT FINDINGS
- Evidence of decreased immune function and decreased inflammatory response (infections without fever, swelling, drainage, redness)
- Thin, fragile skin
- Bruising and petechiae (fragile blood vessels)
- Hypertension (sodium and water retention)
- Tachycardia
- Gastric ulcers due to oversecretion of hydrochloric acid
- Weight gain and increased appetite
- Irregular menses
- Dependent edema: Changes in fat distribution, including the characteristic fat distribution of moon face, truncal obesity, and fat collection on the back of the neck (buffalo hump)
- Fractures (osteoporosis)
- Bone pain and fractures with an increased risk for falls Qs
- Muscle wasting (particularly in the extremities)
- Impaired glucose tolerance
- Frequent infections, poor wound healing
- Hirsutism
- Acne
- Red cheeks
- Striae (reddened lines on the abdomen, upper arms, thighs)
- Clitoral hypertrophy
- Thinning, balding hair
- Hyperglycemia
- Emotional lability

LABORATORY TESTS

Elevated plasma cortisol levels in the absence of acute illness or stress indicate Cushing's disease/syndrome. Urine (24-hr urine collection) contains elevated levels of free cortisol.

Plasma adrenocorticotropic hormone (ACTH) levels
- Hypersecretion of ACTH by the anterior pituitary results in elevated ACTH levels.
- Disorders of the adrenal cortex or medication therapy results in decreased ACTH levels.

Salivary cortisol elevations confirm the diagnosis of Cushing's disease.

Potassium and calcium levels: Decreased

Glucose level: Increased

Sodium level: Increased

Lymphocytes: Decreased

Dexamethasone suppression tests: Tests vary in length and amount of dexamethasone to administer. 24-hr urine collections show suppression of cortisol excretion in clients who do not have Cushing's disease. Nonsuppression of cortisol excretion indicates Cushing's disease. Clients should stop taking medications and try to reduce stress prior to and during testing. False positive results can result for clients who have acute illnesses and alcohol use disorder.

DIAGNOSTIC PROCEDURES

- X-ray, magnetic resonance imaging, and CT scans identify lesions of the pituitary gland, adrenal gland, lung, GI tract, and pancreas.
- Radiological imaging determines the source of adrenal insufficiency (tumor, adrenal atrophy).

NURSING ACTIONS
- Establish IV access.
- Determine allergies.
- Explain the procedure.
- Provide padding, pillows, and/or blankets for comfort. Qs

CLIENT EDUCATION: Explain that the tests are noninvasive and not painful.

PATIENT-CENTERED CARE

NURSING CARE

- Monitor I&O and daily weight.
- Assess for indications of hypervolemia (edema, distended neck veins, shortness of breath, adventitious breath sounds, hypertension, tachycardia).
- Maintain a safe environment to minimize the risk of pathological fractures and skin trauma. Qs
- Prevent infection by performing frequent hand hygiene.
- Encourage physical activity within the client's limitations.
- Provide meticulous skin care.
- Change the client's position at least every 2 hr.
- Monitor for and protect against skin breakdown and infection.
- Use surgical asepsis when performing dressing changes and any invasive procedures.
- Monitor WBC count with differential daily.

MEDICATIONS

Treatment depends on the cause. For Cushing's syndrome, tapering off glucocorticoids and managing symptoms are necessary.

Ketoconazole

An adrenal corticosteroid inhibitor, ketoconazole is an antifungal agent that inhibits adrenal corticosteroid synthesis in high dosages.

NURSING ACTIONS
- Ketoconazole supplements radiation or surgery.
- Monitor liver enzymes and for indications of liver toxicity (yellow sclera, dark-colored urine).
- Monitor fluids and electrolytes for clients who have gastric effects.

CLIENT EDUCATION
- Advise the client that the medication can cause nausea, vomiting, and dizziness.
- Advise the client that relief is temporary. Symptoms will return if he stops taking the medication.
- Inform the client that he may take the medication with food to relieve gastric effects. Qs

Mitotane

Produces selective destruction of adrenocortical cells

NURSING ACTIONS
- Mitotane treats inoperable adrenal carcinoma.
- Monitor for indications of shock, renal damage, and hepatotoxicity.
- Monitor for orthostatic hypotension.

CLIENT EDUCATION
- Advise the client that the purpose of the medication is to reduce the size of the tumor.
- Inform the client to notify the provider if he has weakness, dizziness, nausea, vomiting, or weight loss.
- Advise the client to use caution when driving or operating heavy machinery.
- Inform the client that he will need lifelong replacement with glucocorticoids.

Hydrocortisone

For replacement therapy for clients who have adrenocortical insufficiency

NURSING ACTIONS
- Monitor potassium and glucose levels.
- Measure daily weight. Notify the provider of weight gain greater than 2.3 kg (5 lb)/week.
- Monitor blood pressure and pulse.
- Monitor for manifestations of infection (increased temperature, increased WBC).

CLIENT EDUCATION
- Instruct the client to carry emergency identification about corticosteroid use.
- Advise the client to report abdominal pain or black, tarry stools.
- Inform the client to notify the provider for any signs of infection.
- Instruct the client to take the medication without skipping any doses.
- Advise the client to consume a diet high in calcium and vitamin D.
- Tell the client to consult the provider before taking any OTC medications or supplements.

THERAPEUTIC PROCEDURES

Chemotherapy

With cytotoxic agents for Cushing's disease resulting from a tumor

NURSING ACTIONS
- RNs who have advanced education in the administration of chemotherapy administer IV chemotherapy.
  - Other nurses who provide care to the client must monitor and manage the multitude of adverse effects of medications.
  - For standards of care from the Oncology Nursing Society, see www.ons.org. The Occupational Safety and Health Administration regulations are available at www.osha.gov.
- Monitor for adverse effects, such as thrombocytopenia, nausea, and vomiting, along with other effects specific to the chemotherapeutic agent.
- Monitor WBC, absolute neutrophil count, platelet count, Hgb, and Hct.
- Assess for bruising and bleeding gums.
- Administer an antiemetic.

CLIENT EDUCATION
- Instruct the client to avoid crowds and contact with individuals who have infections.
- Advise the client to watch for bleeding, such as tarry stools or coffee-ground emesis.
- Advise the client that he might have some hair loss.

Radiation therapy

NURSING ACTIONS: Provide skin care and assess for skin damage. ⓠEBP

CLIENT EDUCATION
- Tell the client not to remove radiation markings.
- Advise the client to avoid applying lotions, other than those the radiologist prescribes, to affected areas.
- Advise the client to avoid exposing irradiated areas to sunlight.
- Advise the client to expect fatigue and altered taste due to radiation.

Hypophysectomy

Surgical removal of the pituitary gland (depending on the cause of Cushing's disease)

NURSING ACTIONS
- Monitor and correct electrolytes, especially sodium, potassium, and chloride. Monitor and adjust glucose levels. Monitor ECG.
- Protect the client from developing an infection by using good hand hygiene and making sure the client avoids contact with individuals who have infections. Use caution to prevent a fracture by providing assistance getting out of bed and raising side rails.
- Monitor for bleeding. Monitor nasal drainage for a possible cerebrospinal fluid (CSF) leak. Assess drainage for the presence of glucose or a halo sign (yellow on the edge and clear in the middle), which can indicate CSF.
- Assess neurologic status every hour for the first 24 hr and then every 4 hr.
- Administer glucocorticoids to prevent an abrupt drop in cortisol level.
- Administer stool softeners to prevent straining.

CLIENT EDUCATION
- Advise the client to use caution preoperatively to prevent infection or fractures.
- Inform the client that the surgeon will perform a transsphenoidal hypophysectomy through the sphenoid sinus via the nasal cavity or under the upper lip and to expect nasal packing postoperatively. The client will have a drip pad under his nose for bloody drainage and will need to breathe through his mouth. Advise him to avoid coughing, blowing his nose, and sneezing.
- Teach the client that he might have numbness at the surgical site and a diminished sense of smell for 3 to 4 months after surgery.
- Instruct the client to avoid bending over at the waist and straining to prevent increased intracranial pressure. If he must bend to pick up an object or to tie shoes, he should bend at the knees.

- Instruct the client to avoid brushing his teeth for 2 weeks. Advise the client to floss and rinse his mouth. Q EBP
- Advise the client to notify the provider of sweet-tasting drainage, drainage that makes a halo (yellow on the edge and clear in the middle), or clear drainage from his nose, which can indicate a CSF leak. Another indication is a headache.
- Advise the client to notify the provider of excessive bleeding, confusion, or headache.
- To avoid constipation, which contributes to increased intracranial pressure, the client should eat high-fiber food and take docusate.

Adrenalectomy

Surgical removal of the adrenal gland can be unilateral (one gland) or bilateral (both glands).

NURSING ACTIONS
- Provide glucocorticoid and hormone replacement.
- Monitor for adrenal crisis due to an abrupt drop in cortisol level. Findings include hypotension, tachycardia, tachypnea, nausea, and headache.
- Monitor vital signs and hemodynamic levels initially every 15 min.
- Monitor fluids and electrolytes.
- Monitor the incision site for bleeding.
- Monitor bowel sounds.
- Provide pain medication. Administer stool softeners.
- Slowly reintroduce foods.
- Assess the abdomen for distention and tenderness. Monitor the incision site for redness, discharge, and swelling.

CLIENT EDUCATION
- Teach the client about postoperative pain management, deep breathing, and antiembolism care.
- Advise the client of the need to take glucocorticoids, mineralocorticoids, and hormone replacements.

INTERPROFESSIONAL CARE

Request a dietary consult. Dietary alterations include decreased sodium intake and increased intake of potassium, protein, calcium, and vitamin D.

COMPLICATIONS

Perforated viscera/ulceration

Decreases production of protective mucus in the lining of the stomach due to an increase in cortisol

NURSING ACTIONS
- Monitor for evidence of GI bleeding (tarry, black stool; coffee-ground emesis).
- Administer antiulcer medications.

CLIENT EDUCATION: Advise the client to monitor for GI bleeding and to avoid alcohol, caffeine, and smoking.

Bone fractures due to hypocalcemia

NURSING ACTIONS
- Use caution when moving the client. Qs
- Provide assistance when the client is ambulating.
- Clear floors to prevent falls.

CLIENT EDUCATION
- Encourage a diet high in calcium and vitamin D.
- Advise the client to avoid dangerous activities.

Infection due to immunosuppression

Immunosuppression and reduced inflammatory response occur due to elevated glucocorticoid levels.

NURSING ACTIONS: Monitor for subtle indications of infection (fatigue, fever, localized swelling or redness).

CLIENT EDUCATION
- Instruct the client about minimizing his exposure to infectious organisms. (Avoid people who are ill. Avoid crowds. Use hand hygiene.) Qs
- Report indications of infection to the provider.

Adrenal crisis (acute adrenal insufficiency)

Sudden drop in corticosteroids is due to sudden tumor removal; stress of illness, trauma, surgery, or dehydration; or abrupt withdrawal of steroid medication.

NURSING ACTIONS
- Indications include hypotension, hypoglycemia, hyperkalemia, abdominal pain, weakness, and weight loss.
- Administration of glucocorticoids treats acute adrenal insufficiency.
- Administer insulin with dextrose, a potassium-binding and -excreting resin (sodium polystyrene sulfonate), or loop or thiazide diuretics to treat hyperkalemia.
- Administer glucagon or glucose via IV bolus to treat hypoglycemia.
- Monitor vital signs and glucose levels.
- Monitor ECG.

CLIENT EDUCATION
- Instruct the client to taper the medication.
- During times of stress, the client might need additional glucocorticoids prevent adrenal crisis.

Application Exercises

1. A nurse is planning care for a client who has Cushing's disease. The nurse should recognize that clients who have Cushing's disease are at increased risk for which of the following? (Select all that apply.)

   A. Infection

   B. Gastric ulcer

   C. Renal calculi

   D. Bone fractures

   E. Dysphagia

2. At the beginning of a shift, a nurse is assessing a client who has Cushing's disease. Which of the following findings is the priority?

   A. Weight gain

   B. Fatigue

   C. Fragile skin

   D. Joint pain

3. A nurse is reviewing the laboratory findings of a client who has Cushing's disease. Which of the following findings should the nurse expect for this client? (Select all that apply.)

   A. Sodium 150 mEq/L

   B. Potassium 3.3 mEq/L

   C. Calcium 8.0 mg/dL

   D. Lymphocyte count 35%

   E. Fasting glucose 145 mg/dL

4. A nurse is caring for a client who is 6 hr postoperative following a transsphenoidal hypophysectomy. The nurse should test the client's nasal drainage for the presence of which of the following?

   A. RBCs

   B. Ketones

   C. Glucose

   D. Streptococci

5. A nurse is providing discharge reaching for a client who had a transsphenoidal hypophysectomy. Which of the following instructions should the nurse include? (Select all that apply.)

   A. Brush your teeth after every meal or snack.

   B. Avoid bending at the knees.

   C. Eat a high-fiber diet.

   D. Notify the provider of any sweet-tasting drainage.

   E. Notify the provider of a diminished sense of smell.

PRACTICE Active Learning Scenario

A nurse is teaching a client who has bilateral adrenal hyperplasia and a new prescription for hydrocortisone. Use the ATI Active Learning Template: Medication to complete this item.

THERAPEUTIC USES: Explain why the client needs to take this medication.

CLIENT EDUCATION: Identify three teaching points to include about this medication.

Application Exercises Key

1. A. **CORRECT:** Suppression of the immune system places the client at risk for infection.

   B. **CORRECT:** The overproduction of cortisol inhibits the production of a protective mucus lining in the stomach and causes an increase in the amount of gastric acid. These factors place clients who have Cushing's disease at increased risk for gastric ulcers.

   C. Clients who have Cushing's disease are not at risk for renal calculi, but they are at risk for neurological and cardiovascular problems.

   D. **CORRECT:** Clients who have Cushing's disease are at risk for bone fractures because decreased calcium absorption leads to osteoporosis.

   E. Clients who have Cushing's disease are not at risk for dysphagia, but they are at risk for other gastrointestinal problems, including anorexia, nausea, vomiting, and abdominal pain.

   Ⓝ *NCLEX® Connection: Physiological Adaptation, Pathophysiology*

2. A. **CORRECT:** The greatest risk to a client who has Cushing's disease is fluid retention, which can lead to pulmonary edema, hypertension, and heart failure; therefore, this is the priority finding.

   B. Cushing's disease puts the client at risk for fatigue and weight gain; however, another finding is the priority.

   C. Cushing's disease puts the client at risk for fragile skin and hyperpigmentation; however, another finding is the priority.

   D. Cushing's disease puts the client at risk for muscle atrophy and pathologic fractures; however, another finding is the priority.

   Ⓝ *NCLEX® Connection: Physiological Adaptation, Pathophysiology*

3. A. **CORRECT:** This finding is above the expected reference range. Hypernatremia is an expected finding for clients who have Cushing's disease.

   B. **CORRECT:** This finding is below the expected reference range. Hypokalemia is an expected finding for clients who have Cushing's disease.

   C. **CORRECT:** This finding is below the expected reference range. Hypocalcemia is an expected finding for clients who have Cushing's disease.

   D. This finding is within the expected reference range. A decreased lymphocyte count is an expected finding for clients who have Cushing's disease.

   E. **CORRECT:** This finding is above the expected reference range. Clients who have Cushing's disease have an elevated fasting blood glucose because the disorder affects glucose metabolism.

   Ⓝ *NCLEX® Connection: Reduction of Risk Potential, Laboratory Values*

4. A. Cerebrospinal fluid does not contain RBCs unless the client has a cerebral hemorrhage or the procedure was traumatic.

   B. Cerebrospinal fluid does not contain ketones, although it does contain protein and lactic acid.

   C. **CORRECT:** Cerebral spinal fluid contains glucose. The nurse should test nasal drainage for glucose.

   D. Cerebrospinal fluid does not contain any bacteria unless the client has meningitis or another infection that involves the brain and spinal cord.

   Ⓝ *NCLEX® Connection: Reduction of Risk Potential, Laboratory Values*

5. A. The client should avoid brushing his teeth for 2 weeks to allow time for the incision to heal.

   B. The client should avoid bending at the waist. If bending is necessary, he should bend at the knees.

   C. **CORRECT:** To avoid constipation, which contributes to increased intracranial pressure, the client should eat a high-fiber diet and take docusate.

   D. **CORRECT:** Sweet-tasting fluid is an indication of a cerebrospinal fluid leak. The client should notify the provider.

   E. Diminished sense of smell is an expected finding after surgery.

   Ⓝ *NCLEX® Connection: Reduction of Risk Potential, Therapeutic Procedures*

PRACTICE Answer

Using the ATI Active Learning Template: Medication

THERAPEUTIC USES: Hydrocortisone is a glucocorticoid that treats adrenal insufficiency resulting from adrenalectomy surgery.

CLIENT EDUCATION

- Instruct the client to carry emergency identification about corticosteroid use.
- Advise the client to report abdominal pain or black, tarry stools.
- Inform the client to notify the provider for any signs of infection.
- Tell the client to take the medication without skipping any doses.
- Teach the client to consume a diet high in calcium and vitamin D.
- Advise the client to consult the provider before taking any OTC medications or supplements.

Ⓝ *NCLEX® Connection: Pharmacological and Parenteral Therapies, Medication Administration*

CHAPTER 81 Addison's Disease and Acute Adrenal Insufficiency (Addisonian Crisis)

Addison's disease is an adrenocortical insufficiency. It is caused by damage or dysfunction of the adrenal cortex. With Addison's disease, the production of mineralocorticoids and glucocorticoids is diminished, resulting in decreased aldosterone and cortisol.

Acute adrenal insufficiency, also known as Addisonian crisis, has a rapid onset. It is a medical emergency. If it is not quickly diagnosed and properly treated, the prognosis is poor.

Older adult clients are less able to tolerate the complications of Addison's disease and acute adrenal insufficiency and need more frequent monitoring. ©

PRODUCED BY THE ADRENAL CORTEX

Mineralocorticoids: Aldosterone increases sodium absorption and causes potassium excretion in the kidney.

Glucocorticoids: Cortisol affects glucose, protein, and fat metabolism; the body's response to stress; and the body's immune function.

Sex hormones: Androgens and estrogens

ASSESSMENT

RISK FACTORS

CAUSES OF PRIMARY ADDISON'S DISEASE
- Idiopathic autoimmune dysfunction (majority of cases)
- Tuberculosis
- Histoplasmosis
- Adrenalectomy
- Cancer
- Radiation therapy of the abdomen

CAUSES OF SECONDARY ADDISON'S DISEASE
- Steroid withdrawal
- Hypophysectomy
- Pituitary neoplasm
- High dose radiation of pituitary gland or entire brain

ACUTE ADRENAL INSUFFICIENCY is a life-treating event that left untreated can lead to death. Factors that precipitate acute adrenal insufficiency are the following.
- Sepsis
- Trauma
- Stress (myocardial infarction, surgery, anesthesia, hypothermia, volume loss, hypoglycemia)
- Adrenal hemorrhage
- Steroid withdrawal

EXPECTED FINDINGS
- Weight loss
- Craving for salt
- Hyperpigmentation
- Weakness and fatigue
- Nausea and vomiting
- Abdominal pain
- Constipation or diarrhea
- Dizziness with orthostatic hypotension
- Severe hypotension (acute adrenal insufficiency)
- Dehydration
- Hyponatremia
- Hyperkalemia
- Hypoglycemia
- Hypercalcemia
- Manifestations of chronic Addison's disease develop slowly.
- Manifestations of acute adrenal insufficiency develop rapidly.

LABORATORY TESTS

Serum electrolytes: increased K+, decreased Na+, and increased calcium

BUN and creatinine: increased

Serum glucose: normal to decreased

Serum cortisol: decreased

Adrenocorticotropic hormone (ACTH) stimulation test: ACTH is infused, and the cortisol response is measured 30 min and 1 hr after the injection. With primary adrenal insufficiency, plasma cortisol levels do not rise. With secondary adrenal insufficiency, plasma cortisol levels are increased.

DIAGNOSTIC PROCEDURES

Electrocardiogram (ECG)

Used to assess for ECG changes or dysrhythmias associated with electrolyte imbalance.

CLIENT EDUCATION: Explain procedures to the client.

X-ray, CT scan, and MRI scan

Radiological imaging to determine source of adrenal insufficiency, such as a tumor or adrenal atrophy

CLIENT EDUCATION: Explain to the client that tests are noninvasive and not painful.

PATIENT-CENTERED CARE

NURSING CARE

- Monitor for fluid deficits and electrolyte imbalances. Administer saline infusions to restore fluid volume. Observe for dehydration. Obtain orthostatic vital signs.
- Administer hydrocortisone IV bolus and a continuous infusion or intermittent IV bolus.
- Monitor for and treat hyperkalemia:
  - Obtain serum potassium and ECG.
  - Administer sodium polystyrene sulfonate, insulin, calcium, glucose, and sodium bicarbonate.
  - Assess vital signs frequently, and monitor for dysrhythmias.
- Monitor for and treat hypoglycemia:
  - Perform frequent checks of neurologic status, monitor for hypoglycemia, and check serum glucose.
  - Administer food and/or supplemental glucose.
- Maintain a safe environment. Qs
  - Provide assistance ambulating.
  - Prevent falls by keeping floors clear.

MEDICATIONS

Hydrocortisone, prednisone, and cortisone

Glucocorticoids are used as adrenocorticoid replacement for adrenal insufficiency and as an anti-inflammatory.

NURSING CONSIDERATIONS

- Monitor weight, blood pressure, and electrolytes.
- Increase dosage during periods of stress or illness if necessary.
- Taper dose if discontinuing to avoid acute adrenal insufficiency.
- Administer with food to reduce gastric effects.

CLIENT EDUCATION
Advise the client to do the following. Qpcc
- Take medication as directed.
- Avoid discontinuing the medication abruptly.
- Report manifestations of Cushing's syndrome (round face, edema, weight gain).
- Advise the client to take the medication with food.
- Report manifestations of adrenal insufficiency (fever, fatigue, muscle weakness, anorexia).

Fludrocortisone

A mineralocorticoid used as a replacement in adrenal insufficiency

NURSING CONSIDERATIONS

- Monitor weight, blood pressure, and electrolytes.
- Hypertension is a potential adverse effect.
- Dosage might need to be increased during periods of stress or illness.

CLIENT EDUCATION

- Advise the client to take the medication as directed.
- Inform the client that mild peripheral edema is expected.

INTERPROFESSIONAL CARE

Home assistance for fluid, medication, and dietary management can be required.

CLIENT EDUCATION

- Advise the client to take prescribed medications as instructed and monitor for adverse reactions. Qpcc
- Tell the client to avoid using alcohol and caffeine.
- Teach the client to monitor for indications of gastric bleeding (coffee-ground emesis; tarry, black stool).
- Advise the client to monitor for hypoglycemia (diaphoresis, shaking, tachycardia, headache).
- Instruct the client to report manifestations of adrenal insufficiency (fever, fatigue, muscle weakness, dizziness, anorexia).
- To prevent acute adrenal insufficiency, instruct clients who have Addison's disease to increase corticosteroid doses as prescribed during times of stress.
- Inform the client that medication therapy can be lifelong.

COMPLICATIONS

Acute adrenal insufficiency (Addisonian crisis)

Acute adrenal insufficiency (Addisonian crisis) occurs when there is an acute drop in adrenocorticoids due to sudden discontinuation of glucocorticoid medications or when induced by severe trauma, infection, or stress. Qebp

NURSING ACTIONS

- Administer insulin and dextrose to move potassium into cells.
- Administer calcium to counteract the effects of hyperkalemia and protect the heart; and sodium polystyrene sulfonate, a resin that absorbs potassium.
- If acidosis occurs, administer sodium bicarbonate to promote alkalinity and increase uptake of and move potassium into cells.
- Loop or thiazide diuretics are used to manage hyperkalemia.
- Establish an IV line and initiate a rapid infusion of 0.9% sodium chloride.
- Monitor vital signs. Monitor for manifestations of hyperkalemia, such as bradycardia, heart block, peaked T waves, and prolonged PR interval.
- Monitor electrolytes.
- Administer hydrocortisone sodium succinate as replacement therapy.
- Administer an H2 antagonist, such as ranitidine, intravenously for ulcer prevention.

CLIENT EDUCATION

- Advise the client to notify the provider of any infection, trauma, or stress that can increase the need for adrenocorticoids.
- Advise the client to take the medication as directed.
- Advise the client not to discontinue the medication abruptly. Qs

Hypoglycemia

Insufficient glucocorticoid causes increased insulin sensitivity and decreased glycogen, which leads to hypoglycemia.

NURSING ACTIONS: Monitor glucose levels.

CLIENT EDUCATION
- Advise the client and family to monitor for hypoglycemia. Manifestations can include diaphoresis, shaking, tachycardia, and headache.
- Instruct the client to have a 15 g carbohydrate snack readily available. Q EBP

Hyperkalemia/Hyponatremia

Decrease in aldosterone levels can cause an increased excretion of sodium and a decreased excretion of potassium.

NURSING ACTIONS: Monitor electrolytes and ECG.

CLIENT EDUCATION
- Advise the client to take the medications as directed.
- Instruct the client to report indications of hyperkalemia (muscle weakness, tingling sensation, irregular heartbeat). Qs

Application Exercises

1. A nurse is providing medication teaching for a client who has Addison's disease and is taking hydrocortisone. Which of the following instructions should the nurse include? (Select all that apply.)

   A. Take the medication on an empty stomach.

   B. Notify the provider of any illness or stress.

   C. Report any manifestations of weakness or dizziness.

   D. Do not discontinue the medication suddenly.

   E. Eat a low-sodium diet.

2. A nurse is reviewing laboratory results for a client who has Addison's disease. Which of the following laboratory results should the nurse expect for this client? (Select all that apply.)

   A. Sodium 130 mEq/L

   B. Potassium 6.1 mEq/L

   C. Calcium 11.6 mg/dL

   D. Blood urea nitrogen (BUN) 28 mg/dL

   E. Fasting blood glucose 148 mg/dL

3. A nurse in an acute care facility is admitting a client who has acute adrenal insufficiency. Which of the following prescriptions should the nurse anticipate? (Select all that apply.)

   A. IV therapy with 0.45% sodium chloride

   B. Regular insulin

   C. Hydrocortisone sodium succinate

   D. Sodium polystyrene sulfonate

   E. Furosemide

4. A nurse is planning to teach a client who is being evaluated for Addison's disease about the adrenocorticotropic hormone (ACTH) stimulation test. The nurse should base her instructions to the client on which of the following?

   A. The ACTH stimulation test measures the response by the kidneys to ACTH.

   B. In the presence of primary adrenal insufficiency, plasma cortisol levels rise in response to administration of ACTH.

   C. ACTH is a hormone produced by the pituitary gland.

   D. The client is instructed to take a dose of ACTH by mouth the evening before the test.

PRACTICE Active Learning Scenario

A nurse in provider's office is reviewing the health history of a client who has Addison's disease. Use the ATI Active Learning Template: System Disorder to complete this item.

RISK FACTORS: Identify the most common cause and two additional causes of primary Addison's disease.

EXPECTED FINDINGS: Identify three manifestations of Addison's disease.

Application Exercises Key

1. A. The client should take hydrocortisone with food to decrease GI distress.

   B. **CORRECT:** Physical and emotional stress increase the need for hydrocortisone. The provider may increase the dosage when stress occurs.

   C. **CORRECT:** Weakness and dizziness are indications of adrenal insufficiency. The client should report these indications to the provider.

   D. **CORRECT:** Rapid discontinuation can result in adverse effects, including acute adrenal insufficiency. If hydrocortisone is to be discontinued, the dose should be tapered.

   E. Clients who have Addison's disease are expected to have hyponatremia. A low-sodium diet is not advised.

   Ⓝ *NCLEX® Connection: Pharmacological and Parenteral Therapies, Medication Administration*

2. A. **CORRECT:** This finding is below the expected reference range. In the presence of Addison's disease, insufficient glucose can cause sodium and water excretion. Hyponatremia is an expected finding.

   B. **CORRECT:** This finding is above the expected reference range. Hyperkalemia is an expected finding for a client who has Addison's disease.

   C. **CORRECT:** This finding is above the expected reference range. Hypercalcemia is an expected finding for a client who has Addison's disease.

   D. **CORRECT:** This BUN level is above the expected reference range, which is an expected finding for a client who has Addison's disease due to dehydration.

   E. This finding is above the expected reference range for a fasting blood glucose level. Hypoglycemia or blood glucose in the normal range is an expected finding for a client who has Addison's disease, so this finding is unexpected.

   Ⓝ *NCLEX® Connection: Reduction of Risk Potential, Laboratory Values*

3. A. 0.45% sodium chloride is hypotonic. Clients who have acute adrenal insufficiency are hyponatremic. The nurse should anticipate a prescription for a solution that contains 0.9% sodium chloride.

   B. **CORRECT:** Clients who have acute adrenal insufficiency are hyperkalemic. Insulin is administered to shift potassium into the cells.

   C. **CORRECT:** Hydrocortisone sodium succinate is administered as replacement therapy of both glucocorticoid and mineralocorticoid.

   D. **CORRECT:** Clients who have acute adrenal insufficiency are hyperkalemic. Sodium polystyrene sulfonate is administered because it absorbs potassium.

   E. **CORRECT:** Loop and thiazide diuretics promote potassium excretion and are administered to treat hyperkalemia.

   Ⓝ *NCLEX® Connection: Physiological Adaptation, Alterations in Body Systems*

4. A. The ACTH stimulation test measures the response by the adrenal glands to ACTH.

   B. In the presence of primary adrenal insufficiency, plasma cortisol levels do not rise in response to administration of ACTH.

   C. **CORRECT:** Secretion of corticotropin-releasing hormone from the hypothalamus prompts the pituitary gland to secrete ACTH.

   D. ACTH is administered IV during the testing process, and plasma cortisol levels are measured 30 min and 1 hr after the injection.

   Ⓝ *NCLEX® Connection: Reduction of Risk Potential, Diagnostic Tests*

PRACTICE Answer

Using the ATI Active Learning Template: System Disorder

RISK FACTORS
- Most common: autoimmune dysfunction
- Additional causes: tuberculosis, histoplasmosis, adrenalectomy, cancer

EXPECTED FINDINGS
- Hyperpigmentation
- Weight loss
- Craving for salt
- Weakness
- Fatigue
- Nausea
- Vomiting
- Dizziness upon standing or moving from lying to sitting position

Ⓝ *NCLEX® Connection: Physiological Adaptation, Pathophysiology*

CHAPTER 82 *Diabetes Mellitus Management*

Diabetes mellitus is a metabolic disorder resulting from either an inadequate production of insulin (type 1) or an inability of the body's cells to respond to insulin that is present (type 2).

Type 1 diabetes mellitus is an autoimmune dysfunction involving the destruction of beta cells, which produce insulin in the islets of Langerhans of the pancreas. Immune system cells and antibodies are present in circulation and can also be triggered by certain genetic tissue types or viral infections.

Type 2 diabetes mellitus is a progressive condition due to increasing inability of cells to respond to insulin (insulin resistance) and decreased production of insulin by the beta cells. It is linked to obesity, sedentary lifestyle, and heredity. Metabolic syndrome often precedes type 2 diabetes mellitus.

Diabetes mellitus has wide ranging systemic effects and is a contributing factor to development of cardiovascular disease, hypertension, kidney disease, neuropathy, retinopathy, peripheral vascular disease, and stroke.

Diabetes mellitus is significantly more prevalent in African American, American Indian, and Hispanic populations and is more common in men than women.

HEALTH PROMOTION AND DISEASE PREVENTION

Diabetic screening

- Determine risk factors: obesity, hypertension, sedentary lifestyle, hyperlipidemia, cigarette smoking, genetic history, ethnic group, and women who have polycystic ovary syndrome or delivered infants weighing more than 9 lb.
- The American Diabetes Association recommends screening a client who has a BMI greater than 25 and age greater than 45 years, or if a child is overweight and has additional risk factors.
- Screening is done with fasting serum glucose levels or glycosylated hemoglobin (A1C).

CLIENT EDUCATION

- Teach the client that exercise and good nutrition are necessary for preventing or controlling diabetes.
  - ○ Carbohydrates: 45% of total daily intake
  - ○ Protein: 15% to 20% of total daily intake, depending upon kidney function
  - ○ Unsaturated and polyunsaturated fats: 20% to 35% of total daily intake
- Consistency in the amount of food consumed and regularity in meal times promotes blood glucose control.
- Encourage a diet low in saturated fats to decrease low-density lipoprotein (LDL), assist with weight loss for secondary prevention of diabetes, and reduce risk of heart disease.
- Modify the client's diet to include omega-3 fatty acids and fiber to lower cholesterol, improve blood glucose for clients who have diabetes, for secondary prevention of diabetes, and to reduce the risk of heart disease.
- Encourage physical activity at least three times per week.

ASSESSMENT

RISK FACTORS

Metabolic syndrome: A collection of manifestations that predispose an individual to the development of diabetes mellitus including abdominal obesity, insulin resistance, sedentary lifestyle, hypertension, and elevated lipid and triglyceride levels. It also has an associated risk of cardiovascular disease.

Insulin resistance: Impaired fasting glucose levels 100 to 125 mg/dL, impaired glucose tolerance 140 to 199 mg/dL, or A1C level 5.5% to 6.0%.

- Pancreatitis and Cushing's syndrome are secondary causes of diabetes.
- Vision and hearing deficits can interfere with the understanding of teaching, reading of materials, and preparation of medications.
- Tissue deterioration secondary to aging can affect the client's ability to prepare food, care for self, perform ADLs, perform foot/wound care, and perform glucose monitoring.
- A fixed income can mean that there are limited funds for buying diabetic supplies, wound care supplies, insulin, and medications. This can result in complications.

Age
- Older adult clients might not be able to drive to the provider's office, grocery store, or pharmacy. Assess support systems available for older adult clients. Ⓖ
- Older adults are at risk for altered metabolism of medication due to decreased kidney and liver function because of the aging process.
- Older adults can have vision alterations (yellowing of lens, decreased depth perception, cataracts), which can affect ability to read information and administer mediation.

EXPECTED FINDINGS

Hyperglycemia: Blood glucose level usually greater than 250 mg/dL

Polyuria: Excess urine production and frequency from osmotic diuresis

Polydipsia: Excessive thirst due to dehydration
- Loss of skin turgor, skin warm and dry
- Dry mucous membranes
- Weakness and malaise
- Rapid weak pulse and hypotension

Polyphagia: Excessive hunger and eating caused from inability of cells to receive glucose (because of a lack of insulin or cellular resistance to available insulin) and the body's use of protein and fat for energy (which causes ketosis)
- The client can display weight loss.
- Ketones accumulate in the blood due to breakdown of fatty acids when insulin is not available, resulting in metabolic acidosis.
- Kussmaul respirations: increased respiratory rate and depth in attempt to excrete carbon dioxide and acid due to metabolic acidosis.

OTHER MANIFESTATIONS: Acetone/fruity breath odor (due to accumulation of ketones), headache, nausea, vomiting, abdominal pain, inability to concentrate, fatigue, weakness, vision changes, slow healing of wounds, decreased level of consciousness, seizures leading to coma

LABORATORY TESTS

Diagnostic criteria for diabetes include two findings (on separate days) of at least one of the following.
- Manifestations of diabetes plus casual blood glucose concentration greater than 200 mg/dL (without regard to time since last meal)
- Fasting blood glucose greater than 126 mg/dL
- 2-hr glucose greater than 200 mg/dL with oral glucose tolerance test
- Glycosylated hemoglobin (A1C) greater than 6.5%

Fasting blood glucose

NURSING ACTIONS: Postpone administration of antidiabetic medication until after the level is drawn.

CLIENT EDUCATION: Instruct the client to fast (no food or drink other than water) for the 8 hr prior to the blood test.

Oral glucose tolerance test

- Often used to diagnose gestational diabetes mellitus during pregnancy
- Not generally used for routine diagnosis
- A fasting blood glucose level is drawn at the start of the test. The client is then instructed to consume a specified amount of glucose. Blood glucose levels are obtained every 30 min for 2 hr. The clients must be assessed for hypoglycemia throughout the procedure.

CLIENT EDUCATION
- Instruct the client to consume a balanced diet for 3 days prior to the test. Then instruct the client to fast for 10 to 12 hr prior to the test.
- Only water may be taken during the testing period. Food or other liquids will affect the test results.

Glycosylated hemoglobin (HbA1c)

- The expected reference range is 4% to 6%, but an acceptable reference range for clients who have diabetes can be 6.5% to 8%, with a target goal of less than 7%.
- HbA1c is the best indicator of the average blood glucose level for the past 120 days. It assists in evaluating treatment effectiveness and compliance.

CLIENT EDUCATION
- Instruct the client that the test evaluates treatment effectiveness and compliance.
- Recommended quarterly or twice yearly depending on the glycemic levels.

Urine ketones

High ketones in the urine associated with hyperglycemia (exceed 300 mg/dL) is a medical emergency.

DIAGNOSTIC PROCEDURES

Self-monitored blood glucose (SMBG)

NURSING ACTION: Ensure that the client follows the proper procedure for blood sample collection and use of a glucose meter. Supplemental short-acting insulin may be prescribed for elevated pre-meal glucose levels.

CLIENT EDUCATION
- Instruct the client to check the accuracy of the strips with the control solution provided.
- Instruct the client to use the correct code number in the meter to match the strip bottle number.
- Instruct the client to store strips in the closed container in a dry location.
- Instruct the client to obtain an adequate amount of blood sample when preforming the test.
- Encourage appropriate hand hygiene.
- Encourage use of fresh lancets, and avoid sharing glucose monitoring equipment to prevent infection.
- Advise the client to keep a record of the SMBG that includes time, date, serum glucose level, insulin dose, food intake, and other events that can alter glucose metabolism, such as activity level or illness.

MEDICATIONS

- Insulin regimens are established for clients who have type 1 diabetes mellitus
  - More than 1 type of insulin: rapid-, short-, intermediate-, and long-acting
  - Given one or more times a day based on blood glucose results
- Insulin can be required by some clients who have type 2 diabetes or gestational diabetes if glycemic control is not obtained with diet, exercise, and oral hypoglycemic agents.
  - Continuous infusion of insulin can be accomplished using a small pump that is worn externally. The pump is programmed to deliver insulin through a needle in subcutaneous tissue. The needle should be changed at least every 2 to 3 days to prevent infection.
  - Complications of the insulin pump are accidental cessation of insulin administration, obstruction of the tubing/needle, pump failure, and infection.
- Insulin pens are prefilled cartridges of 150 to 300 units of insulin in a programmable device with disposable needles.
  - Convenient for travel
  - Used for clients who have vision impairment or problems with dexterity
- Oral hypoglycemics are used by clients who have type 2 diabetes, along with diet and exercise, to regulate blood glucose.

Insulin

Also see the **RN PHARMACOLOGY REVIEW MODULE: CHAPTER 39: DIABETES MELLITUS.**

Rapid-acting insulin: Insulin lispro, insulin aspart, insulin glulisine
- Administer before meals to control postprandial rise in blood glucose.
- Onset is rapid (10 to 30 min), depending on which insulin is administered.
- Administer in conjunction with intermediate- or long-acting insulin to provide glycemic control between meals and at night.

Short-acting insulin: Regular insulin
- Administer 30 to 60 min before meals to control postprandial hyperglycemia.
- Regular insulin is available in two concentrations.
  - U-500 is reserved for the client who has insulin resistance. It is never administered IV.
  - U-100 is prescribed for most clients and may be administered IV.

Intermediate-acting insulin: NPH insulin
- Administered for glycemic control between meals and at night.
- Not administered before meals to control postprandial rise in blood glucose.
- Contains protamine (a protein), which causes a delay in the insulin absorption or onset and extends the duration of action of the insulin.
- Administer NPH insulin subcutaneous only and as the only insulin to mix with short-acting insulin.

82.1 Hypoglycemia and hyperglycemia manifestations and management

Hypoglycemia

- Teach the client measures to take in response to manifestations of hypoglycemia (mild shakiness, mental confusion, sweating, palpitations, headache, lack of coordination, blurred vision, seizures, and coma).
- Hypoglycemia preventive measures are to avoid excess insulin, exercise, and alcohol consumption on an empty stomach.
- A decrease in food intake or delay in food absorption can also cause hypoglycemia.
- Check blood glucose level.
- Follow guidelines outlined by the provider or diabetes educator.
- Instruct the client who has hypoglycemia (glucose of 70 mg/dL or less) to take 15 to 20 g of a readily absorbable carbohydrate (4 to 6 oz of fruit juice or regular soft drink, glucose tablets or glucose gel per package instructions, 6 to 10 hard candies, or 1 tbsp of honey) and recheck blood glucose in 15 min.
- Repeat the administration of carbohydrates if not within normal limits, and recheck blood glucose in 15 min.
- If blood glucose is within normal limits, have a snack containing a carbohydrate and protein (if the next meal is more than 1 hr away). Blood glucose increases approximately 40 mg/dL over 30 min following ingestion of 10 g of absorbable carbohydrate.
- If the client is unconscious or unable to swallow, administer glucagon subcutaneous or IM (repeat in 10 min if still unconscious) and notify the provider. Place the client into a lateral position to prevent aspiration.
- In acute care, the nurse should administer 50% dextrose if IV access is available. Consciousness should occur within 20 min.
- Once consciousness occurs and the client is able to swallow, have the client ingest oral carbohydrates.

Hyperglycemia

- Teach the client manifestations of hyperglycemia (hot, dry skin and fruity breath) and measures to take in response to hyperglycemia.
- Encourage oral fluid intake of sugar-free fluids to prevent dehydration.
- Administer insulin as prescribed.
- Restrict exercise when blood glucose levels are greater than 250 mg/dL.
- Test urine for ketones and report if outside of the expected reference range.
- Consult the provider if manifestations progress.

Long-acting insulin: Insulin glargine, insulin detemir
- Administered once daily, anytime during the day but always at the same time each day.
- Glargine insulin forms microprecipitates that dissolves slowly over 24 hr and maintains a steady blood sugar level with no peaks or troughs.
- Insulin detemir has an added fatty-acid chain that delays absorption. Although it does not have a peak, duration is dose-dependent (12 to 24 hr).
- Administer glargine insulin and insulin detemir subcutaneous only. Never administer IV.

NURSING CONSIDERATIONS
- Observe the client perform self-administration of insulin, and offer additional instruction as indicated.
- Monitor for hypoglycemic reactions (sweating, weakness, dizziness, confusion, headache, tachycardia, slurred speech) at insulin peak times.
- Dosage can be adjusted when the client is scheduled for procedures that require fasting.

CLIENT EDUCATION
- Provide information regarding self-administration of insulin.
  - Rotate injection sites (to prevent lipohypertrophy) within one anatomic site (to prevent day-to-day changes in absorption rates).
  - Inject at a 90° angle (45° angle if the client is thin). Aspiration for blood is not necessary.
  - When mixing a rapid- or short-acting insulin with a longer-acting insulin, draw up the shorter-acting insulin into the syringe first and then the longer-acting insulin. This reduces the risk of introducing the longer-acting insulin into the shorter-acting insulin vial.
- Advise the client to eat at regular intervals, avoid alcohol intake, and adjust insulin to exercise and diet to avoid hypoglycemia.
- Encourage the client to wear a medical identification wristband.

82.2 Insulin subcutaneous injection site

Oral hypoglycemics

Biguanides: Metformin
- Reduces the production of glucose by the liver (gluconeogenesis)
- Increases tissue sensitivity to insulin
- Slows carbohydrate absorption in the intestines
- NURSING CONSIDERATIONS
  - Monitor significance of gastrointestinal (GI) effects (flatulence, anorexia, nausea, vomiting).
  - Monitor for lactic acidosis, especially in clients who have kidney disorders or liver dysfunction.
  - Stop medication for 48 hr before any type of elective radiographic test with iodinated contrast dye and restart 48 hr after (can cause lactic acidosis due to acute kidney injury).
- CLIENT EDUCATION
  - Take with food to decrease adverse GI effects.
  - Instruct the client to take vitamin B_{12} and folic acid supplements.
  - Contact the provider if manifestations of lactic acidosis develop (myalgia, sluggishness, somnolence, and hyperventilation).
  - May be taken during pregnancy for gestational diabetes.
  - Never crush or chew the medication.

Second-generation sulfonylureas: Glipizide, glimepiride, glyburide
- Stimulates insulin release from the pancreas causing a decrease in blood sugar levels.
- Increases tissue sensitivity to insulin.
- NURSING CONSIDERATIONS
  - Monitor for hypoglycemia.
  - Beta-blockers can mask tachycardia typically seen during hypoglycemia.
- CLIENT EDUCATION
  - Administer 30 min before meals.
  - Monitor for hypoglycemia and report frequent episodes to the provider.
  - Instruct the client to avoid alcohol due to disulfiram effect.

Meglitinides: Repaglinide, nateglinide
- Stimulates insulin release from pancreas.
- Administered for post-meal hyperglycemia.
- NURSING CONSIDERATIONS
  - Monitor for hypoglycemia.
  - Monitor HbA1c every 3 months to determine effectiveness.
- CLIENT EDUCATION
  - Administer 15 to 30 min before a meal.
  - Must eat with 30 min of administration.
  - Omit the dose if skipped a meal to prevent hypoglycemic crisis.

Thiazolidinediones: Pioglitazone
- Reduces the production of glucose by the liver (gluconeogenesis)
- Increases tissue sensitivity to insulin
- NURSING CONSIDERATIONS
  - Monitor for fluid retention, especially in clients who have a history of heart failure.
  - Monitor for elevation of ALT, LDH, and triglycerides levels.

- CLIENT EDUCATION
  - Report rapid weight gain, shortness of breath, or decreased exercise tolerance.
  - Use additional contraception methods because the medication reduces the blood levels of oral contraceptives and stimulate ovulation.
  - Have liver function tests at baseline and every 3 to 6 months thereafter.

Alpha-glucosidase inhibitors: Acarbose, miglitol
- Slow carbohydrate absorption from the intestinal tract
- Reduces post-meal hyperglycemia
- NURSING CONSIDERATIONS
  - Alert the client that GI discomfort (abdominal distention, cramps, excessive gas, diarrhea) is common with these medications.
  - Monitor liver function every 3 months.
  - Treat hypoglycemia with dextrose, not table sugar (prevents table sugar from breaking down).
- CLIENT EDUCATION
  - Instruct the client to have liver function tests performed every 3 months or as prescribed.
  - Take the medication with the first bite of each meal in order for the medication to be effective.
  - Have available dextrose paste to treat hypoglycemia.

Dipeptidyl peptidase-4 (DPP-4) inhibitors: Sitagliptin, saxagliptin, linagliptin, alogliptin
- Augments naturally occurring intestinal incretin hormones, which promote release of insulin and decrease secretion of glucagon
- Lowers fasting and postprandial glucose levels
- NURSING CONSIDERATIONS
  - Few adverse effects, but upper respiratory manifestations (nasal and throat inflammation) and pancreatitis can occur.
  - Alert the client of GI discomforts (nausea, vomiting, and diarrhea).
- CLIENT EDUCATION
  - Instruct the client to report persistent upper respiratory manifestations.
  - Instruct the client to report severe abdominal pain, with or without emesis.
  - Medication only works when blood sugar is rising.

Sodium-glucose cotransporter 2 inhibitors: Canagliflozin, dapagliflozin
- Blocks reabsorption of glucose from the kidneys
- NURSING CONSIDERATIONS
  - Monitor for development of urinary tract infections, and genital yeast infections in women.
  - Monitor for postural hypotension in older adult clients.
- CLIENT EDUCATION
  - Take the medication before the first meal of the day.
  - Change positions slowly.
  - Monitor and report genital burning, itching, increased drainage.

Non-insulin injectable medications

Incretin mimetic: Exenatide, liraglutide
- Mimics the function of intestinal incretin hormone by decreasing glucagon secretion and gastric emptying.
- Decrease insulin demand by reducing fasting and postprandial hyperglycemia.

- NURSING CONSIDERATIONS
  - Administer subcutaneously 60 min before morning and evening meal.
  - Monitor for gastrointestinal distress.
- CLIENT EDUCATION
  - Do not administer after a meal.
  - Oral antibiotic, oral contraceptive, or acetaminophen should never be given within 1 hr of oral exenatide or 2 hr after an injection of exenatide.
  - Can have decreased appetite and weight loss.
  - Wait for next scheduled dose if the scheduled medication is missed.
  - Instruct the client to report severe abdominal pain, with or without emesis.

Amylin mimetic: Pramlintide
- A synthetic amylin hormone found in the beta cells of the pancreas, it suppresses glucagon secretion and controls postprandial blood glucose levels.
- NURSING CONSIDERATIONS
  - Administer subcutaneously immediately before each major meal.
  - Do not administer if client has hypoglycemia unawareness, or noncompliance/poor adherence to treatment regimens and self-monitoring blood glucose.
  - It may be administered with insulin therapy or oral hypoglycemic agent.
  - Pre-meal doses of rapid- or short-acting insulins should be reduced by 50% to reduce risk of hypoglycemia.
- CLIENT EDUCATION
  - Monitor and report frequent periods of hypoglycemia.
  - Monitor for injection site reactions.

PATIENT-CENTERED CARE

NURSING CARE

Monitor the following.
- Blood glucose levels and factors affecting levels (other medications)
- I&O and weight
- Skin integrity and healing status of any wounds for presence of recurrent infections (feet and folds of the skin should be monitored)
- Sensory alterations (tingling, numbness)
- Visual alterations
- Dietary practices
- Exercise patterns
- SMBG skill proficiency
- Self-medication administration proficiency

CLIENT EDUCATION
- Teach the client appropriate techniques for SMBG, including obtaining blood samples, recording and responding to results, and correctly handling supplies and equipment.
- Provide information regarding self-administration of insulin.
- Rotate injection sites to prevent lipohypertrophy (increased swelling of fat) or lipoatrophy (loss of fat tissue) within one anatomic site (prevents day-to-day changes in absorption rates).

Foot care

- Inspect feet daily. Wash feet daily with mild soap and warm water. Test water temperature with hands before washing feet.
- Pat feet dry gently, especially between the toes, and avoid lotions between toes to decrease excess moisture and prevent infection.
- Use mild foot powder (powder with cornstarch) on sweaty feet.
- Do not use commercial remedies for the removal of calluses or corns, which can increase the risk for tissue injury and infection.
- Consult a podiatrist.
- The best time to perform nail care is after a bath/shower, when toenails are soft and easier to trim.
- Separate overlapping toes with cotton or lamb's wool.
- Avoid open-toe, open-heel shoes. Leather shoes are preferred to plastic. Wear shoes that fit correctly. Wear slippers with soles. Do not go barefoot.
- Wear clean, absorbent socks or stockings that are made of cotton or wool and have not been mended.
- Do not use hot water bottles or heating pads to warm feet. Wear socks for warmth.
- Avoid prolonged sitting, standing, and crossing of legs.
- Teach the client to follow facility policies or recommendations of a podiatrist for nail care. Some protocols allow for trimming toenails straight across with clippers and filing edges with an emery board or nail file to prevent soft tissue injury. If clippers or scissors are contraindicated, the client should file the nails straight across.
- Teach the client to cleanse cuts with warm water and mild soap, gently dry, and apply a dry dressing. Instruct the client to monitor healing and to seek intervention promptly.

Nutritional guidelines

- Consult a dietitian for collaborative education with the client and family on meal planning to include food intake, weight management, and lipid and glucose management. Qrc
- Plan meals to achieve appropriate timing of food intake, activity, onset, and peak of insulin. Calories and food composition should be similar each day. Eat at regular intervals, and do not skip meals.
- Count grams of carbohydrates consumed for glycemic control.
- Recognize that 15 g carbohydrates is equal to 1 carbohydrate exchange.
- Restrict calories and increase physical activity as appropriate to facilitate weight loss (for clients who are obese) or to prevent obesity.
- Include fiber in the diet to increase carbohydrate metabolism and to help control cholesterol levels.
- Use artificial sweeteners.
- Read and interpret fat content information on food labels to keep saturated fats within 7% of the recommendations of the daily total caloric intake.

Illness

Teach the client guidelines to follow when sick.
- Monitor blood glucose every 3 to 4 hr.
- Continue to take insulin or oral hypoglycemic agents.
- Consume 4 oz of sugar-free, noncaffeinated liquid every 30 min to prevent dehydration.
- Meet carbohydrate needs through soft food (custard, cream soup, gelatin, graham crackers) six to eight times per day, if possible. If not, consume liquids equal to usual carbohydrate content.
- Test urine for ketones and report to provider if they are outside the expected reference range. (The level should be negative to small.)
- Rest.
- Call the provider for the following.
  - Blood glucose greater than 240 mg/dL. Test urine for ketones, if prescribed.
  - Fever greater than 38.6° C (101.5° F), does not respond to acetaminophen, or lasts more than 24 hr.
  - Feeling disoriented or confused
  - Experiencing rapid breathing
  - Vomiting that occur more than once
  - Diarrhea that occurs more than five times or for longer than 24 hr
  - Inability to tolerate liquids
  - Illness that lasts longer than 2 days

INTERPROFESSIONAL CARE

Refer the client to a diabetes educator for comprehensive education in diabetes management.

COMPLICATIONS

Consistent maintenance of blood glucose within the expected reference range is the best protection against the complications of diabetes mellitus. Expected reference ranges can vary.

Cardiovascular and cerebrovascular disease

Hypertension, myocardial infarction, and stroke

NURSING ACTIONS: Monitor blood pressure.

CLIENT EDUCATION
- Encourage checks of cholesterol (HDL, LDL, and triglycerides) yearly, and monitoring of blood pressure (less than 130/80 mm Hg) and HbA1c every 3 months.
- Encourage participation in regular activity for weight loss and control.
- Encourage a diet of low-fat meals that are high in fruits, vegetables, and whole grains.
- Teach the client to report shortness of breath, headaches (persistent and transient), numbness in distal extremities, swelling of feet, infrequent urination, and changes in vision.
- Encourage a dietary consult.

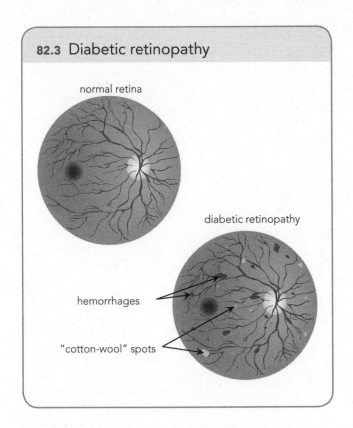

normal retina

diabetic retinopathy

hemorrhages

"cotton-wool" spots

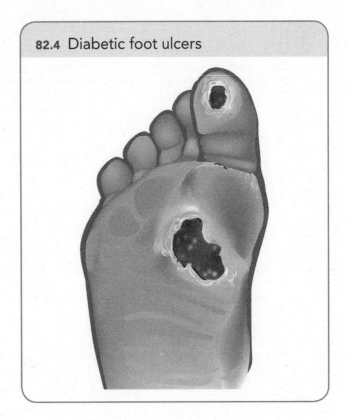

Diabetic retinopathy

Impaired vision and blindness

CLIENT EDUCATION
- Encourage yearly eye exams to ensure the health of the eyes and to protect vision.
- Encourage management of blood glucose levels.

Diabetic neuropathy

- Caused from damage to sensory nerve fibers resulting in numbness and pain
- Is progressive, can affect every aspect of the body, and can lead to ischemia and infection

NURSING ACTIONS
- Monitor blood glucose to keep within an acceptable range to slow progression.
- Provide foot care.

CLIENT EDUCATION
- Encourage annual exams by a podiatrist.
- Encourage regular follow-up with provider to assess and treat neuropathy.

Diabetic nephropathy

Damage to the kidneys from prolonged elevated blood glucose levels and dehydration

NURSING ACTIONS
- Monitor hydration and kidney function (I&O, serum creatinine).
- Report an hourly output less than 30 mL/hr.
- Monitor blood pressure.

CLIENT EDUCATION
- Encourage yearly urine analysis, BUN, microalbumin, and serum creatinine.
- Encourage the client to avoid soda, alcohol, and toxic levels of acetaminophen or NSAIDs.
- Teach the client to consume 2 to 3 L/day of fluid from food and beverages with artificial sweetener, and to drink an adequate amount of water.
- Tell the client to report decrease in output to the provider.

Application Exercises

1. A nurse is caring for a client who has blood glucose 52 mg/dL. The client is lethargic but arousable. Which of the following actions should the nurse perform first?

   A. Recheck blood glucose in 15 min.

   B. Provide a carbohydrate and protein food.

   C. Provide 4 oz grape juice.

   D. Report findings to the provider.

2. A nurse is preparing to administer a morning dose of insulin aspart to a client who has type 1 diabetes mellitus. Which of the following actions should the nurse implement?

   A. Check blood glucose immediately after breakfast.

   B. Administer insulin when breakfast arrives.

   C. Hold breakfast for 1 hr after insulin administration.

   D. Clarify the prescription because insulin should not be administered at this time.

3. A nurse is preparing to administer morning doses of insulin glargine and regular insulin to a client who has a blood glucose 278 mg/dL. Which of the following actions should the nurse take?

   A. Draw up the regular insulin and then the glargine insulin in the same syringe.

   B. Draw up the glargine insulin then the regular insulin in the same syringe.

   C. Draw up and administer regular and glargine insulin in separate syringes.

   D. Administer the regular insulin, wait 1 hr, and then administer the glargine insulin.

4. A nurse is presenting information to a group of clients about nutrition habits that prevent type 2 diabetes mellitus. Which of the following should the nurse include in the information? (Select all that apply.)

   A. Eat less meat and processed foods.

   B. Decrease intake of saturated fats.

   C. Increase daily fiber intake.

   D. Limit saturated fat intake to 15% of daily caloric intake.

   E. Include omega-3 fatty acids in the diet.

5. A nurse is teaching foot care to a client who has diabetes mellitus. Which of the following information should the nurse include in the teaching? (Select all that apply.)

   A. Remove calluses using over-the-counter remedies.

   B. Apply lotion between toes.

   C. Perform nail care after bathing.

   D. Trim toenails straight across.

   E. Wear closed-toe shoes.

PRACTICE Active Learning Scenario

A nurse is providing guidelines to a client who has type 1 diabetes mellitus about self-care during illness. What information should the nurse include in the guidelines? Use the ATI Active Learning Template: System Disorder to complete this item.

LABORATORY TESTS: Discuss parameters for testing urine and notifying the provider.

CLIENT EDUCATION: Describe six teaching points.

Application Exercises Key

1. A. The nurse should recheck the blood glucose in 15 min after a rapidly absorbed carbohydrate is ingested; however, another action is the priority.

   B. The nurse should give the client a carbohydrate and protein food if the next meal is more than 1 hr away after the blood glucose returns to a normal range; however, the nurse should take another action first.

   C. **CORRECT:** The greatest risk to the client is injury from hypoglycemia; therefore, the priority action the nurse should take is to administer a rapidly absorbed carbohydrate, such as grape juice, takes priority when treating the blood glucose of 52 mg/dL.

   D. The nurse should report the findings to the provider; however, the nurse should take another action first.

   Ⓝ *NCLEX® Connection: Physiological Adaptation, Unexpected Response to Therapies*

2. A. Blood glucose should be checked prior to insulin administration to prevent an episode of hypoglycemia.

   B. **CORRECT:** Administer insulin aspart when breakfast arrives to avoid a hypoglycemic episode. Insulin aspart is rapid-acting, and should be administered 5 to 10 min before breakfast.

   C. Insulin aspart is rapid-acting and is administered 5 to 10 min before breakfast. Breakfast should be available at the time of the injection.

   D. Insulin aspart is administered at breakfast time and may be prescribed for administration 2 to 3 times a day.

   Ⓝ *NCLEX® Connection: Pharmacological and Parenteral Therapies, Medication Administration*

3. A. These insulins are not compatible and should not be drawn up in the same syringe.

   B. These insulins are not compatible and should not be drawn up in the same syringe.

   C. **CORRECT:** Administer each insulin as a separate injection. These insulins are not compatible and should not be drawn up in the same syringe.

   D. These insulins should be administered at the same time. Regular insulin is short-acting and should lower the blood glucose level in a short period of time. Insulin glargine is long-acting and administered once a day.

   Ⓝ *NCLEX® Connection: Pharmacological and Parenteral Therapies, Medication Administration*

4. A. **CORRECT:** Healthy nutrition should include decreasing the consumption of meats and processed foods, which can prevent diabetes and hyperlipidemia.

   B. **CORRECT:** Healthy nutrition should include lowering LDL by decreasing intake of saturated fats, which can prevent diabetes and hyperlipidemia.

   C. **CORRECT:** Healthy nutrition should include increasing dietary fiber to control weight gain and decrease the risk of diabetes and hyperlipidemia.

   D. The recommended saturated fat intake is no more than 7% of total daily caloric intake.

   E. **CORRECT:** Healthy nutrition should include omega-3 fatty acids for secondary prevention of diabetes and heart disease.

   Ⓝ *NCLEX® Connection: Basic Care and Comfort, Nutrition and Oral Hydration*

5. A. A podiatrist should remove calluses or corns. Over-the-counter remedies can increase the risk for tissue injury and an infection.

   B. Applying lotion between the toes increases moisture for growth of micro-organisms, which can lead to infection.

   C. **CORRECT:** Perform nail care after bathing, when toenails are soft and easier to trim.

   D. **CORRECT:** Trim toenails straight across to prevent injury to soft tissue of the toes.

   E. **CORRECT:** Wear closed-toe shoes to prevent injury to soft tissue of the toes and feet.

   Ⓝ *NCLEX® Connection: Health Promotion and Maintenance, Health Promotion/Disease Prevention*

PRACTICE Answer

Using the ATI Active Learning Template: System Disorder

LABORATORY TESTS: Test urine for ketones and report to provider if they are outside the expected reference range. (The level should be negative.)

CLIENT EDUCATION

- Monitor blood glucose every 3 to 4 hr.
- Continue to take insulin as prescribed.
- Prevent dehydration by consuming 2 to 3 L/day of fluid obtained from food and beverages with artificial sweetener and drinking an adequate amount of water.
- Call the provider if unable to tolerate liquids.

- If unable to eat soft foods, consume liquids equal to usual carbohydrate content.
- Call the provider for illness longer than 2 days, or diarrhea more than five episodes or for longer than 24 hr.
- Call the provider for fever that is greater than 38.6° C (101.5° F), does not respond to acetaminophen, or lasts more than 24 hr.

Ⓝ *NCLEX® Connection: Physiological Adaptation, Illness Management*

CHAPTER 83 *Complications of Diabetes Mellitus*

Diabetic ketoacidosis (DKA) is an acute, life-threatening condition characterized by uncontrolled hyperglycemia (greater than 300 mg/dL) resulting in the breakdown of body fat for energy, dehydration, metabolic acidosis, and an accumulation of ketones in the blood and urine. The onset is rapid, and the mortality rate is up to 10%.

Hyperglycemic-hyperosmolar state (HHS) is an acute, life-threatening condition characterized by profound hyperglycemia (greater than 600 mg/dL), hyperosmolarity that leads to dehydration, and an absence of ketosis. Onset generally occurs gradually over several days, and if left untreated can lead to coma and death.

ASSESSMENT

RISK FACTORS

Diabetic ketoacidosis

- Lack of sufficient insulin related to undiagnosed or untreated type 1 diabetes mellitus or nonadherence to a diabetic regimen.
- Reduced or missed dose of insulin (insufficient dosing of insulin or error in dosage).
- Any condition that increases carbohydrate metabolism, such as physical or emotional stress, illness, infection (No. 1 cause of DKA), surgery, or trauma that requires an increased need for insulin.
- Increased hormone production (e.g., cortisol, glucagon, epinephrine) stimulates the liver to produce glucose and decreases the effect of insulin.

Hyperglycemic-hyperosmolar state

- Lack of sufficient insulin related to undiagnosed diabetes mellitus. There is sufficient endogenous insulin present to prevent the development of ketosis, but not enough to prevent hyperglycemia.
- Inadequate fluid intake or poor kidney function contribute to the development of HHS.
- Most common in older adult clients (50 to 70 years old).
- Mortality rates in older clients are between 40% to 70% given the older clients seek medical attention later and are sicker than the younger clients.
- Medical conditions such as myocardial infarction, cerebral vascular injury, or sepsis.
- Some medications (glucocorticoids, thiazide diuretics, phenytoin, beta blockers, and calcium channel blockers).
- Infection or stress.

EXPECTED FINDINGS

	DKA	HHS
Polyuria: Osmotic diuresis resulting in excess urine production	✓	✓
Polydipsia (excess thirst): Osmotic diuresis causing excess loss of fluids resulting in dehydration and increased thirst	✓	✓
Polyphagia: Cell starvation due to inability to receive glucose resulting in increased appetite	✓	✓
Weight loss: Cells are unable to use glucose because of insulin deficiency. The body is placed in a catabolic state.	✓	✓
GI effects (nausea, vomiting, abdominal pain): Increased ketones and acidosis lead to nausea, vomiting, and abdominal pain	✓	
Blurred vision, headache, weakness: Fluid volume depletion caused from osmotic diuresis resulting in dehydration	✓	✓
Orthostatic hypotension: Fluid volume depletion caused by osmotic diuresis resulting in dehydration	✓	✓
Fruity odor of breath: Elevated ketone bodies (small fatty acids) used for energy that collect in the blood, which leads to metabolic acidosis	✓	
Kussmaul respirations: Deep rapid respirations occur in an attempt to excrete carbon dioxide and acid when in metabolic acidosis	✓	
Metabolic acidosis: Breakdown of stored glucose, protein, and fat to produce ketone bodies	✓	
Mental status changes: Lack of glucose circulating to the brain can cause neuron dysfunction and even cell death of the brain. The brain cannot produce or store glucose.	✓	✓
Seizures, myoclonic jerking: Related to serum osmolarity greater than 350 mOsm/L		✓
Reversible paralysis: Related to how elevated the serum osmolarity becomes (coma occurs once serum osmolarity is greater than 350 mOsm/L)		✓

LABORATORY TESTS

Therapeutic management is guided by serial laboratory analysis.

Serum glucose

DKA: Greater than 300 mg/dL

HHS: Greater than 600 mg/dL

Serum electrolytes: Sodium (Na⁺) and potassium (K⁺)

DKA
- **Na⁺:** low, normal, or high
- **K⁺:** initial levels depend on how long DKA existed prior to treatment, then decrease with treatment

HHS
- **Na⁺:** normal or low
- **K⁺:** normal to high as a result of dehydration; must monitor for decrease when treatment started

Serum kidney studies: BUN and creatinine

DKA
- Increased secondary to dehydration
- BUN greater than 30 mg/dL
- Creatinine greater than 1.5 mg/dL

HHS
- Increased secondary to dehydration
- BUN greater than 30 mg/dL
- Creatinine greater than 1.5 mg/dL

Ketones: Serum and urine

DKA: Present in serum and urine

HHS: Absent in serum and urine

Serum osmolarity

DKA: High

HHS: Greater than 320 mOsm/L

Serum pH (ABG)

DKA
- Metabolic acidosis with respiratory compensation (Kussmaul respirations)
- pH less than 7.3

HHS
- Absence of acidosis
- pH greater than 7.4

PATIENT-CENTERED CARE

NURSING CARE

- Always treat the underlying cause (infectious process).
  - Provide rapid isotonic fluid (0.9% sodium chloride) replacement to maintain perfusion to vital organs. Monitor for evidence of fluid volume excess (urine output, kidney function, pulmonary status, jugular venous distention, and body weight) due to the need for large quantities of fluid.
  - Physiological changes in cardiac and pulmonary function can place older adult clients at greater risk for fluid overload (precipitate heart failure exacerbation) from fluid replacement therapy. ©
- Follow with a hypotonic fluid (0.45% sodium chloride) to continue replacing losses to total body fluid.
- When serum glucose levels approach 250 mg/dL, add glucose to IV fluids to minimize the risk of cerebral edema associated with drastic changes in serum osmolarity and prevent hypoglycemia.
- Administer regular insulin 0.1 to 0.15 unit/kg as an IV bolus dose and then follow with a continuous IV infusion of regular insulin at 0.1 unit/kg/hr.
- Insulin is administered IV rather than subcutaneously to provide immediate treatment. The client who has DKA will absorb subcutaneous insulin slowly and erratically, making it difficult to adjust dosages of insulin appropriately. Monitor blood glucose hourly. Blood glucose of less than 200 mg/dL is the goal for resolution.
- Monitor serum potassium levels. Potassium levels will initially be increased, but with insulin therapy potassium will shift into cells, and the client will need to be monitored for hypokalemia.
  - Provide potassium replacement therapy in all replacement IV fluids, as indicated by laboratory values.
  - Monitor cardiac rhythm constantly.
  - Make sure urinary output is adequate before administering potassium.
- Administer sodium bicarbonate by slow IV infusion for severe acidosis (pH less than 7.0). Infuse potassium along with bicarbonate because bicarbonate promotes hypokalemia, unless the client has hyperkalemia.
- Monitor for and report changes in neurological status in clients who have HHS. **Qs**

CONSIDERATIONS FOR OLDER ADULT CLIENTS ©
- Teach older adult clients to monitor blood glucose every 1 to 4 hr when ill.
- Emphasize the importance of not skipping an insulin dose when ill.
- Maintain hydration because older adult clients can have a diminished thirst sensation.
- Changes in mental status can prevent older adult clients from seeking treatment.

CLIENT EDUCATION

- Provide the client with education to prevent reoccurrence.
- Encourage all clients to wear a medical alert bracelet.
- Teach clients to take measures to decrease the risk of dehydration.
  - Unless contraindicated by other health problems, consume 2 to 3 L/day of fluid from food and beverages with artificial sweetener, and drink an adequate amount of water.
  - If blood glucose levels are low, consume liquids with sugar.
- Instruct clients to monitor glucose every 4 hr when ill and continue to take insulin.
- Teach clients to check urine for ketones if blood glucose is greater than 240 mg/dL
- Tell clients to consume liquids with carbohydrates and electrolytes (sports drinks) when unable to eat solid food.
- Teach clients to notify the provider for the following.
  - Illness that lasts longer than 24 hr
  - Blood glucose greater than 250 mg/dL
  - Inability to tolerate food or fluids
  - Ketones in urine for more than 24 hr
  - Temperature of 38.6° C (101.5° F) for 24 hr

Application Exercises

1. A nurse is reviewing the health record of a client who has hyperglycemic-hyperosmolar state (HHS). The nurse should identify that which of the following data confirm this diagnosis? (Select all that apply.)

   A. Evidence of recent myocardial infarction

   B. BUN 35 mg/dL

   C. Takes a calcium channel blocker

   D. Age 77 years

   E. No insulin production

2. A nurse is assessing a client who has diabetic ketoacidosis and ketones in the urine. The nurse should expect which of the following findings? (Select all that apply.)

   A. Weight gain

   B. Fruity odor of breath

   C. Abdominal pain

   D. Kussmaul respirations

   E. Metabolic acidosis

3. A nurse is reviewing laboratory reports of a client who has hyperglycemic-hyperosmolar state (HHS). The nurse should expect which of the following findings?

   A. Serum pH 7.2

   B. Serum osmolarity 350 mOsm/L

   C. Serum potassium 3.8 mg/dL

   D. Serum creatinine 0.8 mg/dL

4. A nurse is preparing to administer IV fluids to a client who has diabetic ketoacidosis. Which of the following actions should the nurse take?

   A. Administer an IV infusion of regular insulin at 0.3 unit/kg/hr.

   B. Administer an IV infusion of 0.45% sodium chloride.

   C. Rapidly administer an IV infusion of 0.9% sodium chloride.

   D. Add glucose to the IV infusion when serum glucose is 350 mg/dL.

5. A nurse is providing discharge teaching to a client who has experienced diabetic ketoacidosis. Which of the following information should the nurse include in the teaching? (Select all that apply.)

   A. Drink 2 L fluids daily.

   B. Monitor blood glucose every 4 hr when ill.

   C. Administer insulin as prescribed when ill.

   D. Notify the provider when blood glucose is 200 mg/dL.

   E. Report ketones in the urine after 24 hr of illness.

PRACTICE Active Learning Scenario

A nurse is planning care for a client who has diabetic ketoacidosis. What should the nurse include in the plan of care? Use the ATI Active Learning Template: Basic Concept to complete this item.

RELATED CONTENT: List three treatments. Describe the nursing actions for each treatment.

1. A. **CORRECT:** The client who has type 2 diabetes mellitus and had a myocardial infarction is at risk for developing HHS. This is due to the increased hormone production during illness or stress, which can stimulate the liver to produce glucose and decrease the effects of insulin.

    B. **CORRECT:** The client who has type 2 diabetes mellitus can be at risk for developing HHS when the BUN is 35 mg/dL because it is an indication of decreased kidney function and inability of the kidney to filter high levels of blood glucose into the urine.

    C. **CORRECT:** A calcium channel blocker is one of several medications that increase the risk for HHS in a client who has type 2 diabetes mellitus.

    D. **CORRECT:** The older adult client is at risk for developing type 2 diabetes mellitus and can be unaware of associated manifestations, increasing the risk for HHS.

    E. The client who has type 2 diabetes mellitus can produce enough insulin to prevent ketoacidosis but not enough to control blood glucose, resulting in HHS.

    Ⓝ *NCLEX® Connection: Physiological Adaptation, Pathophysiology*

2. A. Weight loss occurs when the cells are unable to use glucose because of insulin deficiency and places the body in a catabolic state.

    B. **CORRECT:** Fruity odor of breath is a manifestation of elevated ketone levels that lead to metabolic acidosis.

    C. **CORRECT:** Abdominal pain is a GI manifestation of increased ketones and acidosis.

    D. **CORRECT:** Kussmaul respirations are an attempt to excrete carbon dioxide and acid when in metabolic acidosis.

    E. **CORRECT:** Metabolic acidosis is caused by glucose, protein, and fat breakdown, which produces ketones.

    Ⓝ *NCLEX® Connection: Physiological Adaptation, Pathophysiology*

3. A. Serum pH of 7.2 is an indication of diabetic ketoacidosis and is not an expected finding for HHS.

    B. **CORRECT:** A client who has HHS would have a serum osmolarity greater than 320 mOsm/L.

    C. Potassium 3.8 mEq/L is within the expected reference range. A client who has HHS would initially have a decreased serum potassium due to diuresis.

    D. Creatinine 0.8 mg/dL is within the expected reference range. A client who has HHS would have a serum creatinine of greater than 1.5 mg/dL, secondary to dehydration.

    Ⓝ *NCLEX® Connection: Reduction of Risk Potential, Laboratory Values*

4. A. The nurse should administer an IV infusion of regular insulin at 0.1 unit/kg/hr to gradually lower blood glucose to prevent cerebral edema.

    B. The administration of an IV infusion of 0.45% sodium chloride should follow the isotonic fluid and is used as maintenance fluids.

    C. **CORRECT:** The nurse should rapidly administer an IV infusion of 0.9% sodium chloride, an isotonic fluid, as prescribed to maintain blood perfusion to vital organs.

    D. The nurse should add glucose to the IV infusion when the serum glucose is 250 mg/dL, not 350 mg/dL, to prevent hypoglycemia and minimize cerebral edema.

    Ⓝ *NCLEX® Connection: Pharmacological and Parenteral Therapies, Parenteral/Intravenous Therapies*

5. A. **CORRECT:** Drinking 2 L fluids daily can prevent dehydration if the client develops diabetic ketoacidosis.

    B. **CORRECT:** Blood glucose tends to increase during illness. Blood glucose should be monitored every 4 hr.

    C. **CORRECT:** Illness often causes blood glucose to increase. Regular doses of insulin should be administered.

    D. Notify the provider when blood glucose is greater than 250 mg/dL.

    E. **CORRECT:** The provider should be notified if there are ketones in the urine after 24 hr of illness.

    Ⓝ *NCLEX® Connection: Physiological Adaptation, Illness Management*

PRACTICE Answer

Using the ATI Active Learning Template: Basic Concept

RELATED CONTENT

Fluid replacement
- Rapidly infuse the prescribed amount of IV 0.9% sodium chloride.
- Follow with IV infusion of 0.45% sodium chloride as maintenance fluids.
- Monitor laboratory tests.

- Monitor and replace potassium as prescribed.
- Review BUN and creatinine levels for expected improvement.
- Monitor serum osmolarity.
- Evaluate blood glucose hourly.

Insulin administration
- Administer regular insulin IV bolus dose as prescribed.
- Follow with regular insulin IV infusion as prescribed.

Ⓝ *NCLEX® Connection: Physiological Adaptation, Illness Management*

NCLEX® Connections

When reviewing the following chapters, keep in mind the relevant topics and tasks of the NCLEX outline, in particular:

Client Needs: Health Promotion and Maintenance

HEALTH PROMOTION/DISEASE PREVENTION: Educate the client on actions to promote/maintain health and prevent disease.

HEALTH SCREENING: Apply knowledge of pathophysiology to health screening.

HIGH RISK BEHAVIORS: Provide information for prevention and treatment of high risk health behaviors.

Client Needs: Pharmacological and Parenteral Therapies

MEDICATION ADMINISTRATION: Educate client on medication self-administration procedures.

PARENTERAL/INTRAVENOUS THERAPY: Monitor intravenous infusion and maintain site.

PHARMACOLOGICAL PAIN MANAGEMENT: Administer and document pharmacological pain management appropriate for client age and diagnoses.

Client Needs: Physiological Adaptation

ALTERATIONS IN BODY SYSTEMS
Provide care to a client with an infectious disease.

Evaluate client response to treatment for an infectious disease.

CHAPTER 84

UNIT 13   NURSING CARE OF CLIENTS WHO HAVE IMMUNE
SYSTEM AND CONNECTIVE TISSUE DISORDERS
SECTION: DIAGNOSTIC AND THERAPEUTIC PROCEDURES

CHAPTER 84 *Immune and Infectious Disorders Diagnostic Procedures*

Diagnostic procedures for immune and infectious disorders involve identification of pathogenic micro-organisms. The most accurate and definitive way to identify micro-organisms and cell characteristics is by examining blood, body fluids, and tissue samples under a microscope. Effective treatment of infectious disease begins with identification of the pathogenic micro-organism.

White blood cells

- WBCs, or leukocytes, stimulate the inflammatory response and offer protection against various types of infection and foreign antigens.
- There are five types of WBCs. Laboratory analysis of circulating WBCs is the differential, which lists the percentages of the types of WBCs for a total of 100%. The percentages represent the proportion of each type of cell in a sample of WBCs. If the percentage of one type of cell increases, the percentages of other types decrease accordingly.

INTERPRETATION OF FINDINGS

The expected reference range for WBCs is 5,000 to 10,000/mm³.

Leukopenia is a total WBC count less than 4,000/mm³. It can indicate drug toxicity, autoimmune disease, bone marrow failure, and some overwhelming infections.

Leukocytosis is a total WBC count greater than 10,000/mm³. It can indicate inflammation, infection, some malignancies, trauma, dehydration, stress, steroid use, and thyroid storm.

- A client who has had a splenectomy can have a persistently increased WBC count.
- Older adult clients can have a severe bacterial infection without leukocytosis. Manifestations of infection, such as fever, can be absent in an older adult who has an infection. The nurse should monitor older adults clients carefully for infection risks. ©

Neutropenia is a neutrophil count less than 2,000/mm³. Neutropenia occurs in clients who have viral infections, overwhelming bacterial infections, or are undergoing radiation or chemotherapy. A client who has neutropenia is at an increased risk for infection.

- The absolute neutrophil count (ANC) of a client who has neutropenia can help decide the client's real risk for infection. Multiplying the total WBC count by the percentage of neutrophils plus the percentage of bands determines the ANC.
- An ANC less than 1,000 means that neutropenic precautions are essential.
- Neutropenic precautions (a protective environment) include the following.
  - Restricting visitors
  - Prohibiting visits by people who have an infection
  - Restricting exposure to live plants
  - Restricting ingestion of fresh fruits and vegetables
  - Avoiding contamination from the client's own bacterial flora by avoiding the measurement of rectal temperature and administering IM injections. Qᴾᶜᶜ

Left shift is an increase in immature neutrophils (bands or stabs) that occurs with an acute infection. Neutrophil production increases, allowing the release of immature neutrophils that are not capable of phagocytosis (ingesting and destroying bacteria).

TYPES OF WBCs

Neutrophils

The majority of neutrophils are segmented (mature) with others being banded (not fully mature).

PERCENTAGE OF CIRCULATING NEUTROPHILS: 55% to 70%

INCREASED WITH
- Acute bacterial infection
- Myelocytic leukemia
- Trauma
- Rheumatoid arthritis

DECREASED WITH
- Sepsis
- Radiation therapy, aplastic anemia, chemotherapy
- Influenza

Lymphocytes (T cells and B cells)

- T-lymphocytes initiate cell–mediated immunity.
- B-lymphocytes initiate humoral immunity.

PERCENT OF CIRCULATING LYMPHOCYTES: 20% to 40%

INCREASED WITH
- Chronic bacterial or viral infection
- Viruses such as mononucleosis, mumps, and measles
- Bacteria such as hepatitis
- Lymphocytic leukemia, multiple myeloma

DECREASED WITH
- Leukemia
- Sepsis

Monocytes

PERCENT OF CIRCULATING MONOCYTES: 2% to 8%

INCREASED WITH
- Chronic inflammation
- Protozoal infections
- Tuberculosis
- Viral infections such as mononucleosis

DECREASED WITH
- Corticosteroid therapy
- Aplastic anemia
- Hairy cell leukemia

Eosinophils

PERCENT OF CIRCULATING EOSINOPHILS: 1% to 4%

INCREASED WITH
- Allergic reactions
- Parasitic infection
- Eczema
- Leukemia
- Autoimmune diseases

DECREASED WITH
- Stress
- Corticosteroids

Basophils

PERCENT OF CIRCULATING BASOPHILS: 0.5% to 1%

INCREASED WITH: Leukemia

DECREASED WITH
- Acute allergic/hypersensitivity reactions
- Hyperthyroidism
- Stress reactions

Radioallergosorbent test

A radioallergosorbent test (RAST) is a blood test to determine sensitivity to various allergens. It can complement skin testing or be an alternative when the risk of a hypersensitivity reaction to an allergen exists.

ADVANTAGES
- Will not precipitate a dangerous allergic reaction
- Quicker than skin testing

DISADVANTAGES
- Available for fewer antigens
- Can be less sensitive than skin testing

INDICATIONS

POTENTIAL DIAGNOSES: Environmental and food allergies

CLIENT PRESENTATION
- Report of hypersensitivity reactions
- Hives, asthma, gastrointestinal (GI) dysfunction, rhinitis, dermatitis, angioedema

CONSIDERATIONS

INTRAPROCEDURE: Obtain a blood sample.

INTERPRETATION OF FINDINGS

The technician mixes specific allergens with the blood and incubates it with radiolabeled anti-IgE antibodies. Results reflect allergen-specific IgE levels and thus the degree of sensitivity on a 0 to 6 scale.

Skin testing for allergens

- Skin testing for allergens involves the use of intradermal injections or scratching the superficial layer (scratch or prick test) of the skin with small amounts of potential allergens.
- Intradermal testing runs a higher risk of hypersensitivity reactions and follows inconclusive scratch-test results.

INDICATIONS

POTENTIAL DIAGNOSES: Environmental and food allergies

CLIENT PRESENTATION: Hives, asthma, GI dysfunction, rhinitis, dermatitis, angioedema

INTERPRETATION OF FINDINGS

- A localized reaction (wheal and flare) to an allergen is a positive reaction to that allergen.
- The larger the reaction, the more severe the allergy.

CONSIDERATIONS

PREPROCEDURE

NURSING ACTIONS
- Prepare the skin on the client's back or forearm for application of various allergens using soap and water.
- Use alcohol to remove any oil.
- Have equipment available to treat anaphylaxis. Qs

CLIENT EDUCATION: Instruct the client to avoid taking corticosteroids and antihistamines from 48 hr to 2 weeks, depending on their duration of action and other factors, prior to testing.

INTRAPROCEDURE

NURSING ACTIONS
- Scratch or prick the skin with a needle after applying a drop of an allergen.
- Use a standard pattern of application to help identify the allergen. QEBP
- Apply control drops (substances that should not produce a reaction, such as 0.9% sodium chloride irrigation, and substances that should produce a reaction, such as histamine).
- Assess for reactions after 15 to 20 min.

POSTPROCEDURE

NURSING ACTIONS
- Assess the skin for areas of reaction, and document the allergen that is responsible.
- Remove all solutions from the skin.
- Recommend an antihistamine or topical corticosteroid if the client's skin itches after testing.

CLIENT EDUCATION Qpcc
- Teach desensitizing options and avoidance therapies for allergens.
- Advise the client to follow a diet that eliminates allergens some (gluten-free).

PRACTICE Active Learning Scenario

A nurse is caring for a client who will have a radioallergosorbent test (RAST). Use the ATI Active Learning Template: Diagnostic Procedure to complete this item.

INDICATIONS: List two.

INTERPRETATION OF FINDINGS: Describe one.

NURSING INTERVENTIONS (PRE, INTRA, POST): Describe one intraprocedure nursing action.

Application Exercises

1. A nurse is caring for a client who has a WBC count of 20,000/mm³. The nurse should conclude that the client has which of the following?

   A. Neutropenia

   B. Leukocytosis

   C. Left shift

   D. Leukopenia

2. A nurse is reviewing the laboratory findings of a client who has measles. The nurse should expect to find an increase in which of the following types of WBCs?

   A. Neutrophils

   B. Basophils

   C. Lymphocytes

   D. Eosinophils

3. A nurse is preparing to administer a scratch test to a client who has possible food and environmental allergies. Which of the following actions should the nurse perform prior to the procedure? (Select all that apply.)

   A. Cleanse the client's skin with povidone-iodine.

   B. Ask the client about previous reactions to allergens.

   C. Ask the client about medications she took over the past several days.

   D. Inform the client to expect itching at one site.

   E. Obtain emergency resuscitation equipment.

Application Exercises Key

1.   A. Neutropenia is a neutrophil count less than 2,000/mm³.

    B. **CORRECT:** Leukocytosis is a WBC count greater than 10,000/mm³, which can indicate inflammation or infection.

    C. A left shift is an increase in immature neutrophils (bands or stabs) that occurs with acute infection.

    D. Leukopenia is a total WBC count of less than 4,000/mm³, which can indicate overwhelming infection or drug toxicity.

    Ⓝ *NCLEX® Connection: Reduction of Risk Potential, Laboratory Values*

2.   A. Neutrophils increase with an acute bacterial infection. Measles is a viral infection.

    B. Basophils increase with leukemia.

    C. **CORRECT:** Lymphocytes increase with viral infections, such as measles, mumps, and mononucleosis.

    D. Eosinophils increase with allergic reactions, leukemia, eczema, and parasitic infections.

    Ⓝ *NCLEX® Connection: Reduction of Risk Potential, Laboratory Values*

3.   A. The nurse should use soap and water to cleanse the skin. Povidone-iodine could interfere with an allergen and elicit a response.

    B. **CORRECT:** The nurse should ask the client about any previous reactions to allergens, which could indicate an increased risk of an anaphylactic reaction.

    C. **CORRECT:** The nurse should ask the client about medications she took over the past several days. Antihistamines and corticosteroids can suppress reactions.

    D. **CORRECT:** The nurse will apply histamine at a control site so the client will probably have itching at this site.

    E. **CORRECT:** Emergency equipment should be available, even if the client denies previous anaphylactic reactions.

    Ⓝ *NCLEX® Connection: Reduction of Risk Potential, Diagnostic Tests*

PRACTICE Answer

Using the ATI Active Learning Template: Diagnostic Procedure

INDICATIONS
- Possible environmental and food allergies
- Report of hypersensitivity reactions
- Hives, asthma, gastrointestinal dysfunction, rhinitis, dermatitis, angioedema

INTERPRETATION OF FINDINGS: The technician mixes specific allergens with the blood and incubates it with anti-IgE antibodies. Results reflect allergen-specific IgE levels and thus the degree of sensitivity on a 0 to 6 scale.

NURSING INTERVENTIONS (PRE, INTRA, POST): Obtain a blood sample.

Ⓝ *NCLEX® Connection: Reduction of Risk Potential, Diagnostic Tests*

CHAPTER 85 *Immunizations*

Administration of a vaccine causes production of antibodies that prevent illness from a specific microbe. Vaccines can be made from killed viruses or live, attenuated (weakened) viruses.

IMMUNITY

ACTIVE IMMUNITY is an adaptive process that allows the body to make antibodies in response to the entry of antigens into the body.

- **Active-natural immunity** develops when the body produces antibodies in response to exposure to a live pathogen that enters the body naturally. ⓠEBP
- **Active-artificial immunity** develops when a vaccine is given and the body produces antibodies in response to exposure to a killed or attenuated virus.

PASSIVE IMMUNITY develops when antibodies that are created by another human or animal are transferred to the client. Because the client does not independently develop antibodies passive immunity is temporary.

- **Passive-natural immunity** occurs when antibodies are passed from the mother to the fetus/newborn through the placenta and breast milk.
- **Passive-artificial immunity** occurs after antibodies in the form of immune globulins are administered to an individual who requires immediate protection against a disease where exposure has already occurred, such as following a bite from a poisonous snake or an animal who has rabies. After several weeks or months, the individual is no longer protected.

ADMINISTRATION

The 2016 Centers for Disease Control and Prevention (CDC) immunization recommendations for adults (19 years and older) follows. Go to www.cdc.gov/vaccines for updates.

Tetanus, diphtheria (Td) booster: Give booster every 10 years. For adults 19 and older who did not receive a dose of tetanus, diphtheria, pertussis (Tdap) previously, substitute one dose with Tdap.

- Pregnant women should receive the vaccine between 27 and 36 weeks gestation. Pregnant women should get Tdap vaccine with each pregnancy to protect the fetus from pertussis.

Measles, mumps, and rubella (MMR) vaccine: Follow recommendations for administering one or two doses to clients between the ages of 19 and 49 who lack documentation of immunization or prior infection, or laboratory proof of immunity. People born before 1957 are considered immune to measles and mumps.

Varicella vaccine: Give two doses to adults who do not have evidence of a previous infection. A second dose should be given to adults who have had only one previous dose. Pregnant women needing protection against varicella should wait until the postpartum period for immunization.

Pneumococcal vaccine: Two types are available: 13-valent pneumococcal conjugate vaccine (PCV-13) and 23-valent pneumococcal polysaccharide vaccine (PPSV23).

- Follow recommendations for administration to adults who are immunocompromised, have specific chronic diseases, smoke cigarettes, or live in long-term care facilities.
- For adults 65 years and older who have not been immunized with PCV13 or PPSV23, administer PCV13 first and then give PPSV23 in 6 to 12 months; do not administer both during the same visit. For adults who received a dose of PPSV23 at age 65 or older, an additional dose is not indicated. Ⓖ

Hepatitis A: Two doses for high-risk individuals.

Hepatitis B: Administer three doses to high-risk individuals who lack completion of the series. There must be at least 1 month between doses one and two, and at least 2 months between doses two and three. A minimum of 4 months are required between doses one and three.

Influenza vaccine

- Recommended for all adults annually.
- Inactivated influenza vaccine (IIV) is approved for clients who are pregnant.
- Recombinant influenza vaccine (RIV) is approved for adults 18 years and older.
- The live attenuated vaccine (LAIV), given as a nasal spray, is indicated only for adults under age 50 who are not pregnant or immunocompromised.

Meningococcal polysaccharide vaccine (MPSV4) and Meningococcal 4-valent conjugate (MenACWY) vaccine

- Administer a dose of MenACWY to students up to age 21 years entering college and living in dormitories if a dose was not received on or after the 16th birthday. Two doses of MenACWY at least 2 months apart are recommended for individuals who have anatomical or functional asplenia, and one dose is recommended for military recruits and those traveling to or living in areas of hyperendemic or epidemic rates of meningococcal disease.
- MPSV4 is preferred for adults who are 56 years of age or older, require a single dose, and have not had MenACWY previously.
- Reimmunization with MenACWY is recommended every 5 years for adults who remain at high risk for infection and were previously immunized with MenACWY or MPSV4.

Human papilloma virus HPV2, HPV4, or HPV9: Three doses are recommended for female clients up to age 26 years who were not immunized as children. Female clients can receive HPV2, HPV4, or HPV9. If not immunized as children, HPV4 or HPV9 is recommended for male clients age 19 to 21 years, and for male clients age 22 to 26 years who have a high risk for human papilloma virus.

Zoster vaccine: Recommended as a one-time dose for all adults older than 60 years. Ⓖ

PURPOSE

EXPECTED PHARMACOLOGICAL ACTION

Immunizations produce antibodies that provide active immunity. Immunizations can take months to have an effect, but they provide long-lasting protection against infectious diseases.

THERAPEUTIC USES

- Eradication of infectious diseases
- Prevention of childhood and adult infectious diseases and their complications (tetanus, pneumococcal pneumonia, hepatitis)

CONTRAINDICATIONS/PRECAUTIONS

- An anaphylactic reaction to a vaccine is a contraindication to further doses of that vaccine. Qs
- An anaphylactic reaction to a vaccine is a contraindication to use of other vaccines containing the same substance.
- Moderate or severe illnesses with or without fever are precautions to receiving immunizations. The common cold and other minor illnesses are not contraindications.
- Do not administer live virus vaccines, such as varicella or MMR, to a client who is severely immunocompromised. Severe febrile illness is a contraindication to all immunizations.
- Precautions to immunizations require the provider to analyze data and weigh the risks that come with and without immunizations.

Td, DTaP

ADVERSE EFFECTS
- Mild: Redness, swelling, and tenderness at the injection site; low fever; behavioral changes (drowsiness, irritability, anorexia)
- Moderate: Fever 40.6° C (105° F) or greater; seizures (with or without fever); shock-like state
- Severe: Acute encephalopathy (rare)

CONTRAINDICATIONS: Occurrence of encephalopathy within 7 days following prior dose of the vaccine

PRECAUTIONS
- Occurrence of Guillain-Barré syndrome within 6 weeks of prior dose of tetanus toxoid
- Progressive neurologic disorders; uncontrolled seizures
- Fever 40.6° C (105° F) or greater within 48 hr of prior dose
- Shock-like state within 48 hr of prior dose
- Seizures within 3 days of prior dose

MMR

ADVERSE EFFECTS
- Mild: Local reactions (rash; fever; swollen glands in cheeks or neck)
- Moderate: Joint pain and stiffness lasting for days to weeks, febrile seizure, low platelet count
- Severe: Transient thrombocytopenia, deafness, long-term seizures, brain damage

CONTRAINDICATIONS: Pregnancy

PRECAUTIONS
- History of thrombocytopenia or thrombocytopenic purpura
- Anaphylactic reaction to eggs, gelatin, or neomycin
- Transfusion with blood product containing antibodies within the prior 11 months
- Simultaneous tuberculin skin testing

Varicella

ADVERSE EFFECTS
- Mild: Tenderness and swelling at injection site, fever, rash (mild) for up to 1 month after immunization
- Moderate: Seizures
- Severe: Pneumonia, low blood count (extremely rare), severe brain reactions (extremely rare)

CONTRAINDICATIONS
- Pregnancy
- Anaphylactic reaction to gelatin or neomycin

PRECAUTIONS
- Transfusion with blood product containing antibodies within the prior 11 months
- Treatment with antiviral medication within 24 hr prior to immunization (avoid taking antivirals for 14 days following immunization)
- Extended use (2 weeks or longer) of corticosteroids or other medications that affect the immune system
- Cancer

Pneumococcal conjugate vaccine

ADVERSE EFFECTS
- Swelling, redness and tenderness at site of injection
- Fever
- Irritability
- Drowsiness
- Anorexia

CONTRAINDICATIONS: Anaphylactic reaction to any vaccine containing diphtheria toxoid

Pneumococcal polysaccharide vaccine

ADVERSE EFFECTS
- Redness and tenderness at site of injection
- Fever
- Myalgia

PRECAUTION: Pregnancy

Hepatitis A

ADVERSE EFFECTS
- Local reaction at injection site
- Headache
- Loss of appetite
- Mild fatigue

CONTRAINDICATIONS: Severe allergy to latex

PRECAUTION: Pregnancy

Hepatitis B

ADVERSE EFFECTS
- Local reaction at injection site
- Temperature of 37.7° C (99.9° F) or greater

CONTRAINDICATIONS: Severe allergy (anaphylaxis) to yeast

Inactivated influenza vaccine

ADVERSE EFFECTS
- Swelling, redness and tenderness at the injection site
- Hoarseness
- Fever
- Malaise
- Headache
- Cough
- Aches
- Increased risk for Guillain-Barré syndrome

PRECAUTIONS: Occurrence of Guillain-Barré syndrome within 6 weeks of prior influenza vaccine

Live, attenuated influenza vaccine

ADVERSE EFFECTS
- Vomiting, diarrhea
- Cough
- Fever
- Headache
- Myalgia
- Nasal congestion/runny nose

CONTRAINDICATIONS
- Age 50 years or older
- Pregnancy

PRECAUTIONS
- Occurrence of Guillain-Barré syndrome within 6 weeks of prior influenza vaccine
- Treatment with antiviral medication within 48 hr prior to immunization (avoid taking antivirals for 14 days following immunization)
- Some chronic conditions

The Advisory Committee on Immunization Practices recommends the option of the live-attenuated influenza vaccine to clients regardless of the severity of egg allergy. Clients who have a history of an egg allergy, other than a hive-only reaction, should receive the immunization where a provider is present and emergency equipment is available. (At the time of publication, these recommendations are awaiting approval by the CDC. Please refer to www.cdc.gov for current approval status.)

Meningococcal ACWY

ADVERSE EFFECTS
- Mild local reaction and rare risk of allergic response
- Possible mild fever

Zoster

ADVERSE EFFECTS
- Local reaction at injection site
- Headache

CONTRAINDICATIONS
- Clients who are immunocompromised
- Pregnancy
- Treatment with medications that alter the immune system

Human papilloma virus (HPV4 and HPV9)

ADVERSE EFFECTS
- Mild local reaction and fever
- Mild to moderate fever
- Headache
- Fainting has occurred shortly after receiving vaccine

CONTRAINDICATIONS
- Pregnancy
- Severe allergy (anaphylaxis) to yeast

Human papilloma virus (HPV2)

ADVERSE EFFECTS
- Redness, swelling and tenderness at the injection site
- Temperature 37.7° C (99.9° F) or greater
- Headache
- Fatigue
- Nausea, vomiting, abdominal pain
- Myalgia
- Fainting (shortly after receiving the vaccine)

CONTRAINDICATIONS
- Pregnancy
- Severe allergy to latex

INTERACTIONS

None significant

NURSING ADMINISTRATION

- Have emergency medications and equipment on standby in case the client experiences an allergic response such as anaphylaxis (rare) or serious reaction at injection site. Qs
- Follow storage and reconstitution directions.
- Provide written, vaccine information sheets (VIS), and review the content with clients. Document the publication date of each VIS given to the client.
- Administer antipyretic for fever, apply cool compress for localized tenderness, and mobilize the affected extremity.
- Instruct clients to observe for complications and to notify the provider if adverse effects occur.
- Document administration of vaccines including date, route, site, type, manufacturer, lot number, and expiration date. Also document the client's name, address, and signature. Include the name, title of the person administering the vaccine, and the address of the facility where the permanent record is located. Qʟ

ADULTS

- Give subcutaneous immunizations in outer aspect of the upper arm or anterolateral thigh.
- Give IM immunizations into the deltoid muscle.

NURSING EVALUATION OF MEDICATION EFFECTIVENESS

Depending on therapeutic intent, effectiveness can be evidenced by the following.
- Improvement of local reaction to immunization with absence of pain, fever, and swelling at the site of injection
- Development of immunity

Application Exercises

1. A nurse is preparing to administer an IM injection of immune globulin to a client who has been exposed to hepatitis A. Which of the following statements by the nurse is appropriate?

   A. "This medication offers permanent immunity to hepatitis A."

   B. "This medication involves three injections over several months."

   C. "This medication provides you with an immune response more quickly than your body can produce it."

   D. "This medication contains an attenuated virus to help your body create antibodies."

2. A nurse is preparing to administer a varicella immunization to a client. Which of the following questions by the nurse is appropriate?

   A. "Are you allergic to eggs?"

   B. "Are you allergic to baker's yeast?"

   C. "Are you pregnant?"

   D. "Do you have a history of Guillain-Barré syndrome?"

3. A nurse is reviewing strategies to promote comfort with a client who received an immunization. Which of the following information should the nurse include? (Select all that apply.)

   A. Massage the injection site.

   B. Apply a cool compress to the injection site.

   C. Take acetaminophen or ibuprofen.

   D. Use the affected extremity.

   E. Apply an antimicrobial ointment to the injection site.

4. A nurse is preparing to document administration of a meningococcal vaccine to a client. Which of the following information should the nurse include in the documentation? (Select all that apply.)

   A. Age of client receiving the vaccine

   B. Name of vaccine manufacturer

   C. Vaccine expiration date

   D. Date of administration

   E. Serial number of the vaccine

5. A nurse in a clinic is caring for a client who is to receive an immunization. The client asks about contraindications to immunizations. Which of the following is an appropriate response by the nurse?

   A. "The use of insulin is a contraindication."

   B. "An anaphylactic reaction is a contraindication for administration of any type of immunization."

   C. "The common cold is a contraindication for receiving an immunization."

   D. "Your provider will weigh the risks if you have experienced any adverse effects."

PRACTICE Active Learning Scenario

A nurse at a community health clinic is administering influenza vaccines for a group of clients. What information should the nurse take into consideration when selecting the type of vaccine to administer? Use the ATI Active Learning Template: Medication to complete this item.

NURSING INTERVENTIONS: Identify the three types of influenza vaccine and which clients should receive each of the three types.

Application Exercises Key

1. A. This medication produces passive-artificial immunity that lasts only several weeks or months.

   B. This medication produces passive-artificial immunity and is given one time after exposure to hepatitis A.

   C. **CORRECT:** This medication produces passive-artificial immunity and contains antibodies to help protect against hepatitis A for several weeks or months.

   D. This medication contains antibodies, not an attenuated virus.

   Ⓝ *NCLEX® Connection: Pharmacological and Parenteral Therapies, Parenteral/Intravenous Therapies*

2. A. Allergy to eggs should be reviewed if the client is to receive an influenza immunization.

   B. Allergy to yeast should be reviewed if the client is to receive HPV immunization.

   C. **CORRECT:** The nurse should ask whether the client is pregnant because the varicella immunization is contraindicated during pregnancy.

   D. Guillain-Barré syndrome is not a contraindication for varicella immunization.

   Ⓝ *NCLEX® Connection: Pharmacological and Parenteral Therapies, Adverse Effects/Contraindications/Side Effects/Interactions*

3. A. Massaging the injection site for any extended period of time can increase localized discomfort.

   B. **CORRECT:** Applying a cool compress to the injection site can relieve discomfort from the localized reaction.

   C. **CORRECT:** Taking an antipyretic can relieve a low-grade fever and localized discomfort at the injection site.

   D. **CORRECT:** Mobilizing the affected extremity will help relieve discomfort due to a localized reaction.

   E. Applying an antimicrobial ointment at the injection site is not indicated.

   Ⓝ *NCLEX® Connection: Pharmacological and Parenteral Therapies, Parenteral/Intravenous Therapies*

4. A. Age of the person receiving an immunization is not included.

   B. **CORRECT:** The nurse should document the name of the vaccine manufacturer.

   C. **CORRECT:** The nurse should document the expiration date of the vaccine.

   D. **CORRECT:** The nurse should document the date the vaccine was administered.

   E. The nurse should document the lot number, not the serial number, of the vaccine.

   Ⓝ *NCLEX® Connection: Pharmacological and Parenteral Therapies, Adverse Effects/Contraindications/Side Effects/Interactions*

5. A. The client who takes insulin is able to receive immunizations unless other contraindications are present.

   B. The client who has experienced an anaphylactic reaction can receive other immunizations that contain different substances.

   C. The client who has a common cold may receive an immunization because the client is not immunosuppressed.

   D. **CORRECT:** The client who has experienced adverse effects should inform the provider, who can weigh the risks of an immunization.

   Ⓝ *NCLEX® Connection: Pharmacological and Parenteral Therapies, Adverse Effects/Contraindications/Side Effects/Interactions*

PRACTICE Answer

Using the ATI Active Learning Template: Medication

NURSING INTERVENTIONS

- Inactivated influenza vaccine (IIV) is approved for clients who are pregnant.
- Recombinant influenza vaccine (RIV) is approved for adults 18 years of age and older.
- The live attenuated vaccine (LAIV), given as a nasal spray, is indicated only for adults under age 50 who are not pregnant or immunocompromised.

Ⓝ *NCLEX® Connection: Health Promotion and Maintenance, Aging Process*

CHAPTER 86 *HIV/AIDS*

Human immunodeficiency virus (HIV) is a retrovirus that is transmitted through blood and body fluids (semen, vaginal secretions).

HIV targets CD4+ lymphocytes, also known as T-cells or T-lymphocytes. T-cells work in concert with B-lymphocytes. Both are part of specific acquired (adaptive) immunity. HIV integrates its RNA into host cell DNA through reverse transcriptase, reshaping the host's immune system.

HIV is found in feces, urine, tears, saliva, cerebrospinal fluid, cervical cells, lymph nodes, corneal tissue, and brain tissue, but epidemiologic studies indicate that these are unlikely sources of infection.

All women who are pregnant should be screened for HIV. Q EBP

DISEASE PROCESS STAGES

HIV infection is one continuous disease process with three stages.

Progression of HIV infection

- Manifestations occur within 2 to 4 weeks of infection.
- Manifestations are similar to those of influenza and can include a rash and a sore throat.
- This stage is marked by a rapid rise in the HIV viral load, decreased CD4+ cells, and increased CD8 cells.
- The resolution of manifestations coincides with the decline in viral HIV copies.
- Lymphadenopathy persists throughout the disease process.

Chronic asymptomatic infection

- This stage can be prolonged and clinically silent (asymptomatic).
- The client can remain asymptomatic for 10 years or more.
- Anti–HIV antibodies are produced (HIV positive).
- Over time, the virus begins active replication using the host's genetic machinery.
  - CD4+ cells are destroyed.
  - The viral load increases.
  - Dramatic loss of immunity begins.

AIDS

- This stage is characterized by life–threatening opportunistic infections.
- This is the end stage of HIV infection. Without treatment, death occurs within 5 years.
- All people with AIDS have HIV, but not all people who have HIV have AIDS.

86.1 HIV infection stages

A confirmed case classification meets the laboratory criteria for a diagnosis of HIV infection and one of the four HIV infection stages.

To read more about HIV, go to www.cdc.gov.

Stage 1
DEFINING CONDITIONS: None

CD4+ T-LYMPHOCYTE COUNT:
500 cells/mm^3 or more

CD4+ T-LYMPHOCYTE PERCENTAGE OF TOTAL LYMPHOCYTES: 29% or more

Stage 2
DEFINING CONDITIONS: None

CD4+ T-LYMPHOCYTE COUNT:
200 to 499 cells/mm^3

CD4+ T-LYMPHOCYTE PERCENTAGE OF TOTAL LYMPHOCYTES: 14% to 28%

Stage 3 (AIDS)
Documentation of an AIDS-defining condition supersedes a CD4+ T-lymphocyte count of 200 cells/mm^3 or more and a CD4+ T-lymphocyte percentage of total lymphocytes of more than 14%.

DEFINING CONDITIONS: One or more of the following

- Candidiasis of the esophagus, bronchi, trachea, or lungs
- Herpes simplex: Chronic ulcers (more than 1 month duration)
- HIV-related encephalopathy
- Disseminated or extrapulmonary histoplasmosis
- Kaposi's sarcoma
- Burkitt's lymphoma

- Mycobacterium tuberculosis of any site
- *Pneumocystis jirovecii* pneumonia
- Recurrent pneumonia
- Progressive multifocal leukoencephalopathy
- Recurrent salmonella septicemia
- Wasting syndrome attributed to HIV

CD4+ T-LYMPHOCYTE COUNT: Less than 200 cells/mm^3

CD4+ T-LYMPHOCYTE PERCENTAGE OF TOTAL LYMPHOCYTES: Less than 14%

Stage 4
No information available

HEALTH PROMOTION AND DISEASE PREVENTION

- Teach the client how the virus is transmitted and ways to prevent infection, such as the use of condoms, abstinence, and avoiding sharing needles.
- Encourage the client to maintain up-to-date immunizations, including yearly seasonal influenza and pneumococcal polysaccharide vaccine.
- Providers should use standard precautions when caring for the client.

ASSESSMENT

RISK FACTORS

- Unprotected sex (vaginal, anal, oral)
- Multiple sex partners
- Occupational exposure (health care workers)
- Perinatal exposure
- Blood transfusions (not a significant source of infection in the U.S.)
- IV drug use with a contaminated needle
- Older adult clients
  - HIV infection can go undiagnosed in older adult clients due to the similarity of its manifestations to other illnesses that are common in this age group. ⓖ
  - Older adults are more susceptible to fluid and electrolyte imbalances, malnutrition, skin alterations, and wasting syndrome than younger adults.
  - Older adult women experience vaginal dryness and thinning of the vaginal wall, increasing their susceptibility to HIV infection.

EXPECTED FINDINGS

- Chills
- Rash
- Anorexia, nausea, weight loss
- Weakness and fatigue
- Headache and sore throat
- Night sweats

LABORATORY TESTS

CBC and differential: Abnormal (anemia, thrombocytopenia, leukopenia)

Platelet count: Decreased less than 150,000/mm^3

DIAGNOSTIC PROCEDURES

- Positive result from an HIV antibody screening test (enzyme-linked immunosorbent assay [ELISA]) confirmed by a positive result from a supplemental HIV antibody test (Western blot or indirect immunofluorescence assay [IFA])
- Home test kits are also available using a drop of blood. These provide anonymous registration and counseling before the test via a telephone call.
- Two non-invasive tests are available using either mucosal fluid or urine.
- Client who has a positive result from a confirmatory test (e.g., Western blot) should then be tested for viral load.

HIV RNA quantification (HIV viral load test)

- Determines viral load before beginning treatment
- Can be repeated at intervals to monitor disease progression, identify compliance with treatment and determine HIV medication resistance.

HIV drug resistance testing (HIV genotype or HIV tropism)

- Guides changes in medication therapy when resistance occurs
- Useful with CD4 counts fall despite therapy

Liver profile, biopsies, and testing of stool for parasites

NURSING ACTIONS: Prepare the client for the test.

CLIENT EDUCATION ⓠpcc
- Inform the client about the details of the test, such as length and what to expect.
- Explain that a positive Western blot or IFA test means the client has been exposed to and has the AIDS virus in her body but does not mean the client has clinical AIDS.
- Allow the client time to ask questions or express emotions.
- Provide education regarding safe sexual practices.

Brain or lung MRI or CT scan

Detailed image of the brain or lung to detect abnormalities

NURSING ACTIONS: Prepare the client for the procedure.

CLIENT EDUCATION: Inform the client about the length of time the test takes (up to 1 hr).

PATIENT-CENTERED CARE

NURSING CARE

- Assess risk factors (sexual practices, IV drug use).
- Monitor fluid intake/urinary output.
- Obtain daily weights to monitor weight loss.
- Monitor nutritional intake.
- Monitor electrolytes.
- Assess skin integrity (rashes, open areas, bruising).
- Assess pain status.
- Monitor vital signs (especially temperature).
- Assess lung sounds/respiratory status (diminished lung sounds).
- Assess neurological status (confusion, dementia, visual changes).
- Encourage activity alternated with rest periods.
- Administer supplemental oxygen as needed.
- Provide analgesia as needed.
- Provide skin care as needed.

MEDICATIONS

Highly active antiretroviral therapy involves using three to four HIV medications in combination with other antiretroviral medications to reduce medication resistance, adverse effects, and dosages.

Fusion inhibitors: Enfuvirtide blocks the fusion of HIV with the host cell

Entry inhibitors: Maraviroc

Nucleoside reverse transcriptase inhibitors: Zidovudine interferes with the virus's ability to convert RNA into DNA.

Non-nucleoside reverse transcriptase inhibitors: Delavirdine and efavirenz inhibit viral replication in cells.

Protease inhibitors: Atazanavir, nelfinavir, saquinavir, and indinavir inhibit an enzyme needed for the virus to replicate.

Integrase inhibitors: Raltegravir

Antineoplastic medication: Interleukin is an immunostimulant that enhances the immune response and reduces the production of cancer cells (used commonly with Kaposi's sarcoma).

NURSING CONSIDERATIONS

- Monitor laboratory results (CBC, WBC, liver function tests). Antiretroviral medications can increase alanine aminotransferase, aspartate aminotransferase, bilirubin, mean corpuscular volume, high-density lipoproteins, total cholesterol, and triglycerides. Q_{EBP}
- Monitor total CD4+ T lymphocyte count as well as CD4 percentage and ratio of CD4 to CD8 cells.
  - Normal CD4-to-CD8 ratio is 2:1. A ratio of less than 1 indicates more severe disease manifestations
  - Low CD4 T lymphocyte counts and steadily decreasing counts indicate poor prognosis or medication resistance.

CLIENT EDUCATION Q_{PCC}

- Educate the client about the adverse effects of the medications and ways to decrease the severity of adverse effects.
- Educate the client about the need to take medications on a regular schedule and to not miss doses. Missed medication doses can cause drug resistance.

INTERPROFESSIONAL CARE

- Infectious disease services may be consulted to manage HIV.
- Respiratory services may be consulted to improve respiratory status and provide portable oxygen.
- Nutritional services may be consulted for dietary supplementation. Food services can be indicated for clients who are homebound and need meals prepared.
- Rehabilitation services may be consulted for strengthening and improving the client's level of energy.
- Refer the client to local AIDS support groups as appropriate. Q_{TC}
- Home health service can be indicated for clients who need help with strengthening and assistance regarding ADLs. Home health services may also provide assistance with IVs, dressing changes, and total parenteral nutrition (TPN).
- Long-term care facilities can be indicated for clients who have chronic HIV.
- Hospice services can be indicated for clients who have a late stage of HIV.

Alternative therapy

Vitamins, herbal products, and shark cartilage can help alleviate manifestations of HIV. Ask the client if she is taking herbal products. These can alter the effects of prescribed medications.

CLIENT EDUCATION

- Instruct the client to practice good hygiene and frequent hand hygiene to reduce the risk of infection.
- Instruct the client to avoid crowded areas or traveling to countries with poor sanitation.
- Encourage the client to avoid raw foods, such as fruits or vegetables, and undercooked foods such as meats, fish, or eggs.
- Instruct the client to avoid cleaning pet litter boxes to reduce the risk of toxoplasmosis.
- Encourage the client to keep the home environment clean and to avoid being exposed to family and friends who have colds or flu viruses.
- Instruct the client to wash dishes in hot water using a dishwasher if available.
- Encourage the client to bathe daily using antimicrobial soap.
- Provide client teaching. Qpcc
  - Transmission, infection control measures, and safe sex practices
  - Importance of maintaining a well-balanced diet
  - Self-administration of prescribed medications and potential adverse effects
  - Findings that need to be reported immediately (infection)
- Instruct the client to adhere to the antiretroviral dosing schedules.
- Instruct the client about the need for frequent follow-up monitoring of CD4+ and viral load counts.
- Encourage the use of constructive coping mechanisms.
- Assist the client with identifying primary support systems.
- Teach the client to report manifestations of infection immediately to the provider.

COMPLICATIONS

Opportunistic infections

- **Bacterial diseases,** such as tuberculosis, bacterial pneumonia, and septicemia (blood poisoning)
- **HIV-associated malignancies,** such as Kaposi's sarcoma, lymphoma, and squamous cell carcinoma
- **Viral diseases,** such as those caused by cytomegalovirus, herpes simplex, and herpes zoster virus
- **Fungal diseases,** such as pneumocystis jirovecii pneumonia (PCP), candidiasis, cryptococcosis, and penicilliosis
- **Protozoal diseases,** such as PCP, toxoplasmosis, microsporidiosis, cryptosporidiosis, isosporiasis, and leishmaniasis

NURSING ACTIONS

- Implement and maintain antiretroviral medication therapy as prescribed.
- Administer antineoplastics, antibiotics, analgesics, antifungals, and antidiarrheals as prescribed.
- Administer appetite stimulants (to enhance nutrition).
- Monitor for skin breakdown.
- Maintain fluid intake.
- Maintain nutrition.

CLIENT EDUCATION: Teach the client to report indications of infection immediately to the provider. Qpcc

Wasting syndrome

NURSING ACTIONS

- Maintain nutrition orally or by TPN if indicated.
- Monitor weight, calorie counts, and I&O.
- Provide between-meal supplements/snacks.
- Decrease fat content of foods to prevent complications of fat intolerance.
- Rinse the client's mouth several times daily with saline or sodium bicarbonate and sterile water to reduce mouth pain and increase appetite.
- Serve at least six small feedings with high protein value. Qebp

Fluid/electrolyte imbalance

NURSING ACTIONS

- Monitor fluid/electrolyte status.
- Report abnormal laboratory data promptly.
- Encourage the client to drink 2,000 to 3,000 mL of fluid daily.
- Make dietary adjustments to reduce diarrhea.

Seizures (HIV encephalopathy)

NURSING ACTIONS

- Maintain client safety.
- Implement seizure precautions. Qs

Application Exercises

1. A nurse in an outpatient clinic is assessing a client who reports night sweats and fatigue. He states he has had a cough along with nausea and diarrhea. His temperature is 38.1° C (100.6° F) orally. The client is afraid he has HIV. Which of the following actions should the nurse take? (Select all that apply.)

   A. Perform a physical assessment.

   B. Determine when manifestations began.

   C. Teach the client about HIV transmission.

   D. Draw blood for HIV testing.

   E. Obtain a sexual history.

2. A nurse is caring for a client who is suspected of having HIV. The nurse should identify that which of the following diagnostic tests and laboratory values are used to confirm HIV infection? (Select all that apply.)

   A. Western blot

   B. Indirect immunofluorescence assay

   C. CD4+ T-lymphocyte count

   D. HIV RNA quantification test

   E. Cerebrospinal fluid (CSF) analysis

3. A nurse is providing teaching for a client who has stage 3 HIV disease. Which of the following statements by the client should indicate to the nurse an understanding of the teaching?

   A. "I will wear gloves while changing the pet litter box."

   B. "I will rinse raw fruits with water before eating them."

   C. "I will wear a mask when around family members who are ill."

   D. "I will cook vegetables before eating them."

4. A nurse is assessing a client for HIV. The nurse should identify that which of the following are risk factors associated with this virus? (Select all that apply.)

   A. Perinatal exposure

   B. Pregnancy

   C. Monogamous sex partner

   D. Older adult woman

   E. Occupational exposure

5. A nurse is providing teaching for a client who has stage 2 HIV disease and is having difficulty maintaining a normal weight. Which of the following statements by the client should indicate to the nurse an understanding of the teaching.

   A. "I will choose a diet high in fat to help gain weight."

   B. "I will be sure to eat three large meals daily."

   C. "I will drink up to 1 liter of liquid each day."

   D. "I will add high-protein foods to my diet."

PRACTICE Active Learning Scenario

A nurse is planning care for a client who has AIDS. Use the ATI Active Learning Template: System Disorder to complete this item.

NURSING CARE: Describe at least three nursing actions.

Application Exercises Key

1. A. **CORRECT:** The nurse should perform a physical assessment to gather data about the client's condition.

   B. **CORRECT:** The nurse should gather more data to determine whether the manifestations are acute or chronic.

   C. Teaching the client about HIV transmission is not an appropriate action by the nurse at this time.

   D. Drawing blood for HIV testing is not an appropriate action by nurse at this time.

   E. **CORRECT:** The nurse should obtain a sexual history to determine how the virus was transmitted.

   Ⓝ *NCLEX® Connection: Physiological Adaptation, Illness Management*

2. A. **CORRECT:** Positive results of a Western blot test confirm the presence of HIV infection.

   B. **CORRECT:** Positive results of an indirect immunofluorescence assay confirm the presence of HIV infection.

   C. CD4+ T-lymphocyte count assists with classifying the stage of HIV infection.

   D. HIV RNA quantification tests are used to determine vial level and to monitor treatment.

   E. CSF analysis can be used to confirm meningitis.

   Ⓝ *NCLEX® Connection: Reduction of Risk Potential, Diagnostic Tests*

3. A. A client who has AIDS should avoid changing the litter box to prevent acquiring toxoplasmosis.

   B. A client who has AIDS should avoid consuming raw fruits due to the presence of bacteria that can cause opportunistic infections.

   C. Due to compromised immune response, a client who has AIDS should avoid contact with family members who are ill.

   D. **CORRECT:** A client who has AIDS should cook vegetables before eating to kill bacteria that cause opportunistic infections.

   Ⓝ *NCLEX® Connection: Physiological Adaptation, Illness Management*

4. A. **CORRECT:** Perinatal exposure is a risk factor associated with HIV. Women who are pregnant should take precautionary measures to prevent HIV exposure.

   B. Women who are pregnant should be tested for HIV, but pregnancy is not a risk factor associated with this virus.

   C. Having a monogamous sex partner is not a risk factor associated with the HIV virus.

   D. **CORRECT:** Being an older adult woman is a risk factor associated with the HIV virus due vaginal dryness and the thinning of the vaginal wall.

   E. **CORRECT:** Occupational exposure, such as being a health care worker, is a risk factor associated with the HIV virus.

   Ⓝ *NCLEX® Connection: Health Promotion and Maintenance, Health Promotion/Disease Prevention*

5. A. The client should be taught to avoid high-fat foods to gain weight because fat intolerance—causing flatus, bloating, and diarrhea—is common in clients who have HIV/AIDS.

   B. The client should be taught that small frequent meals (such as six meals daily) are better tolerated than three large meals.

   C. The client should be taught to drink 2 to 3 L of liquids daily to maintain nutrition status.

   D. **CORRECT:** The client should be taught to add high-protein, high-calorie foods to the diet daily as the best way to gain weight and maintain health.

   NCLEX® Connection: Physiological Adaptation, Illness Management

---

PRACTICE Answer

Using ATI Active Learning Template: System Disorder

NURSING CARE
- Assess risk factors (sexual practices, IV drug use).
- Monitor fluid intake/urinary output.
- Obtain daily weights to monitor weight loss.
- Monitor nutritional intake.
- Monitor electrolytes.
- Assess skin integrity (rashes, open areas, bruising).
- Assess pain status.
- Monitor vital signs (especially temperature).
- Assess lung sounds/respiratory status (diminished lung sounds).
- Assess neurological status (confusion, dementia, visual changes).

Ⓝ *NCLEX® Connection: Physiological Adaptation, Alterations in Body Systems*

UNIT 13 — NURSING CARE OF CLIENTS WHO HAVE IMMUNE SYSTEM AND CONNECTIVE TISSUE DISORDERS
SECTION: CONNECTIVE TISSUE DISORDERS

CHAPTER 87 *Lupus Erythematosus, Gout, and Fibromyalgia*

Lupus erythematosus (lupus) is an autoimmune disorder in which an atypical immune response results in chronic inflammation and destruction of healthy tissue. Other autoimmune disorders include rheumatoid arthritis, vasculitis, multiple sclerosis, scleroderma (including Raynaud's phenomenon), and psoriasis.

In autoimmune disorders, small antigens can bond with healthy tissue. The body then produces antibodies that attack the healthy tissue. This can be triggered by toxins, medications, bacteria, and viruses. Control of manifestations and a decrease in the number and frequency of exacerbations is the goal of treatment, because there is no cure for autoimmune disorders.

Gout, also known as gouty arthritis, is a systemic disorder caused by hyperuricemia (increase in serum uric acid). Urate levels can be affected by medications, diet, and overproduction in the body. This can cause uric crystal deposits to form in the joints, and a gout attack can occur.

Fibromyalgia is a chronic pain syndrome that involves stiffness, sleep disturbance, generalized muscle weakness and chronic fatigue. It is estimated that 25% to 65% of people who have fibromyalgia have another form of a rheumatologic disorder, such as RA or SLE.

Occurrence of autoimmune disorders increases with age. ⓖ

Lupus erythematosus

- Lupus varies in severity and progression. It is generally characterized by periods of exacerbations (flares) and remissions.
- Lupus is classified as discoid or systemic. A temporary form of lupus can be medication-induced.
  - **Discoid lupus erythematosus (DLE)** only affects the skin.
  - **Systemic lupus erythematosus (SLE)** affects the connective tissues of multiple organ systems and can lead to major organ failure.
  - **Medication-induced lupus erythematosus** can be caused by medications (procainamide, hydralazine, isoniazid). Findings resolve when the medication is discontinued.
- Lupus can be difficult to diagnose because of the vague nature of early manifestations.

ASSESSMENT

RISK FACTORS

- Women between the ages of 20 and 40
- African American, Asian, or Native American descent
- The incidence of lupus declines in women following menopause but remains steady in men.
- Diagnosis of lupus can be delayed in older adult clients because many of the manifestations mimic other disorders or can be associated with reports common to the normal aging process. ⓖ
  - Joint pain and swelling can significantly limit ADLs in older adult clients who have comorbidities.
  - Older adult clients are at an increased risk for fractures if corticosteroid therapy is used.

EXPECTED FINDINGS

- Fatigue/malaise
- Alopecia
- Blurred vision
- Pleuritic pain
- Anorexia/weight loss
- Depression
- Joint pain, swelling, tenderness

PHYSICAL ASSESSMENT FINDINGS Qᴱᴮᴾ

- Fever (also a major indication of exacerbation)
- Anemia
- Lymphadenopathy
- Pericarditis (presence of a cardiac friction rub or pleural friction rub)
- Raynaud's phenomenon (arteriolar vasospasm in response to cold/stress)
- Findings consistent with organ involvement (kidney, heart, lungs, and vasculature)
- Erythematous "butterfly" rash over the nose and cheeks (raised, dry, and scaly)
- Alopecia

LABORATORY TESTS

Skin biopsy: Used to diagnose DLE by confirming the presence of lupus cells and cellular inflammation.

Immunologic tests: Used to diagnose SLE
- Antinuclear antibodies (ANAs): antibodies produced against one's own DNA; positive titers in 95% of clients who have lupus
  - SLE prep
  - dsDNA (very specific for SLE; assists with differentiation between SLE and medication-induced lupus)
  - ssDNA
  - Anti-DNP
  - SS-A
- Serum complement (C3, C4): decreased
  - The complement system is made of proteins (there are nine major complement proteins). These proteins work with the immune system and play a role in the development of inflammation. C3 and C4 are diagnostic for SLE because they decrease due to depletion secondary to an exaggerated inflammatory response.
- Erythrocyte sedimentation rate (ESR): elevated due to systemic inflammation

BUN and serum creatinine: Increased (with kidney involvement)

Urinalysis: Positive for protein and RBCs (kidney involvement)

CBC: Pancytopenia

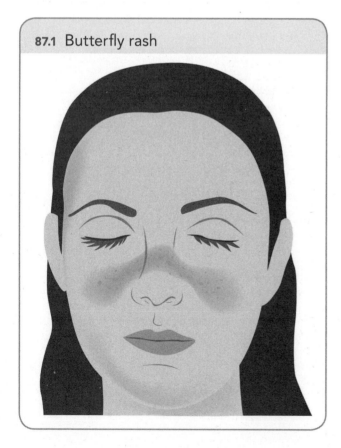

87.1 Butterfly rash

PATIENT-CENTERED CARE

NURSING CARE

- Assess/monitor the following.
  - Pain, mobility, and fatigue
  - Vital signs (especially blood pressure)
  - Systemic manifestations
    - Hypertension and edema (renal compromise)
    - Urine output (renal compromise)
    - Diminished breath sounds (pleural effusion)
    - Tachycardia and sharp inspiratory chest pain (pericarditis)
    - Rubor, pallor, and cyanosis of hands/feet (vasculitis/vasospasm, Raynaud's phenomenon)
    - Arthralgias, myalgias, and polyarthritis (joint and connective tissue involvement)
    - Changes in mental status that indicate neurologic involvement (psychoses, paresis, seizures)
    - BUN, serum creatinine, and urinary output for renal involvement
    - Nutritional status
- Provide small, frequent meals if anorexia is a concern. Offer between-meal supplements. Ⓠ EBP
- Encourage the client to limit salt intake for fluid retention secondary to steroid therapy.
- Provide emotional support to the client and family.

MEDICATIONS

NSAIDs

Used to reduce inflammation and arthritic pain.

NURSING CONSIDERATIONS
- NSAIDs are contraindicated for clients who have impaired kidney function.
- Monitor for NSAID-induced hepatitis.

Corticosteroids

Prednisone used for immunosuppression and to reduce inflammation.

NURSING CONSIDERATIONS: Monitor for fluid retention, hypertension, and impaired kidney function.

CLIENT EDUCATION: Do not stop taking steroids abruptly. Gradually taper the dosage as prescribed.

Immunosuppressant agents

Methotrexate and azathioprine used to suppress the immune response. Ⓠ PCC

NURSING CONSIDERATIONS: Monitor for toxic effects (bone marrow suppression, increased liver enzymes).

Antimalarial

Hydroxychloroquine used for suppression of synovitis, fever, and fatigue.

NURSING CONSIDERATIONS: Encourage frequent eye examinations.

INTERPROFESSIONAL CARE

- Physical and occupational therapy services can be used for strengthening exercises and adaptive devices as needed.
- Refer clients to support groups as appropriate.

CLIENT EDUCATION

- Avoid UV and prolonged sun exposure. Use sunscreen when outside and exposed to sunlight.
- Use mild protein shampoo and avoid harsh hair treatments.
- Use steroid creams for skin rash.
- Report peripheral and periorbital edema promptly.
- Report evidence of infection related to immunosuppression.
- Avoid crowds and individuals who are sick, because illness can precipitate an exacerbation.
- Educate client of childbearing age regarding risks of pregnancy with lupus and treatment medications. Qs

COMPLICATIONS

Lupus nephritis

Clients whose SLE cannot be managed with immunosuppressants and corticosteroids can experience chronic kidney disease resulting in the possible need for a kidney transplant. Lupus nephritis is the leading cause of death related to SLE.

NURSING ACTIONS: Monitor for periorbital and lower extremity swelling and hypertension. Monitor renal status (creatinine, BUN).

CLIENT EDUCATION
- Teach the client the importance of taking immunosuppressants and corticosteroids as prescribed.
- Teach the client the importance of avoiding stress and illness.

Pericarditis and myocarditis

Inflammation of the heart, its vessels, and the surrounding sac can occur secondary to SLE.

NURSING ACTIONS: Monitor for chest pain, fatigue, arrhythmias, and fever.

CLIENT EDUCATION
- Instruct the client to report chest pain.
- Remind the client to take immunosuppressants and corticosteroids as prescribed.
- Teach the client to avoid stress and illness.
- Tell the client to report chest pain to the provider.

Gout

Gout or gouty arthritis is the most common inflammatory arthritis. Gout is a systemic disease caused by a disruption in purine metabolism in which uric acid crystals are deposited in joints and body tissues. Gout is classified as either primary or secondary.

Primary gout

- Most common.
- Uric acid production is greater than excretion of it by the kidneys.
- Can have genetic component.
- Middle- and older-adult males (peak onset between ages 40 and 50), as well as postmenopausal women are commonly affected.

Secondary gout

- Caused by another disease or condition (chronic kidney failure, excessive diuretic use) that causes excessive uric acid in the blood.
- Treatment is based on treating the underlying condition.
- Can affect people of any age.

ASSESSMENT

RISK FACTORS

- Obesity
- Cardiovascular disease
- Trauma
- Alcohol ingestion
- Starvation dieting
- Diuretic use
- Some chemotherapy agents
- Chronic kidney failure

EXPECTED FINDINGS

- Severe joint pain, especially in the metatarsophalangeal joint of the great toe
- Redness, swelling, and warmth of affected joint

PHYSICAL ASSESSMENT FINDINGS
- Painful, swollen joint that is very painful if touched or moved
- Appearance of tophi (chronic gout)

LABORATORY TESTS

Erythrocyte sedimentation rate (ESR): Elevated

Serum uric acid: Repeated measurements obtained due to effect of dietary intake on results. Consistent elevation above 6.5 mg/dL is associated with gout.

Urinary uric acid: Elevated

Blood urea nitrogen (BUN), serum creatinine: Elevated

PATIENT-CENTERED CARE

NURSING CARE

Assess/monitor the following.
- Pain
- Redness/swelling of affected joint
- Serum uric acid levels

MEDICATIONS

Acute gout

Antigout agent
- Colchicine (PO or parenteral) is used to decrease pain and inflammation.
- NURSING CONSIDERATIONS: Use cautiously in clients who have impaired kidney function.

NSAIDs
- Indomethacin or ibuprofen is used to decrease pain and inflammation.
- NURSING CONSIDERATIONS: Contraindicated for clients who have impaired kidney function.
- CLIENT EDUCATION: Do not take on an empty stomach.

Corticosteroids
- Prednisone used to treat inflammation.
- NURSING CONSIDERATIONS: Monitor for fluid retention, hypertension, and impaired kidney dysfunction.
- CLIENT EDUCATION: Do not stop taking the medication abruptly. Gradually taper dosage as prescribed.

Chronic gout

Xanthine oxidase inhibitor
- Allopurinol is used as a maintenance medication to promote uric acid excretion and decrease its production.
- NURSING CONSIDERATIONS: Increase fluid intake.
- CLIENT EDUCATION: Take after meals and with a full glass of water.

Uricosuric
- Probenecid is used as a maintenance medication to promote uric acid excretion.
- NURSING CONSIDERATIONS: Monitor uric acid levels.
- CLIENT EDUCATION: Do not use aspirin because it will decrease the effectiveness of the medication.

CLIENT EDUCATION

- Remind the client to stay on a low-purine diet, which includes no organ meats or shellfish. Q EBP
- Teach the client to limit alcohol intake.
- Tell the client to avoid starvation diets, aspirin, and diuretics.
- Teach the client to limit physical or emotional stress.
- Remind the client to increase fluid intake.
- Encourage medication adherence.

Fibromyalgia

- Fibromyalgia, also known as fibromyalgia syndrome, is a chronic pain syndrome which manifests as pain, stiffness, and tenderness at certain "trigger points" in the body.
- The pain is typically described as a burning a gnawing pain that can be elicited by palpating "trigger points".
- The client can also experience chronic fatigue, sleep disturbances, and functional impairment.
- Pain and tenderness vary depending on stress, activity, and weather conditions.

ASSESSMENT

RISK FACTORS

- Females between ages of 30 and 50
- History of rheumatologic conditions, chronic fatigue syndrome, or Lyme disease
- Deep sleep deprivation

EXPECTED FINDINGS

- Mild to severe fatigue
- Sleep disturbances
- Numbness/tingling of extremities
- Sensitivity to noxious smells, loud noises, and bright lights
- Headaches
- Jaw pain
- Depression
- Concentration and memory difficulties
- GI manifestations: abdominal pain, heartburn, constipation, diarrhea
- Genitourinary manifestations: frequency, urgency, dysuria, pelvic pain
- Visual changes

PATIENT-CENTERED CARE

NURSING CARE

- Assess/monitor pain, mobility, and fatigue.
- Provide emotional support to the client and family

MEDICATIONS

Serotonin-norepinephrine reuptake inhibitors (SNRIs) and anticonvulsants

Pregabalin (anticonvulsant) and duloxetine (SNRI) are used to increase the release of serotonin and norepinephrine, resulting in decreased nerve pain.

NURSING CONSIDERATIONS: Can cause drowsiness/sleepiness.

NURSING CONSIDERATIONS: Remind the client not to drink alcohol while on this medication.

NSAIDs

Used to decrease pain and inflammation

NURSING CONSIDERATIONS: Contraindicated for clients who have impaired kidney function.

CLIENT EDUCATION: Do not take on an empty stomach.

Tricyclic antidepressants

Amitriptyline, nortriptyline, and trazodone are used to help induce sleep and decrease pain.

NURSING CONSIDERATIONS: Amitriptyline and nortriptyline can cause confusion and orthostatic hypotension in older adult clients. Trazodone is often the medication of choice for the older adult clients due to decreased adverse effects. Ⓒ

INTERPROFESSIONAL CARE

- Physical therapy can be helpful to decrease pain.
- Refer the client to national foundations and local support groups.
- Complementary and alternative therapies can be helpful (acupuncture, stress management).

CLIENT EDUCATION

- Teach the client to limit intake of caffeine, alcohol, and other substances that interfere with sleep.
- Teach the client to develop a routine for sleep.

Application Exercises

1. A nurse is reviewing the plan of care for a client who has systemic lupus erythematosus (SLE). The client reports fatigue, joint tenderness, swelling, and difficulty urinating. Which of the following laboratory findings should the nurse anticipate? (Select all that apply.)
   - A. Positive ANA titer
   - B. Increased hemoglobin
   - C. 2+ urine protein
   - D. Increased serum C3 and C4
   - E. Elevated BUN

2. A nurse is teaching a client who has SLE about self-care. Which of the following statements by the client indicates an understanding of the teaching?
   - A. "I should limit my time to 10 minutes in the tanning bed."
   - B. "I will apply powder to any skin rash."
   - C. "I should use a mild hair shampoo."
   - D. "I will inspect my skin once a month for rashes."

3. A nurse is discussing gout with a client who is concerned about developing the disorder. Which of the following findings should the nurse identify as risk factors for this disease? (Select all that apply.)
   - A. Diuretic use
   - B. Obesity
   - C. Deep sleep deprivation
   - D. Depression
   - E. Cardiovascular disease

4. A nurse is assessing a client who has a new diagnosis of SLE. Which of the following findings should the nurse expect?
   - A. Weight gain
   - B. Petechiae on thighs
   - C. Systolic murmur
   - D. Alopecia

5. A nurse is caring for a client who has SLE and is experiencing an episode of Raynaud's phenomenon. Which of the following findings should the nurse anticipate?
   - A. Swelling of joints of the fingers
   - B. Pallor of toes with cold exposure
   - C. Feet that become reddened with ambulation
   - D. Client report of intense feeling of heat in the fingers

Application Exercises Key

1. A. **CORRECT:** A positive antinuclear antibody (ANA) titer is an expected finding in a client who has SLE. The ANA test identifies the presence of antibodies produced against the client's own DNA.

   B. Pancytopenia, rather than an elevated hemoglobin, is an expected finding in a client who has SLE.

   C. **CORRECT:** Increased urine protein is an expected finding due to kidney injury as a result of SLE.

   D. The client who has SLE is expected to have a decreased level of serum C3 and C4.

   E. **CORRECT:** Elevated BUN is an expected finding due to kidney injury in a client who has SLE.

   Ⓝ *NCLEX® Connection: Reduction of Risk Potential, Laboratory Values*

2. A. A client who has SLE should avoid the use of tanning beds, as well as prolonged sun exposure.

   B. A client who has SLE should apply steroid-based creams to skin rashes, not a powder.

   C. **CORRECT:** A client who has SLE should use a mild hair shampoo that does not irritate the scalp.

   D. A client who has SLE should inspect her skin daily for any open areas or rashes.

   Ⓝ *NCLEX® Connection: Physiological Adaptation, Illness Management*

3. A. **CORRECT:** The use of diuretics is a risk factor for gout.

   B. **CORRECT:** Obesity is a risk factor for gout.

   C. Deep sleep deprivation is a manifestation of fibromyalgia and is not a risk factor for gout.

   D. Depression is a manifestation of SLE and is not a risk factor for gout.

   E. **CORRECT:** Cardiovascular disease is a risk factor for gout.

   Ⓝ *NCLEX® Connection: Physiological Adaptation, Pathophysiology*

4. A. Weight loss, rather than weight gain, is an expected finding in a client who has a new diagnosis of SLE.

   B. A butterfly rash on the face is a finding in a client who has lupus.

   C. A cardiac friction rub is an expected finding of SLE.

   D. **CORRECT:** Alopecia (hair loss) is an expected finding in a client who has SLE.

   Ⓝ *NCLEX® Connection: Physiological Adaptation, Pathophysiology*

5. A. Swelling, pain, and joint tenderness are findings in a client who has SLE and is not specific to an episode of Raynaud's phenomenon.

   B. **CORRECT:** Pallor of the extremities occurs in Raynaud's phenomenon in a client who has SLE and has been exposed to cold or stress.

   C. The extremities becoming red, white, and blue when exposed to cold or stress is characteristic of an episode of Raynaud's phenomenon in a client who has SLE.

   D. A client report of intense pain in the hands and feet is characteristic of an episode of Raynaud's phenomenon in a client who has SLE.

   Ⓝ *NCLEX® Connection: Physiological Adaptation, Pathophysiology*

PRACTICE Active Learning Scenario

A nurse is teaching a client who has a new diagnosis of fibromyalgia. What should the nurse include in the teaching? Use the ATI Active Learning Template: System Disorder to complete this item.

ALTERATION IN HEALTH (DIAGNOSIS)

RISK FACTORS: Describe two.

EXPECTED FINDINGS: Include three findings.

MEDICATIONS: Identify two types of medications used to treat fibromyalgia along with their purpose and specific nursing considerations.

PRACTICE Answer

Using the ATI Active Learning Template: System Disorder

ALTERATION IN HEALTH (DIAGNOSIS)

- Fibromyalgia, also known as fibromyalgia syndrome, is a chronic pain syndrome which manifests as pain, stiffness, and tenderness at certain "trigger points" in the body.
- The pain is typically described as a burning or gnawing pain that can be elicited by palpating "trigger points".
- The client can also experience chronic fatigue, sleep disturbances, and functional impairment.
- Pain and tenderness vary depending on stress, activity, and weather conditions.

RISK FACTORS

- Females between ages of 30 and 50
- History of rheumatologic conditions, chronic fatigue syndrome, or Lyme disease
- Deep sleep deprivation

EXPECTED FINDINGS

- Mild to severe fatigue
- Sleep disturbances
- Numbness/tingling of extremities
- Sensitivity to noxious smells, loud noises, and bright lights
- Headaches
- Jaw pain
- Depression
- Concentration and memory difficulties
- GI manifestations: abdominal pain, heartburn, constipation, diarrhea
- Genitourinary manifestations: frequency, urgency, dysuria, pelvic pain
- Visual changes

MEDICATIONS

Serotonin-norepinephrine reuptake inhibitors (SNRIs) and anticonvulsants
- Pregabalin (anticonvulsant) and duloxetine (SNRI) are used to increase the release of serotonin and norepinephrine, resulting in decreased nerve pain.
- Nursing Considerations: Can cause drowsiness/sleepiness.
- Client Education: Remind the client not to drink alcohol while on this medication.

NSAIDs
- Used to decrease pain and inflammation.
- Nursing Considerations: Contraindicated for clients who have impaired kidney function.
- Client Education: Do not take on an empty stomach.

Tricyclic antidepressants
- Amitriptyline, nortriptyline, and trazodone are used to help induce sleep and decrease pain.
- Nursing Considerations: Amitriptyline and nortriptyline can cause confusion and orthostatic hypotension in older adult clients. Trazodone is often the medication of choice for the older adult client due to decreased adverse effects.

Ⓝ *NCLEX® Connection: Physiological Adaptation, Illness Management*

UNIT 13   NURSING CARE OF CLIENTS WHO HAVE IMMUNE SYSTEM AND CONNECTIVE TISSUE DISORDERS
SECTION: CONNECTIVE TISSUE DISORDERS

CHAPTER 88   *Rheumatoid Arthritis*

Rheumatoid arthritis (RA) is a chronic, progressive inflammatory disease that can affect tissues and organs but principally attacks the joints, producing an inflammatory synovitis. It involves joints bilaterally and symmetrically, and typically affects several joints at one time. RA typically affects upper joints first.

RA is an autoimmune disease that is precipitated by WBCs attacking synovial tissue. The WBCs cause the synovial tissue to become inflamed and thickened. The inflammation can extend to the cartilage, bone, tendons, and ligaments that surround the joint. Joint deformity and bone erosion can result from these changes, decreasing the joint's range of motion and function.

RA is also a systemic disease that can affect any connective tissue in the body. Common structures affected are the blood vessels, pleura surrounding the lungs, and pericardium. Iritis and scleritis can also develop in the eyes.

The natural course of the disease is one of exacerbations and remissions.

88.1 Rheumatoid arthritis changes

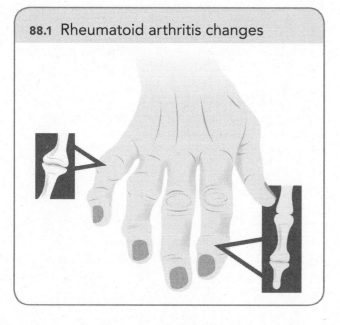

HEALTH PROMOTION AND DISEASE PREVENTION

- Use adaptive devices that prevent development of deformity of inflamed joints during ADLs.
- Continue using affected joints and ambulating to maintain function and range of motion.

ASSESSMENT

RISK FACTORS

- Female gender (3:1 compared to male clients)
- Age 20 to 50 years
- Genetic predisposition
- Epstein-Barr virus
- Stress
- Environmental factors
- Older age
  - Early signs of RA (fatigue, joint discomfort) are vague and can be attributed to other disorders in older adult clients. Ⓒ
  - Joint pain and dysfunction can have a greater effect on older adult clients than on younger adult clients due to the presence of other chronic conditions.
  - Older adult clients can be less able to overcome and/or cope with joint pain/deformity.

EXPECTED FINDINGS

Findings depend on the area affected by the disease process.
- Pain at rest and with movement
- Morning stiffness
- Pleuritic pain (pain upon inspiration)
- Xerostomia (dry mouth)
- Anorexia/weight loss
- Fatigue
- Paresthesias
- Recent illness/stressor
- Joint pain
- Lack of function
- Joint swelling and deformity
  - Joint deformities are late signs of RA.
  - Joint swelling, warmth, and erythema are common.
  - Finger, hands, wrists, knees, and foot joints are generally affected.
  - Finger joints affected are the proximal interphalangeal and metacarpophalangeal joints.
  - Joints can become deformed merely by completing ADLs.
  - Ulnar deviation, swan neck, and boutonnière deformities are common in the fingers.
- Subcutaneous nodules
- Fever (generally low-grade)
- Muscle weakness/atrophy
- Reddened sclera and/or abnormal shape of pupils
- Lymph node enlargement

LABORATORY TESTS

Anti-CCP antibodies

This test detects antibodies to cyclic citrullinated peptide (anti-CCP). The result is positive in most people who have rheumatoid arthritis, even years before symptoms develop. The test is more sensitive for RA than rheumatoid factor (RF) antibodies.

Rheumatoid factor antibody

Diagnostic level for rheumatoid arthritis is 1:40 to 1:60 (expected reference range 1:20 or less).
- High titers correlate with severe disease.
- Other autoimmune diseases also can increase RF antibody.

Erythrocyte sedimentation rate (ESR)

Elevated ESR is associated with the inflammation or infection in the body.
- 20 to 40 mm/hr is mild inflammation.
- 40 to 70 mm/hr is moderate inflammation.
- 70 to 150 mm/hr is severe inflammation.
- Other autoimmune diseases also can increase ESR antibody.

C-reactive protein: Positive

- This test may be done in place of ESR.
- This test is useful for diagnosing disease or monitoring disease activity, and for monitoring the response to anti-inflammatory therapy.

Antinuclear antibody (ANA) titer

Antibody produced against one's own DNA
- A positive ANA titer is associated with RA. (It is normally negative at 1:20 dilution.)
- Other autoimmune diseases also can increase ANA.

Elevated WBCs

- WBC count can be elevated during an exacerbation secondary to the inflammatory response.
- Decreased RBCs due to anemia.

DIAGNOSTIC PROCEDURES

Arthrocentesis

- Arthrocentesis is synovial fluid aspiration by needle.
- With RA, increased WBCs and RF are present in fluid.

NURSING ACTIONS: Monitor for bleeding or a synovial fluid leak from the needle biopsy site.

CLIENT EDUCATION: Take acetaminophen for pain.

X-ray

X-rays are used to determine the degree of joint destruction and monitor its progression. They can provide adequate visualization and reveal bony erosions and narrowed joint spaces. This negates the need for more expensive radiologic tests, such a CT scan or magnetic resonance imaging (MRI).

NURSING ACTIONS: Assist the client into position.

CLIENT EDUCATION: Instruct the client about the need to minimize movement during the procedure.

PATIENT-CENTERED CARE

NURSING CARE

- Apply heat or cold to the affected areas as indicated based on client response.
  - Morning stiffness (hot shower)
  - Pain in hands/fingers (heated paraffin)
  - Edema (cold therapy)
- Assist with and encourage physical activity to maintain joint mobility (within the capabilities of the client).
- Monitor for indications of fatigue.
- Teach the client measures to do the following.
  - Maximize functional activity.
  - Minimize pain.
  - Monitor skin closely.
  - Conserve energy (space out activities, take rest periods, ask for additional assistance when needed).
  - Promote coping strategies.
  - Encourage routine health screenings.
- Provide a safe environment. Qs
  - Provide referrals for physical therapy and occupational therapy.
  - Provide information for support organizations.
  - Facilitate the use of assistive devices.
  - Remove unnecessary equipment and supplies.
- Use progressive muscle relaxation.
- Administer medications and proper positioning as prescribed.
- Monitor for medication effectiveness (reduced pain, increased mobility).
- Teach the client regarding signs/symptoms that need to be reported immediately (fever, infection, pain upon inspiration, pain in the substernal area of the chest).

Nutritional teaching

- Encourage foods high in vitamins, protein, and iron.
- Eat small, frequent meals.

MEDICATIONS

NSAIDs

- Treatment begins with NSAIDs.
- NSAIDs provide analgesic, antipyretic, and anti-inflammatory effects.
- NSAIDs can cause considerable gastrointestinal (GI) distress.

NURSING CONSIDERATIONS

- Request a concurrent prescription for a GI-acid lowering agent (histamine$_2$-receptor antagonist, proton pump inhibitor) if GI distress is reported.
- Monitor for fluid retention, hypertension, and renal dysfunction.

CLIENT EDUCATION

- Instruct the client to take the medication with food or with a full glass of water or milk. If taking routinely, an H$_2$-receptor antagonist can also be prescribed.
- Instruct the client to observe for GI bleeding (coffee-ground emesis; dark, tarry stools).
- Instruct the client to avoid alcohol, which can increase the risk of GI complications.

COX-2 enzyme blockers

Cause less GI distress but carry a risk of cardiac disease.

Corticosteroids

Corticosteroids (prednisone) are strong anti-inflammatory medications that can be given for acute exacerbations or advanced forms of the disease.

They are not given for long-term therapy due to significant adverse effects (osteoporosis, hyperglycemia, immunosuppression, cataracts).

NURSING CONSIDERATIONS

- Observe for Cushingoid changes.
- Monitor weight and blood pressure.

CLIENT EDUCATION

- Instruct the client to observe for changes in vision, blood glucose, and impaired healing.
- Instruct the client to avoid crowds.
- Instruct the client to follow the prescription, such as alternate-day dosing, tapering, and discontinuing medication.

Disease modifying anti-rheumatic drugs (DMARDs)

DMARDs work in a variety of ways to slow the progression of RA and suppress the immune system's reaction to RA that causes pain and inflammation. Relief of symptoms might not occur for several weeks.

- **Antimalarial agent:** Hydroxychloroquine
- **Antibiotic:** Minocycline
- **Sulfonamide:** Sulfasalazine
- **Biologic response modifiers:** Etanercept, infliximab, adalimumab, and chelator penicillamine
- **Cytotoxic medications:** Methotrexate, leflunomide, cyclophosphamide, and azathioprine can cause severe adverse effects.

THERAPEUTIC PROCEDURES

Plasmapheresis

- Removes circulating antibodies from plasma, decreasing attacks on the client's tissues
- May be done for a severe, life-threatening exacerbation

Total joint arthroplasty

Surgical repair and replacement of a joint may be done for a severely deformed joint that has not responded to medication therapy.

INTERPROFESSIONAL CARE

- Refer the client to support groups as appropriate.
- Refer the client to occupational therapy for adaptive devices that can facilitate carrying out ADLs and prevent deformities.
- A home health aide can be necessary for assistance with ADLs.

COMPLICATIONS

Sjögren's syndrome

- Triad of symptoms: dry eyes, mouth, and vagina
- Caused by obstruction of secretory ducts and glands

NURSING ACTIONS

- Provide eye drops and artificial saliva, and recommend vaginal lubricants as needed.
- Provide fluids with meals.

Secondary osteoporosis

Immobilization caused by arthritis can contribute to the development of osteoporosis.

NURSING ACTIONS: Encourage weight-bearing exercises as tolerated.

Vasculitis (organ ischemia)

Inflammation of arteries can disrupt blood flow, causing ischemia. Smaller arteries in the skin, eyes, and brain are most commonly affected in RA.

NURSING ACTIONS: Monitor for skin lesions, decrease in vision, and symptoms of cognitive dysfunction.

PRACTICE Active Learning Scenario

A nurse is providing information about the adverse effects of prednisone to a client who has rheumatoid arthritis. Use the ATI Active Learning Template: Medication and the ATI Pharmacology Review Module to complete this item.

COMPLICATIONS: Identify three adverse effects of this medication, as well as related client education.

Application Exercises

1. A nurse working in an outpatient clinic is assessing a client who has rheumatoid arthritis (RA). The client reports increased joint tenderness and swelling. Which of the following findings should the nurse expect? (Select all that apply.)

   A. Recent influenza
   B. Decreased range of motion
   C. Hypersalivation
   D. Increased blood pressure
   E. Pain at rest

2. A nurse is teaching a client who has a new diagnosis of rheumatoid arthritis. Which of the following statements should the nurse include in the teaching?

   A. "You can experience morning stiffness when you get out bed."
   B. "You can experience abdominal pain."
   C. "You can experience weight gain."
   D. "You can experience low blood sugar."

3. A nurse is caring for a client who has rheumatoid arthritis. Which of the following laboratory tests are used to diagnose this disease? (Select all that apply.)

   A. Urinalysis
   B. Erythrocyte sedimentation rate (ESR)
   C. BUN
   D. Antinuclear antibody (ANA) titer
   E. WBC count

Application Exercises Key

1. A. **CORRECT:** Exacerbating factors, such as a recent illness like influenza, are indicative in clients who have RA.
   B. **CORRECT:** A decrease in range of motion is indicative in clients who have RA.
   C. Clients who have RA can experience xerostomia, not hypersalivation.
   D. Increased blood pressure is not indicative of RA.
   E. **CORRECT:** Pain at rest is indicative of RA.

   Ⓝ NCLEX® Connection: Physiological Adaptation, Pathophysiology

2. A. **CORRECT:** The nurse should include in the teaching that the client who has RA can experience stiffness in her joints upon rising.
   B. The client who has RA can experience pleuritic pain upon inspiration, not abdominal pain.
   C. The client who has RA can experience weight loss, not weight gain.
   D. The client who has RA does not experience a low blood sugar.

   Ⓝ NCLEX® Connection: Physiological Adaptation, Illness Management

3. A. A urinalysis is not a laboratory test used to diagnose RA. This test can used for detecting kidney failure.
   B. **CORRECT:** ESR is a laboratory test used to diagnose RA. This laboratory test will show an elevated result in clients who have RA.
   C. A BUN is not a laboratory test used to diagnose RA. This test can be used for detecting kidney failure.
   D. **CORRECT:** ANA titer is a laboratory test used to diagnose RA. This laboratory test will show a positive result in clients who have RA.
   E. **CORRECT:** WBC count is a laboratory test used to diagnose RA. This laboratory test will show a decreased result in clients who have RA.

   Ⓝ NCLEX® Connection: Reduction of Risk Potential, Diagnostic Tests

PRACTICE Answer

Using the ATI Active Learning Template: Medication

COMPLICATIONS

- Risk of infection (fever and/or sore throat): Advise clients to notify the provider immediately if symptoms occur.
- Osteoporosis: Advise clients to take calcium supplements, vitamin D, and/or bisphosphonate.
- Fluid retention: Monitor for signs of fluid excess, such as crackles, weight gain, and edema.

- Adrenal suppression
  - Advise clients to observe for symptoms and to notify the provider if symptoms occur.
  - Administer fluids such as normal saline, salt, and hydrocortisone IV.
  - Advise clients not to discontinue the medication suddenly.

- GI discomfort
  - Advise clients to observe for symptoms and to notify the provider if symptoms occur.
  - H₂ antagonists can be used prophylactically.
  - Advise clients to report symptoms of GI bleeding (coffee-ground emesis; black, tarry stools).

- Hyperglycemia: Monitor blood glucose level. Clients who have diabetes mellitus can need to adjust hypoglycemic agent.
- Hypokalemia
  - Monitor serum potassium levels.
  - Advise clients to eat potassium-rich foods.
  - Administer potassium supplements.

Ⓝ NCLEX® Connection: Pharmacological and Parenteral Therapies, Medication Administration

CHAPTER 89

UNIT 13   NURSING CARE OF CLIENTS WHO HAVE IMMUNE
SYSTEM AND CONNECTIVE TISSUE DISORDERS
SECTION: CANCER-RELATED DISORDERS

CHAPTER 89 General Principles of Cancer

Cancer is a neoplastic disease process that involves abnormal cell growth and differentiation. Normal body cells grow, divide, and die in an orderly fashion. In cancer, dying cells grow and form new abnormal cells. The exact cause of cancer is unknown, but viruses, physical and chemical agents, hormones, genetics, and diet are thought to be factors that trigger abnormal cell growth.

Cancer cells can invade surrounding tissues and spread to other areas of the body through lymph and blood vessels (metastasis). No matter where cancer spreads, it always is named based on the origin in which it started. For example, colon cancer that spreads to the liver is called metastatic colon cancer. Metastasis is usually diagnosed when there is onset of new findings (bone pain indicative of bone metastasis; change in bowel or bladder tone indicative of nervous system involvement).

Screening and early diagnosis are the most important aspects of health education and care. The nurse should prevent, recognize, and treat complications associated with carcinoma.

Tumors are not cancer. A tumor is an abnormal collection of cells, but not all tumors are cancers. Non-cancerous tumors are benign. They do have the potential of growing large and pressing on healthy organs and tissues but they do not invade other tissues and they do not metastasize.

BODY TISSUES

Cancers can arise from almost any tissue in the body.
- Epithelial tissue: carcinomas
- Glandular organs: adenocarcinomas
- Mesenchymal tissue: sarcomas
- Blood-forming cells: leukemias
- Lymph tissue: lymphomas
- Plasma cells: myelomas

HEALTH PROMOTION AND DISEASE PREVENTION

- Consume a healthy diet (low-fat with increased consumption of fruits, vegetables, and lean protein).
- Limit intake of sugar and salt.
- Maintain a healthy body weight/body mass index.
- Avoid smoking, tobacco, and alcohol consumption.
- Avoid risky lifestyle choices (recreational drug use, needle sharing, unprotected sexual intercourse).
- Avoid exposure to environmental hazards (radiation, chemicals). Use personal protective equipment when available.
- Breastfeed infants exclusively for the first 6 months of life.
- Engage in physical activity or exercise routinely.
- Protect skin and eyes from UVA and UVB rays.
- Remove at-risk tissue such as moles to prevent conversion to skin cancer.
- Chemoprevention is the use of medications or other substances to disrupt cancer development.
  - Aspirin and celecoxib to reduce the risk of colon cancer
  - Vitamin D and tamoxifen to reduce the risk of breast cancer.
- Immunization to prevent human papilloma virus (HPV), which is associated with cervical cancer.

Screening prevention

Mammogram: Annually for women older than 40

Clinical breast exam: Annually for women older than 40 (every 3 years for women 20 to 39 years old)

Colonoscopy: At age 50 and then every 10 years

Fecal occult blood: Annually for adults of all ages

Digital rectal exam: For men older than 50 years

Screening for gene mutations: For clients who have a strong family history of breast or colon cancer

ASSESSMENT

RISK FACTORS

Age: Highest incidence of cancer occurs in older adults. ⓖ
- Older adult women most commonly develop colorectal, breast, lung, pancreatic, and ovarian cancers.
- Older adult men most commonly develop lung, colorectal, prostate, pancreatic, and gastric cancers.

Immune function: Cancer incidence increases among clients who are immunosuppressed.

Chronic irritation and tissue trauma: Incidence of skin cancer is higher in people who have burn scars or other types of severe skin injury.

Race
- Caucasian women older than 40 are more likely to develop breast cancer than are African-American, American-Indian, and Hispanic women. However, the death rate for each of these groups is higher than for Caucasian women.
- Caucasian men are at an increased risk for testicular cancer, whereas African-American men are at an increased risk for prostate cancer.

Genetic predisposition

Exposure to chemicals, tobacco, and alcohol

Exposure to some viruses and bacteria
- Liver cancer can develop after many years of infection with hepatitis B or hepatitis C.
- Infection with human T-cell leukemia virus increases the risk of lymphoma and leukemia.
- Infection with Epstein-Barr virus has been linked to an increased risk of lymphoma.
- HPV infection is the main cause of cervical cancer.
- HIV increases the risk of lymphoma and Kaposi's sarcoma.
- *Helicobacter pylori* can increase the risk of stomach cancer and lymphoma of the stomach lining.

Diet: A diet high in fat, red meat, processed meat, preservatives, and additives, and low in fiber

Sun, ultraviolet light, or radiation exposure: Ionizing (radon, x-ray) and UV (sun, tanning beds)

Sexual lifestyles: Multiple sexual partners or STIs

Poverty, obesity, and chronic GERD

Chronic disease

Air pollution

EXPECTED FINDINGS

Staging of cancer

The tumor-node-metastasis (TNM) system is used to stage cancer.

TUMOR (T)
- **TX:** Unable to evaluate the primary tumor
- **T0:** No evidence of primary tumor
- **Tis:** Tumor in situ
- **T1, T2, T3, and T4:** Size and extent of tumor

NODE (N)
- **NX:** Unable to evaluate regional lymph nodes
- **N0:** No evidence of regional node involvement
- **N1, N2, and N3:** Number of nodes that are involved and/or extent of spread

METASTASIS (M)
- **MX:** Unable to evaluate distant metastasis
- **M0:** No evidence of distant metastasis
- **M1:** Presence of distant metastasis

Grading QEBP

Grading is needed because some cancer cells are more malignant than others. **Well-differentiated** means the cells look much like normal cells and tend to grow slowly. **Undifferentiated**, or poorly differentiated, means the cells do not look like normal cells and tend to grow quickly and spread.
- **GX:** Grade cannot be determined.
- **G1:** Tumor cells are well differentiated.
- **G2:** Tumor cells are moderately differentiated.
- **G3:** Tumor cells are poorly differentiated but the tissue of origin can be established.
- Tumor cells are poorly differentiated, and determination of the tissue of origin is difficult.

Prognosis

- Early diagnosis of cancer usually results in a better prognosis. Many cancers spread or metastasize before any manifestations are noted.
- Minority populations tend to have a worse prognosis for cancer related to several factors (low socioeconomic status, lack of access to health care, or reluctance to seek treatment).

COMPLICATIONS

Malnutrition

Clients who have cancer are at increased risk for weight loss and anorexia.
- The presence of carcinoma in the body increases the amount of energy required for metabolic function.
- Cancer can impair the body's ability to ingest, digest, and absorb nutrients.
- Adverse effects of cancer treatment can affect the desire for food or the ability to eat. Findings include nausea, vomiting, changes in taste, anorexia, pain, diarrhea, early satiety, dry mouth, thickened saliva, and irritation to the gastrointestinal tract.

NURSING CONSIDERATIONS
- Educate the client about managing the expected effects of treatment.
- Administer antiemetics and antacids as prescribed.
- Monitor relevant laboratory data (albumin, ferritin, and transferrin).
- Encourage frequent oral hygiene.
- Incorporate client preferences into meal planning when possible.
- Avoid early satiety by limiting liquids during meals.
- Teach the client to consume adequate protein, carbohydrates, and calories.
- Collaborate with dietary services. QTC

Constipation/gastric stasis/intestinal obstruction

NURSING CONSIDERATIONS

- Can be related to cancer or cancer treatment.
- Opioids can cause delayed emptying, slowed bowel motility.
- Administer stool softener or laxative as needed.
- Encourage fluids, fiber and activity as tolerated.

Paraneoplastic syndromes

- Paraneoplastic syndromes result when T cells in the body attack normal cells rather than cancerous ones. They result in changes in neurological function (movement, sensation, mental function).
- Management includes minimizing the immune system response by administration of steroids, immune factors, plasmapheresis, or irradiation.

NURSING CONSIDERATIONS

- Recognize manifestations of paraneoplastic syndrome.
- Administer medications as prescribed.
- Provide a safe environment until client returns to baseline mental status.
- Use aids for vision or hearing deficits, as indicated.

ONCOLOGIC EMERGENCIES

Syndrome of inappropriate antidiuretic hormone (SIADH)

SIADH occurs when excessive levels of antidiuretic hormones are produced. Because antidiuretic hormones help the kidneys and body to conserve the correct amount of water, SIADH causes the body to retain water. This results in a dilution of electrolytes (such as sodium) in the blood. It is most commonly associated with lung and brain cancers. Key findings include nausea and vomiting (early); lethargy, hostility, seizures, and coma.

NURSING CONSIDERATIONS

- Monitor for hyponatremia and low serum osmolality.
- Administer furosemide, 0.9% sodium chloride IV, and hypertonic sodium chloride solution as prescribed for severe hyponatremia.
- Monitor vital signs and serum sodium because furosemide promotes sodium excretion and hypertonic sodium chloride can cause fluid overload.

Hypercalcemia

A common complication of breast, lung, head, and neck cancers; leukemias and lymphomas; multiple myelomas; and bony metastases of any cancer

MANIFESTATIONS: Anorexia, nausea, vomiting, shortened QT interval, kidney stones, bone pain, and changes in mental status

NURSING CONSIDERATIONS: Administer 0.9% sodium chloride IV, furosemide, pamidronate, and phosphates as prescribed.

Superior vena cava syndrome

Results from obstruction (metastases from breast or lung cancers) of venous return and engorgement of the vessels from the head and upper body

MANIFESTATIONS: Periorbital and facial edema, erythema of the upper body, dyspnea, and epistaxis

NURSING CONSIDERATIONS

- Position the client in a high-Fowler's position initially to facilitate lung expansion.
- Use high-dose radiation therapy for emergency temporary relief.

Hematologic disorders

Hematologic problems can be caused by the cancer itself or chemotherapy.

Anemia: When cancer invades the bone marrow, it decreases the number of red blood cells, platelets (thrombocytopenia) and white blood cells (neutropenia).

Disseminated intravascular coagulation: Secondary to leukemia or adenocarcinomas

NURSING CONSIDERATIONS

- Observe for bleeding, and apply pressure as needed.
- Be prepared to administer blood clotting factors that have been lost through bleeding and can need to be replaced with plasma transfusions. Heparin also can be used to slow the cascade of events that makes the body overuse its blood clotting factors.

Application Exercises

1. A nurse is caring for a client who has lung cancer and is exhibiting manifestations of syndrome of inappropriate antidiuretic hormone (SIADH). Which of the following findings should the nurse report to the provider? (Select all that apply.)

   A. Behavioral changes

   B. Client report of headache

   C. Urine output 40 mL/hr

   D. Client report of nausea

   E. Increased urine specific gravity

2. A nurse is teaching a female adult client about screening prevention for cancer. Which of the following statements by the client indicates an understanding of the teaching?

   A. "I will need to have a mammogram every 2 years beginning at age 45."

   B. "I should have a colonoscopy every 15 years beginning at age 60."

   C. "I will need to have an annual breast examination every year after 40."

   D. "I should have a fecal occult test done every 3 years."

3. A nurse is planning care for a client who has malnutrition due to cancer. Which of the following interventions should the nurse include in the plan of care? (Select all that apply.)

   A. Advise the client to keep a food diary.

   B. Encourage the client to brush teeth before and after meals.

   C. Assess the laboratory report of ferritin.

   D. Eat nutrient-dense foods last at meal time.

   E. Encourage the client to limit drinking fluids during meals.

4. A nurse in is reviewing the health record of a client who had surgery to stage ovarian cancer. The nurse reviews the following diagnostic notation on the pathology report: T2-N3-MX. Which of the following findings should the nurse identify as a supporting diagnosis?

   A. The tumor is 4 cm in size involving the ovary and adjacent tissues.

   B. No lymph nodes contain cancer cells.

   C. The tumor is receptive to current medication therapy.

   D. The cancer has metastasized to other areas in the body.

PRACTICE Active Learning Scenario

A nurse is preparing an in-service about identifying risk factors for cancer to a group of adults at a community health fair. What information should the nurse include in the in-service? Use the ATI Active Learning Template: System Disorder to complete this item.

RISK FACTORS
- Identify two types of cancer with increased incidence in older adult women.
- Identify two types of cancer with increased incidence in older adult men.
- Identify one type of cancer with increased risk in Caucasian men.
- Identify one type of cancer with increased risk in Caucasian women.
- Describe three diet-related risk factors.
- Describe at least three lifestyle-related risk factors.

PATHOPHYSIOLOGY RELATED TO CLIENT PROBLEM: Describe at least three viruses/bacteria and the type of cancer they can cause.

Application Exercises Key

1. A. **CORRECT:** Behavioral changes indicate cerebral edema due to SIADH. This finding should be reported to the provider.

   B. **CORRECT:** A client report of headache indicates cerebral edema due to SIADH. This finding should be reported to the provider.

   C. Urine output of 40 mL/hr is a finding consistent with suspected SIADH and does not need to be reported to the provider.

   D. **CORRECT:** A client report of nausea can indicate cerebral edema due to SIADH and should be reported to the provider.

   E. An increased urine specific gravity is a finding consistent with SIADH and does not need to be reported to the provider.

   Ⓝ *NCLEX® Connection: Physiological Adaptation, Illness Management*

2. A. The client should begin annual mammograms beginning at age 40.

   B. The client should begin to have a colonoscopy at age 50 and then every 10 years thereafter.

   C. **CORRECT:** The nurse should instruct the client that after the age of 40, she should have annual clinic breast exams.

   D. The client should have a fecal occult test done every year.

   Ⓝ *NCLEX® Connection: Health Promotion and Maintenance, Health Promotion/Disease Prevention*

3. A. **CORRECT:** The use of a food diary assists in monitoring changes in eating habits that occur in malnutrition due to cancer.

   B. **CORRECT:** Oral hygiene before and after meals promotes increased salivation and improves taste perception.

   C. **CORRECT:** Ferritin is an indicator of the protein intake of a client who has malnutrition due to cancer.

   D. The nurse should instruct the client to eat nutrient-dense foods first to increase adequate nutritional intake to treat malnutrition.

   E. **CORRECT:** The nurse should encourage the client to limit drinking fluids with meals because fluids can cause early satiety and decrease adequate intake of food, causing malnutrition, when the client has cancer. Some fluids are needed to treat dry moutn and thickened saliva.

   Ⓝ *NCLEX® Connection: Basic Care and Comfort, Nutrition and Oral Hydration*

4. A. **CORRECT:** A T2 designation describes the size and extent of the ovarian tumor using the tumor-node-metastasis (TNM) staging system.

   B. A N3 designation indicates that three adjacent lymph nodes show evidence of spread of cancer using the TNM staging system.

   C. The TNM diagnostic notation of the staging system is not used to indicate the response of a tumor to a medication therapy regimen used for treatment.

   D. The MX designation indicates there is no evidence of distant metastasis to other areas of the body using the TNM staging system.

   Ⓝ *NCLEX® Connection: Physiological Adaptation, Pathophysiology*

PRACTICE Answer

Using the ATI Active Learning Template: System Disorder

RISK FACTORS
- Older adult women: Colorectal, breast, lung, pancreatic, and ovarian cancers
- Older adult men: Lung, colorectal, prostate, pancreatic and gastric cancers
- Caucasian men: Testicular cancer
- Caucasian women: Breast cancer

- Diet-related: Diet high in fat and red meat, low in fiber
- Lifestyle-related
  - Multiple sexual partners or STIs
  - Sun, ultraviolet light, and radiation exposure
  - Use of tobacco and alcohol

PATHOPHYSIOLOGY RELATED TO CLIENT PROBLEM
- Hepatitis B or C: Liver cancer
- Human T-cell leukemia virus: Lymphoma and leukemia
- Epstein-Barr virus: Lymphoma
- Human papilloma virus: Cervical cancer
- HIV: Lymphoma and Kaposi's sarcoma
- *Helicobacter pylori*: Stomach cancer and lymphoma of the stomach lining

Ⓝ *NCLEX® Connection: Health Promotion and Maintenance, Health Promotion/Disease Prevention*

CHAPTER 90

UNIT 12   NURSING CARE OF CLIENTS WHO HAVE IMMUNE
SYSTEM AND CONNECTIVE TISSUE DISORDERS
SECTION: CANCER-RELATED DISORDERS

CHAPTER 90 ## Cancer Screening and Diagnostic Procedures

Screening and diagnostic procedures provide objective and subjective client data. Screening and diagnosis for cancer can involve the use of hands-on assessment techniques, invasive procedures, radiography and imaging studies, and laboratory testing. The type and location of the suspected cancer dictate which methods are used. Identification of tumor cells is required for definitive diagnosis and the development of a targeted treatment plan.

INDICATIONS

CLIENT PRESENTATION

Cancer
- Altered body function (fatigue, weakness, anorexia)
- Change in body structure (weight loss, masses)
- Change in body symmetry or onset of recent findings (pain, nausea, vomiting)

Metastasis
- Secondary sites of discomfort
- Swelling and/or tenderness of lymph nodes or areas of the body
- Presence of masses
- Altered function of another body system
- Bone pain

CONSIDERATIONS

- Complete a health history and physical assessment including client report of findings and family history of cancer or genetic disorder.
- Provide privacy.
- Consider the client's cultural preference for examination (e.g., the health professional's gender). Qᴘᴄᴄ
- Inspect for changes in color, symmetry, movement, or body function.
- Auscultate for adventitious sounds that indicate altered body system function.
  - Heart, lung, and bowel sounds
  - Main arteries (carotid, femoral, renal, iliac)
  - Masses or areas of discomfort

- Palpate to detect masses or tissue abnormalities.
  - Use light, medium, and deep pressure as appropriate.
  - Some palpation assessments should be performed by the provider only (digital rectal exam for colorectal cancer).
- Percuss for changes in expected sound over organs.
  - Dullness in the lungs or bowel can indicate areas of consolidation or tumor.
  - Increased liver size (noted by measurement of borders [dullness]) can indicate inflammation or tumor.

CLIENT EDUCATION
- Explain all procedures prior to assessment.
- Report unexpected findings to the provider.
- Provide explanation when there is need for further testing or evaluation of unexpected findings.
- Instruct the client on self-examination practices to continue at home (breast or testicular self-examination).
  - Testicular cancer is rare and most common in men between the ages of 20 and 35 years of age.
  - With early detection, testicular cancer has a 95% cure rate.
  - Testicular self-examination is best performed during or after a bath or shower when the scrotum is relaxed.
  - Move the penis to the side, and examine one testicle at a time.
  - Hold the testicle between the thumb and fingers of both hands, and roll it gently between the fingers.
  - Look and feel for any hard lumps; smooth rounded bumps; or change in size, shape, or consistency of the testicle.
  - It is normal for one testicle to be larger or hang lower than the other.
  - Palpation of the epididymis can feel like a lump.
  - Noncancerous conditions, such as hydrocele or varicocele, cause testicular lumps or swelling.
- Instruct the client on seven warning signs (CAUTION) clients should watch for.
  - **C:** Change in bowel or bladder habits
  - **A:** A sore that doesn't heal
  - **U:** Unusual bleeding or discharge
  - **T:** Thickening or lump in the breast or elsewhere
  - **I:** Indigestion or difficulty swallowing
  - **O:** Obvious change in warts or moles
  - **N:** Nagging cough or hoarseness

BIOPSY

Provides definitive diagnosis indicating the site of origin (specific cell type) and cell characteristics (specific receptors on cell surface). Qᴇʙᴘ

Can be obtained during other procedures (endoscopy, laparoscopy, thoracotomy).

Shave biopsy (basal or squamous cell skin cancer): Sampling of outer skin layers (raised lesions) using a scalpel or razor blade.

Needle biopsy (fine or core): Aspiration of tumor close to the skin surface for fluid and tissue sampling. Bone marrow aspiration is a form of needle biopsy used to diagnose leukemia and lymphoma.

Incisional or excisional (open) biopsy: Cutting through skin to remove part (incisional) or all (excisional) of a tumor. Punch biopsy is a form of excisional biopsy used to diagnose skin cancer. A circular instrument punches a 2 to 6 mm sample of subcutaneous fat.

Sentinel lymph node biopsy: Removal of lymph node in proximity to the cancer. Dye is used to create a map of affected nodes.

- If lymph nodes are negative, the cancer has not likely spread.
- If lymph nodes are positive, surgical excision of remaining lymph nodes in the area is performed (lymph node dissection).

NURSING CONSIDERATIONS
- Obtain a signed informed consent form from the client.
- Assemble supplies and facilitate aseptic technique.
- Prevent bleeding. Withhold anticoagulants as prescribed. Monitor findings of coagulation studies.
- Monitor for bleeding (visible staining of dressing, hypotension, tachycardia).
- Provide a safe environment until effects of sedation are minimal. (Maintain bed rest. Withhold oral intake.)
- Ensure adequate oxygenation during the recovery period.
- Position the client in a recovery position appropriate to the procedure (lay on right side following liver biopsy).

LABORATORY TESTS

Performed to assess for possible cancer or effects on the body (electrolyte imbalance, altered function)

Liver function tests: Elevation can indicate primary liver cancer or metastasis of another cancer (colorectal cancer).

Tumor marker assays: Detect the presence of normal body proteins at higher than expected levels (carcinoembryonic antigen, prostate-specific antigen [PSA], alpha fetoprotein).
- Samples of urine, stool, tissue, blood, or other body fluids: are tested for an excess of specific proteins or DNA patterns.
- Used to detect cancer, measure the severity of cancer, or monitor for a positive response to the cancer treatment regimen (expected finding is a decrease in the tumor marker or return to expected reference range).

Other testing: Can be done in addition to biopsy to identify tumor cell type (sputum analysis, cytology of fluid sampling).

NURSING CONSIDERATIONS: Explain the purpose of testing, as appropriate.

CLIENT EDUCATION: Inform the client that laboratory testing can continue throughout treatment (to monitor progress) and following treatment (to screen for return of cancer).

GENETIC TESTS

To identify the presence of certain genes in a sample of blood or saliva
- Genetic overexpression or the existence of extra genes can increase the risk of cancer or cause rapid tumor growth.
- Genetic mutations can be inherited. Positive results indicate the client is at high risk for development of certain types of cancer (presence of BRCA1 and BRCA2 genes associated with breast cancer). Q EBP
- In most states, informed consent is required for genetic testing to protect the client from discrimination by providers or insurance company.

NURSING CONSIDERATIONS: Consult a genetic counselor to clarify misconceptions regarding positive results and cancer risk.

CLIENT EDUCATION: Assure the client that genetic information is protected.

IMAGING STUDIES

Common imaging techniques are used as secondary tools to assist in treatment of cancer. Imaging is completed around the time of diagnosis to measure the severity of cancer.

CT scan, MRI, PET scan, ultrasound, and x-ray

- Provide visualization of tumors and their borders.
- Detect metastasis to organs and other body structures.
- Monitor the client during remission.

Digital imaging: Usually more accurate than x-ray. Digital storage of images and results allows for information to be easily shared among members of the interprofessional treatment team. Q

X-rays: Provide visualization of body structures (chest x-ray, mammogram)
- Clients can be given dye (IV pyelogram) or contrast (barium enema) to enhance visualization.
- With angiography, the client is injected with dye and then x-rays are taken to map vascular structures, such as arterial, venous, or lymphatic mapping.
- NURSING CONSIDERATIONS
  - Obtain signed informed consent form.
  - Monitor for allergic reaction to contrast dye (dyspnea, tachycardia, restlessness).
  - Monitor incision or puncture site for infection or bleeding.
  - Instruct the client about wound care.

Computerized axial tomography (CT) scanning: Combines x-ray images taken from different angles and uses computer processing to create cross-sectional images. Can be performed with or without contrast. Contrast can be administered orally or intravenously.

MRI: Uses magnetic field and radio waves rather than radiation to generate pictures of tissue and organs. Contrast can be added to enhance the images. Clients who have any type of metal inside the body (clips, pacemaker, metal implants) should not have a MRI.

Ultrasound: High-energy sound waves bounce off internal tissues and organs to produce an echo pattern that can be seen as an ultrasound image. A biopsy can be performed during the ultrasound.

Nuclear imaging: Evaluates the function of organs and structures by detecting the presence of radiation in the body after the client is given a radioactive tracer (IV or oral). Used for detection and staging of cancer. Cancerous tissues can absorb more or less tracer than expected. These tissues are distinguishable by nuclear imaging.

Positron emission tomography (PET): Measures positrons released with tissue uptake of radioactive sugar (more rapid in cancer). Mammography (PEM) can be performed this way. CT can be used with PET scans.

Electrocardiogram, echocardiogram, or multigated acquisition scan: Used to evaluate heart function prior to cancer treatment or to identify damage following chemotherapy or radiation to the upper body.

Other types of imaging: Bone scan, gallium scan, and thyroid scan

NURSING CONSIDERATIONS: Prepare the client as indicated according to the type of procedure.

Endoscopy

Permits visualization inside the body using flexible scopes and cameras. Tumors can be visualized in the joints (arthroscopy), respiratory system (laryngoscopy, bronchoscopy), body cavity (mediastinoscopy, thoracoscopy), or gastrointestinal system (enteroscopy, sigmoidoscopy). Organs can be visualized as well (hysteroscopy, cystoscopy).

NURSING CONSIDERATIONS
- Obtain signed informed consent form.
- Prepare the client as indicated for the type of procedure to be performed.
- Provide a safe environment until effects of sedation are minimal (maintain bed rest, withhold oral intake).
- Ensure adequate oxygenation during the recovery period.

INTERPRETATION OF FINDINGS

- Findings that indicate or increase suspicion of cancer must be further evaluated.
- A variety of imaging and laboratory tests can be used to detect the following.
  - Degree of tumor involvement
  - Type of tumor
  - Areas of metastasis
  - Complications of cancer

NURSING CONSIDERATIONS
- Maintain knowledge of screening and diagnostic procedures.
- Educate the client about routine cancer screenings as part of health promotion and disease prevention.
- Prepare the client for testing, as indicated.
  - Withhold or restrict food or fluids.
  - Withhold medications that can alter test results or harm the client.
  - Administer preprocedure medication (sedatives, IV or PO fluids, analgesics, barium).
  - Maintain appropriate monitoring, as indicated (ECG, arterial line).
  - Position the client and promote comfort.

CLIENT EDUCATION
- Provide education to the client regarding the purpose and process of procedures.
- Provide a safe environment pre-, intra-, and postprocedure.
- Provide teaching and resources for client about self-care in the home environment.

PRACTICE Active Learning Scenario

A nurse manager is discussing collection of findings as part of screening for cancer with a group of nurses. What information should the nurse manager include in the discussion? Use the ATI Active Learning Template: Diagnostic Procedure to complete this item.

INTERPRETATION OF FINDINGS
- Describe at least three findings indicating the presence of metastasis.
- Describe four assessment techniques and possible findings.

CLIENT EDUCATION: Describe two self-assessment techniques that can identify data.

PRACTICE Answer

Using the ATI Active Learning Template: Diagnostic Procedure

INTERPRETATION OF FINDINGS
Metastasis
- Discomfort at secondary sites
- Swelling and/or tenderness of lymph nodes or areas of the body
- Presence of masses
- Altered function of another body system
- Bone pain
Assessment techniques
- Inspection for changes in color, symmetry, movement, or body function
- Auscultation for adventitious sounds, which can indicate altered body system function
- Palpation to detect masses or tissue abnormalities
- Percussion to detect changes in expected sound over organs, which can indicate inflammation or tumor

CLIENT EDUCATION: Testicular and breast self-examinations

Ⓝ *NCLEX® Connection: Health Promotion and Maintenance, Health Promotion/Disease Prevention*

Application Exercises

1. A nurse in a clinic is caring for a client who has suspected uterine cancer. Which of the following assessment techniques should the nurse anticipate the provider will perform?

   A. Bimanual pelvic examination

   B. Papanicolaou (Pap) test with cultures

   C. Digital rectal examination

   D. Percussion of upper abdominal quadrants for tympany

2. A nurse is teaching a client who is scheduled for nuclear imaging for suspected cancer. Which of the following statements should the nurse give?

   A. "The presence of a liver enzyme will be identified."

   B. "You will be given an injection of a radioactive substance."

   C. "An endoscope will be inserted through your mouth."

   D. "The tumor will be aspirated."

3. A nurse is assessing a client for suspected cancer. Which of the following findings should the nurse expect? (Select all that apply.)

   A. Temperature 102° F (38.9° C) for more than 48 hr

   B. Sore that does not heal

   C. Difficulty swallowing

   D. Unusual discharge

   E. Weight gain 4 lb (1.8 kg) in 2 weeks

4. A nurse is teaching a client who is scheduled for a shave biopsy for suspected cancer. Which of the following client statements indicates understanding of the procedure?

   A. "A test of my bone marrow will be performed."

   B. "A lymph node will be removed."

   C. "A needle will be inserted into the mass."

   D. "A small skin sample will be obtained."

5. A nurse is planning care for a client who is scheduled for genetic testing for suspected cancer. Which of the following interventions should the nurse include in the plan of care?

   A. Obtain a signed informed consent form.

   B. Withhold all medications prior to the procedure.

   C. Verify the prescription for a tumor marker assay.

   D. Ensure the client is placed in a recovery position after testing.

Application Exercises Key

1. A. **CORRECT:** Due to the location of uterine cancer, the provider should perform a bimanual pelvic examination to assess for uterine size, shape, and contour, which can be altered by a mass.

   B. A Pap test with cultures is performed when screening for cervical cancer.

   C. A digital rectal examination is performed when screening for prostate or rectal cancer.

   D. Percussion of the upper abdominal quadrants for tympany is a screening tool for detecting an abdominal mass.

   Ⓝ *NCLEX® Connection: Health Promotion and Maintenance, Health Promotion/Disease Prevention*

2. A. Liver function tests involve the identification of altered liver enzymes, which can be present in a client who has cancer. They are not nuclear imaging tests.

   B. **CORRECT:** Nuclear imaging involves the administration of an oral or IV radioactive tracer to identify cancerous tissue.

   C. Endoscopy permits visualization inside the body. It is not a form of nuclear imaging.

   D. A needle biopsy is performed to aspirate fluid and tissue samples for cancer cells. It is not a form of nuclear imaging.

   Ⓝ *NCLEX® Connection: Physiological Adaptation, Pathophysiology*

3. A. Presence of a fever for an extended period is not a warning sign for cancer.

   B. **CORRECT:** A sore that does not heal is a warning sign for cancer.

   C. **CORRECT:** Difficulty swallowing is a warning sign for cancer.

   D. **CORRECT:** The presence of unusual discharge is a warning sign for cancer.

   E. Weight gain is not a warning sign for cancer.

   Ⓝ *NCLEX® Connection: Health Promotion and Maintenance, Health Promotion/Disease Prevention*

4. A. Bone marrow aspiration is a type of needle biopsy.

   B. Sentinel node biopsy involves excision of a lymph node.

   C. Needle biopsy involves aspiration of a tumor for fluid and tissue sampling.

   D. **CORRECT:** A shave biopsy is a sampling of the outer skin layer using a scalpel or razor blade.

   Ⓝ *NCLEX® Connection: Physiological Adaptation, Illness Management*

5. A. **CORRECT:** A signed informed consent form should be obtained prior to the procedure.

   B. Medication does not affect the results of genetic testing.

   C. A tumor marker assay is a laboratory test to identify the presence of specific body proteins in blood, body secretions, and tissue. It is not a component of genetic testing.

   D. Genetic testing involves collection of blood or saliva. Recovery positioning is not required following testing.

   Ⓝ *NCLEX® Connection: Basic Care and Comfort, Nutrition and Oral Hydration*

CHAPTER 91

UNIT 13   NURSING CARE OF CLIENTS WHO HAVE IMMUNE
SYSTEM AND CONNECTIVE TISSUE DISORDERS
SECTION: CANCER-RELATED DISORDERS

CHAPTER 91 *Cancer Treatment Options*

Cancer treatment is based on the cell of origin of the cancer. When metastasis occurs, treatment is still based on the primary tumor origin even though the malignancy is located elsewhere in the body. Many cancers are curable when diagnosed early.

Cancer treatment options focus on removing or destroying cancer cells and preventing the continued abnormal cell growth and differentiation. Treatment can be curative or palliative. The treatment plan is guided by client factors (age, childbearing desire, pregnancy, current state of health expected lifespan) and can involve several treatment methods.

Adjuvant treatment is what is given in addition to the primary treatment standard, and can include hormone, radiation, and targeted therapies; immunotherapy; and chemotherapy.

Nursing care for clients who have cancer should include collaboration with supportive therapies and services, counseling, and transfer of care to another provider at discharge. Qᴛᴄ

PROCEDURES

Cancer treatment includes manipulation or removal of the tumor.

Tumor reduction can be done through topical procedures (cryosurgery, laser therapy, ablation) or by destruction of the main arteries that provide blood flow to the tumor (artery embolization).

Tumor excision can be open or endoscopic (curettage and electrodissection for skin cancer).
- The tumor and tissue immediately surrounding it (tumor margin) are removed. The goal is that all of the outermost tissue that was removed does not contain cancer cells (a negative margin).
- Surgery can be done for excision, biopsy (diagnosis and staging), or relief (palliation) based on findings.
- Lymph node dissection or sentinel lymph node biopsy is done to determine if the cancer has spread or there is added risk of spread.
- More extensive surgeries (tumors involving multiple organs or structures, lymph node involvement, deep lesions) increase the risk of complications and typically require longer recovery periods. Intensive care can be required.

NURSING ACTIONS
- Obtain a signed informed consent form.
- Prepare the client for procedures (NPO status, withholding or administering medications as prescribed, monitoring laboratory findings).
- Provide postoperative care as indicated by tumor location and procedure type.
- Prevent general postoperative complications (infection, fluid or electrolyte imbalance, hemorrhage, thromboembolism, inadequate oxygenation, shock).
- Prevent and treat pain as prescribed using pharmacological and nonpharmacological measures.
- Educate the client on care for drains, wounds, and implanted devices.
- Teach the client to monitor for complications after discharge.

Chemotherapy

Chemotherapy involves administration of systemic or local cytotoxic medications that damage a cell's DNA or destroy rapidly dividing cells.

- Chemotherapeutic agents are often selected in relation to their effect on various stages of cell division. Subsequently, combinations of anticancer medications are used to enhance destruction of cancer cells.
- Most chemotherapy agents are cytotoxic. The adverse effects of these agents are related to the unintentional harm done to normal rapidly proliferating cells, such as those found in the mucous membranes of the gastrointestinal (GI) tract, hair follicles, and bone marrow.
- For some cancer medications, agents that protect healthy cells (cytoprotectants or chemoprotectants) are given before or with chemotherapy to decrease the effect on normal tissues. Examples include amifostine and mesna.
- Chemotherapy can be administered in a health care setting, provider's office, clinic, or home.
- Most chemotherapy medications, including oral, are absorbed through the skin and mucous membranes. Anyone preparing, giving or disposing of these medications must wear proper personal protective equipment.

ROUTE

- Depending on the agent, it can be given by the topical (for skin lesions); oral; parenteral; IV; intra-arterial; intraventricular (into the ventricles of the brain); intracavitary, which includes intraperitoneal (into the abdominal cavity), intravesicular (into the bladder), and intrapleural (into the pleural space); or intrathecal (into the spinal cavity) route. Specialized training/certification is necessary for the administration of some agents.
- Oral anticancer medications are just as toxic to the client taking the medication and the nurse handling the medication as are standard chemotherapy medications.
- Oral medications should not be crushed, split, broken or chewed.

CATHETERS

- A central catheter is usually placed for chemotherapy administration or laboratory blood testing. Some medications can cause serious damage to the skin and muscle tissue if they leak outside a vein (vesicants). Getting these through a central venous catheter rather than a short-term peripheral IV reduces the risk that the medication will leak and damage tissues. Many different types of central venous catheters can be used. Two of the more commonly used included the peripherally inserted central catheter and implanted port. (Refer to **CHAPTER 27: CARDIOVASCULAR DIAGNOSTIC AND THERAPEUTIC PROCEDURES**.)
- Implanted port is used when therapy is intended to be given on a long-term basis. The port is comprised of a small reservoir that is covered by a thick septum.

CATEGORIES OF MEDICATIONS

- There are several categories of chemotherapy medications based on how they work and the chemical structure. Medications are selected based on the sensitivity of cancer cells to the medications and the stage of the cancer. How the medication works is important in predicting side effects.
- Categories include alkylating agents, antimetabolites, antimitotic agents, antitumor antibiotics, Topoisomerase inhibitors and other miscellaneous medications.

NURSING CONSIDERATIONS

- Instruct the client/family in the proper use of vascular access devices.
- Extravasation of agents that are vesicants requires specific, immediate attention to minimize tissue damage. Selection of a neutralizing solution is dependent on vesicant. Closely monitor the infusion site for evidence of infiltration. Qs

INTRACAVITARY CHEMOTHERAPY

Involves the administration of chemotherapy directly into a body cavity (abdomen, pleural space, or bladder)

- A small catheter can be used.
- Local irritation can be increased, but systemic adverse effects are usually prevented.
- In some cases, the medication can be removed following a dwell time.

NURSING CONSIDERATIONS

- Inform client that some discomfort can be present during infusion.
- Instruct the client to monitor for evidence of infection at the site of administration.

INDICATIONS

- Chemotherapy can be used to cure a disease, help control its progression, or as palliative treatment for individuals who have a terminal disease.
- Chemotherapy is most commonly used for treatment of cancer. It may also be used for other disorders, such as autoimmune diseases.

CONSIDERATIONS

PREPROCEDURE

- Because administration of chemotherapeutic medications is limited to certified individuals, management of adverse effects is the primary focus of health care personnel.
- Instruct the client on findings that indicate potential complications. The client should report findings immediately.

COMPLICATIONS

Immunosuppression/neutropenia

- Due to bone marrow suppression by cytotoxic medications
- The most significant adverse effect of chemotherapy

NURSING CONSIDERATIONS

- Monitor temperature, white blood cell (WBC) count, and absolute neutrophil count (ANC).
- A fever greater than 37.8° C (100° F) should be reported to the provider immediately.
- Clients who have neutropenia might not develop a high fever or have purulent drainage even when an infection is present.
- Monitor skin and mucous membranes for infection (breakdown, fissures, and abscess).
- Cultures should be obtained prior to initiating antimicrobial therapy.
- The risk of serious infection increases as the (ANC falls. An ANC less than 1,000/mm³ indicates a weak immune system. The nurse should implement neutropenic precautions, including placing the client in a private room.

NEUTROPENIC PRECAUTIONS

- Have the client remain in the room unless he needs to leave for a diagnostic procedure or therapy. In this case, place a mask on him during transport.
- Protect the client from possible sources of infection (plants, change water in equipment daily).
- Have client, staff, and visitors perform frequent hand hygiene. Restrict visitors who are ill.
- Avoid invasive procedures that could cause a break in tissue (rectal temperatures, injections, indwelling urinary catheters) unless necessary.
- Keep dedicated equipment (blood pressure machine, thermometer, stethoscope) in the client's room.
- Administer colony-stimulating factors (filgrastim) as prescribed to stimulate WBC production.

CLIENT EDUCATION

- Encourage the client to avoid crowds while undergoing chemotherapy.
- Take temperature daily. Report elevated temperature to the provider.
- Avoid food sources that could contain bacteria (fresh fruits and vegetables; undercooked meat, fish, and eggs; pepper and paprika).
- Avoid yard work, gardening, or changing a pet's litter box.
- Avoid fluids that have been sitting at room temperature for longer than 1 hr.
- Wash all dishes in hot, soapy water or a dishwasher. Wash glasses and cups after each use.
- Wash toothbrush daily in the dishwasher or rinse in a bleach solution.
- Do not share toiletry or personal hygiene items with others.
- Report fever greater than 37.8° C (100° F) or other manifestations of bacterial or viral infections immediately to the provider.

Nausea, vomiting, anorexia

- Many medications used for chemotherapy are emetogenic (induce vomiting) or cause anorexia and an altered taste in the mouth.
- Serotonin blockers, such as ondansetron, have been found to be effective and are often administered with corticosteroids, phenothiazines, and antihistamines. Q⃝EBP
- Neurokinin receptor antagonists (aprepitant); corticosteroids (dexamethasone, methylprednisolone); dopamine antagonists (promethazine, prochlorperazine); histamine blockers and proton pump inhibitors (omeprazole, ranitidine); prokinetic agents (metoclopramide), benzodiazepines (lorazepam); and cannabinoids (dronabinol, nabilone) are other examples of medications used for chemotherapy-induced nausea and vomiting (CINV).

NURSING CONSIDERATIONS

- Ensure antiemetics are given before chemotherapy and repeated based on the response and duration of CINV.
- Administer antiemetic medications for several days after each treatment, even when CINV appears to be controlled.
- Remove vomiting cues, such as odor and supplies associated with nausea.
- Implement nonpharmacological methods to reduce nausea (visual imagery, relaxation, acupuncture, distraction).
- Perform calorie counts to determine intake. Provide liquid nutritional supplements as needed. Add protein powders to food or tube feedings.
- Administer megestrol to increase appetite if prescribed.
- Assess for findings of dehydration or fluid and electrolyte imbalance.
- Perform mouth care prior to serving meals to enhance appetite.

CLIENT EDUCATION

- Instruct the client about the administration of antiemetics and schedule them prior to meals.
- Encourage the client to eat several small meals a day if better tolerated. Low-fat dry foods (crackers, toast) and avoiding drinking liquids during meals can prevent nausea.
- Suggest that the client select foods that are served cold and do not require cooking. Cooking food can emit odors that stimulate nausea.
- Encourage consumption of high-protein, high-calorie, nutrient-dense foods and avoidance of low- or empty-calorie foods. Use meal supplements as needed.
- Encourage the use of plastic eating utensils, sucking on hard candy, and avoiding red meats to prevent or reduce the sensation of metallic taste.
- Teach the client to create a food diary to identify items that can trigger nausea.

Alopecia

An adverse effect of certain chemotherapeutic medications related to their interference with the life cycle of rapidly proliferating cells

NURSING CONSIDERATIONS

- Discuss the effect of alopecia on self-image.
- Discuss options such as hats, turbans, and wigs to deal with hair loss. Qᴘᴄᴄ
- Hair loss can occur throughout the body or as mild as thinning hair of the scalp.
- Recommend soliciting information from the American Cancer Society regarding products for clients experiencing alopecia.
- Inform clients that hair loss occurs 7 to 10 days after treatment begins (for some agents). Encourage the client to select hairpiece before treatment starts.
- Reinforce that alopecia is temporary, and hair should return about 1 month after chemotherapy is discontinued. The new hair can differ from the original hair in color, texture, and thickness.

CLIENT EDUCATION

- Instruct the client to avoid the use of damaging hair care measures, such as electric rollers, curling irons, hair dye, and permanent waves. A soft hair brush or wide-tooth comb for grooming is preferred.
- Suggest that the client cut hair short before treatment to decrease weight on the hair follicle.
- If a client chooses to wear a wig, collaborate with a hairdresser to assist with selection. Suggest that the wig be worn before therapy begins to reduce appearance changes.
- After hair loss, the client should protect the scalp from sun exposure and use a diaper rash ointment/cream for itching. Qs
- Educate the client regarding the use of head coverings to reduce body heat loss and protect skin while wearing helmets, headphones, headsets, or wigs.

Oral effects

Mucositis refers to inflammation in the mucous lining of the upper GI tract from the mouth to the stomach.

Stomatitis refers to inflammation of tissues in the oral cavity, such as the gums, tongue, roof and floor of the mouth, and inside the lips and cheeks.

NURSING CONSIDERATIONS

- Examine the client's mouth several times a day, and inquire about the presence of oral lesions.
- Document the location and size of lesions. Lesions should be cultured and reported to the provider.
- Avoid using glycerin-based mouthwashes or mouth swabs. Nonalcoholic, anesthetic mouthwashes are recommended. Qᴇʙᴘ
- Administer a topical anesthetic prior to meals.
- Discourage consumption of salty, acidic, or spicy foods.
- Offer oral hygiene before and after each meal. Use lubricating or moisturizing agents to counteract dry mouth.

CLIENT EDUCATION

- Encourage the client to rinse the mouth with a solution of 0.9% sodium chloride, room-temperature tap water, or salt and soda water. Frequency is guided by the intensity of the mucositis.
- Encourage gentle flossing and brushing using a soft-bristled toothbrush or foam swabs to avoid traumatizing the oral mucosa.
- Rinse the mouth before and after meals. Avoid mouthwash that contains alcohol or other irritants
- Instruct the client to take medications to control infection as prescribed (nystatin suspension, acyclovir).
- Instruct the client regarding the use of coating agents, topical analgesics, topical anesthetics, or oral or parenteral analgesics that may be prescribed.
- Encourage the client to eat soft, bland foods and supplements that are high in calories (mashed potatoes, scrambled eggs, cooked cereal, milk shakes, ice cream, frozen yogurt, bananas, and breakfast mixes). Avoid spicy, salty, acidic food.
- Teach the client to avoid drinking alcohol and the use of tobacco.

Anemia and thrombocytopenia

Secondary to bone marrow suppression (myelosuppression)

Anemia
- NURSING CONSIDERATIONS
  - Monitor for fatigue, pallor, dizziness, and shortness of breath.
  - Help the client manage anemia-related fatigue by scheduling activities with rest periods in between and using energy saving measures (sitting during showers and ADLs).
  - Administer erythropoietic medications (e.g., darbepoetin alfa, epoetin alfa) and antianemic medications (e.g., ferrous sulfate) as prescribed.
  - Monitor Hgb values to determine response to medications. Be prepared to administer blood if prescribed.

Thrombocytopenia
- NURSING CONSIDERATIONS
  - Monitor for petechiae, ecchymosis, bleeding of the gums, nosebleeds, and occult or frank blood in stools, urine, or vomitus.
  - Institute bleeding precautions.
    - Avoid IVs and injections.
    - Apply pressure for approximately 10 min after blood is obtained.
    - Handle client gently and avoid trauma.
  - Administer thrombopoietic medications such as oprelvekin to stimulate platelet production. Monitor platelet count, and be prepared to administer platelets if the count falls below 10,000/mm^3.

- CLIENT EDUCATION
  - Instruct the client and family how to manage active bleeding.
  - Instruct the client about measures to prevent bleeding (use electric razor and soft-bristled toothbrush, avoid blowing nose vigorously, ensure that dentures fit appropriately).
  - Instruct the client to avoid the use of NSAIDs.
  - Teach the client to prevent injury when ambulating (wear closed-toes shoes, remove tripping hazards in the home) and apply cold if injury occurs. Qs

Chemotherapy-induced peripheral neuropathy

Loss of sensory or motor function of peripheral nerves is caused by exposure to certain anticancer medications. Higher doses of medication lead to greater neuropathy.

NURSING CONSIDERATIONS
- Monitor for loss of sensation in hands and feet, orthostatic hypotension, loss of taste, and constipation.
- Monitor for orthostatic hypotension.
- Monitor for early symptoms including numbness, tingling, and redness.

CLIENT EDUCATION
- Teach the client how to prevent injury, including falls.
- Educate the client regarding the need to protect skin because loss of sensation makes the client unaware of heat, cold, or pressure.
- Inform regarding risk of erectile dysfunction and treatment options.

Radiation therapy

Radiation therapy involves ionizing radiation to target tissues and destroy cells.
- Adverse effects on tissues within the radiation path include skin changes, hair loss, and debilitating fatigue.
- Radiation therapy is usually given as a series of divided small doses on a daily basis for a set period of time.
- Cytoprotectants, such as amifostine, are sometimes used to protect against harmful effects of radiation therapy, such as dryness of the mouth caused by radiation treatment for head and neck cancer.
- Radiation therapy can be administered internally (brachytherapy) with an implant or externally (teletherapy) with a radiation beam. The type used depends on the health of the client and shape, size, and location of the tumor.
- External beam radiation therapy does not cause the client to become radioactive.
- Internal radiation causes body fluids to be contaminated with radiation, and body wastes should be disposed of appropriately, as directed by the facility.
- Radiation therapy can be given preoperatively to decrease the size of a tumor.
- Radiation exposure to health care personnel and visitors is reduced by limiting indirect contact time, maintaining indicated distances from sources of radiation, and preventing direct contact with the source.

Internal radiation therapy

Brachytherapy describes internal radiation that is placed close to the target tissue. This is done via placement in a body orifice (vagina) or body cavity (abdomen) or delivered via IV such as with radionuclide iodine, which is absorbed by the thyroid.
- Brachytherapy provides radiation to the tumor and a limited amount to surrounding normal tissues.
- Waste products are radioactive until the isotope has been completely eliminated from the body. Waste products should not be touched by anyone.

NURSING CONSIDERATIONS
- Place the client in a private room away from other clients when possible. Keep door closed as much as possible.
- Place a sign on the door warning of the radiation source. Qs
- Wear a dosimeter film badge that records personal amount of radiation exposure.
- Limit visitors to 30-min visits, and have visitors maintain a distance of 6 feet from the source.
- Visitors and health care personnel who are pregnant or under the age of 18 should not come into contact with the client or radiation source.
- Wear a lead apron while providing care keeping the front of the apron facing the source of radiation.
- Keep a lead container in the client's room if the delivery method could allow spontaneous loss of radioactive material. Tongs are available for placing radioactive material into this container.
- Follow protocol for proper removal of dressings and bed linens from the room.

CLIENT EDUCATION

- Inform the client of the need to remain in an indicated position to prevent dislodgement of the radiation implant.
- Instruct the client to call the nurse for assistance with elimination.
- Instruct the client and family about radiation precautions needed in health care and home environments.

External radiation therapy

External radiation or teletherapy is delivered in relatively small doses over the course of several weeks and aimed at the body from an external source. Unlike internal radiation, the client is not radioactive and is not hazardous to others.

NURSING CONSIDERATIONS

- The skin over the targeted area is marked with "tattoos" that guide the positioning of the external radiation source.
- Provide a well-balanced diet that does not contain red meat. Radiation can cause dysgeusia (altered taste), making foods such as red meat unpalatable.
- Help the client manage fatigue by scheduling activities with rest periods in between and using energy-saving measures (sitting during showers and ADLs).
- Monitor for radiation injury to skin and mucous membranes and implement a skin care regimen.
  - Skin: blanching, erythema, desquamation, sloughing, hemorrhage
  - Mouth: mucositis, xerostomia (dry mouth)
  - Neck: difficulty swallowing
  - Abdomen: gastroenteritis
- Monitor CBC (possible decreased platelets and WBCs).

CLIENT EDUCATION

- Adverse effects depend on which part of the body is being exposed to the radiation and how much radiation is being administered.
- Review nutrition considerations related to mucositis.
  - Avoid spicy, salty, acidic foods.
  - Hot foods might not be tolerated.
- Gently wash the skin over the irradiated area with mild soap and water. Dry the area thoroughly using patting motions. Q EBP
- Do not remove or wash off radiation tattoos (markings) used to guide therapy. Do not apply powders, ointments, lotions, deodorants, or perfumes to the irradiated skin.
- Wear soft clothing. Avoid tight or constricting clothes.
- Do not expose the irradiated skin to sun or a heat source.
- Inspect skin for evidence of damage and report to the provider.

Hormone therapy

Hormone therapy is effective against tumors that are supported or suppressed by hormones, such as in breast or prostate cancer.

- By giving a similar hormone, uptake of the support hormone is blocked, or production reduced. Luteinizing hormone-releasing hormone (LH-RH) agonists like leuprolide and goserelin are effective against tumors that require a particular hormone for support.
  - The use of androgenic hormones in a client who has estrogen-dependent cancer can suppress growth of this type of cancer.
  - The use of estrogenic hormones for a testosterone-dependent cancer can suppress growth of this type of cancer.
- Hormone antagonists compete with the support hormone for binding sites on or in the tumor cell and are effective against tumors that require a particular hormone for support.
  - The use of an anti-estrogen hormone in a client who has estrogen-dependent cancer can suppress growth of this type of cancer. The same is true for anti-testosterone hormones.

LH-RH agonists

NURSING CONSIDERATIONS: Monitor cardiac status and blood pressure and for pulmonary edema.

CLIENT EDUCATION

- Inform male clients about the impact on sexual functions (decreased libido, erectile dysfunction) and feminizing effects of hormone therapy (gynecomastia, hot flashes, bone loss). Q PCC
- Instruct the client to increase intake of calcium and vitamin D.
- Inform female clients of masculinizing effects (chest and facial hair growth, amenorrhea, decreased breast tissue).

Androgen antagonists (bicalutamide)

NURSING CONSIDERATIONS: Monitor laboratory findings (CBC [anemia], calcium, increased liver enzymes).

CLIENT EDUCATION

- Alert male clients about feminizing effects of hormone therapy (gynecomastia, erectile dysfunction).
- Advise the client to notify the provider of sore throat or bruising.

Estrogen receptor down-regulators

Estrogen receptor down-regulators (e.g., fulvestrant) induce degradation of estrogen receptors.

Estrogen antagonists

Tamoxifen, anastrozole, trastuzumab

NURSING CONSIDERATIONS
- Monitor CBC, clotting times, lipid profiles, calcium and cholesterol serum levels, and liver function for medication-related changes.
- Monitor neurologic and cardiovascular functioning for changes.

CLIENT EDUCATION
- Inform the client of adverse effects, which include nausea, vomiting, hot flashes, weight gain, vaginal bleeding, and increased risk of thrombosis.
- Reinforce the need for yearly gynecologic exams and the need to take calcium and vitamin D supplements.

Immunotherapy

Immunotherapy (biotherapy) uses biologic response modifiers, which alter a client's biological response to cancerous tumor cells. Antibodies, cytokines, and other immune substances normally produced by the immune system are administered to increase the body's defense against cancer.
- Interleukins and interferons are the two primary cytokines (immune response modulators) used in immunotherapy.
- **Interleukins** help coordinate the inflammatory and immune responses of the body, particularly the lymphocytes.
- **Interferons**, when stimulated, can exert an antitumor effect by activating a variety of responses.

NURSING CONSIDERATIONS
- **Interleukins:** Monitor for influenza-like symptoms and edema.
- **Interferons:** Monitor for altered mental status and lethargy.
- Monitor for peripheral neuropathy that can affect vision, hearing, balance, and gait.
- Take precautions for orthostatic hypotension.

CLIENT EDUCATION
- Instruct the client to immediately report influenza-like manifestations or changes consistent with peripheral neuropathy.
- Alert the client that skin rashes are common. Use of a perfume-free moisturizer can be helpful.
- Instruct the client to avoid sun exposure and swimming if skin manifestations develop.

Photodynamic therapy

Photodynamic therapy involves injection of a photosensitizing agent that is absorbed by all cells in the body. One to three days later when the agent remains in only the cancer cells, the tumor is exposed to a specific wavelength of light via an endoscope. Cells are subsequently destroyed, and tumors are eliminated or reduced in size.
- Used to treat non-small cell lung cancer and esophageal cancer.
- Effective with small tumors close to body surface (within 1 cm).
- Adverse effects are related to the area of the body being treated.

NURSING CONSIDERATIONS: Instruct the client to avoid sun exposure for 6 weeks. (Limit time outdoors, and wear sunglasses.)

Supportive treatment

In addition to cancer treatment, the client can require assistance for altered body function or to meet emotional and spiritual needs.
- Facilitate safe activity, providing assistive devices when necessary for clients who have altered mobility or require assistance with self-care activities. Qs
- Coordinate transfer of client care to home health, hospice, or a tertiary care setting (rehabilitation center) as appropriate.
- Provide alternate means of communication for clients who have cancer affecting the mouth, throat, larynx, or vocal cords.
- Use assistive aids and devices for clients who have visual or hearing impairments.
- Consult physical therapy, and genetic or other counseling services as indicated.
- Consult pain management for persistent or uncontrolled pain. (See **CHAPTER 93: PAIN MANAGEMENT FOR CLIENTS WHO HAVE CANCER.**)

Inadequate nutrition

Clients who have cancer are at risk for inadequate nutrition related to diagnosis or treatment. (Refer to the **NUTRITION FOR NURSING REVIEW MODULE: CHAPTER 16: CANCER AND IMMUNOSUPPRESSION DISORDERS.**)

NURSING CONSIDERATIONS
- Administer nutritional supplements or substitutes as prescribed.
- Monitor feeding tube or central line as appropriate.
- Encourage the addition of protein- and calorie-dense foods.
- Monitor for effectiveness of nutrition modifications (laboratory values, urine and bowel elimination, absence of GI upset).
- Monitor weight.
- Consult nutrition services.

Altered elimination.

NURSING CONSIDERATIONS

- Assist with alternate means of elimination as indicated.
  - Insert indwelling or intermittent urinary catheter.
  - Apply drainage devices.
- Monitor urine and bowel output.
- Instruct the client on self-management of elimination.

Body image changes

Body image changes are a factor in clients for whom surgery is disfiguring, especially cancers of the face or sexual organs (breasts or genitalia).

NURSING CONSIDERATIONS

- Encourage the client to express feelings.
- Encourage the client to look at or touch affected body areas.
- Assist the client with prosthetic devices as indicated.
- Encourage the client to use positive measures to promote proper body image (makeup, clothing).

Altered sexuality

Altered sexuality can result from functional impairment or body image changes related to cancer treatments. Pain with sexual intercourse can also be a factor.

NURSING CONSIDERATIONS

- Encourage the client and partner to communicate feelings to each other.
- Administer hormone therapy as prescribed.
- Instruct the client about medications to promote erection or manage pain sensation.

Ineffective coping

The client's ability to cope with the diagnosis and prognosis can be ineffective.

NURSING CONSIDERATIONS Qpcc

- Administer medications as prescribed for anxiety or depression.
- Encourage the client to express feelings verbally or through journaling and blogging.
- Encourage the client to participate in a support group (physical or online) for clients who have similar cancers. Make a referral to a community resource.
- Make a referral to counseling services for the client and family as needed.
- Educate the client on anticipatory grief and the stages of grief.
- Consult palliative services as indicated.
- Incorporate the client's beliefs and preferences regarding spirituality and illness/death.

Immunocompromise

Cancer or cancer treatment can place the client in an immunocompromised state.

NURSING CONSIDERATIONS: Teach the client to avoid individuals who have colds/infections/viruses.

Application Exercises

1. A nurse is planning care for a client who has a platelet count of 10,000/mm³. Which of the following interventions should the nurse include in the plan of care?

   A. Apply prolonged pressure to puncture site after blood sampling.

   B. Administer epoetin alfa as prescribed.

   C. Place the client in a private room.

   D. Have the client use an oral topical anesthetic before meals.

2. A nurse is caring for a client who is receiving chemotherapy and has mucositis. Which of the following actions should the nurse take?

   A. Use a glycerin-soaked swab to clean the client's teeth.

   B. Encourage increased intake of citrus fruit juices.

   C. Obtain a culture of the lesions.

   D. Provide an alcohol-based mouthwash for oral hygiene.

3. A nurse is planning care for a client who is undergoing chemotherapy and is on neutropenic precautions. Which of the following interventions should be included in the plan of care? (Select all that apply.)

   A. Encourage a high-fiber diet.

   B. Remove plants from the room.

   C. Have the client wear a mask when leaving the room.

   D. Have client-specific equipment remain in the room.

   E. Eliminate raw foods from the client's diet.

4. A nurse is caring for a client who is undergoing chemotherapy and reports severe nausea. Which of the following statements should the nurse make?

   A. "Your nausea will lessen with each course of chemotherapy."

   B. "Hot food is better tolerated due to the aroma."

   C. "Try eating several small meals throughout the day."

   D. "Increase your intake of red meat as tolerated."

5. A nurse is caring for a client who has cervical cancer and is scheduled for brachytherapy. Which of the following actions should the nurse take? (Select all that apply.)

   A. Permit visitors to stay with the client 30 min at a time.

   B. Place the client on bed rest.

   C. Insert an indwelling urinary catheter.

   D. Administer fiber laxatives.

   E. Dispose soiled linens in hamper outside client's room.

PRACTICE Active Learning Scenario

A nurse is teaching a female client who is receiving chemotherapy and has alopecia. What should the nurse include in the teaching? Use the Active Learning Template: System Disorder to complete this item.

PATHOPHYSIOLOGY RELATED TO CLIENT PROBLEM

CLIENT EDUCATION: Describe at least four teaching points.

NURSING CARE: Describe at least two nursing actions.

Application Exercises Key

1. A. **CORRECT:** The nurse should implement bleeding precautions for the client who has thrombocytopenia.

   B. Epoetin alfa is administered to the client who has anemia.

   C. The client who has neutropenia is placed in a private room.

   D. A topical oral anesthetic is used for the client who has mucositis.

   Ⓝ *NCLEX® Connection: Reduction of Risk Potential, Therapeutic Procedures*

2. A. Glycerin-based swabs should be avoided when providing oral hygiene to a client who has mucositis.

   B. Acidic foods should be discouraged for a client who has oral mucositis.

   C. **CORRECT:** The nurse should obtain a culture of the oral lesions to identify pathogens and determine appropriate treatment.

   D. Nonalcoholic mouthwashes are recommended for a client who has mucositis.

   Ⓝ *NCLEX® Connection: Physiological Adaptation, Unexpected Response to Therapies*

3. A. There is no benefit to a high-fiber diet for a client who has neutropenia.

   B. **CORRECT:** Neutropenic precautions include the client not having contact with flowers and plants due to the presence of surface infectious agents in the water and soil.

   C. **CORRECT:** Neutropenic precautions include having the client wear a mask when leaving the room to reduce the incidence of infection.

   D. **CORRECT:** Neutropenic precautions include having equipment available that is only for use in caring for the client to reduce the incidence of infection.

   E. **CORRECT:** A client who has neutropenia should avoid consuming raw foods due to the presence of surface infectious agents on peeling and rind.

   Ⓝ *NCLEX® Connection: Pharmacological and Parenteral Therapies, Pharmacological Pain Management*

4. A. Nausea usually occurs to the same extent with each session of chemotherapy.

   B. Cold foods are better tolerated than warm or hot foods because odors from heated foods can induce nausea.

   C. **CORRECT:** Several small meals a day are usually better tolerated by the client who has nausea.

   D. Red meat is not tolerated well by the client undergoing chemotherapy because the taste of meat is frequently altered and unpalatable.

   Ⓝ *NCLEX® Connection: Pharmacological and Parenteral Therapies, Pharmacological Pain Management*

5. A. **CORRECT:** The client who has cervical cancer will have a vaginal radiation implant. Visitors should remain for no more than 30 min at a time and maintain a distance of at least 6 ft.

   B. **CORRECT:** The client who has cervical cancer will have a vaginal radiation implant. Bed rest is needed to prevent displacement of the implant.

   C. **CORRECT:** The client who has cervical cancer will have a vaginal radiation implant. A catheter is needed to prevent displacement of the implant during ambulation.

   D. Fiber laxatives, which stimulate bowel movements, are not used to prevent displacing the vaginal radiation implant.

   E. The nurse should dispose all the client's linens in a metal container inside the client's room due to the exposure of radiation.

   Ⓝ *NCLEX® Connection: Physiological Adaptation, Alterations in Body Systems*

PRACTICE Answer

Using the Active Learning Template: System Disorder

PATHOPHYSIOLOGY RELATED TO CLIENT PROBLEM: Alopecia occurs as an adverse effect of chemotherapy medications. The medications interfere with the life cycle of rapidly proliferating cells, such as those found in hair follicles, resulting in hair loss.

CLIENT EDUCATION
- Wear hats, turbans, and wigs.
- Avoid the use of damaging hair-care measures, such as electric rollers and curling irons, hair dye, and permanent waves.
- Use a soft hair brush or wide-tooth comb for grooming.
- Avoid sun exposure. Use a diaper rash ointment or cream for itching.
- Alopecia is temporary, and hair will return when chemotherapy is discontinued.

NURSING CARE
- Discuss the effect of alopecia on self-image. Encourage the client to express feelings.
- Recommend use of information from the American Cancer Society on managing alopecia.
- Provide referral to a cancer support group.

Ⓝ *NCLEX® Connection: Physiological Adaptation, Alterations in Body Systems*

CHAPTER 92 *Cancer Disorders*

The various types of cancer share general cancer principles: abnormal cell growth, tumor formation, and potential for invasion to other locations. Each type of cancer has distinguishing characteristics related to risk, manifestations, screening, and diagnosis. The prognosis and treatment varies by type.

Skin cancer

- Sunlight exposure is the leading cause of skin cancer. The most effective strategy for prevention of skin cancer is avoidance or reduction of skin exposure to sunlight.
- Precancerous skin lesions, called actinic keratoses, are common in people who have chronically sun-damaged skin, such as older adults. Ⓖ

TYPES OF SKIN CANCER

Squamous cell (epidermis)

CHARACTERISTICS
- Rough, scaly lesion with central ulceration and crusting
- Bleeding (possible)

COURSE: Localized; can metastasize.

Basal cell (basal epidermis or nearby dermal cells)

CHARACTERISTICS
- Small, waxy nodule with superficial blood vessels, well-defined borders
- Erythema and ulcerations

COURSE: Invades local structures (nerves, bone, cartilage, lymphatic and vascular tissue); rarely metastatic but high rate of recurrence.

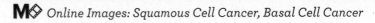 *Online Images: Squamous Cell Cancer, Basal Cell Cancer*

Malignant melanoma (cancer of melanocytes) (92.1)

CHARACTERISTICS
- Irregular shape and borders with multiple colors
- New moles or change in an existing mole (can occur in intestines or any other body structure that contains pigment cells)
- Itching, cracks, ulcerations, or bleeding (possible)

COURSE: Rapid invasion and metastasis with high morbidity and mortality

HEALTH PROMOTION AND DISEASE PREVENTION

- Limit exposure to sunlight, especially between 1000 and 1500.
- Apply sunscreen when near reflective surfaces (sand, snow, water, concrete).
- Use sunblock that has an SPF of at least 15, with both UVA and UVB protection. Apply 30 min before exposure to sun. Sunblock should be reapplied at least every 2 hr.
- Wear protective clothing, hats, sunglasses, and lip balm that has an SPF of at least 15.
- Avoid indoor tanning (tanning beds, booths, sunlamps).
- Teach clients the "ABCDE" system to evaluate moles.
  - **A: Asymmetry:** One side does not match the other
  - **B: Borders**: Ragged, notched, irregular, or blurred edges
  - **C: Color:** Lack of uniformity in pigmentation (shades of tan, brown, or black)
  - **D: Diameter:** Width greater than 6 mm, or about the size of a pencil eraser or a pea
  - **E: Evolving:** Or change in appearance (shape, size, color, height, texture) or condition (bleeding, itching)
- Because of the cumulative effects of sun damage over the lifespan, screening for suspicious lesions is an essential part of the routine physical assessment of older adult clients. Ⓖ

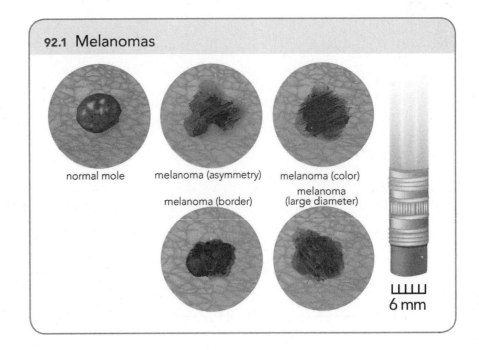

92.1 Melanomas

normal mole

melanoma (asymmetry)

melanoma (color)

melanoma (border)

melanoma (large diameter)

6 mm

ASSESSMENT

RISK FACTORS

- Occupational history of chemical carcinogens
- History of severe skin injury
- Immunosuppression therapy
- Exposure to ultraviolet light (natural light or indoor tanning) over long periods of time
- Chronic skin inflammation, burns, or scars
- Fair complexion (blonde or red hair, fair skin, freckles, blue eyes) with a tendency to burn easily
- Presence of several large or many small moles
- Family or personal history of melanoma
- Residing in higher elevations or in close proximity to equator (thinner layer of ozone)
- Age older than 50 years

EXPECTED FINDINGS

Report of change in appearance of mole or lesion

DIAGNOSTIC PROCEDURES

Assessment (self or clinician)

EXPECTED FINDINGS
- New or suspicious lesions
- Recent changes in size, color, or sensation of any mole, birthmark, wart or scar

NURSING ACTIONS: Instruct client to develop a body map (diagram of scars or lesions) and monitor monthly for changes. Inspect skin between fingers and toes and on scalp.

Biopsy (punch, shave, or excisional)

EXPECTED FINDINGS: Cancerous cells

NURSING ACTIONS
- Instruct client to monitor for infection.
- Teach client wound care, including care of sutures (punch, excisional biopsy).

Lymph node biopsy/dissection

EXPECTED FINDINGS: Tissue examined microscopically for the spread of cancer

NURSING ACTIONS
- Monitor site of lymph node biopsy or removal for bleeding or infection.
- If melanoma is diagnosed, blood tests are prescribed (CBC, CMP, liver) to check for organ involvement.

PATIENT-CENTERED CARE

THERAPEUTIC PROCEDURES

Chemotherapy

Topical chemotherapy with 5-fluorouracil cream
- For treatment of actinic keratoses or for widespread superficial basal cell carcinoma.
- CLIENT EDUCATION
  - Prepare the client for extended treatment that will cause the lesion to weep, crust, and erode.
  - Reassure the client that the appearance of the lesion will improve after treatment.

Interferon therapy
- For postoperative treatment of stage III or greater melanomas.
- NURSING CONSIDERATIONS
  - Report and provide relief for adverse or toxic effects of chemotherapy.
  - Encourage adequate nutrition and fluid intake.
  - Instruct clients on self-injection procedure.

Targeted therapy (92.2)

- Blocks or slows the spread of cancer by interfering with specific molecules (targets) that are involved in growth, progression, and spread of cancer.
- Vemurafenib is an oral medication used for targeted therapy to treat melanoma.

Radiation

- Limited to older clients who have large, deeply invasive tumors and those who are poor surgical candidates.
- Melanoma is relatively resistant to radiation therapy.

Cryosurgery

- Freezes and destroys isolated lesions by applying liquid nitrogen (−200° C).
- Skin becomes edematous and tender.
- CLIENT EDUCATION: Teach the client to cleanse with hydrogen peroxide and apply a topical antimicrobial until healed.

Curettage and electrodessication

Removes cancerous cells with the use of a curette to scrape away cancerous tissue, followed by the application of an electric probe to destroy remaining tumor tissue.

Excision

The incision will be closed with sutures if possible. A skin graft can be necessary for large areas.
- CLIENT EDUCATION: Advise the client about postoperative wound care and care of the skin graft if used.

Mohs surgery

- Used with basal and squamous cell carcinoma
- Tissue is sectioned horizontally in layers and each layer is examined for presence of residual cancer; the process is continued until the samples are free of cancer
- COMPLICATIONS: Skin abscess and cellulitis

Leukemias and lymphomas

LEUKEMIAS

- Leukemias are cancers of white blood cells or of cells that develop into white blood cells. In leukemia, the white blood cells are not functional. They invade and destroy bone marrow, and they can metastasize to the liver, spleen, lymph nodes, testes, and brain.
- Leukemias are divided into acute (acute lymphocytic leukemia and acute myelogenous leukemia) and chronic (chronic lymphocytic leukemia and chronic myelogenous leukemia) and are further classified by the type of white blood cells primarily affected.
- The goal of treatment is to eliminate all leukemic cells.
- The exact cause of leukemia is not known.
- Overgrowth of leukemic cells prevents growth of other blood components (platelets, erythrocytes, mature leukocytes). **Qs**
  - Lack of mature leukocytes leads to immunosuppression. Infection is the leading cause of death among clients who have leukemia.
  - Lack of platelets increases the client's risk of bleeding.

Incidence and cure rates

Acute lymphocytic leukemia (ALL): Various factors influence the prognosis for children, but the 5-year survival rate is approximately 85% (age at diagnosis, gender, cell type involved); less than 50% of adults can be cured.

Acute myelogenous leukemia (AML): Most common leukemia among adults; prognosis is poor.

Acute promyelocytic leukemia (APL): Subtype of AML. Most curable of adult leukemias.

Chronic lymphocytic leukemia (CLL): Most cases involve people older than 50 years of age. This disease does not occur in children.

Chronic myelogenous leukemia (CML): Most cases involve young adults. The disease is uncommon in children. Prognosis is less than 2 years of survival from the time of diagnosis. Three phases: chronic (slow growing with mild manifestations); accelerated (more rapid growing with severe manifestations and failure to respond to therapy); blast (very aggressive with metastasis to organs).

92.2 Cancer therapies at a glance

Ablation procedures
Can be used to destroy cancerous cells.

Radiofrequency ablation delivers an electric current directly to the tumor via thin needles. This current is converted into heat waves that kill the cancer cells.

Cryotherapy (cryoablation) uses liquid nitrogen injected directly into the tumor to destroy the tumor.

Microwave thermotherapy uses microwaves transmitted through a probe to heat and destroy the abnormal tissue

Chemotherapy
Chemotherapy uses anti-cancer drugs administered orally or intravenously to destroy cancer cells.

Photodynamic therapy
Photodynamic therapy involves the injection of a photosensitizing agent that is absorbed by all the cells in the body. One to three days later when the agent remains in only the cancer cells, the tumor is exposed to a laser light via an endoscope. Cells are subsequently destroyed and tumors are eliminated or reduced in size. Used with small, noninvasive lesions.

Radiation
With extensive disease, radiation is combined with chemotherapy

Brachytherapy is radiation delivered inside the body.

External beam radiation therapy (EBRT) uses radiation from a source outside of the body to destroy cancer cells.

Intensity-modulated radiation uses thousands of beams and angles of varying intensity that are even more controlled to target the cancer tissues and reduce exposure of radiation to healthy tissue.

Targeted therapy
Targeted therapy is a newer molecular-based medication therapy that targets specific receptors or other processes that produce cancer cells. Because this therapy has specific targets, it often causes less adverse effects than regular cancer chemotherapy, which typically kills large numbers of normal cells along with cancer cells.

Examples of targeted therapy includes biologic response modifiers, monoclonal antibodies, cytokines, growth factors, and gene therapy.

Immunotherapy (biotherapy) uses biologic response modifiers (BRMs), which alter a client's biological response to cancerous tumor cells. Cytokines work to enhance the immune system. They help the client's immune system recognize cancer cells and use the body's natural defenses to destroy them. Interleukins and interferons are the two primary cytokines (immune response modulators) used in immunotherapy.

- Interleukins help coordinate the inflammatory and immune responses of the body, in particular, the lymphocytes.
- Interferons, when stimulated, can exert an antitumor effect by activating a variety of responses.
- Tumor necrosis factor

LYMPHOMAS

- Lymphomas are cancers of lymphocytes (a type of white blood cell) and lymph nodes (which produce antibodies and fight infection).
- Lymphomas can metastasize to almost any organ.

Types of lymphoma

Hodgkin's lymphoma (HL)

- Peaks in two age groups: teens and young adults; adults in their 50s and 60s.
- Possible causes include viral infections and exposure to chemical agents.
- Typically starts in a single node or chain of nodes that contain the Reed-Sternberg cell.
- HL spreads predictably from one group of lymph nodes to the next
- One of the most treatable types of cancer

Non-Hodgkin's lymphoma (NHL)

- More common in men and older adults.
- Possible causes include gene damage, viral infections, autoimmune disease, and exposure to radiation or toxic chemicals.
- Includes all lymphoid cancers that do not have the Reed-Sternberg cell; there are 60 subtypes.
- Generally spreads through the lymphatic system in an erratic pattern.
- There is an increased incidence in clients exposed to pesticides, insecticides, and dust.

HEALTH PROMOTION AND DISEASE PREVENTION

- Use protective equipment, such as a mask, and ensure proper ventilation while working in environments that contain carcinogens or particles in the air.
- Influenza and pneumonia vaccinations are important for all clients who are immunosuppressed.

ASSESSMENT

RISK FACTORS

- Immunosuppression
- Exposure to chemotherapy agents or medications that suppress bone marrow
- Genetic factors (hereditary)
- Ionizing radiation (radiation therapy, environmental)

OLDER ADULT CLIENTS Ⓖ

- Often have diminished immune function and decreased bone marrow function, which increase the risk of complications of leukemia and lymphoma.
- Have decreased energy reserves and can tire more easily during treatment. Safety is a concern with ambulation.

EXPECTED FINDINGS

Acute leukemia

- Bone pain
- Joint swelling
- Enlarged liver and spleen
- Weight loss
- Fever
- Poor wound healing (infected lesions)
- Manifestations of anemia (fatigue, pallor, tachycardia, dyspnea on exertion)
- Evidence of bleeding (ecchymoses, hematuria, bleeding gums)

Hodgkin's and non-Hodgkin's lymphoma

- Most clients only experience an enlarged lymph node (usually in the neck with HL), which is a typical finding in clients who have indolent (slow-growing) lymphomas.
- Other possible manifestations include fever, night sweats, unplanned weight loss, fatigue, and infections.

DIAGNOSTIC PROCEDURES

Staging of lymphoma involves extensive testing to ensure proper treatment is prescribed. HL has two main subtypes; "classic" HL is further distinguished into four categories. NHL has more than 60 subtypes. Treatment must be specific to the client's needs.

CBC

EXPECTED FINDINGS
- WBC can be high, low, or normal (leukemia)
- Hemoglobin, hematocrit, and platelets decreased

NURSING ACTIONS: Explain unexpected findings to client.

Coagulation time

EXPECTED FINDINGS: Increased with acute leukemia

NURSING ACTIONS: Monitor for bleeding.

Biopsy of bone marrow (core or fine-needle aspiration)

EXPECTED FINDINGS
- Large quantities of immature leukemic blast cells (confirms diagnosis)
- Typing of protein markers (to differentiate myeloid or lymphoid leukemia)

NURSING ACTIONS
- Administer pain medication as prescribed.
- Apply pressure for 5 to 10 min, then a pressure dressing.
- Monitor for bleeding and infection for 24 hr.

CT scan (always used for HL staging)

EXPECTED FINDINGS: Guide for lymphoma staging procedures: identify presence, size, and shape of nodes, tumors.

NURSING ACTIONS: Prepare the client for the procedure.

Biopsy of lymph nodes

EXPECTED FINDINGS
- **Hodgkin's lymphoma:** presence of Reed-Sternberg cells (cancerous B-lymphocytes)
- **Non-Hodgkin's lymphoma:** any other lymph node malignancy

CLIENT EDUCATION: Provide information specific to the diagnosis.

Chest x-ray, CT scan, PET scan, bone scan

EXPECTED FINDINGS: Confirms diagnosis or metastatic disease

CLIENT EDUCATION: Provide information specific to the diagnosis.

PATIENT-CENTERED CARE

NURSING CARE

- Monitor for evidence of infection. Assess for other physiological indicators of infection (lung crackles, cough, urinary frequency or urgency, oliguria, lesions of skin or mucous membrane).
- Manifestations that stem from the immune response (increased WBC, fever, pus, redness, inflammation) are not likely due to immunosuppression.
- Prevent infection. (Implement neutropenic precautions.) These interventions are especially important during chemotherapy induction and for clients who have received a bone marrow transplant. Qs
  - Frequent, thorough hand hygiene is a priority intervention.
  - Place the client in a private room.
  - Allow only healthy visitors; when unavoidable, visitors who are ill must wear a mask.
  - Screen visitors carefully.
  - Restrict foods that can be contaminated with bacteria (no fresh or raw fruits, vegetables).
  - Monitor WBC.
  - Prevent transmission of bacteria and viruses (no live plants, flowers; use high-efficiency particulate air [HEPA] filtration). Eliminate standing water (humidifiers, denture cups, vases) to prevent bacteria breeding.
  - Encourage good personal hygiene.
  - Avoid crowds.

- Prevent injury.
  - Monitor platelets.
  - Assess frequently for obvious and occult bleeding.
  - Protect the client from trauma (avoid injections and venipunctures, apply firm pressure, increase vitamin K intake).
  - Teach the client how to avoid trauma (use electric shaver, soft bristled toothbrush, avoid contact sports).
- Conserve the client's energy.
  - Encourage rest, adequate nutrition, and fluid intake.
  - Ensure the client gets adequate sleep.
  - Assess the client's energy resources/capability.
  - Plan activities as appropriate.

THERAPEUTIC PROCEDURES

Chemotherapy

- Chemotherapy can be used to treat lymphoma in combination with other therapies.
- There are three phases of chemotherapy used to treat leukemia. **(92.3)**

CLIENT EDUCATION: Report manifestations of infection or illness immediately to the provider.

Colony-stimulating medications

Medications such as filgrastim stimulate the production of leukocytes.

NURSING CONSIDERATIONS: Monitor for report of bone pain. Monitor CBC twice weekly to check leukocytes. Use cautiously with clients who have bone marrow cancer.

CLIENT EDUCATION: Encourage the client to report bone discomfort.

Immunotherapy (92.2)

Monoclonal antibodies are man-made proteins attack a specific target to treat lymphoma. Includes such medications as ofatumumab and alemtuzumab used for CLL.

92.3 Phases of chemotherapy to treat leukemia

	GOAL	PROCEDURE	LENGTH OF TIME
Induction therapy: intensive combination therapy	Induce remission: absence of all findings of leukemia, including less than 5% blasts in bone marrow.	Aggressive treatment (possible continuous infusion); IV infusion; CNS and CSF infusion prophylaxis (ALL)	4 to 6 weeks (hospitalization required due to increased risk for infection and hemorrhage)
Consolidation or intensification therapy	Cure by eradicating any residual leukemic cells.	Same medications as induction phase at lower dosage or different combination of medications	About 6 months
Maintenance therapy	Prevent relapse.	Lower doses of oral or IV chemotherapy	Months to years
Reinduction therapy: for a client who relapses	Place the client back in remission.	Combinations of chemotherapy used to achieve remission	Probability of relapse occurring decreases over time

Targeted therapy (92.2)

Radiation

- External lymph node radiation is the primary form of treatment for HL. Radiation therapy or radiolabeled antibodies can be used as part of treatment for NHL.
- With extensive disease, radiation is combined with chemotherapy
- Radiation is not typically a treatment used for clients who have leukemia.

Bone marrow transplantation

Bone marrow is destroyed or ablated using radiation or chemotherapy and later replaced with healthy stem cells. The body is able to resume normal production of blood cells.

- Autologous cells are the client's own cells that are collected before chemotherapy.
- Matching of donor to recipient stem cells compares certain human leukocyte antigens (HLA) to reduce risk of rejection.
  ○ Syngeneic cells are donated from the client's identical twin (HLA identical).
  ○ Allogeneic cells are obtained from an HLA-matched donor, such as a relative or from umbilical cord blood (closely matched HLA).
- Without transplantation, the client will likely die from infection or bleeding.
- Following transplantation, the client is at high risk for infection and bleeding until the transfused stem cells begin producing white blood cells again.

COMPLICATIONS

Pancytopenia

Decrease in white and red blood cells and platelets
- Neutropenia secondary to disease or treatment greatly increases the client's risk for infection.
- The risk of serious infection increases as the ANC falls. An ANC less than 1,000/mm³ indicates a weak immune system. The nurse should implement neutropenic precautions, including placing the client in a private room.

NURSING ACTIONS
- Maintain a hygienic environment and encourage the client to do the same.
- Monitor for infection (cough, alterations in breath sounds, urine, or feces). Report temperature greater than 37.8° C (100° F).
- Administer antimicrobial, antiviral, and antifungal medications as prescribed.
- Administer blood products (granulocytes) as needed.

Thrombocytopenia

- Secondary to disease and/or treatment; greatly increases the client's risk for bleeding.
- The greatest risk is at platelet counts less than 50,000/mm³, and spontaneous bleeding can occur at less than 20,000/mm³. Qs

NURSING ACTIONS
- Monitor for petechiae, ecchymosis, bleeding of the gums, nosebleeds, and occult or frank blood in stool, urine, or vomitus.
- Institute bleeding precautions. (Avoid IVs and injections; apply pressure for approximately 10 min after blood is obtained; and handle client gently and avoid trauma.)
- Minimize the risk of trauma (safe environment).
- Administer blood products (platelets) if platelet count is less than 10,000/mm³.

Hypoxemia

Anemia secondary to disease or treatment significantly increases the client's risk for hypoxemia.

NURSING ACTIONS
- Plan client care to balance rest and activity and use assistive devices, as indicated.
- Monitor RBC.
- Provide a diet high in protein and carbohydrates.
- Administer colony-stimulating factors, such as epoetin alfa, as prescribed.
- Administer blood products (packed red blood cells) as needed.

BONE MARROW TRANSPLANT COMPLICATIONS

Failure of stem cells to engraft (grow)

Bone marrow transplant must be repeated.

Graft-versus-host disease (graft rejection)

NURSING ACTIONS: Administer immunosuppressants as prescribed.

Phlebitis

Blockage/inflammation of veins in the liver can occur up to 1 month after bone marrow transplant.

NURSING ACTIONS
- Monitor for jaundice, abdominal pain, and liver enlargement.
- Monitor daily weights and abdominal girth to assess for fluid retention.

Thyroid cancer

As thyroid tumors increase in size or spread, they impact the function of surrounding structures (larynx, pharynx, esophagus).

The four types of thyroid cancer

Papillary carcinoma grows slowly and is the most common form.

Follicular carcinoma affects blood vessels, bone, and lung tissues. It often attaches to the trachea, muscles, vasculature, and skin.

Medullary carcinoma is often the result of an endocrine disorder, which causes multiple tumors, most common in clients older than 50.

Anaplastic carcinoma replicates quickly, invading the area surrounding the tumor. It usually metastasizes before diagnosis.

HEALTH PROMOTION AND DISEASE PREVENTION

- Avoid or stop smoking.
- Wear a thyroid guard to protect the neck during upper body x-rays.

ASSESSMENT

RISK FACTORS

- Female gender
- Diet low in iodine (follicular carcinoma)
- Radiation exposure
- Older adults have higher incidence of follicular and medullary carcinoma. Ⓖ

EXPECTED FINDINGS

- Dyspnea
- Hoarse voice
- Dysphasia
- Stridor
- Change in size, shape of thyroid
- Palpable nodules or irregularities
- Dehydration (hormone imbalance)
- Thyroid bruits (possible with enlargement)

DIAGNOSTIC PROCEDURES

Serum thyroglobulin

EXPECTED FINDINGS: Elevated

NURSING ACTIONS: Inform the client that the result can indicate remaining cancer cells after treatment or return of cancer.

TSH, T_3, T_4

EXPECTED FINDINGS
- Indicates function of the thyroid
- T_3, T_4 levels, and TSH are usually normal in thyroid cancer

CLIENT EDUCATION: Inform the client that results indicate the function of the thyroid. Instruct regarding additional testing needed.

Calcitonin

EXPECTED FINDINGS: Elevated

CLIENT EDUCATION: Inform client that this can indicate medullary carcinoma of the thyroid.

24-hr urine

EXPECTED FINDINGS: Altered TSH, T_3, T_4, or iodine levels

CLIENT EDUCATION: Instruct the client to discard the first void, then save all urine for the next 24 hr.

Other laboratory testing

EXPECTED FINDINGS: Adrenocorticotropic hormone, prostaglandins, serotonin (medullary carcinoma)

CLIENT EDUCATION: Explain unexpected findings to the client.

BRAF gene mutation

EXPECTED FINDINGS: Presence indicates carcinoma, possible thyroid papillary cancer.

NURSING ACTIONS: Consult genetic counseling services, if indicated.

RET/PTC gene alterations

EXPECTED FINDINGS: Presence indicates high probability of papillary carcinoma.

NURSING ACTIONS: Consult genetic counseling services, if indicated.

Carcinoembryonic agent (CEA)

EXPECTED FINDINGS: Positive indicates cancer, possible medullary carcinoma

CLIENT EDUCATION: Inform the client that CEA can represent many types of cancer.

Biopsy (fine-needle plus open or core, if indicated)

EXPECTED FINDINGS: To identify presence of cancer cells in thyroid nodules or lymph nodes

NURSING ACTIONS
- Instruct client that lesions greater than 1 cm and suspicious lymph nodes are tested.
- Administer pain medication as prescribed.
- Apply pressure for 5 to 10 min, then a pressure dressing.
- Monitor for bleeding and infection for 24 hr.

Laryngoscopy

EXPECTED FINDINGS: Presence of cancer on vocal cords

CLIENT EDUCATION: Instruct the client to not eat or drink after midnight prior to the procedure.

Ultrasound

EXPECTED FINDINGS
- Used to guide biopsy
- Reveals whether nodules are fluid-filled (typically benign) or solid (typically cancerous).

NURSING ACTIONS: Instruct and prepare client for the procedure.

Radioiodine scan

EXPECTED FINDINGS
- Presence of radioactive cells (cells that retained radioiodine)
- Not useful with medullary carcinoma

CLIENT EDUCATION: Inform the client that dye will be administered (injection or oral) then the thyroid and other suspicious areas are scanned.

Chest x-ray, MRI, PET scan, CT scan

EXPECTED FINDINGS: Presence of disease or metastatic disease

PATIENT-CENTERED CARE

NURSING CARE

- Monitor airway patency in client who has a tumor affecting or compressing the trachea.
- Assess swallowing in client who has a tumor affecting or compressing the esophagus.
- Administer medications as prescribed to treat hypertension, dysrhythmia, or tachycardia.

MEDICATIONS

Thyroid suppression therapy

- Involves administration of synthetic thyroxine (T_4, levothyroxine sodium).
- Suppression therapy replaces T_4 needed for body function. It also prevents or slows growth of cancerous thyroid cells.
- Therapy is typically prescribed for several months following thyroid surgery.

CLIENT EDUCATION
- Instruct the client to never stop taking levothyroxine sodium, unless instructed by the provider. Qs
- Instruct the client to take levothyroxine sodium on an empty stomach.

THERAPEUTIC PROCEDURES

Radiation

Used to treat anaplastic carcinoma.

Radioactive iodine (RAI) therapy

Used to destroy papillary or follicular carcinoma and can be used to treat hyperthyroidism.
- RAI therapy works similarly to radioactive scanning (used to diagnose thyroid cancer).
- The client ingests RAI in liquid or tablet form, which is absorbed by thyroid cells which are then destroyed.
- Client can benefit from RAI therapy following thyroid suppression therapy.

NURSING ACTIONS
- Teach the client about radioactive precautions to reduce risk of radiation exposure.
- Instruct the client to chew gum or suck on hard candy to relieve dry mouth or reduced salivation.
- Provide information on nutrition supplements for client experiencing altered taste. Consult nutrition services.

Surgical interventions

Papillary, follicular, and medullary carcinoma are treated surgically.
- **Thyroidectomy** (total or partial) or **thyroid lobectomy** is the treatment of choice for papillary carcinoma that is limited to the thyroid gland.
- Involved lymph nodes in the neck are removed during surgery.
- During surgery, the parathyroid glands or laryngeal nerve can be damaged.
- A wound drain can be placed intraoperatively.

NURSING ACTIONS
- Monitor and treat cardiac abnormalities as prescribed.
- Support neck with pillows or sandbags.
- Maintain a humidifier to promote airway clearance.
- Monitor for hemorrhage (incision site, hypotension, tachycardia, increased swallowing or throat "tickling").
- Monitor for respiratory distress (caused by tetany, swelling, or laryngeal nerve damage).
- Monitor for parathyroid injury (decreased PTH, hypocalcemia, tetany).
- Monitor for thyroid storm (excessive release of thyroid hormone).

CLIENT EDUCATION
- Teach the client to place both hands behind the neck when moving or coughing (reduces strain on the incision).
- Teach the client that suppressive therapy with thyroid hormone is typically prescribed.

CLIENT EDUCATION

CARE AFTER DISCHARGE: Teach client strategies for managing hypothyroidism (e.g., importance of thyroid hormone replacement therapy).

NURSING ACTIONS
- Monitor vital signs for impaired oxygenation, hypotension, or bradycardia.
- Use ECG monitoring to detect dysrhythmias.
- Assess mental status and provide a safe environment.

COMPLICATIONS

Myxedema coma

A rare, potentially lethal form of hypothyroidism resulting in decreased respiratory function (respiratory depression and cerebral hypoxia), altered cardiovascular function (bradycardia, hypotension, decreased cardiac output), endocrine abnormalities (hypoglycemia and hyponatremia), hypothermia, and stupor.

NURSING ACTIONS
- Notify provider of suspected myxedema coma.
- Provide continuous monitoring of telemetry and vital signs.
- Administer fluids, electrolytes, and medications as prescribed.

Thyroid storm

- Caused by excess thyroid hormone release following surgery. This is a life-threatening emergency.
- Key findings are fever, tachycardia, and systolic hypertension. Other manifestations include GI disturbance (nausea, vomiting, diarrhea, abdominal pain), anxiety, restlessness, confusion (progresses to psychosis), and neurological alterations (tremors or seizure).

NURSING ACTIONS
- Notify the provider immediately.
- Administer antithyroid drugs, sodium iodide, beta-adrenergic blocking agents, and glucocorticoids as prescribed.
- Monitor cardiac rhythm and central venous pressure.
- Reduce fever (administer antipyretics, apply cooling blanket).

Lung cancer

- Lung cancer is one of the leading causes of cancer-related deaths for both men and women.
- Prognosis of lung cancer is poor because it is often diagnosed in an advanced stage, when metastasis has occurred. Palliative care is often the focus at the advanced stage (III, IV).
- Most lung cancers arise from bronchogenic carcinomas (arising from the bronchial epithelium)
- Most lung cancers are non-small cell lung cancer (NSCLC), which includes squamous, adeno, and large cell carcinomas.
- Small cell lung cancer (SCLC) is fast-growing and is consistently linked to a history of cigarette smoking.

HEALTH PROMOTION AND DISEASE PREVENTION

- Promote smoking cessation.
- Use protective equipment (mask) and ensure proper ventilation while working in environments that can contain carcinogens or particles in the air.
- Screening (annual CT) for early detection for those at high risk for lung cancer development

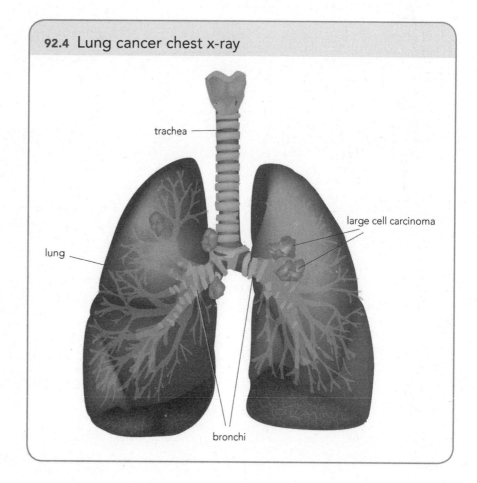

92.4 Lung cancer chest x-ray

trachea

large cell carcinoma

lung

bronchi

ASSESSMENT

RISK FACTORS

- Cigarette smoking (including secondhand smoke)
- Radiation exposure
- Chronic exposure to inhaled environmental irritants (air pollution, asbestos, other talc dusts)
- Older adult clients have decreased pulmonary reserves due to normal lung changes (decreased lung elasticity and thickening alveoli), contributing to impaired gas exchange. Ⓒ
- Structural changes in the skeletal system decrease diaphragmatic expansion, thereby restricting ventilation.

EXPECTED FINDINGS

- Orthopnea
- Chronic cough
- Chronic dyspnea
- Chest wall pain
- Fatigue, weight loss, or anorexia
- Clients can experience few manifestations early in the disease. Monitor for manifestations that often appear late in the disease.
  - Fever (pneumonitis or bronchitis that occurs with obstruction)
  - Persistent cough, with or without hemoptysis (rust-colored or blood-tinged sputum)
  - Hoarseness
  - Altered breathing pattern: dyspnea, prolonged exhalation alternated with shallow breaths (obstruction), rapid, shallow breaths (pleuritic chest pain, elevated diaphragm)
  - Altered breath sounds (wheezing)
  - Diminished or absent breath sounds (obstruction)
  - Chest pain or tightness
  - Chest wall masses
  - Muffled heart sounds
  - Pleural friction rub
  - Clubbing of fingers
  - Increased work of breathing (retractions, use of accessory muscle, stridor, nasal flaring)
  - Decreased bone density

DIAGNOSTIC PROCEDURES

Cytologic testing; thoracentesis (if pleural effusion is present)

EXPECTED FINDINGS: Sputum specimen contains cancer cells

NURSING ACTIONS: Instruct regarding sputum specimen collection. Advise cancer cells might not always be found in sputum specimens if when cancer is present.

Thoracoscopy

EXPECTED FINDINGS: Presence of cancer cells

NURSING ACTIONS: Keep client NPO after midnight.

Biopsy (bronchoscopy)

EXPECTED FINDINGS: Presence of tumor

NURSING ACTIONS

- Keep client NPO after midnight.
- Provide throat lozenges or sprays for report of a sore throat once the gag reflex returns following the procedure.

X-ray, CT scan (92.4)

EXPECTED FINDINGS: Presence of tumor

NURSING ACTIONS: Explain and prepare client for the procedure.

Needle biopsy of lymph nodes, thoracentesis with pleural biopsy; MRI, PET scan

EXPECTED FINDINGS: Presence of cancer and metastatic disease

NURSING ACTIONS: Explain and prepare client for the procedure.

Pulmonary function tests and arterial blood gases

EXPECTED FINDINGS: Compromised respiratory status

NURSING ACTIONS: Explain and prepare client for the procedure.

PATIENT-CENTERED CARE

NURSING CARE

- Determine the pack-year history (number of packs of cigarettes smoked per day times the number of years smoked) for clients who smoke. ⒬EBP
- Evaluate use of other tobacco products (cigars, pipes, and chewing tobacco).
- Ask about exposure to secondhand smoke.
- Monitor for a cough that changes in pattern.
- Monitor nutritional status, weight loss, and anorexia.
  - Promote adequate nutrition to provide needed calories for increased work of breathing and prevention of infection.
  - Encourage fluids to promote adequate hydration.
- Maintain a patent airway and suction as needed.
- Position the client in Fowler's position to maximize ventilation.

MEDICATIONS

Bronchodilators and corticosteroids can be given to help decrease inflammation and to dry secretions.

THERAPEUTIC PROCEDURES

Chemotherapy

Chemotherapy is the primary choice of treatment for lung cancers. It is often used in combination with radiation and/or surgery. Platinum compounds such as cisplatin are commonly used.

ADVERSE EFFECTS include nausea, vomiting, hair loss, mucositis, neutropenia, thrombocytopenia, and peripheral neuropathy.

Photodynamic therapy (92.2)

Photodynamic therapy is performed through bronchoscopy to treat small, accessible tumors.

Radiation therapy (92.2)

Radiation therapy is effective for lung cancer that has not spread beyond the chest wall and is used as an adjuvant therapy.

Radiofrequency ablation (92.2)

Most commonly used with NSCLC.

Targeted therapy (92.2)

Surgical interventions

- The goal of surgery is to remove all tumor cells, including involved lymph nodes.
- Often involves removal of a lung (pneumonectomy), lobe (lobectomy), segment (segmentectomy), or peripheral lung tissue (wedge resection).

NURSING ACTIONS
- Monitor vital signs, oxygenation (SaO$_2$, ABG values), and for evidence of hemorrhage.
- Manage the chest tube and drainage system.
- Administer oxygen and manage the ventilator if appropriate.
- Manage pain. Teach the client regarding PCA use if prescribed.

CLIENT EDUCATION: Teach the client about the surgical procedure and chest tube placement.

Palliative procedures

- Thoracentesis or pleurodesis to ease breathing
- Laser therapy and photodynamic therapy can be used in treatment and palliative therapy to open airways blocked by tumors.
- Pericardiocentesis or pericardial window to improve cardiac function

INTERPROFESSIONAL CARE

- Respiratory services should be consulted for inhalers, breathing treatments, and suctioning for airway management.
- Rehabilitation care may be consulted if the client has prolonged weakness and needs assistance with increasing the level of activity.

CLIENT EDUCATION

- Encourage the client to take rest periods as needed.
- Encourage the client to eat high-calorie foods to promote energy.
- Promote smoking cessation if the client smokes.
- Provide information for psychosocial support. Q𝗣𝗖𝗖

COMPLICATIONS

Superior vena cava syndrome

- Results from pressure placed on the vena cava by a tumor. It is a medical emergency.
- Radiation and stent placement provide temporary relief. Prepare the client for radiation and stent placement.

NURSING ACTIONS
- Monitor for manifestations of superior vena cava syndrome and report to the provider immediately.
  - Early findings include facial edema, edema in neck, nosebleeds, peripheral edema, and dyspnea.
  - Late findings include mental status changes, cyanosis, hemorrhage, and hypotension.
- Monitor vital signs and oxygenation during and after the procedure.

Oropharyngeal cancer

- Oral and pharyngeal carcinoma are more lethal than many types of cancer (cervical, testicular, thyroid, Hodgkin's lymphoma).
- Mouth lesions that do not heal within 2 weeks can be cancerous and should be reported to a provider.
- Oropharyngeal cancer has a high rate of recurrence.

The three main types of oropharyngeal cancer

Squamous cell carcinoma is the most common oral cancer and can be present on the lips, tongue, buccal mucosa, and oropharynx.

Basal cell carcinoma affects the lips and skin around the mouth.

Kaposi's sarcoma can be found on the hard palate, gums, tongue, or tonsils. Lesions appear as raised, purple nodules or plaques.

HEALTH PROMOTION AND DISEASE PREVENTION

- Schedule dental visits twice yearly for cleaning and inspection of mouth tissues.
- Limit exposure to ultraviolet rays (mid-day sun exposure, indoor tanning).
- Eliminate tobacco use.

ASSESSMENT

RISK FACTORS

- Male gender
- Tobacco use
- Alcohol consumption (alcohol use combined with tobacco use significantly increases risk)
- Radiation exposure, including x-rays of head and neck
- Inadequate oral hygiene
- Lack of fruits and vegetables in the diet
- Occupation in textile, coal, metal, and plumbing industries
- Age older than 40 years
- Human papilloma virus (HPV16) infection
- Periodontal disease with mandibular bone loss
- TP53 gene mutation
- Weakened immune system

EXPECTED FINDINGS

- Mucosal erythroplasia (red patches): earliest finding
- Oral bleeding
- Difficulty chewing or swallowing
- Speech changes
- Thick or absent saliva
- Palpable masses
- Facial paresthesia

DIAGNOSTIC PROCEDURES

Biopsy: fine-needle, incisional, excisional

EXPECTED FINDINGS: Presence of cancer

CLIENT EDUCATION: Provide diagnosis-specific information.

Cell brushing

EXPECTED FINDINGS: Presence of cancer

CLIENT EDUCATION: Inform client that a brush will be used to collect cells from suspicious areas in the mouth.

Toluidine blue 1% staining

EXPECTED FINDINGS: Malignant oral lesions retain blue stain

CLIENT EDUCATION: Inform client that false positives are possible with inflammatory lesions.

MRI

EXPECTED FINDINGS
- Presence of cancer
- Thickness of lesion
- Presence of nerve involvement

CLIENT EDUCATION: Instruct and prepare client for procedure.

PATIENT-CENTERED CARE

Protecting the airway and providing adequate nutrition are priority interventions in managing oropharyngeal cancer. Qs

NURSING CARE

- Monitor for adequate clearance of secretions (have the client turn, cough, deep breathe; suction as needed).
- Auscultate for adventitious lung sounds: wheezes (due to aspiration) or stridor (due to obstruction).
- Consult respiratory therapy to provide chest physiotherapy, as indicated.
- Position the client in semi- or high-Fowler's position to promote chest expansion.
- Use a cool mist face tent to promote clearance of secretions and reduce inflammation.
- Assess for difficulty swallowing.
- Administer steroids to reduce inflammation; administer antibiotic if infection is present
- Perform oral hygiene every 2 hr (use an ultra-soft brush or foam brush for a client who has a platelet count less than 40,000/mm³).

MEDICATIONS

- Medications that block growth factor receptors prevent tumor growth (cetuximab, erlotinib).
- Antibiotics for infection as indicated

INTERPROFESSIONAL CARE

- Provide alternate means of communication for clients who have impaired communication (pen and paper, picture boards). Consult speech therapy, as indicated.
- Consult nutrition services to assess swallowing and provide nutrition recommendations, as needed.

THERAPEUTIC PROCEDURES

Radiation and/or chemotherapy is used to treat oral lesions.

Targeted therapy (92.2)

Ablation (cryotherapy, photodynamic therapy) (92.2)

Used to remove lesions.

Radiation (external, implanted, or both)

Commonly used prior to surgery to reduce tumor size.
- **External radiation** is used cautiously to minimize radiation dose to the brain and spinal cord.
- **Implanted radiation** is used to cure early lesion on the floor of the mouth or anterior tongue.
- Hospitalization is typically required until radiation dosing is complete.
- Place client on radiation transmission precautions. See **CHAPTER 91: CANCER TREATMENT OPTIONS.**
- Provide tracheostomy care if needed. Tracheostomy can be required due to edema and increased oral secretions.

Photodynamic therapy (92.2)

Tumor excision

Used to remove lesions through the inside of the mouth or through external entry into the head and neck.

- The larger the tumor, the greater the risk to the client for disfigurement and loss of function.
- Composite resections are the most extensive form of oral carcinoma surgery. They can include partial or total glossectomy and partial mandibulectomy.
- Combined neck dissection, mandibulectomy, and oropharyngeal resection can be used ("commando" procedure).
- Radical neck dissection can include removal of the sternocleidomastoid muscle, internal jugular vein, cranial nerve XI (accessory nerve), and all cervical lymph nodes on the affected side.
- Surgery to remove large lesions can also include placement of a tracheostomy or wound drain.

NURSING ACTIONS

- Provide clear liquid diet for 24 hr (clients having small lesions removed locally).
- Maintain NPO status until intraoral suture lines heal (clients who have large tumors).
- Provide routine tracheostomy care and suctioning, as appropriate.
- Monitor wounds, incision sites, and donor grafting sites for evidence of infection.
- Consult a speech language pathologist for clients who have slurred speech or difficulty speaking.
- Provide comfort to clients who have permanent loss of voice or disfigurement. Make a referral to counseling services, as indicated.
- Teach clients to avoid mouthwashes containing alcohol or lemon-glycerin swabs (acidic) to prevent pain and worsening of condition. Q EBP
- Encourage the client to rinse mouth frequently with warm sodium bicarbonate or 0.9% sodium chloride solution.

CLIENT EDUCATION

- Teach the client about the need and options for alternate communication following surgery.
- Teach the client to keep the head of the bed elevated to reduce edema.
- Instruct the client to report leakage of fluid from the suture line, swallowing difficulty, or coughing once oral intake is resumed.
- Encourage the client to perform swallowing exercises regularly, as prescribed.
- Teach the client and family how to thicken liquids prior to consumption, as indicted.
- Instruct the client and family to continue thorough, frequent oral hygiene at home, cleansing the toothbrush after each use.
- Instruct the client about possible temporary or permanent loss or changes in taste (dislike of meats, metallic taste).
- Instruct clients that some people who are cured will later develop cancer of the lung, mouth, or throat and will need follow-up exams for the rest of their life

COMPLICATIONS

Osteonecrosis (bone death) and issues related to motor impairment of jaw structure

Colorectal cancer

- Colorectal cancer (CRC) is cancer of the rectum or colon. Most CRCs are adenocarcinoma, a tumor that arises from a gland in the epithelial layer of the colon.
- CRC occurs in stages from 0 to IV according to the tissue depth of the lesion and whether it has spread to local or distant sites.
- Adenocarcinoma begins as a polyp and is benign in the early stages. If left untreated, the polyp will grow and the risk of malignancy increases.
- CRC can metastasize (through blood or lymph) to the liver (most common site), lungs, brain, or bones. Spreading can occur as a result of peritoneal seeding (during surgical resection of tumor).
- The most common location of CRC is the rectosigmoidal region.

HEALTH PROMOTION/ DISEASE PREVENTION

- Consume a diet rich in calcium (calcium binds to free fatty acids and bile salts in the lower gastrointestinal tract).
- Consume diet low in fat and simple carbohydrates but high in fiber.
- Age-specific regular colorectal cancer screening
- Genetic testing for familial adenomatous polyposis and hereditary nonpolyposis colorectal cancer for those whose family members have had hereditary colorectal cancer
- Engage in healthy lifestyle including regular physical exercise, and no smoking or excessive alcohol use.

ASSESSMENT

RISK FACTORS

- CRC is more common in women; rectal cancer is more common in men.
- Adenomatous colon polyps
- African American descent
- Inflammatory bowel disease (ulcerative colitis, Crohn's disease)
- High-fat, low-fiber diet
- Age older than 50 years; incidence in younger clients related to HPV infections
- Long-term smoking
- Physical inactivity
- Heavy alcohol consumption
- Infection exposure to *Helicobacter pylori*, *Streptococcus bovis*, John Cunningham virus, and human papilloma virus
- History of breast, ovarian, or endometrial cancer

EXPECTED FINDINGS

- Changes in stool consistency or shape (with or without noticeable blood)
- Blood in stool (many times the only finding)
  - Left-sided tumors are more likely to produce frank bleeding and change in bowel pattern, consistency.
  - Right-sided tumors cause stools to be darker due to ulceration of the colon and intermittent bleeding.
- Cramps and/or gas
- Palpable mass (elicited by provider only through abdominal palpation or digital rectal exam)
- Weight loss and fatigue
- Vomiting
- Abdominal fullness, distention or pain
- Abnormal bowel sounds indicative of obstruction (high-pitched tinkling bowel sounds)

DIAGNOSTIC PROCEDURES

- Virtual colonoscopy can be performed using CT scan or MRI. Imaging is performed after air is injected into the colon. The procedure is otherwise noninvasive. No sedation is required.
- Screening guidelines for individuals with polyps or a family history of CRC should be initiated at an earlier age and possibly performed more frequently.

Fecal occult blood testing (FOBT)

EXPECTED FINDINGS: Two positive stools within 3 days

NURSING ACTIONS

- Do not use stool from digital rectal examination to avoid false-positive results.
- Instruct client to avoid red meat, anti-inflammatory medications, and vitamin C for 48 hr prior to testing (to prevent false positives).
- Negative results to not completely rule out the possibility of CRC.
- Recommend annual FOBT for clients ages 50 to 75.

Biopsy (endoscopic)

EXPECTED FINDINGS: Definitive diagnosis

CLIENT EDUCATION: Provide client with diagnosis-specific information.

Traditional or CT guided colonoscopy

EXPECTED FINDINGS: Visualization of lesions (CT guided scan more accurate)

NURSING ACTIONS

- Prepare client for procedure.
- Instruct client on diet regimen (clear liquids then NPO after midnight) and bowel preparation for colonoscopy.

Endoscopy: colonoscopy, sigmoidoscopy

EXPECTED FINDINGS: Visualization of polyps or lesions

CLIENT EDUCATION: Recommend screening between ages 50 and 75 (colonoscopy every 10 years, sigmoidoscopy every 5 years).

Double contrast (air and barium) barium enema

EXPECTED FINDINGS: Visualization and location of tumor

NURSING ACTIONS: Administer stimulant laxative following procedure as prescribed (facilitates evacuation of barium, which can harden in the intestine).

CBC

EXPECTED FINDINGS: Decreased hemoglobin, hematocrit

CLIENT EDUCATION: Explain unexpected findings.

Carcinoembryonic antigen (CEA)

EXPECTED FINDINGS: Positive (denotes malignancy; not specific to CRC)

CLIENT EDUCATION: Inform the client that positive CEA can be indicative of many types of cancer.

CT, MRI

EXPECTED FINDINGS: Visualization and location of tumor and/or metastasis

PATIENT-CENTERED CARE

THERAPEUTIC PROCEDURES

Colon resection (colectomy): Involves the removal of a portion of the colon to excise the tumor. Open surgical or laparoscopic methods can be used. The remaining colon can be reconnected by (end-to-end) anastomosis or a colostomy can be created (temporary or permanent).

Colectomy: Removal of the colon with a temporary or permanent colostomy or ileostomy

Abdominal-perineal (AP) resection

NURSING ACTIONS

- Assess the stoma (should be reddish pink, moist, small amount of blood postoperatively) and report ischemia, necrosis, or frank bleeding. **(92.5)**
- Manage pain and teach the client regarding PCA.
- Maintain nasogastric suction (decompression).
- Progress the diet slowly after suctioning is discontinued and monitor the client's response (bowel sounds present, no nausea or vomiting).
- Instruct the client to avoid heavy lifting.
- Instruct the client on the use of stool softeners as prescribed to avoid straining.
- Provide ostomy teaching (findings of ischemia to be reported to the provider, expected output, appliance management) if applicable.
- Management of a colostomy can be more difficult for the older adult client due to impaired vision and a decline in fine motor skills. Ⓖ

PREOPERATIVE CLIENT EDUCATION

- Educate the client regarding preoperative diet (clear liquids several days prior to surgery).
- Instruct the client to complete bowel prep with cathartics as prescribed.
- Inform the client of the administration of antibiotics (neomycin, metronidazole) to eradicate intestinal flora.

POSTOPERATIVE CLIENT EDUCATION

- Teach client regarding turning and deep breathing
- Educate the client regarding the care of the incision, activity limits, and ostomy care, if applicable.
- Provide instructions regarding management of postoperative complications, including incontinence or sexual dysfunction (most likely to occur with AP resection).

Chemotherapy

Given for stage IV cancer.

Adjuvant therapy

Given to decrease the chance of metastases for stage II and distant metastases for type III cancers.

Targeted medication therapy (92.2)

Monoclonal antibodies
- Angiogenesis inhibitors (inhibit growth of new blood vessels to tumors): bevacizumab
- Tyrosine kinase inhibitors (decrease cell proliferation and increase cell death of certain cancers): cetuximab and panitumumab

Radiation therapy

Radiation therapy is given in conjunction with chemotherapy to improve prognosis (usually used for rectal cancer to prevent lymph node involvement and recurrence). Radiation can also be used as a palliative measure to control pain, hemorrhage, bowel obstruction, or metastatic disease.

INTERPROFESSIONAL CARE

- Ostomy nurse referral for instruction on care of colostomy
- Referral to ostomy support group
- Case manager or social worker for ongoing patient and family support

COMPLICATIONS

Second primary colorectal tumor or complete intestinal obstruction.

Pancreatic cancer

- Pancreatic carcinoma has vague manifestations and is usually diagnosed in late stages after liver or gall bladder involvement.
- Tumors are usually adenocarcinoma, originate in the pancreatic head, and grow rapidly in glandular patterns.
- It has a high mortality rate. Five year survival rates are low.

ASSESSMENT

RISK FACTORS

- Possible inherited risk
- Older than 45 years of age, male gender
- More likely in African American clients
- Tobacco use
- Chronic pancreatitis
- Cirrhosis
- High intake of red meat (especially processed)
- Long-term exposure to gasoline and pesticides
- Diabetes mellitus
- Family history of pancreatic cancer
- Metastatic from another cancer, such as breast, lung, kidney, or skin

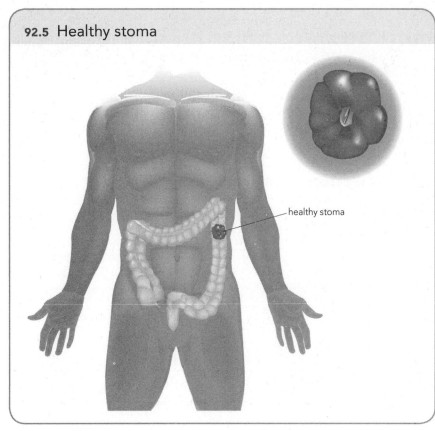

92.5 Healthy stoma

healthy stoma

EXPECTED FINDINGS

- Pain that radiates to the back and is unrelieved by change in position, and is more severe at night
- Fatigue
- Anorexia
- Pruritus

PHYSICAL ASSESSMENT FINDINGS
- Weight loss
- Palpable abdominal mass, enlarged gallbladder and liver
- Hepatomegaly
- Jaundice (late finding)
- Clay colored stools
- Dark, frothy urine
- Ascites
- Pruritus (buildup of bile salt)
- Early satiety or anorexia

DIAGNOSTIC PROCEDURES

Biopsy (percutaneous or laparoscopic)

EXPECTED FINDINGS: Presence of cancer cells; holds some risk of seeding (not always performed if imaging shows tumor can be surgically removed)

CLIENT EDUCATION: Provide diagnosis-specific information.

Endoscopic retrograde cholangiopancreatography (ERCP)

EXPECTED FINDINGS: Definitive diagnosis of tumor

CLIENT EDUCATION: Inform client that a biliary drain or stent can be placed during the procedure.

Abdominal paracentesis

EXPECTED FINDINGS: Presence of malignant cells in abdominal fluid

CLIENT EDUCATION: Instruct client on care of dressing at puncture site and activity restrictions, as prescribed.

Tumor markers

CA 19-9

Carcinoembryonic antigen (CEA)

EXPECTED FINDINGS: Positive (denotes non-specific malignancy)

CLIENT EDUCATION: Inform client that CA 19-9 or CEA can indicate many types of cancer.

Other laboratory testing

EXPECTED FINDINGS: Amylase, lipase, alkaline phosphatase, and bilirubin-elevated

NURSING ACTIONS: Elevated liver enzymes, albumin, and bilirubin can indicate primary or metastatic cancer.

Imaging

EXPECTED FINDINGS: Ultrasound or computerized tomography-visualization of the tumor during biopsy

NURSING ACTIONS: Prepare client and explain unexpected findings.

Endoscopic ultrasound

EXPECTED FINDINGS: Visualization of tumor in clients who have strong family history or genetic syndrome that increases risk.

NURSING ACTIONS: Prepare client and explain unexpected findings.

PATIENT-CENTERED CARE

NURSING CARE

- Care of a client who has pancreatic cancer usually focuses on palliation and not curative measures. Pain management is the priority intervention. Advise client to ask for analgesics before the pain becomes severe.
- Monitor blood glucose and administer insulin as prescribed.
- A jejunostomy is often placed to provide enteral feedings (prevents reflux, promotes absorption). Provide nutritional support (enteral supplements, TPN).

NURSING ACTIONS: Increase feeding as tolerated, monitoring frequency of diarrhea.

THERAPEUTIC PROCEDURES

Chemotherapy

Chemotherapy can be used to shrink tumor size. Several medications are given to improve the results.
- **Targeted therapy** can be included.
- **Radiation** can be used to shrink tumor size.

Surgical interventions

Can be open or laparoscopic. ⓠEBP

Surgical interventions can be considered potentially curative or palliative.

Partial pancreatectomy: Used to remove tumors less than 3 cm in diameter.

Total pancreatectomy: Removes the entire pancreas.

Whipple procedure (pancreaticoduodenectomy): Removal of the head of the pancreas, duodenum, parts of the jejunum and stomach, gallbladder, and possibly the spleen. The pancreatic duct is connected to the common bile duct, and the stomach is connected to the jejunum.

NURSING ACTIONS
- Monitor NG tube and surgical drains for color and amount.
- Monitor for bloody or bile-tinged drainage, which could indicate anastomotic disruption.
- Place the client in semi-Fowler's position to facilitate lung expansion and to prevent stress on the suture line.
- Monitor blood glucose and administer insulin as needed.

CLIENT EDUCATION: Instruct the client about support measures for pain, anorexia, weight loss, and community resources.

Palliative to relieve or prevent symptoms

Stent placement: A stent is placed to keep the bile duct open and resists compression form the surrounding cancer.

Bypass surgery: Reroutes the flow of bile from the common bile duct, bypassing the pancreas and into the small intestines.

COMPLICATIONS

Fistulas

Breakdown of a site of anastomosis

NURSING ACTIONS: Report drainage that is not serosanguineous from the drain, or drainage from the wound to the provider immediately.

Peritonitis

Internal leakage of corrosive pancreatic fluid

NURSING ACTIONS
- Monitor for manifestations of peritonitis (elevated fever, WBC, abdominal pain, abdominal tenderness/rebound tenderness, alteration in bowel sounds, shoulder pain).
- Administer antibiotics as prescribed.

Thromboembolism

Due to hypercoagulable state caused by release of necrotic products from the tumor, immobility postoperatively

NURSING ACTIONS
- Report findings of thromboembolism to the provider.
- Administer anticoagulants as prescribed.
- Maintain bed rest as indicated.

Liver cancer

Hepatocellular carcinoma (HCC) is the most frequently occurring type of primary liver cancer. Primary liver cancer can also originate in the bile duct or liver vasculature.

Cancers can be primary tumors originating in the liver or metastatic cancers that spread from other organ to the liver.

Intrahepatic cholangiocarcinomas: Cancer that starts in the cells that line the small bile ducts

Angiosarcoma/hemangioma: Rare cancer that starts in cells lining the blood vessels of the liver

Hepatoblastoma: Rare cancer that develops in children, typically younger than 4 years old

HEALTH PROMOTION AND DISEASE PREVENTION

- Avoid excessive alcohol intake.
- Eat a low-fat diet and maintain a BMI less than 30.
- Receive a hepatitis B vaccination.
- Take precautions against hepatitis B and C. (Recognize that multiple sexual partners, IV drug use, and the sharing of needles all increase risk.)

ASSESSMENT

RISK FACTORS

- Older age ©
- Cirrhosis
  - Chronic hepatitis B or C infection
  - Alcohol-related liver disease
  - Hemochromatosis (inability to breakdown iron)
- Male gender
- Tobacco use
- Mediterranean or Asian heritage (particularly Vietnamese)
- African American or Hispanic clients

EXPECTED FINDINGS

- Abdominal pain
- Loss of appetite
- Weakness and fatigue

PHYSICAL ASSESSMENT FINDINGS
- Weight loss
- Enlarged liver upon palpation
- Jaundice
- Ascites
- Pruritus
- Encephalopathy
- Bleeding or bruising

DIAGNOSTIC PROCEDURES

Biopsy

Percutaneous or through the jugular to the hepatic veins (via fluoroscopy)

EXPECTED FINDINGS: Presence of cancerous cells

NURSING ACTIONS
- Inform client that biopsy through venous route reduces the risk of hemorrhage.
- Position the client to the right side for 1 to 2 hr to ensure hemostasis.
- Monitor for hemorrhage (coagulation studies, frank bleeding).

Alpha-fetoprotein (AFP)

EXPECTED FINDINGS: Elevated AFP: high probability of cancer (false positive: cirrhosis, hepatitis); elevated CEA along with elevated AFP can discriminate metastatic from primary cancer.

CLIENT EDUCATION: Educate client about potential for false positives.

Other laboratory testing

EXPECTED FINDINGS: Alkaline phosphatase (ALP), serum aspartate aminotransferase (AST), albumin, and bilirubin: elevated

CLIENT EDUCATION: Educate client about other reasons liver function tests might be elevated.

Imaging: contrast-enhanced ultrasound or CT scan

EXPECTED FINDINGS: Visualization of tumor

NURSING ACTIONS: Educate and prepare the client for procedure.

PATIENT-CENTERED CARE

NURSING CARE

- Observe for potential bleeding complications (frank bleeding, decreased hemoglobin and hematocrit, altered coagulation findings). Q_{PCC}
- Administer blood products (packed red blood cells and fresh frozen plasma) to replace blood volume and clotting factors as prescribed by the provider.
- Encourage the client to consume small, frequent meals that are high-calorie, moderate fat.
- Replace vitamins due to the inability of the liver to store them (vitamin pills or vitamin-enriched supplements).
- Restrict fluids for clients who have ascites.
- Instruct the client on the benefits of avoiding alcohol (prevents further damage, allows for healing and regeneration of the liver, decreases risk of bleeding and other life-threatening complications).
- Measure abdominal girth daily (indicates increased ascites).

- Assess for adequate nutrition (fluid and electrolytes, weight loss, anorexia).
- Monitor for worsening hepatic function (liver function tests, jaundice).
- Assess and treat pain and abdominal discomfort.
- Provide medications as prescribed. Medications are administered sparingly (especially opioids, sedatives, and barbiturates) due to impaired liver function (reduced ability to metabolize medications).

MEDICATIONS

Targeted therapy (sorafenib)
- A multi-tyrosine kinase inhibitor taken orally and used to treat advanced liver cancer.
- CLIENT EDUCATION: Teach the client to report bleeding, heart palpitations, chest pain.

Hepatic arterial infusion
- The direct infusion of chemotherapy via a catheter into the tumor. The client can go home with a catheter in place if continuous infusion is desired. Systemic adverse effects of chemotherapy are avoided through this delivery method. Q_{EBP}
- CLIENT EDUCATION: Instruct the client to watch for evidence of infection at the catheter site, hepatic toxicity (jaundice, liver function tests), and immunosuppression (fatigue, decreased WBC).

Systemically delivered chemotherapy has been found to be largely ineffective in treating tumors of the liver or prolonging life. Therefore, more direct delivery methods are used.

THERAPEUTIC PROCEDURES

Hepatic artery embolization

Using a catheter threaded through the femoral artery and up to the liver, particles are injected into the arteries that supply blood to the tumor to block blood flow. If a chemotherapeutic drug is included, this procedure is called **chemoembolization**. If radiation is included, this procedure is called **radioembolization**.

NURSING ACTIONS: Monitor for bleeding.

Ablation procedures

Can be used to destroy cancerous cells.
- Radiofrequency ablation delivers an electric current directly to the tumor via thin needles. This current is converted into heat waves that kill the cancer cells.
- Percutaneous alcohol (ethanol) injections directly into the tumor mass cause cell death.
- Cryotherapy uses liquid nitrogen injected directly into the tumor to destroy the tumor.
- Microwave thermotherapy uses microwaves transmitted through a probe to heat and destroy the abnormal tissue

NURSING ACTIONS
- Monitor for hypothermia, bile leak, and hemorrhage.
- Monitor urine for myoglobinuria.

Tunneled abdominal drain

Can be placed and used at home to remove excess ascetic fluid.

CLIENT EDUCATION

- Teach client and family how to empty the drain and maintain the system.
- Instruct the client and family not to remove more than 2,000 mL at one time to prevent hypovolemia shock.

External radiation

Although liver cancer cells are sensitive to radiation, the treatment cannot be used at very high doses because normal liver tissue is also easily damaged.

Surgical Interventions

Surgical resection or liver transplantation is required for long-term survival. Q𝐄𝐁𝐏

Surgical resection: If liver cancer involves only one lobe of the liver, surgical removal can be indicated. A liver-lobe resection can result in a survival rate of up to 5 years. Most liver tumors are not resectable.

Liver transplantation: can be an option for clients who have small primary tumors.

- Immunosuppressants that are given after the transplant can increase the risk for recurrence of cancer and for development of secondary infection.
- For interprofessional care, see **CHAPTER 91: CANCER TREATMENT OPTIONS**.

NURSING ACTIONS

- Inform the client about diagnostic tests that are done to determine if the liver cancer has metastasized (chest x-ray, PET scan, MRI, laparoscopy).
- Monitor for altered blood glucose due to stress on the liver caused by surgery.
- Monitor for bleeding, and replace fluids and blood as necessary.

COMPLICATIONS

- Acute graft rejection following liver transplantation
- Liver failure or kidney failure (due to impaired blood flow to the kidneys)

Kidney and renal pelvis cancer

- Adenocarcinoma of the kidney, or renal cell cancer (RCC), is the most common form of kidney cancer.
- Paraneoplastic syndromes (syndromes resulting from cancer in the body) can occur with RCC. The tumor can produce hormones or prevent hormone production, causing imbalance in the body. Effects include:
  - Anemia (reduced erythropoietin)
  - Erythrocytosis (excess erythropoietin)
  - Hypercalcemia (tumor production of parathyroid hormone)
  - Liver dysfunction
  - Increased sedimentation rate
  - Hypertension (increased renin)
- RCC can be discovered when imaging studies or exploratory surgery are performed for other reasons.
- RCC that spreads to the inferior vena cava has a poor prognosis.

HEALTH PROMOTION AND DISEASE PREVENTION

Minimize exposure to chemicals (environmental).

ASSESSMENT

RISK FACTORS

- Von Hippel-Lindau syndrome
- Exposure to lead, cadmium, or phosphate
- Age (55 to 60 years: highest incidence)
- Family history of kidney, bladder, ureter, prostate gland, uterus, ovary, or appendix cancer.
- Genetic and hereditary risk factors
- African American and American Indian clients

EXPECTED FINDINGS

- Smoky or cola-colored urine Q𝐄𝐁𝐏
- Hematuria (late finding)
- Hormonal changes: darkening of nipples or gynecomastia in men
- Inability to urinate or weak urine stream (urinary tract obstruction)
- Abdominal or flank pain (often dull, aching)
- Palpable mass
- Renal bruit (possible)
- Weight loss
- Fever
- Hypertension
- Hypercalcemia

DIAGNOSTIC PROCEDURES

Biopsy (percutaneous through the flank)

EXPECTED FINDINGS: Positive for cancer

NURSING ACTIONS
- Provide the client with diagnosis-specific information.
- Maintain client activity restrictions as prescribed (bed rest laying prone for at least 6 hr).

Urinalysis

EXPECTED FINDINGS: Hematuria (possible)

CLIENT EDUCATION
- Inform the client of other reasons for hematuria.
- Teach the client about the role of the kidneys in red blood cell production.
- Inform the client of other reasons for elevated ESR.

Nuclear imaging: IV urogram with nephrograms

EXPECTED FINDINGS
- Presence of tumor
- Increased (possible)

NURSING ACTIONS
- Prepare the client for the procedure (keep NPO, assess for contrast dye allergy).
- Inform the client of other reasons for increased LFTs.

Imaging: CT, MRI, PET scans

EXPECTED FINDINGS: Identify tumor borders and presence in surrounding tissue

NURSING ACTIONS: Prepare the client for imaging.

Hematologic studies

EXPECTED FINDINGS
- **Hgb/Hct:** decreased
- **Ca:** elevated
- **ESR:** elevated
- **ACTH:** elevated
- **hCG:** elevated
- **BUN/creatinine:** elevated
- **LFTs:** increases

NURSING ACTIONS: Inform client regarding lab-specific findings.

PATIENT-CENTERED CARE

NURSING CARE

Monitor urine output and laboratory findings (BUN, serum creatinine, urinalysis) to assess renal function of the unaffected kidney.

THERAPEUTIC PROCEDURES

External beam radiation

External beam radiation uses radiation from a source outside of the body to destroy cancer cells.

Targeted therapy (92.2)

Immunotherapy (biotherapy) (92.2)

Ablation therapy for kidney cancer

- Cryoablation uses a probe to deliver cold gases to the tumor
- Radiofrequency ablation uses high-energy radio waves to heat and destroy the tumor
- Arterial embolization uses a catheter to deliver material to block the artery that feeds the kidney with the tumor

Chemotherapy

Chemotherapy uses anti-cancer drugs administered orally or intravenously to destroy cancer cells. Kidney cancer cells are usually resistant to chemotherapy. However, chemotherapy can be used after targeted medication or immunotherapy.

Surgical interventions

Clients undergoing surgery for RCC are at increased risk for bleeding due to the highly vascular nature of RCC.

Nephrectomy is the standard of treatment for RCC.
- Ribs can be removed during surgery to allow better access to the kidney or tumor.
- Surgical entry can be transthoracic, lumbar, or abdominal. A wound drain can be placed.
- Adrenal glands are left intact, when possible.
- The unaffected kidney must be able to sustain adequate renal function.

NURSING ACTIONS
- Monitor vital signs and daily weight.
- Monitor lung sounds, respiratory effort, or presence of sputum production.
  - Monitor for evidence of bleeding (hypotension, decreased urine output, altered level of consciousness). Blood can pool under the client's back.
  - Monitor for adrenal insufficiency (nausea, vomiting, diarrhea, hypoglycemia, hypotension).
  - Monitor hemoglobin, hematocrit, and WBC every 6 to 12 hr for first 24 to 48 hr.
  - Monitor urine output to evaluate remaining kidney function (25 to 30 mL/hr).
  - Monitor incision, drain, and drainage
- Administer opioid analgesics for pain, as prescribed.

CLIENT EDUCATION
- Avoid lifting more than 5 lb or engaging in strenuous activity.
- Teach the client about measures to protect the function of the remaining kidney (control blood pressure, drink adequate fluids, limit NSAID use, stop smoking). Qs

COMPLICATIONS

Adrenal insufficiency

Manifestations of adrenal insufficiency are similar to those of hemorrhage (hypotension, decreased urine output, altered level of consciousness). This is a life-threatening emergency.
- Hypotension and decreased volume of urine output are preceded by an increased volume of urine output.
- Other manifestations include hyperkalemia, abdominal pain, and weakness.

NURSING ACTIONS
- Notify the provider of suspected adrenal insufficiency.
- Administer corticosteroids, as prescribed.
- Monitor ECG for dysrhythmia.
- Administer medications to remove excess potassium, and avoid potassium-sparing medications.
- Monitor capillary blood glucose hourly.
- Prevent and treat hypoglycemia (administer glucose, glucagon, or IV fluids containing dextrose) as prescribed.
- Administer IV fluids to offset volume depletion.

Spinal cord decompression

- RCC can expand and compress the spinal cord.
- Key manifestations include sharp, severe, band-like pain.

NURSING ACTIONS
- Report pain findings to the provider.
- Prepare the client for imaging studies to assess for spinal cord decompression.

Urinary bladder cancer

- Bladder cancer begins most often in the cells that line the bladder called urothelium or transitional epithelium layer.
- There are four layers of the bladder wall: transitional epithelium (innermost layer), lamina propria, muscularis propria, and fatty connective tissue. As cancer advances, it grows through the next layer.
- Bladder cancer can be invasive (cancer cells grow outside of the transitional epithelium) or noninvasive (cancer cells remain in the transitional epithelium layer). Bladder cancer is often described based on how far it invades the bladder wall.
- Transitional cell carcinoma can be further classified as papillary or flat based on how it grows.

HEALTH PROMOTION AND DISEASE PREVENTION

- Use personal protective equipment (PPE) when handling chemicals, paints, fertilizers, gases, or items that contain certain environmental chemicals.
- When working with chemicals is unavoidable, shower and don clean clothing after task completion.

ASSESSMENT

RISK FACTORS

- Frequent contact with rubber, paint, or electric cable
- Inhalation of gas, fumes, or chemical compounds
- Tobacco use
- Schistosoma haematobium (parasite) infection
- Long-term cyclophosphamide use
- Male gender
- Chronic urinary tract inflammation
- Caucasian clients, male clients, and clients older than 55

CAUSES OF CHRONIC BLADDER IRRITATION: UTI, kidney and bladder stones, or chronic bladder catheters

EXPECTED FINDINGS

- Hematuria
- Dysuria, frequency, urgency (infection or obstruction present)
- Weight loss
- Anorexia

DIAGNOSTIC PROCEDURES

Biopsy (cystoscopic)

EXPECTED FINDINGS: Presence of cancer

NURSING ACTIONS: Prepare the client for cystoscopy.

Bladder wash

EXPECTED FINDINGS: Presence of cancerous cells in saline "wash" solution (definitive diagnosis)

CLIENT EDUCATION: Inform the client that saline will be instilled into the bladder, then retrieved for microscopic examination.

Imaging: CT, MRI scan

EXPECTED FINDINGS
- CT scan: extent of tumor invasion
- MRI: depth and spread of tumor

NURSING ACTIONS: Prepare the client for imaging.

Nuclear imaging

IV (excretory) urography and pyelography

EXPECTED FINDINGS: Possible changes in structure or function of the urinary tract

NURSING ACTIONS: Prepare the client for the procedure (keep NPO, assess for contrast allergy).

Urinalysis

EXPECTED FINDINGS: Microscopic or gross hematuria

CLIENT EDUCATION: Inform the client of other possible reasons for hematuria.

PATIENT-CENTERED CARE

THERAPEUTIC PROCEDURES

Intravesical treatments

Intravesical chemotherapy: Chemotherapy medications are put directly into the bladder. Many of these same medications are administered systemically during chemotherapy.

Intravesical immunotherapy (92.2)
- Interferon are substances infused into the bladder to stimulate the immune system
- Bacillus Calmette-Guérin (BCG)
  - BCG is a live virus compound commonly used to vaccinate high-risk individuals against tuberculosis.
  - BCG is infused into the bladder and retained for 2 hr.

NURSING ACTIONS Qpcc
- Have the client void, then insert an indwelling urinary catheter for therapy infusion.
- After infusion, position the client on the back, abdomen, and each side for 15 min in each position.
- Assist the client to a standing position. Ensure the client can safely stand for the second hour.
- After the 2 hr dwell time, the urinary catheter is removed and the client is instructed to sit to void. This position prevents urine splashing, reducing the risk of contamination.
- Provide or assist in perineal cleansing.

CLIENT EDUCATION
- Restrict fluids for 4 hr prior to infusion therapy.
- Teach the client precautions to prevent exposure of others to BCG over the following 24 hr. After each voiding (sitting position), the client should do the following.
  - Cleanse the genitals.
  - Disinfect the urine by pouring 10% bleach solution (in an amount equal to the void) into the toilet prior to flushing.
  - Cleanse the seat and toilet surfaces.
- Teach the client to wash clothing and linen that comes in contact with urine for 24 hr following infusion.
- Instruct the client to avoid sexual intercourse for 24 hr following the infusion.

Systemic chemotherapy

Can be used alone or in combination with radiation. Chemotherapy can be given before surgery (neoadjuvant) or after surgery (adjuvant).

External beam radiation (92.2)

This can cause radiation cystitis.

Surgical interventions

- Surface excision, transurethral resection of bladder tumors, and partial cystectomy (removal of part of the bladder) are used to treat small, confined tumors.
- Radical cystectomy with removal of surrounding tissue or muscle is used for large, invasive, or recurrent tumors. Intensive care can be required following extensive bladder repair. Ureters are diverted to another location. (92.6)
- Internal or external drains or catheters can be placed intraoperatively.
- Clients who have neobladder surgery are at risk for extreme weight loss.
- Radical cystectomy with lymph node dissection includes the removal of other pelvic structures.
  - In males, the removal of the seminal vesicles and prostate with possible urethrectomy
  - In females, the removal of the ovaries, fallopian tubes, uterus, cervix, anterior vaginal wall, and urethra

NURSING ACTIONS
- Consult enterostomal therapy to assist with management and client/family education related to urinary diversion. Qpcc
- Provide adequate nutrition, snacks, and supplements to clients who have bladder reconstruction. Consult nutrition services as needed.
- Monitor output from drains or catheters for expected color and amount.
- Notify the provider if urine is decreased or absent in a client who has an external pouch.
- Secure the client's external drainage catheter. Notify the provider if it becomes dislodged or removed.

CLIENT EDUCATION
- Instruct the client to self-catheterize and plan procedure at timed intervals since there is no sensation of bladder fullness (neobladder, continent pouch).
- Teach the client to monitor peristomal skin for redness, excoriation, or infection (ileal conduit, continent pouch).

92.6 Urinary diversions

	URETER DIVERSION	PORTAL OF EXIT	URINARY ELIMINATION
Ileal conduit	Ileum	Abdominal stoma	Continuous drainage into external pouch
Continent pouch	Pouch created from large intestine	Abdominal stoma	Penrose drain and catheter might be present until sutures heal. Client performs intermittent urinary catheterization.
Bladder reconstruction (neobladder)	Pouch created from small intestine	Urethra	Client performs intermittent urinary catheterization.
Ureterosigmoidostomy		Anus	During bowel movement

COMPLICATIONS

Hydronephrosis

- Inability to eliminate urine causes dilation of the renal pelvis.
- A tumor that blocks the urinary tract can prevent urinary elimination.

NURSING ACTIONS: Notify the provider if urine output is decreased or absent.

Breast cancer

- Breast cancer is the second-leading cause of cancer deaths in women in the U.S.
- Breast cancer in males is rare. Average onset age 68 years. Can present as a hard, painless mass. Gynecomastia can be present.
- Breast cancer can be noninvasive or invasive (most common). Common sites of metastasis are bone, lung, brain, and liver. ⓠEBP

Noninvasive breast cancers

Ductal carcinoma in situ (DCIS)
- Cancer cells are located in the duct and have not invaded surrounding tissue.
- DCIS cells lack the biologic capacity to metastasize

Lobular carcinoma in situ (LCIS)
- Abnormal cell growth occurs in the milk-producing glands
- Can increase risk of developing a separate breast cancer at a later time
- Managed with observation
- When other risk factors exist, prophylactic treatment (tamoxifen, raloxifene, or mastectomy) can be considered: cancer originates in the mammary ducts and grows in the epithelial cells lining the ducts

Invasive breast cancers

Infiltrating ductal carcinoma
Can present as a lump, skin dimpling or edematous thickening and pitting of breast skin (orange peel)

Inflammatory breast cancer (IBC)
- Can present as swelling, skin redness, and breast pain.
- Seldom presents as a lump and might not be present on a mammogram

HEALTH PROMOTION AND DISEASE PREVENTION

- Consume at least five servings of fruits and vegetables daily.
- Obtain screening mammography.
- Maintain healthy weight.
- Engage in regular physical exercise.
- Minimize alcohol intake.
- Breast feeding for a year or more decreases breast cancer risk.
- Avoid hormone replacement therapy.
- Avoid environmental estrogens.

ASSESSMENT

RISK FACTORS

- High genetic risk
  - Inherited mutations of BRCA1 and BRCA2
  - History of previous breast cancer
  - Dense breast tissue ⓠEBP
  - Biopsy confirmed atypical hyperplasia
  - Early age at diagnosis
  - Female gender (less than 1% of males develop breast cancer)
- Age over 65
- First-degree relative who has breast cancer
- Early menarche
- Late menopause
- Childlessness or first pregnancy after age 30
- Early or prolonged use of oral contraceptives
- High-fat diet (possible risk)
- Low-fiber diet (possible risk)
- Excessive alcohol intake (possibly related to folic acid depletion)
- Cigarette smoking
- Exposure to low-level radiation
- Hormone replacement therapy
- Recent oral birth control use
- Obesity
- Breast cancer rates are expected to increase over the next 50 years due to the increase of the older adult population. Ⓖ
- Older adult clients are at greater risk of complications following surgery for cancer.

EXPECTED FINDINGS

- Breast change (appearance, texture, presence of lumps)
- Breast pain or soreness

PHYSICAL ASSESSMENT FINDINGS
- Skin changes (*peau d'orange*) **(92.7)**
- Dimpling
- Breast tumors (usually small, irregularly shaped, firm, nontender, and nonmobile)
- Increased vascularity
- Nipple discharge
- Nipple retraction or ulceration
- Enlarged lymph nodes

DIAGNOSTIC PROCEDURES

MEN: Breast cancer in men is often diagnosed later, with a poorer prognosis. Males at increased risk should discuss a screening plan with the provider.

WOMEN who have breast changes or at high risk should be screened earlier and more frequently. These clients should also have an MRI performed.

Self-breast exam (SBE), clinical breast exam (CBE)

EXPECTED FINDINGS: Palpable tumors or lesions

CLIENT EDUCATION
- Instruct client to perform SBE monthly.
- Instruct client to have regular CBE (every 3 years age 20 to 39; yearly over 40 years of age).

Biopsy (open or fine-needle)

EXPECTED FINDINGS: Definitive diagnosis of cancer cell type

CLIENT EDUCATION: Provide diagnosis-specific information.

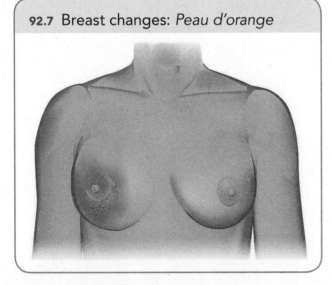

92.7 Breast changes: *Peau d'orange*

Genetic testing

EXPECTED FINDINGS
- **BRCA1 and BRCA2:** presence of gene mutation increases breast cancer risk
- **HER2:** presence of excess HER2 (normal gene that causes cell replication) indicates the need for targeted therapy.

CLIENT EDUCATION: Recommend genetic testing for BRCA1 and BRCA2 to clients at risk (two first-degree relatives diagnosed with breast cancer prior to age 50 or family history of breast and ovarian cancer).

MRI

EXPECTED FINDINGS: Better visualization of lesions in clients who have dense breasts.

NURSING ACTIONS: Prepare client for imaging.

Nuclear imaging: breast-specific gamma imaging

EXPECTED FINDINGS: Visualization of the lesion

CLIENT EDUCATION: Inform client that scanning will display the "uptake" of the radioactive substance injected prior to the procedure.

Positron emission mammography (PEM)

Type of PET scan

EXPECTED FINDINGS: Visualization of the lesion

CLIENT EDUCATION: Inform client that PEM provides consistent images despite hormone fluctuations.

Ultrasound (US)

EXPECTED FINDINGS: Visualization of the lesion

CLIENT EDUCATION: Inform client that US provides better visualization of lesions in clients who have dense breasts.

X-ray

EXPECTED FINDINGS: Visualization of the lesion (digital mammography is more accurate)

CLIENT EDUCATION: Instruct clients older than 40 years to schedule an annual mammogram.

Mammography

EXPECTED FINDINGS: Visualization of the lesion

CLIENT EDUCATION: Instruct clients regarding additional diagnostic testing.

Other tests

Chest x-ray, CT scan, MRI, liver enzymes, serum calcium and alkaline phosphatase

EXPECTED FINDINGS: Metastatic disease

CLIENT EDUCATION: Provide diagnosis-specific information.

PATIENT-CENTERED CARE

THERAPEUTIC PROCEDURES

Adjuvant therapy follows surgery to decrease the risk of reoccurrence.

Hormone therapy

Most effective in cancer cells with estrogen or progesterone receptors. This type of cancer has a better prognosis.

Ovarian ablation: Luteinizing releasing hormone (LH–RH): leuprolide or goserelin
- Inhibits estrogen synthesis.
- Can be used in premenopausal women to stop or prevent the growth of breast tumors.

Selective estrogen receptor modulators (SERMs): toremifene (tamoxifen and raloxifene)
- Used in women who are at high risk for breast cancer or who have advanced breast cancer. Q EBP
- Suppress the growth of remaining cancer cells postmastectomy or lumpectomy.
- Tamoxifen has been found to increase the risk of endometrial cancer, deep-vein thrombosis, and pulmonary embolism. Raloxifene does not share these adverse effects.

Chemotherapy/radiation therapy

- Chemotherapy and/or radiation can augment or replace a mastectomy, depending on several factors (client's age, hormone status related to menopause, genetic predisposition, and staging of disease).
- Clients who undergo chemotherapy are usually given a combination of several medications (cyclophosphamide, doxorubicin, and fluorouracil).

- Radiation therapy is usually reserved for clients who had a lumpectomy or breast-conserving procedure.
  - Whole or partial breast radiation may be prescribed. Skin care is a priority concern due to radiation damage and generalized fatigue.
  - Brachytherapy with radioactive seeds can also be an option.
  - Intraoperative radiation therapy allows an intense dose of radiation to be delivered directly to the surgical site.
- Target therapy is most effective in breast cancer with HER2/neu gene. Trastuzumab, pertuzumab, and ado-trastuzumab emtansine (a) are signal transduction inhibitors. They inhibit proteins that are signals for cancer cells to grow.
- Clients who have metastatic cancer can receive a vascular endothelial growth factor inhibitor, such as bevacizumab (v). This medication reduces blood flow to the growing tumor.

Surgical interventions

Surgical procedures include lumpectomy (breast-conserving), wide excision or partial mastectomy, total mastectomy, modified radical mastectomy (lymph nodes removed), radical mastectomy (lymph nodes and muscle removed), and reconstructive surgery. **(92.8)**

NURSING ACTIONS
- Have the client sit with the head of the bed elevated 30° when awake and support her arm on a pillow. Lying on the unaffected side can relieve pain.
- Have the client wear a sling while ambulating (to support arm).
- Avoid administering injections, taking blood pressure, or obtaining blood from the client's affected arm. Place a sign above the client's bed regarding these precautions. Qs
- Emphasize the importance of a well-fitted breast prosthesis for a client who had a mastectomy.
- Provide emotional support to the client and her family.
- Encourage the client to express feelings related to perception of sexuality and body image.

92.8 Total mastectomy with lymph node dissection

lymph nodes

CLIENT EDUCATION

- Teach the client how to care for her incision and drainage tubes. (Drains are usually left in for 1 to 3 weeks.)
- Advise the client to avoid placing her arm in a dependent position. This position will interfere with wound healing.
- Encourage early arm and hand exercises (squeezing a rubber ball, elbow flexion and extension, and hand-wall climbing) to prevent lymphedema and to regain full range of motion.
- Teach the client not to wear constrictive clothing and to avoid cuts and injuries to the affected arm.
- Teach/reinforce teaching regarding BSE.
- Instruct the client to report numbness, pain, heaviness, or impaired motor function of the affected arm to the surgeon.
- Encourage the client to discuss breast reconstruction alternatives with the surgeon.
  - Reconstruction can begin during the original breast removal procedure or after some healing has occurred.
  - A tissue expander (a saline-filled implant that has a port through which additional saline can be injected, gradually expanding the tissue prior to permanent implant) is often placed during the original procedure.
  - Saline or silicone implants are used for permanent placement.
  - Autologous flaps can also be used for reconstruction.
  - Nipple reconstruction can be done using tissue from the labia, abdomen, or inner thigh.
- Genetic counseling for clients who test positive for the BRCA1/BRCA2 genetic mutation includes recommendation of bilateral mastectomy and oophorectomy to prevent cancer occurrence. Clients who do not choose this option should have early, frequent, thorough screening for breast and ovarian cancer. **Q**ᵀᶜ

Other procedures

Stem cells (autologous or allogeneic) can be used to treat clients who are at high risk of recurrence or have advanced disease.

COMPLICATIONS

Destruction of part of the chest wall and mastitis.

Ovarian cancer

- Ovarian cancers are epithelial tumors that grow on the surface of the ovaries.
- The tumors grow quickly and are often bilateral.
- Metastases frequently occur before the primary ovarian malignancy is diagnosed.
- Ovarian cancer is the leading cause of death from female reproductive cancers.
- The exact etiology of ovarian cancer is unknown. However, the more times a woman ovulates in her lifetime seems to be a risk factor because ovarian cancer is more prevalent in women with early menarche, late-onset menopause, nulliparity, and those who use infertility agents.

HEALTH PROMOTION AND DISEASE PREVENTION

- Birth control pills and pregnancy can offer protection against ovarian cancer (reduced estrogen exposure).
- Risk-reducing or prophylactic bilateral salpingo-oophorectomy helps protect women with BRCA1 or BRCA2 mutations against ovarian cancer
- Although regular exams are recommended, it is difficult to palpate ovarian tumors during a pelvic exam

ASSESSMENT

RISK FACTORS

- Age greater than 40 years
- Nulliparity or first pregnancy after 30 years of age
- Family history of ovarian, breast, or genetic mutation for hereditary nonpolyposis colon cancer (HNPCC)
- BRCA1 or BRCA2 gene mutations
- Diabetes mellitus
- Early menarche/late menopause
- History of dysmenorrhea or heavy bleeding
- Endometriosis
- High-fat diet (possible risk)
- Hormone replacement therapy
- Use of infertility medications
- Older adult clients following surgery for cancer **Ⓖ**

EXPECTED FINDINGS

- Abdominal pain or swelling
- Abdominal discomfort (dyspepsia, indigestion, gas, distention) **Q**ᴱᴮᴾ
- Abdominal mass
- Urinary frequency
- Unexpected weight loss
- Vaginal bleeding
- Urinary frequency or incontinence

DIAGNOSTIC PROCEDURES

- There is no specific test for ovarian cancer.
- Staging of ovarian cancer is determined at the time of the hysterectomy or exploratory laparotomy when the tumor is removed and examined by the pathologist.

Physical assessment

EXPECTED FINDINGS: Enlarged ovary (possible if tumor is at least 4 inches)

CLIENT EDUCATION: Inform the client of possible causes of an enlarged ovary.

Biopsy

EXPECTED FINDINGS: Presence of cancer cells

CLIENT EDUCATION: Inform the client that biopsy is usually performed during surgery to remove the tumor.

Genetic testing

EXPECTED FINDINGS: **BRCA1** and **BRCA2**: Presence of gene mutation increases ovarian cancer risk.

CLIENT EDUCATION: Inform clients that genetic testing can be used to determine risk of developing ovarian cancer but it is not used to diagnose or monitor treatment.

Tumor markers

EXPECTED FINDINGS
- **Germ cell tumors:** Human chorionic gonadotropin (hCG), alpha-fetoprotein (AFP), and lactate dehydrogenase (LDH) elevated
- **Epithelial tumor:** Cancer antigen-125 (CA-125) elevated (greater than 35 units/mL)

CLIENT EDUCATION
- Inform clients that unexpectedly high hCG levels may occur in germ cell ovarian cancer.
- Inform clients that unexpected AFP findings indicate probability of cancer (false positive: cirrhosis, hepatitis).
- Inform clients that unexpected CA-125 findings indicate possible cancer (false positive: endometriosis, pregnancy, fibroids, and menses). More testing or surgery will likely be required.

Transvaginal ultrasound, chest x-ray, CT or PET scan

EXPECTED FINDINGS: Metastatic disease

CLIENT EDUCATION: Inform clients regarding implications of metastatic disease and offer emotional support.

PATIENT-CENTERED CARE

THERAPEUTIC PROCEDURES

Chemotherapy (traditional or intraperitoneal)

- Chemotherapy is always given for ovarian cancer, even if surgery was performed. Cisplatin and carboplatin are the most common chemotherapeutic medications used for ovarian cancer.
- Intraperitoneal therapy with dwell time, a form of intracavitary chemotherapy, can be used.

NURSING ACTIONS
- Instruct the client to report findings of infection, including peritonitis.
- Monitor temperature, white blood cell (WBC) count, and absolute neutrophil count.

CLIENT EDUCATION: Teach clients regarding side effects of chemotherapy, including nausea, vomiting, loss of appetite, mouth and vaginal sores, and hair loss.

Surgical interventions

Exploratory laparotomy can be performed to diagnose, treat, and stage ovarian tumors. Debulking (cytoreduction) of very large tumors can be done laparoscopically.

A total abdominal hysterectomy (TAH) with bilateral salpingectomy and oophorectomy (BSO) is the usual treatment for ovarian cancer. TAH with BSO also helps determine the extent of the disease as well as local and distant metastases. Staging of the cancer is done at this time.

NURSING ACTIONS
- Observe for urinary retention and difficulty voiding.
- Assess bowel sounds. Paralytic ileus can occur due to manipulation of the bowel during surgery.
- Discuss sexuality, surgically induced menopause, and other self-image issues with the client.

CLIENT EDUCATION
- Instruct the client to avoid straining, driving, lifting more than 5 lb, douching, and participating in sexual intercourse until the provider gives release.
- Instruct the client to immediately report evidence of infection, as well as vaginal discharge that is excessive or has a foul odor.

COMPLICATIONS

Abdominal ascites and intestinal obstruction

Uterine (endometrial) cancer

- Endometrial cancer is the most common gynecological cancer.
- Endometrial cancer is more common in older adult women (related to prolonged exposure to estrogen). Ⓖ
- Estrogen therapy in postmenopausal women who have a uterus should include progesterone to decrease the risk of endometrial cancer.

HEALTH PROMOTION AND DISEASE PREVENTION

Avoid the use of unopposed estrogen when considering postmenopausal hormone replacement therapy.

ASSESSMENT

RISK FACTORS

- Family history of endometrial or colorectal cancer
- Personal history of breast or ovarian cancer
- Diabetes
- Genetic mutation for HNPCC
- Over 50 years of age
- Obesity (due to fat cell production of estrogen)
- Unopposed estrogen hormone replacement therapy
- Nulliparity
- Use of tamoxifen to prevent or treat breast cancer
- Late menopause (longer-term exposure to significant estrogen levels)

EXPECTED FINDINGS

- Irregular and/or postmenopausal bleeding
- Low-back, abdominal, or low pelvic pain

DIAGNOSTIC PROCEDURES

Biopsy

EXPECTED FINDINGS: Endometrial biopsy: presence of carcinoma

CLIENT EDUCATION: Inform clients that biopsy is usually performed through transvaginal ultrasound.

Pathology testing for staging

EXPECTED FINDINGS: Extent, size of tumor, and metastasis

CLIENT EDUCATION: Inform the client that this occurs after exploratory laparotomy or hysterectomy following tumor removal.

Genetic testing

EXPECTED FINDINGS: HNPCC testing: presence of the gene

CLIENT EDUCATION: Inform the client that presence of HNPCC increases the risk of carcinoma.

Tumor markers

EXPECTED FINDINGS
- **Alpha-fetoprotein (AFP):** elevated
- **Cancer antigen-125 (CA-125):** positive

CLIENT EDUCATION: Inform client that results indicate some type of carcinoma.

Transvaginal ultrasound and endometrial biopsy

Endometrial thickness and presence of carcinoma

Other assessments to determine metastatic cancer

Chest x-ray, intravenous pyelography, abdominal ultrasound, CT of the pelvis, MRI of abdomen/pelvis, and liver and bone scans

PATIENT-CENTERED CARE

THERAPEUTIC PROCEDURES

Radiation therapy

- Given as adjuvant therapy, usually after a hysterectomy.
- Brachytherapy and external radiation therapy can be options for cancer that is no longer limited to the uterus.

Brachytherapy: delivered inside the body
- Low dose rate involves the use radioactive implants which are left in place for about 1 to 4 days. Activity is restricted to prevent dislodgement of the radiation source. Immobility increases the risk of deep-vein thrombosis.
- High dose rates are more intense. The radiation source is left in place for less than 1 hour. Hospitalization and bed rest are not required.
- CLIENT EDUCATION
  - Instruct to report vaginal bleeding, urethral burning, hematuria, fatigue, diarrhea, fever or abdominal pain
  - Instruct client she is not radioactive between treatments and there are no restrictions on interactions with others.

External beam radiation therapy (EBRT): delivered outside the body
- Can be used in combination with surgery, brachytherapy, and/or chemotherapy
- Often given 5 days a week for 4 to 6 weeks on an outpatient basis
- Treatment area marked with permanent ink or injected dye
- A mold of the pelvis and lower back is used to maintain the exact position for treatment
- CLIENT EDUCATION
  - Teach clients regarding side effects, including fatigue, nausea, vomiting, loose stool, and vaginal dryness.
  - Educate clients regarding radiation cystitis and proctitis. Ⓠpcc
  - Instruct clients to monitor for signs of skin breakdown in the perineal area.
  - Advise clients to avoid sunbathing.
  - Advise clients to avoid washing treatment areas marked with ink.

Chemotherapy

- Often given in cycles: a period of treatment, followed by a rest period.
- Combination treatment is better than one medication alone.
- Common chemotherapy agents for endometrial cancer include doxorubicin, cisplatin, paclitaxel, and carboplatin.

CLIENT EDUCATION: Teach clients regarding side effects of chemotherapy, including nausea, vomiting, loss of appetite, mouth and vaginal sores, and hair loss.

NURSING ACTIONS: Monitor temperature, WBC count, and absolute neutrophil count.

Surgical interventions

Total hysterectomy with bilateral salpingectomy/oophorectomy is the standard treatment. The vagina is spared, allowing for sexual intercourse to continue.
- An open, laparoscopic, or vaginal approach can be used.
- Peritoneal fluid sampling during this procedure allows for testing of metastasis to the peritoneal cavity.

NURSING ACTIONS
- Observe for urinary retention and difficulty voiding due to proximity to the urethra (more common after vaginal hysterectomy).
- Monitor bowel sounds for paralytic ileus (more common due to manipulation of the bowel during surgery).
- Discuss sexuality, surgically induced menopause, and other self-image issues with the client.

CLIENT EDUCATION
- Instruct the client to avoid straining, driving, lifting more than 5 lb, douching, and sexual intercourse until the provider gives release.
- Instruct the client to immediately report evidence of infection, excess vaginal discharge, or foul-smelling drainage.
- Discuss hormone replacement therapy options with the client if she is premenopausal.

COMPLICATIONS

Anemia and uterine perforation

Cervical cancer

Cervical cancer is a slow-growing cancer. With proper screening, it can be detected early and treated with good results.

Early cervical cancer is often undetected. Manifestations do not occur until the cancer has become invasive.

HEALTH PROMOTION AND DISEASE PREVENTION

- Vaccination series with HPV vaccine between 9 and 26 years of age before first sexual contact Qs
- Pap and pelvic exams for cervical cancer screening
- HPV screening (co-testing) every 5 years for women aged 30 to 65 years
- Limit the number of sexual partners.
- Use condoms during sexual intercourse.

ASSESSMENT

RISK FACTORS

- Infection with high-risk HPV types (strains 16 and 18), which is associated in 90% of cases QEBP
- Chronic cervical inflammation/infections
- Infection with HIV or other immunosuppressive disorder
- History of sexually transmitted infections
- Early sexual activity (before 18 years of age)
- Client or male partner who had multiple sexual partners
- Male partner who had a female partner with cervical cancer
- Low economic status
- Family history of cervical cancer
- African American descent
- Cigarette smoking

EXPECTED FINDINGS

- Painless vaginal bleeding between menses
- Dysuria, hematuria
- Watery, blood-tinged vaginal discharge
- Unexplained weight loss
- Pelvic pain
- Pain during and after vaginal sexual intercourse
- Rectal bleeding
- Chest pain, coughing

DIAGNOSTIC PROCEDURES

Simultaneous PAP test and HPV testing improves the accuracy of the reading.

Papanicolaou (Pap) test

EXPECTED FINDINGS: Abnormal cells

CLIENT EDUCATION
- Instruct clients to begin Pap screening by 21 years of age (or 3 years following first sexual intercourse). Frequency of screening depends on many factors (age, results, presence of a cervix).
- Inform clients that the Pap is a screening tool and not diagnostic. An abnormal Pap requires additional testing.

Biopsy

EXPECTED FINDINGS: Abnormal cells (follow-up to Pap test)

CLIENT EDUCATION: Provide diagnosis-specific information to the client.

HPV typing: DNA test

EXPECTED FINDINGS: Presence of HPV on cervical cells

CLIENT EDUCATION: Inform the client that HPV increases the risk of cervical cancer.

Chest x-ray, MRI, CT, PET

EXPECTED FINDINGS: Metastatic/advanced disease

CLIENT EDUCATION: Inform the client regarding preprocedure instructions

PATIENT-CENTERED CARE

NURSING CARE

Administer antibiotics for pelvic, vaginal, or urinary tract infections.

THERAPEUTIC PROCEDURES

Removal of the lesion

- By conization, cryotherapy, laser ablation, hysterectomy, or a loop electrosurgical excision procedure.
- Conization can be used as either a diagnostic procedure or treatment in early cancer.

CLIENT EDUCATION
- Teach the client to report heavy vaginal bleeding, foul-smelling drainage, or fever to the provider. Qᴾᶜᶜ
- Remind the client that vaginal discharge is normal.
- Tell the client to take showers rather than tub baths.
- Teach the client to avoid heavy lifting, vaginal penetration, douches, and tampons for the prescribed time (typically 3 weeks).

Radiation

Brachytherapy and external radiation therapy can be options for cancer that is no longer limited to local invasion.

NURSING ACTIONS
- Monitor for skin damage, especially in the perineal area.
- Chemotherapy can be used along with radiation.

Surgical interventions

Hysterectomy: Clients who have early stage cervical cancer can require a **simple hysterectomy** (removes the uterus and cervix) or a **radical hysterectomy** (removes the uterus, upper third of the vagina, uterosacral uterovesical ligaments, and pelvic nodes). The choice to have a hysterectomy is guided by the client's condition and desire for future childbearing.

Exenteration: Clients who have more extensive cancer can require this more extensive pelvic surgery.
- **Anterior exenteration** involves removal of the uterus, cervix, fallopian tubes, vagina, ovaries, bladder, urethra, and pelvic lymph nodes. An ileal conduit is established for urinary diversion.
- **Posterior exenteration** involves removal of the uterus, cervix, fallopian tubes, vagina, ovaries, anal canal, rectum, and descending colon. A colostomy is established for bowel diversion.
- **Total exenteration** involves removal of all of the above organs and establishment of both urinary and bowel diversions.

NURSING ACTIONS
- Manage drains as well as urinary and bowel diversions.
- Assess for body image disturbance and encourage the client to speak openly about it.

CLIENT EDUCATION
- Teach the client about findings of wound infection and how to care for drains that can remain after discharge.
- Instruct the client about how to care for urinary and bowel diversion.
- Instruct the client about how to care for perineal wounds and expectations regarding discharge.

COMPLICATIONS

- Fistula development can occur after pelvic exenteration.
- Kidney infections are also common secondary to the urinary diversion.

Prostate cancer

- Second most common type of cancer in men
- Prostate cancer is a slow-growing cancer. Conservative treatment can be the treatment of choice for a client, based on how fast the cancer is growing, if the cancer has spread, and the client's age and life expectancy. Treatment can be delayed up to 10 years following diagnosis.
- The posterior lobe or outer gland epithelium are sites of origin for most prostate cancer. It is usually slow-growing in response to androgen (testosterone and dihydrotestosterone).
- Manifestations are often similar to those of benign prostatic hyperplasia.

HEALTH PROMOTION AND DISEASE PREVENTION

- Consume a diet low in animal fat and include omega-3 fatty acids (fish), fruits, and vegetables.
- Engage in regular exercise.
- Discuss PSA screening with a provider.

ASSESSMENT

RISK FACTORS

- History of vasectomy
- Age greater than 65 years (risk increases with age) Ⓖ
- Family history
- African-American heritage
- High-fat, complex carbohydrates or low-fiber diet
- BRCA2 mutation can be associated with an increased risk
- Rapid growth of the prostate (benign high-grade prostatic intraepithelial neoplasia)
- Exposure to environmental toxins such as arsenic

EXPECTED FINDINGS

- Urinary symptoms: hesitancy, weak stream, urgency, frequency, nocturia
- Recurrent bladder infections
- Urinary retention
- Blood in urine and semen (late manifestation)
- Painful ejaculation
- Pain, particularly bone (pelvis, spine, hips, ribs)
- Unexplained weight loss
- Loss of sexual desire or function
- Penile discharge or scrotal pain/swelling
- Significant residual urine after voiding a small amount of urine
- Swollen lymph nodes, especially in the groin

DIAGNOSTIC PROCEDURES

- Regular screening can begin as early as age 40 for individuals with high risk.
- PSA levels should reduce within a few days postoperatively.
- EPCA-2 is highly sensitive; if positive, biopsy can be excluded.

Digital rectal examination (DRE)

EXPECTED FINDINGS: Hard prostate with palpable irregularities

CLIENT EDUCATION: Instruct the client to discuss prostate screening after age 50.

Biopsy

EXPECTED FINDINGS
- Presence of cancer
- Staging is based on biopsy result.
  - Gleason score of 7 or higher: moderately differentiated
  - Gleason score 8 to 10: poorly differentiated

CLIENT EDUCATION
- Inform the client that PSA, age, race and family history are used to determine if biopsy is needed.
- Provide diagnosis-specific information to the client.

Genetic testing

EXPECTED FINDINGS: BRCA2 positive

CLIENT EDUCATION: Inform the client that presence of the gene increases cancer risk.

Prostate specific antigen (PSA)

EXPECTED FINDINGS: Elevation (greater than 4 ng/mL) indicates possible prostate disease (not specific to carcinoma).

CLIENT EDUCATION
- Instruct clients to discuss prostate screening after age 50.
- Insure that the client's PSA is assessed prior to DRE to promote accuracy of results.

Early prostate cancer antigen (EPCA-2)

EXPECTED FINDINGS: Positive (possible serum maker for prostate cancer)

CLIENT EDUCATION: Inform clients that positive results are highly indicative for prostate cancer.

Other laboratory testing

EXPECTED FINDINGS: BUN and serum creatinine elevated (renal damage)

CLIENT EDUCATION: Explain unexpected findings to the client.

Transrectal ultrasonography (TRUS)

EXPECTED FINDINGS: Visualization of lesions

CLIENT EDUCATION
- Instruct the client regarding possible complications and postprocedure care (extra fluids, no strenuous exercise, symptoms to report).
- Inform the client that an enema will be administered prior to procedure.

Urinalysis

EXPECTED FINDINGS: Hematuria, bacteriuria

CLIENT EDUCATION: Inform the client about causes of hematuria and bacteriuria.

PATIENT-CENTERED CARE

MEDICATIONS

Hormone therapy

Leuprolide acetate, goserelin, triptorelin: luteinizing hormone-releasing hormone (LH–RH) agonists
- Used in advanced prostate cancer to produce chemical castration.
- CLIENT EDUCATION
  ○ Warn the client that hot flashes are an adverse effect.
  ○ Tell the client that impotence and decreased libido can also be adverse effects.
  ○ Inform the client that he should be monitored for osteoporosis, which can occur due to testosterone suppression.

Flutamide, flutamide, bicalutamide, nilutamide: androgen receptor blocker
- Used alone or in conjunction with a LH–RH agonist.
- CLIENT EDUCATION
  ○ Alert the client that gynecomastia is an adverse effect.
  ○ Inform the client that liver function tests should be periodically monitored.

> If primary medications are not successful, high-dose ketoconazole, an antifungal that blocks androgen production, or estrogen (diethylstilbestrol) can be given.

Chemotherapy

Can be used on clients whose cancer has spread or who have had minimal improvement with other therapies.

CLIENT EDUCATION: Tell the client to have routine blood tests performed to monitor for neutropenia, leukopenia, thrombocytopenia, and anemia.

THERAPEUTIC PROCEDURES

Radiation

Internal (brachytherapy) or external beam (EBRT)
- External comes from a source of radiation outside the body.
- Intensity-modulated radiation uses thousands of beams and angles of varying intensity that are even more controlled to target the cancer tissues and reduce exposure of radiation to healthy tissue.
- Not likely to be beneficial if the cancer has spread to the lymph nodes, bones, or other organs

Surgical interventions

Radical prostatectomy is the treatment of choice.
- Not likely to be beneficial if the cancer has spread to the lymph nodes, bones, or other organs.
- Involves the removal of the prostate gland, along with the seminal vesicles, the cuff at the bladder neck, and the regional lymph nodes.
- Open or laparoscopic surgery can be done using a suprapubic, perineal, or retropubic approach.
- Laparoscopic can be used if PSA less than 10 ng/mL, no previous hormone therapy or abdominal surgery.
- Perineal nerves are seldom disrupted, so the client should not experience sexual dysfunction. However, dry climax can occur. Removal of tissue at the bladder neck allows seminal fluid to travel upward rather than down the urethral tract, resulting in retrograde ejaculation.

NURSING ACTIONS
- PREOPERATIVE: Ensure the client understands the procedure and what to expect postoperatively. Qᴾᶜᶜ
- POSTOPERATIVE
  ○ Provide care consistent with other types of abdominal surgery.
  ○ Manage pain with analgesics and cold therapy.
  ○ Observe for evidence of infection.
  ○ If the client has a suprapubic surgical approach, a suprapubic catheter is inserted (in addition to the urethral catheter).
    ▪ Provide catheter care and administer bladder antispasmodics to the client as prescribed.
    ▪ Monitor suprapubic catheter output (usually removed when residual urine measurements are less than 75 mL).

CLIENT EDUCATION
- Instruct the client to report manifestations of infection.
- Teach catheter care if the client is home with a catheter in place.
- Tell the client to avoid heavy lifting (up to 6 weeks), strenuous activity (up to 12 weeks), or straining during bowel movements as prescribed.
- Instruct the client to avoid tub baths for at least 2 to 3 weeks (open radical surgery).
- Teach the client Kegel exercises to reduce urinary incontinence.
- Provide information regarding availability of a sex therapist or intimacy counselor if needed.

COMPLICATIONS

Urinary incontinence

Erectile dysfunction

Radiation cystitis or proctitis
- Some clients can have a transurethral resection of the prostate if obstruction occurs in the early stages of cancer before treatment is initiated.
- Bilateral orchiectomy palliative measures can slow the rate of tumor growth (decreases testosterone levels).
- Active surveillance is an option for older clients who are asymptomatic. Treatment is given only when symptoms become bothersome.

PRACTICE Active Learning Scenario

A nurse is teaching a client who has a new diagnosis of prostate cancer. What information should the nurse include in the teaching? Use the Active Learning Template: System Disorder to complete this item.

MEDICATIONS: Describe at least four medications and their uses.

THERAPEUTIC PROCEDURES: Describe a prostatectomy.

NURSING INTERVENTIONS: Describe at least three nursing actions.

Application Exercises

1. A nurse is caring for a client who has leukemia and has developed thrombocytopenia. Which of the following actions should the nurse take first?

   A. Plan for the client to take rest periods throughout the day.

   B. Encourage the client to cough, turn, and deep breath every 2 hr.

   C. Assess temperature every 4 hr.

   D. Monitor platelet counts.

2. A nurse is reviewing the health record of a client who has suspected ovarian cancer. Which of the following findings supports this diagnosis? (Select all that apply.)

   A. Previous treatment for endometriosis

   B. Family history of colon cancer

   C. First pregnancy at age 24

   D. Report of scant menses

   E. Use of oral contraceptives for 10 years

3. A nurse is caring for a client 24 hr following a liver lobectomy for hepatocellular carcinoma. Which of the following laboratory reports should the nurse monitor?

   A. Urine specific gravity

   B. Blood glucose

   C. Serum amylase

   D. D-dimer

4. A nurse is providing teaching about colon cancer to a group of women 45 to 65 years of age. Which of the following statements should the nurse include in the teaching?

   A. "Colonoscopies for individuals with no family history of cancer should begin at age 40."

   B. "A sigmoidoscopy is recommended every 5 years beginning at age 60."

   C. "Fecal occult blood tests should be done annually beginning at age 50."

   D. "An endoscopy provides a definitive diagnosis of colon cancer."

5. A nurse is caring for a client who has multiple types of skin lesions. Which of the following skin lesions are indicative of a malignant melanoma? (Select all that apply.)

   A. Diffuse vesicles

   B. Uniformly colored papule

   C. Area with asymmetric borders

   D. Rough, scaly patch

   E. Irregular colored mole

Application Exercises Key

1. A. The nurse should offer the client rest periods throughout the day. However, another action is the priority.

   B. The nurse should encourage the client to cough, turn and deep breathe every 2 hr. However, another action is the priority.

   C. The nurse should assess the client's temperature every 4 hr. However, another action is the priority.

   D. **CORRECT:** The greatest risk to the client who has thrombocytopenia is injury due to bleeding. The priority action for the nurse to take is to initiate bleeding precautions, such monitoring platelet count.

2. A. **CORRECT:** Endometriosis is a risk factor for ovarian cancer.

   B. **CORRECT:** A family history of breast, ovarian, or colon cancer is a risk factor for ovarian cancer.

   C. A first pregnancy after 30 years of age or nulliparity is a risk factor for ovarian cancer.

   D. Dysmenorrhea or heavy bleeding is a risk factor for ovarian cancer.

   E. Birth control pills offer protection against ovarian cancer.

3. A. Alterations in urine specific gravity following a liver lobectomy are not expected.

   B. **CORRECT:** Blood glucose should be monitored during the first 24 to 48 hr following a liver lobectomy due to decreased gluconeogenesis and stress to the liver from surgery.

   C. Alterations in serum amylase following a liver lobectomy are not expected.

   D. Alterations in the D-dimer following a liver lobectomy are not expected.

4. A. A colonoscopy is recommended every 10 years beginning at age 50 for a client who has no family history of cancer.

   B. A sigmoidoscopy is recommended every 5 years beginning at age 50.

   C. **CORRECT:** Fecal occult blood tests should be done annually by clients ages 50 to 75.

   D. A biopsy performed during an endoscopic procedure confirms this diagnosis.

5. A. Diffuse vesicles are consistent with an allergic reaction.

   B. A uniformly colored papule is consistent with a birthmark or skin injury.

   C. **CORRECT:** A lesion with asymmetric borders is considered suspicious for a melanoma.

   D. A rough, scaly patch is consistent with skin irritation due to friction.

   E. **CORRECT:** A lack of uniformity of pigmentation of a mole is considered suspicious for a melanoma.

PRACTICE Answer

Using the Active Learning Template: System Disorder

MEDICATIONS
- Hormone therapy: luteinizing hormone-releasing hormone agonists: leuprolide acetate
- Androgen receptor blocker: flutamide
- Chemotherapy: docetaxel
- Antifungal: ketoconazole
- Estrogen: diethylstilbestrol

THERAPEUTIC PROCEDURES:
Prostatectomy is the surgical removal of the prostate gland, seminal vesicles, bladder cuff, and regional lymph nodes. It can be done by an open surgery or laparoscopic approach in the suprapubic, perineal, or retropubic area. Perineal nerves are usually not disrupted, so the client should not experience sexual dysfunction.

NURSING INTERVENTIONS
- Provide preoperative teaching.
- Implement care consistent with abdominal surgery.
- Monitor pain. Administer analgesics and cold therapy.
- Monitor for evidence of infections.
- Provide catheter care (suprapubic or urethral). Administer bladder antispasmodics.

CHAPTER 93 *Pain Management for Clients Who Have Cancer*

Management of cancer pain is necessary to optimize quality of life for a client who has cancer. Not all clients who have cancer have pain.

Either the tumor or the treatment can cause cancer pain. Tumor pressure or cell invasion can cause direct tissue, bone, and nerve pain. Surgery, radiation, chemotherapy, and inactivity can also cause cancer pain.

PAIN

- Pain is subjective and can indicate tissue injury or impending tissue injury.
- Pain can have physical and emotional components.
- The reaction to pain varies from person to person. Age, gender, and culture can influence it.
- Pain can be acute or chronic.
  - **Acute pain** occurs suddenly and is short-term. Acute cancer pain can be the result of surgery.
  - **Chronic pain** results from nerve changes and lasts longer than 3 months. Tumor growth and the effects on surrounding tissue (destruction or pressure) cause chronic cancer pain.

TYPES OF PAIN

Neuropathic
- Due to nerve damage
- Numb, tingling, shooting, burning, or radiating

Visceral/Deep
- Occurs in internal organs
- Can be difficult to identify
- Deep, sharp pain

Somatic
- Occurs in bone or connective tissues
- Throbbing or dull

ASSESSMENT

- The most reliable indicator of pain is the client's verbal expression of pain.
- Use standard pain measures (location, quality, intensity, timing, setting, associated symptoms, aggravating or relieving factors) to assess pain.
- Pain assessment also involves observing and documenting nonverbal indicators and physiological changes.

NONVERBAL INDICATORS OF ACUTE PAIN
- Agitation, grimacing
- Elevated heart rate, respiratory rate, blood pressure
- Diaphoresis, pupil dilation
- Splinting of an area

NONVERBAL INDICATORS OF CHRONIC PAIN
- Depression
- Lethargy
- Anger
- Weakness

BARRIERS TO EFFECTIVE PAIN MANAGEMENT
- Inadequate pain assessment
- Inadequate education of the client about analgesic use
- Knowledge of the health care professional regarding pharmacological pain management
- Reluctance by the client to report pain
- Fear of addiction leading to nonadherence
- Inadequate dosing

MANAGEMENT

Palliative cancer pain management provides comfort and reduce pains rather than to curing the cancer.

The goal of palliative pain management is to reduce pain to improve quality of life while maintaining dignity and mental clarity.

METHODS OF PAIN MANAGEMENT: Surgery, chemotherapy, and radiation therapy can reduce pain by removing the tumor or reducing its size, which can alter pressure on adjacent tissues or organs.

NURSING ACTIONS: Specific to each surgery or procedure

CLIENT AND FAMILY EDUCATION Qpcc
- Include information regarding the specific procedure or treatment.
- Include the family in care and management.
- Provide information about support groups and professional organizations, such as the American Cancer Society.
- **Radiation:** Instruct the client about specific skin care and to avoid sun exposure.
- **Chemotherapy:** Include information about avoiding infection and managing other adverse effects.

MEDICATIONS

Pharmacological management of pain includes NSAIDs, opioids, antidepressants, anticonvulsants, corticosteroids, and local anesthetics. Some clients who have cancer pain require regular use of analgesics for pain control.

Nonopioid medications and NSAIDs

- Acetaminophen
- Ketorolac
- Aspirin (acetylsalicylic acid)
- Ibuprofen
- Celecoxib

THERAPEUTIC INTENT: For mild to moderate pain

NURSING ACTIONS
- Monitor for gastrointestinal (GI) bleeding, such as bloody stools or coffee-ground emesis.
- Monitor for bruising and bleeding.
- Do not administer acetaminophen to clients who have liver disease. Clients who have a healthy liver should take no more than 4 g/day. For long-term treatment, adults should take no more than 3 g/day.
- Monitor for tinnitus and hearing loss with NSAIDs.

CLIENT EDUCATION
- Tell the client to take with food to prevent GI upset.
- Teach the client to be alert to GI or other bleeding and bruising.
- Instruct the client not to crush or chew enteric-coated products.

Opioids

- Morphine
- Meperidine
- Hydromorphone
- Oxycodone
- Fentanyl (available for transdermal use as well as a lozenge/sucker, buccal film and tablets, and nasal and sublingual spray)
- Combinations, such hydrocodone with acetaminophen, for breakthrough pain

THERAPEUTIC INTENT
- Moderate to severe pain
- Breakthrough pain

NURSING ACTIONS
- Use with caution for older adult clients.
- Manage acute severe pain with short-term (24 to 48 hr) around-the-clock administration of opioids rather than following a PRN schedule.
- The parenteral route is best for immediate, short-term relief of acute pain. The oral route is better for chronic, nonfluctuating pain.
- Monitor and intervene for adverse effects of opioid use: constipation, orthostatic hypotension, urinary retention, nausea, vomiting, and sedation.
- Monitor for respiratory depression.
- Have naloxone available to reverse effects.
- Administer stimulant laxatives to prevent opioid-induced constipation.

CLIENT EDUCATION
- Teach clients to avoid driving and using hazardous equipment until they know the effects of the opioid. Qpcc
- Tell the client not to take medications with alcohol.
- Teach the client to prevent constipation with diet changes and stool softeners.
- Inform the client that nausea can subside after a few days.
- Reduce the risk of orthostatic hypotension by teaching the client to rise slowly from a lying or sitting position.

Antidepressants

Tricyclic antidepressants (TCAs)
- Amitriptyline
- Desipramine
- Imipramine

Selective norepinephrine reuptake inhibitors (SNRIs)
- Venlafaxine
- Duloxetine

Selective serotonin reuptake inhibitors (SSRIs)
- Fluoxetine
- Paroxetine
- Sertraline

THERAPEUTIC INTENT
- Reduce depression
- Promote sleep
- Increase serotonin levels to improve feelings of well-being
- Decrease neuropathic pain

NURSING ACTIONS
- Use with caution for older adult clients.
- Use with caution for young adult clients and those who are at risk for suicide, because antidepressants can increase suicide risk.
- **TCAs**
  - Do not administer to clients who have seizure disorders or a history of cardiac problems.
  - Adverse effects include dry mouth, dizziness, mental clouding, weight gain, and constipation.
- **SNRIs:** Adverse effects include nausea, headache, sedation, insomnia, weight gain, impaired memory, sweating, and tremors.
- **SSRIs:** Adverse effects include nausea, vomiting, nervousness, agitation, decreased libido, and insomnia.

CLIENT EDUCATION
- Tell the client to notify the provider if depression increases or if thoughts of suicide occur.
- Inform the client that therapeutic effects can take 2 to 3 weeks.

Anticonvulsants

- Gabapentin
- Valproic acid
- Pregabalin
- Carbamazepine

THERAPEUTIC INTENT: Neuralgia and neuropathic pain

NURSING ACTIONS
- Monitor electrolytes.
- Monitor liver function.
- Monitor blood cell counts.
- Monitor medication levels.
- Monitor for tremors.
- Monitor for rash (life-threatening)

CLIENT EDUCATION
- Inform the client that medication can cause sleepiness and dizziness.
- Tell the client to avoid alcohol.
- Remind the client not to drive at the start of therapy.
- Instruct the client to notify the provider if rash or tremors occur.

Corticosteroids

- Prednisolone (syrup)
- Dexamethasone

THERAPEUTIC INTENT: Reduce pain by reducing swelling

NURSING ACTIONS
- Reduce dosage gradually.
- Monitor for muscle weakness, joint pain, or fever.
- Monitor glucose levels.
- Monitor for changes in behavior or confusion.

CLIENT EDUCATION
- Teach the client not to discontinue the medication suddenly.
- Tell the client to take the medication with food.
- Inform the client that the medication weakens the immune system.
- Remind the client to report any signs of infection.

Adjunctive agents: Sympatholytic agents

Clonidine

THERAPEUTIC INTENT
- Neuropathic pain
- Administer with bupivacaine in epidural or other local infusions.

NURSING ACTIONS: Monitor for hypotension.

CLIENT EDUCATION: Change positions slowly, because these medications can cause orthostatic hypotension.

Adjunctive agents: Skeletal muscle relaxants

Baclofen

THERAPEUTIC INTENT: With other pain medications for muscle spasms accompanying cancer pain

NURSING ACTIONS: Monitor for seizure activity.

CLIENT EDUCATION
- Tell the client to take the medication with food.
- Teach the client to use caution when driving or operating machinery.
- Inform the client that these medications can cause drowsiness and dizziness.

Systemic local anesthetics

- Lidocaine
- Bupivacaine
- Ropivacaine

THERAPEUTIC INTENT: Administer via an infusion pump directly into the area of pain (intrathecal, intra-articular, intrapleural) to provide pain relief.

NURSING ACTIONS
- Monitor for hypotension.
- Monitor for infection at the catheter insertion site.
- Evaluate pain status.
- Monitor for motor impairment and level of sedation.
- Administer with an opioid or another medication, such as clonidine.

CLIENT EDUCATION
- Tell the client to observe the infusion site for indications of infection, such as redness and swelling.
- Teach the client to watch for fever.
- Tell the client to notify the provider of increased pain or decreased movement that can indicate a motor block.
- Teach the client to care for and protect the external part of the catheter.

Topical local anesthetics

Lidocaine (patch)

THERAPEUTIC INTENT: Block generation and conduction of nerve impulses that transmit pain

NURSING ACTIONS: Monitor for pain relief and local skin reactions.

CLIENT EDUCATION: Teach the client to use the medication only on intact skin.

ADMINISTRATION METHODS

Oral

- First choice for administration
- Short- and long-acting formulations available

Transdermal

Fentanyl
- Easy to administer
- Slow onset, consistent dosing
- Long duration (48 to 72 hr)

Rectal

Low WBC and platelet counts are contraindications.

Subcutaneous infusion

Morphine or hydromorphone
- Slow infusion rate (2 to 4 mL/hr)
- Requires nursing support
- Risk of infiltration
- Rapid onset

Intravenous

- Requires nursing support
- Risk of infiltration
- Rapid onset

Epidural or intrathecal

- Risk of infection, pruritus, and urinary retention
- Requires nursing care to monitor, especially with increases in dosage
- More effective than IV analgesia during the immediate postoperative period

Sublingual/buccal

- Place sublingual forms under the tongue for absorption.
- Place buccal forms between the gum and cheek.
- Forms include tablets, films, and sprays.
- The client should refrain from drinking, eating, or smoking when taking the medication.

Topical/local

- Place patches directly over or adjacent to the painful area.
- Produces minimal systemic absorption and adverse effects
- Lidocaine patch on for 12 hr, off for 12 hr
- Monitor for local skin reactions.

ANESTHETIC INTERVENTIONS

Regional nerve blocks

Involves injecting an anesthetic agent, such as bupivacaine, and/or a corticosteroid directly into a nerve root to provide pain relief.

- For identifying or treating an isolated area of pain. For example, an intercostal nerve block treats chest or abdominal wall pain.
- The procedure can take from 15 min to 1 hr, depending on the area receiving the block.

NURSING ACTIONS

- Measure baseline vital signs. Monitor blood pressure and vital signs during the procedure and for at least 1 hr following the procedure (follow established guidelines).
- Establish IV access before the procedure.
- Monitor for manifestations of systemic infusion (metallic taste, ringing in ears, perioral numbness, seizures).
- Assess the insertion site for redness and swelling.
- Assess the level of nerve block and pain.
- Protect the area of numbness from injury.

CLIENT EDUCATION

- Advise the client to observe the injection site for swelling, redness, or drainage.
- Advise the client to protect the area of numbness from injury and to notify the provider of increased pain or manifestations of systemic infusion.

Epidural or intrathecal catheters

- Involves injecting a local anesthetic or analgesic into the epidural space (the area outside the dura mater of the spinal cord) or intrathecal space (the subarachnoid area within the spinal cord sheath that contains cerebrospinal fluid).
- Involves surgically placing an external catheter under the skin with an external port for long-term use.
  - For chronic pain management
  - Allows administration of a continuous infusion or injection PRN
  - For upper abdominal pain, thoracic pain, and pain below the umbilicus

NURSING ACTIONS

- Monitor during and for at least 1 hr following insertion or injection for hypotension, anaphylaxis, muscle weakness, seizures, and dura puncture. Qs
- Monitor for respiratory depression and sedation.
- Monitor the insertion site for hematoma and infection.
- Assess the level of sensory block.
- Evaluate leg strength prior to ambulating.
- Local anesthetics block the sympathetic nervous system, causing peripheral vasodilation and hypotension. This can cause reduced stroke volume, cardiac output, and peripheral resistance. Increase the rate of IV fluid infusion to compensate for the sympathetic blocking effects of regional anesthetics.

CLIENT EDUCATION

- Advise the client to notify the provider of manifestations of infection (fever, swelling, and redness; increase in pain or severe headache; sudden weakness of the lower extremities; decreases in bowel or bladder control).
- Advise the client to notify the provider of manifestations of systemic infusion.
- Long-term reactions can include sexual dysfunction and amenorrhea.

OTHER INVASIVE TECHNIQUES

Neurolytic ablation

Involves interrupting the nerve pathway or destroying the nerve roots that are causing pain; usually involves a CT-guided probe and injection of chemicals, such as phenol or ethanol.

- For example, celiac plexus nerve ablation can be effective for pancreatic, stomach, abdominal, small bowel, and proximal colon pain.
- The procedure is irreversible.
- Nerve ablation can provide relief for several months until nerve fibers regenerate.
- Nerve ablation can cause loss of sensory, motor, and autonomic function.
- Use only when noninvasive methods are ineffective.

Radiofrequency ablation

Electrical current creates heat on a probe that the provider guides to the tumor or nerves to destroy cancer cells or ablate nerve endings (for lung and bone tumors).

Cryoanalgesia

Uses a needlelike probe to deliver extreme cold to interfere with pain conduction via nerve pathways

NURSING ACTIONS

- Monitor vital signs, especially blood pressure, during and for at least 1 hr following the procedure.
- Monitor for manifestations of bleeding, such as tachycardia and hypotension.
- Monitor for skin irritation.
- Monitor for other effects such as diarrhea, loss of bladder or bowel control, and extremity weakness.
- Assess pain relief.

CLIENT EDUCATION

- Instruct the client to apply cold for pain at the insertion site.
- Tell the client to continue to use pain medications PRN.
- Teach the client to notify the provider of an increase in pain or weakness of extremities.

ALTERNATIVE APPROACHES

Use alternative approaches to pain management in addition to pain medications or other techniques. Many of these provide some pain reduction with minimal adverse effects. Qтс

Transcutaneous electrical nerve stimulation (TENS)

Skin electrodes near or over the area of pain transmit low-voltage electrical impulses. The client regulates the voltage to achieve the perception of pins and needles (sensory perception) rather than pain.

NURSING ACTIONS

- Use with conductive gel.
- Monitor electrode sites for burns and rash.
- Offer other pain medications.
- Do not use for clients who have pacemakers, infusion pumps, or cardiac dysrhythmias.

CLIENT EDUCATION

- Instruct the client to place the electrodes on clean, intact skin.
- Advise the client to inspect the skin under the electrodes for burns or irritation.
- Advise the client not to use if pregnant.
- Advise the client not to use near the head or over the heart.

Relaxation techniques and imagery QEBP

Useful during a procedure or a period of increased pain.
- Relaxation techniques include deep breathing, progressive relaxation, and meditation.
- Positive imagery involves visualizing a peaceful image with or without audio recordings.
- Relaxation and imagery can reduce anxiety, stress, and pain, and they can assist the client to feel more in control of the pain.

Distraction

Music, television, exercise, and family and friends can be effective distractions from pain and stress. Other distractions include repetitive actions or movements, focused breathing, or use of a visual focal point. A change of scenery can offer a distraction from pain.

Heat or cold, pressure, massage, or vibration

- Heat increases blood flow, relaxes muscles, and reduces joint stiffness.
- Cold decreases inflammation and causes local analgesia.
- Do not use heat or cold directly on skin that has radiation damage. Qs
- Massage and vibration can cause relaxation, distraction, and increased surface circulation.

Acupuncture

Acupuncture uses vibration or electrical stimulation by inserting small needles into the skin and subcutaneous tissues at different depths to stimulate and alter nerve pathways. It can also increase the client's pain threshold.

Hypnosis

Hypnosis involves using an altered state of awareness to redirect the perception of pain. It can help induce positive imagery, reduce anxiety, and improve coping.

Peer group support

A support group helps provide emotional support for the client and family. Other benefits include the presence of a social network, availability of information, and help in strengthening coping skills.

Application Exercises

1. A nurse is caring for a client who has chronic cancer pain and has a permanent epidural catheter for administration of a fentanyl/bupivacaine solution. The nurse should monitor the client for which of the following findings? (Select all that apply.)

   A. Respiratory depression

   B. Hypotension

   C. Sedation

   D. Muscle spasticity

   E. Sensory blockage

2. A nurse is caring for a client who will undergo a neurolytic ablation. The client asks the nurse the reason for this procedure. Which of the following responses should the nurse make?

   A. "It attempts to provide permanent pain relief."

   B. "It treats adverse effects of your pain medication."

   C. "It treats decreases in immunity."

   D. "It treats decreases in cells that stop bleeding."

3. A nurse is caring for a client who has cancer and has a prescription for transcutaneous electrical nerve stimulation (TENS) for pain management. Which of the following actions should the nurse take?

   A. Apply a conductive gel before applying the electrodes from the TENS unit on the client's skin.

   B. Apply alcohol to the client's skin before attaching the electrodes from the TENS unit.

   C. Attach the electrodes from the TENS unit over painful incisions or skin damage.

   D. Avoid other pain medications when using the TENS unit.

   E. Apply cold to the skin where electrodes are applied.

4. A nurse is planning care for a client who has cancer and will undergo cryoanalgesia. Which of the following interventions should the nurse include in the plan of care?

   A. Monitor oxygen saturation during the procedure.

   B. Instruct the client to apply heat to the insertion site.

   C. Assess for irritation of the mucous membranes in the mouth following the procedure.

   D. Evaluate bladder control after the procedure.

PRACTICE Active Learning Scenario

An nurse manager is leading a discussion with a group of nurses on the oncology unit about alternative approaches to pain management. What information should the nurse manager include in the discussion? Use the ATI Active Learning Template: Basic Concept to complete this item.

RELATED CONTENT

- Describe four approaches.
- Describe two nursing interventions for each approach.
- Describe one teaching point for each approach.

Application Exercises Key

1. A. **CORRECT:** Respiratory depression is an adverse effect of epidural analgesics. Other adverse effects include seizures and dura puncture.

   B. **CORRECT:** Hypotension is an adverse effect of epidural analgesics that can be corrected by administration of fluids. Other adverse effects include hematoma and infection.

   C. **CORRECT:** Sedation is an adverse effect of epidural analgesics. Other adverse effects include anaphylaxis and severe headache.

   D. Muscle weakness, not spasticity, is an adverse effect of epidural analgesics.

   E. **CORRECT:** Sensory blockage is an adverse effect of epidural analgesics. Other adverse effects include decreases in bowel and bladder control.

   Ⓝ *NCLEX® Connection: Pharmacological and Parenteral Therapies, Pharmacological Pain Management*

2. A. **CORRECT:** The nurse should inform the client that neurolytic ablation causes permanent destruction of the nerves that transmit pain from a specific area and is a last resort after other methods have been unsuccessful.

   B. Neurolytic ablation should reduce the need for analgesics and therefore the adverse effects that result from them. However, it is not a treatment for the adverse effects themselves.

   C. Neurolytic ablation does not treat myelosuppression (which reduces immunity). The procedure can cause complications, such as mild paralysis, but it does not affect immunity.

   D. Neurolytic ablation does not treat thrombocytopenia. The procedure can cause complications, such as disruption of bladder and bowel function, but it does not affect clotting mechanisms.

   Ⓝ *NCLEX® Connection: Reduction of Risk Potential, Therapeutic Procedures*

3. A. **CORRECT:** The nurse should apply a conductive gel before applying the electrodes from the TENS unit to the skin.

   B. The skin should be clean and intact before applying the electrodes but the nurse does not have to cleanse it with alcohol.

   C. The nurse should apply the electrodes over intact skin that is over or near the site of pain, but not over incisions or areas of damage.

   D. The nurse may administer pain medication while the client is using the TENS unit.

   Ⓝ *NCLEX® Connection: Basic Care and Comfort, Non-Pharmacological Comfort Interventions*

4. A. Blood pressure is the focus of vital sign monitoring to identify hypotension during and after cryoanalgesia.

   B. The client should apply cold to the insertion site for pain after cryoanalgesia.

   C. The nurse should monitor the skin for irritation following cryoanalgesia.

   D. **CORRECT:** Loss of bladder or bowel control is an adverse effect of cryoanalgesia.

   Ⓝ *NCLEX® Connection: Reduction of Risk Potential, Potential for Alterations in Body Systems*

PRACTICE Answer

Using the ATI Active Learning Template: Basic Concept

RELATED CONTENT

Transcutaneous electrical nerve stimulation (TENS)
- Use with conductive gel.
- Monitor electrode sites for burns or rash.
- Offer pain medications.
- Do not use on clients who have pacemakers, infusion pumps, or dysrhythmias.
- Place electrodes on clean, intact skin. Inspect skin under the electrodes for burns or irritation.
- Do not use if the client is pregnant.
- Do not use near the head or over the heart.

Relaxation and imagery
- Use during a procedure or during a period of increased pain. Encourage deep breathing, progressive relaxation, meditation, or a focus on a peaceful image.
- Use with or without audio recordings.
- Reduces stress, anxiety, and pain, and promotes a feeling of control of the pain.

Application of heat or cold, pressure, massage, or vibration
- Apply heat to increase blood flow, relax muscles, and reduce joint stiffness.
- Apply cold to decrease inflammation and produce local analgesia.
- Massage can cause relaxation, distraction, and increased surface circulation.
- Do not apply heat or cold directly to skin that has radiation damage.
- Avoid further skin irritation with excessive massage or vibration.

Distraction
- Offer music.
- Encourage watching television, exercising, and activities with family and friends.
- Use repetitive actions or movements, focused breathing, a visual focal point, and a change of scenery.

Acupuncture
- Offer to increase the client's pain threshold. Make referrals to community resources.
- Involves inserting small needles into the skin at different depths to stimulate and alter nerve pathways. This affects the pain threshold.

Hypnosis
- Helps redirect the client's perception of pain. Make referrals to community resources.
- Use to induce positive imagery, reduce anxiety, and improve coping.

Peer group
- Make referrals to community resources. Encourage family participation.
- Groups provide emotional support for family members and clients.
- Groups offer the presence of a social network, availability of information, and strengthening of coping skills.

Ⓝ *NCLEX® Connection: Basic Care and Comfort, Non-Pharmacological Comfort Interventions*

When reviewing the following chapters, keep in mind the relevant topics and tasks of the NCLEX outline, in particular:

Client Needs: Reduction of Risk Potential

POTENTIAL FOR COMPLICATIONS FROM SURGICAL PROCEDURES AND HEALTH ALTERATIONS: Evaluate the client's response to postoperative interventions to prevent complications.

THERAPEUTIC PROCEDURES
Provide preoperative and postoperative education.

Provide preoperative care.

Manage the client during and following a procedure with moderate sedation.

Client Needs: Physiological Adaptation

ALTERATIONS IN BODY SYSTEMS: Provide postoperative care.

CHAPTER 94 *Anesthesia and Moderate Sedation*

An anesthetic is a chemical agent clients receive prior to a surgical procedure to induce loss of consciousness, amnesia, and analgesia. There are different types of anesthesia for use in the surgical setting, and the nurse should be familiar with their adverse effects.

Moderate sedation is a type of anesthesia. A client does not lose consciousness, but still receives induction of amnesia and analgesia.

Anesthesia

Anesthesia is a state of depressed central nervous system (CNS) activity, with depression of consciousness, loss of responsiveness to stimulation, and muscle relaxation. Anesthesia is general or local.

General anesthesia causes loss of sensation, consciousness, and reflexes when a client is undergoing major surgery, or one that requires complete muscle relaxation.

Local anesthesia causes loss of sensation without loss of consciousness. Local anesthetics block transmission along nerves, thus achieving loss of autonomic function and muscle paralysis in a specific area of the body.

ASSESSMENT

RISK FACTORS: Older adult clients are more susceptible than any other population to anesthetic agents. ⓖ
- Careful titration of medications helps control the incidence of unwanted effects.
- Airway patency is the main priority in all situations, but cardiac problems can arise much more quickly in older adult clients.
- Pay specific attention when an older adult is undergoing a procedure, because the client's condition can deteriorate quickly.
- **General anesthesia**
  ○ Family history of malignant hyperthermia
  ○ Respiratory disease (hypoventilation)
  ○ Cardiac disease (dysrhythmias, altered cardiac output)
  ○ Gastric contents (aspiration)
  ○ Alcohol or substance use disorder
- **Local anesthesia**
  ○ Allergy to ester-type anesthetics
  ○ Alterations in peripheral circulation

General anesthesia

Anesthetics for general anesthesia are either injectable or for inhalation. Anesthetics for inhalation are volatile gases or liquids in combination with oxygen. Anesthetists give injectable anesthetics IV.
- Inhalation anesthetic agents include halothane, isoflurane, and nitrous oxide in combination with oxygen.
- IV anesthetic agents include benzodiazepines, etomidate, propofol, ketamine, and short-acting barbiturates such as methohexital.
  ○ Propofol is the most common anesthetic agent.
  ○ Clients receive propofol during mechanical ventilation, radiation therapy, and diagnostic procedures.
  ○ Allergies to eggs and soybean oil are contraindications for receiving propofol.
- Exhalation eliminates inhalation anesthetics. The rate of elimination depends on pulmonary ventilation and blood flow to the lungs. Postoperative administration of oxygen and encouraging the client to take deep breaths are important interventions.

PHASES OF GENERAL ANESTHESIA

Induction: Initiation of IV access, administration of preoperative medications given, securing of airway patency

Maintenance: Performance of surgery, airway maintenance

Emergence: Completion of surgery, removal of assistive airway devices

PATIENT-CENTERED CARE

MEDICATIONS

During administration of anesthetics, clients also receive adjunct medications to achieve further reactions.

Opioids

- Fentanyl
- Sufentanil
- Alfentanil

USES
- Sedation
- Analgesics to relieve preoperative and postoperative pain

ADVERSE EFFECTS
- Depresses the CNS, resulting in respiratory depression or distress
- Delays awakening following surgery or a procedure
- Can result in postoperative constipation and urinary retention
- Can trigger nausea and vomiting

Benzodiazepines

- Diazepam
- Midazolam

USES
- Reduce anxiety preoperative
- Promote amnesia
- Produce mild sedation (unconsciousness) with little to moderate respiratory depression with careful titration

ADVERSE EFFECTS: Can result in cardiac and respiratory arrest with rapid administration or without waiting for the full effect to develop

Antiemetics

- Ondansetron
- Metoclopramide
- Promethazine

USES
- Decrease postanesthetic nausea and vomiting
- Enhances gastric emptying (metoclopramide)
- Induces sedation (promethazine)
- Decrease the risk for aspiration

ADVERSE EFFECTS
- Dry mouth
- Dizziness
- Extrapyramidal symptoms and tardive dyskinesia (metoclopramide)
- Respiratory depression and apnea (promethazine)

Anticholinergics

- Atropine
- Glycopyrrolate

USES
- Decrease the risk of bradycardia during surgery and, at times, vagal slowing of the heart due to the parasympathetic response to surgical manipulation
- Block the muscarinic response to acetylcholine by decreasing salivation, bowel movement, and GI secretions
- Slow motility of the GI tract
- Decrease saliva, perspiration, and gastric and pancreatic secretions
- Decrease the risk for aspiration

ADVERSE EFFECTS
- Urinary retention, difficulty starting urination
- Tachycardia
- Dry mouth
- Decreased levodopa effects

CONTRAINDICATION: Glaucoma

Sedatives

- Pentobarbital
- Secobarbital

USES
- Sedative effect for preanesthesia sedation or amnesia
- Induction of general anesthesia

ADVERSE EFFECTS: Respiratory depression

! Avoid giving within 14 days of starting or stopping an MAOI.

Neuromuscular blocking agents

- Succinylcholine
- Vecuronium

USES
- Skeletal muscle relaxation for surgery
- Airway placement
- In conjunction with IV anesthetic agents (propofol, opioids, benzodiazepines)

ADVERSE EFFECTS
- Total flaccid paralysis
- Requires mechanical ventilation because it blocks contraction of all muscles, including the diaphragm and respiratory system

CONSIDERATIONS

- Ensure that the client has signed a consent form, because an adult who has received sedation may not give legal consent.
- Have the client urinate before receiving medication so he will not need to get out of bed.
- Ensure that the bed is in the low position and that the side rails are up for safety.
- Monitor airway and oxygen saturation.
- Monitor and report laboratory values (ABGs, CBC, and electrolytes).
- Monitor cardiac status (rhythm, heart rate, blood pressure).
- Monitor temperature.
- Monitor drains, tubes, catheters, and IV access throughout anesthesia and surgery.
- Assess level of sedation and anesthesia (level of consciousness, vital signs).
- If hypotension occurs as an adverse effect of medication or dehydration, lower the head of bed, administer an IV fluid bolus, and monitor.
- Notify the surgeon and anesthesiologist of abnormalities.

COMPLICATIONS

Malignant hyperthermia

MANIFESTATIONS
- Acute life-threatening medical emergency
- Inherited muscle disorder, that anesthesia induces chemically
- Hypermetabolic condition causing an alteration in calcium activity in muscle cells (muscle rigidity, hyperthermia, and damage to the CNS)
- Triggering agents include inhalation anesthetic agents and succinylcholine.
- Increased carbon dioxide level, decreased oxygen saturation level, and tachycardia occur first, followed by dysrhythmias, muscle rigidity, hypotension, tachypnea, skin mottling, cyanosis, and muscle-cell protein in the urine (myoglobinuria).
- Extremely elevated temperature is a late manifestation: increasing as high as 44° C (111.2° F).

NURSING ACTIONS
- Terminate surgery.
- Administer IV dantrolene, a muscle relaxant.
- Administer 100% oxygen.
- Obtain specimens for ABGs to monitor metabolic acidosis and serum chemistry to evaluate potassium level.
- Infuse iced IV 0.9% sodium chloride.
- Apply a cooling blanket; ice to axillae, groin, neck, and head; and iced lavage.
- Insert an indwelling urinary catheter to monitor output and the presence of blood.

Overdose of anesthetic

MANIFESTATIONS
- Anesthetics and other medications can cause complications and interactions.
- Overdose can occur in an older client who has pre-existing conditions or a client who has poor liver or kidney function.

NURSING ACTIONS: Complete preoperative screening and documentation, and inform the provider or surgeon of pre-existing medical conditions, medications, and allergies.

Unrecognized hypoventilation

MANIFESTATIONS: Cardiac arrest, hypoxia, brain damage, and death can result from failure to oxygenate and exchange gases during surgery.

NURSING ACTIONS
- Monitor end-tidal carbon dioxide levels.
- For equipment malfunction, manually ventilate the client.

Intubation problems

MANIFESTATIONS
- Injury to teeth, lips, and vocal cord during intubation if the mouth is too small, inability to open the mouth wide, and mouth tumors
- Neck injury from improper neck extension during intubation
- Sore throat

NURSING ACTIONS
- Nurses may assist the anesthesiologist with the intubation.
- Have tracheostomy supplies available.

Local anesthesia

- Examples of local anesthetic agents are procaine and lidocaine.
- Concurrent administration of a vasoconstrictor, usually epinephrine, prolongs effects and decreases the risk of systemic toxicity. Distal injuries (fingers) are a contraindication due to decreased circulation. Prolonged vasoconstriction can lead to tissue necrosis.

MAIN METHODS OF ADMINISTRATION

Topical: Apply directly to the skin or mucous membranes.

Local infiltration: Inject directly into tissues through which the surgeon will make an incision.

Regional nerve block: Injection into or around specific nerves
- **Spinal:** Anesthetic injection into the cerebrospinal fluid (CSF) in the subarachnoid space to provide autonomic, sensory, and motor blockade below the level of innervation
- **Epidural:** Anesthetic injection into the epidural space in the thoracic or lumbar areas of the spine to block sensory pathways, but leave motor function intact
- **Nerve block:** Injection of anesthetic around or into an area of nerves to block sensation often for surgery on an extremity or for chronic pain
- **Field block:** Injection of anesthetic around the operative field for procedures of the chest, plastic surgery, dental, and hernia repairs

CONSIDERATIONS

- Observe for a systemic toxic reaction due to CNS stimulation (headache, blurred vision, metallic taste). Without treatment, it leads to unconsciousness, hypotension, apnea, cardiac arrest, and death.
  - Establish airway patency, administer oxygen, and monitor oxygen saturation. Then notify the anesthesiologist and surgeon.
  - Monitor the client following administration of a fast-acting barbiturate.
  - Monitor and report laboratory values (ABGs, CBC, and electrolytes).
- Monitor cardiac status (rhythm, heart rate, blood pressure).
- Monitor drains, tubes, catheters, and IV access throughout anesthesia and surgery
- Assess motor function to ensure paralysis does not ensue (sense of touch returns first followed by pain, warmth, cold, and finally the ability to move).
- With epidural and spinal anesthesia, monitor for autonomic nervous system blockade (hypotension, bradycardia, nausea, vomiting). Lower the head of the bed, increase IV fluid infusion rate if no restrictions, and monitor vital signs.
- CSF leakage (spinal and epidural) manifests with a severe headache when the head of the bed is elevated.
  - Keep the head of the bed flat to promote the dura tear to seal.
  - Provide a quiet environment.
  - Keep the client well hydrated to help replace CSF loss.

Moderate sedation

Moderate sedation is the administration of sedatives and/or hypnotics and opioids to the point where the client relaxes enough that the surgeon can perform minor procedures without discomfort for the client, yet the client can respond to verbal stimuli, retains protective reflexes (gag reflex), is easily arousable, and—most importantly—independently maintains a patent airway.

- Only a qualified provider may administer moderate sedation: anesthesiologists, certified registered nurse anesthetists, attending providers, or RNs with certification in advanced cardiac life support (ACLS) and are under the supervision of a qualified provider.
- Continuously monitor a client who is undergoing moderate sedation. During the procedure, an RN who has no other responsibilities at that time must be present to monitor the client. This nurse must remain with the client at all times before, during, and immediately after the procedure.

PROCEDURES

Minor surgical procedures: dental, podiatric, plastic, ophthalmic procedures

Diagnostic procedures: various types of endoscopy, bone marrow aspiration, lumbar puncture

Cardioversion

Wound care: suturing, dressing changes, incision and drainage of abscesses, burn debridement

Reduction and immobilization of fractures

Placement and removal of implanted devices, catheters, and tubes

ASSESSMENT

RISK FACTORS: Older adult clients are at an increased risk for adverse reactions to sedation because of decreased liver and kidney function. ⓒ

- Older adult clients have less physiologic reserve than younger clients, which can cause decreased immune system response and decreased wound healing.
- Reduction of muscle mass and the amount of body water places older adult clients at risk for dehydration.
- Be aware and maintain a safe environment for older adult clients, due to sensory limitations.
- Pay careful attention to cardiac and respiratory status of older adult clients, as problems can arise faster.

CONSIDERATIONS

PREPROCEDURE

- Obtain a full history, including allergies, medication usage, and pre-existing medical conditions (pulmonary disease). Report any previous experiences with sedation or anesthesia, especially any adverse reactions. Note the last dose of each medication, especially if it could alter the client's response (diuretic, antihypertensive, opioid).
- Provide education about the procedure and the medications the client will receive.
- Perform a full assessment, including baseline vital signs, cardiac rhythm, and level of consciousness.
- Determine the last time the client ate or drank (generally NPO for 6 hr or more before the procedure).
  - The client may have clear liquids up to 2 hr before the surgery or procedure.
  - Instruct the client to adhere to the instructions to remain NPO, or the surgeon might cancel the procedure.
- Establish IV access and administer fluids.
- Verify that the client signed the informed consent.
- Attach monitoring equipment.
- Remove dentures in case intubation becomes necessary.

INTRAPROCEDURE

- Remain with the client at all times. Allow other staff to assist the provider with the procedure.
- Continually assess and monitor level of consciousness (Glasgow coma scale score), cardiac rhythm, respiratory status, and vital signs.
- Maintain a safe environment for the older adult client due to sensory limitations. ⓒ
- Pay careful attention to cardiac and respiratory status for older adult clients, as problems can arise faster.
- The following equipment must be present within immediate reach for routine monitoring and in case deep sedation with respiratory depression occurs.
  - Emergency cart with emergency medications, airway and ventilatory equipment, defibrillator, and IV supplies
  - A 100% oxygen source and administration supplies, airways, manual resuscitation bag, and suction equipment
  - ECG monitor and display, noninvasive blood pressure monitor, pulse oximeter, thermometer, and stethoscope

POSTPROCEDURE

Monitor and document vital signs and level of consciousness until the client is fully awake and all assessment criteria return to presedation levels.

TYPICAL DISCHARGE CRITERIA
- Level of consciousness as on admission
- Vital signs stable for 30 to 90 min
- Ability to cough and breathe deeply
- Ability to tolerate oral fluids
- Ability to urinate
- No nausea, vomiting, shortness of breath, or dizziness
- No obvious bleeding

PATIENT-CENTERED CARE

MEDICATIONS

Opioids: Morphine, fentanyl, alfentanil

Anesthetics: Etomidate, propofol

Benzodiazepines: Midazolam, diazepam

Dosages required for light sedation are highly individual and require careful titration.

When a client receives moderate sedation, use naloxone to reverse the adverse effects of the opioid. Administer flumazenil to reverse the adverse effects of benzodiazepines.

CONSIDERATIONS

Before, during, and after the procedure, keep emergency equipment at the client's bedside.

Most hospitals and facilities require that for moderate sedation, an RN has certification in ACLS or pediatric advanced life support in case of an emergency. For complications, stop or reverse sedation and provide care to alleviate the problem.

COMPLICATIONS

Airway obstruction, cardiac dysrhythmias, hypotension, anaphylaxis

NURSING ACTIONS: Insert an oral airway and suction.

Respiratory depression

NURSING ACTIONS
- Administer oxygen and reversal agents, such as naloxone and flumazenil.
- Insert an oral airway and suction.

Cardiac arrhythmias

NURSING ACTIONS: Obtain a 12-lead ECG and provide antidysrhythmics and fluids.

Hypotension

NURSING ACTIONS: Provide fluids and vasopressors.

Anaphylaxis

NURSING ACTIONS: Administer epinephrine.

Application Exercises

1. A nurse administered midazolam IV bolus to a client before a procedure. His blood pressure is 86/40 mm Hg, and his pulse is 134/min. Which of the following IV medications should the nurse administer?

   A. Naloxone

   B. Morphine

   C. Flumazenil

   D. Atropine

2. A nurse is assisting an anesthesiologist in the delivery of nitrous oxide by face mask to a client during the induction of anesthesia. Which of the following is the priority nursing action?

   A. Assess oxygen saturation.

   B. Measure blood pressure.

   C. Palpate pulse rate.

   D. Check temperature.

3. A nurse is caring for a client who develops malignant hyperthermia. Which of the following actions should the nurse take? (Select all that apply.)

   A. Infuse iced IV fluids.

   B. Provide 100% oxygen.

   C. Place the client on a cooling blanket.

   D. Treat the complication while continuing surgery.

   E. Administer IV dantrolene.

4. A nurse is caring for a client who develops a systemic toxic reaction following a regional block. Which of the following actions should the nurse take?

   A. Monitor serum creatinine levels.

   B. Provide airway support.

   C. Turn the client to the right side.

   D. Administer 0.9% sodium chloride 500 mL IV bolus.

5. A nurse is caring for a client who reports a headache following an epidural regional nerve block. Which of the following actions should the nurse take?

   A. Decrease the client's fluid intake.

   B. Apply pressure to the puncture site.

   C. Place the head of bed flat.

   D. Instruct the client to lie prone.

Application Exercises Key

1. A. Naloxone reverses respiratory depression resulting from an opioid medication.

   B. Morphine relieves pain and can cause hypotension and respiratory depression.

   C. **CORRECT:** Midazolam is a benzodiazepine. The nurse should administer flumazenil to reverse its effects.

   D. Atropine sulfate treats bradycardia.

   Ⓝ *NCLEX® Connection: Physiological Adaptation, Unexpected Response to Therapies*

2. A. **CORRECT:** The greatest risk for the client is injury from hypoxia. Therefore, this is the priority finding.

   B. Measuring blood pressure is important for assessing the client's cardiovascular status. However, another finding is the priority.

   C. Palpating pulse rate is important for assessing the client's cardiovascular status. However, another finding is the priority.

   D. Checking temperature at the time of induction is important for identifying hypothermia. However, another finding is the priority.

   Ⓝ *NCLEX® Connection: Reduction of Risk Potential, Therapeutic Procedures*

3. A. **CORRECT:** Infusing iced IV fluids should help lower the client's rapidly rising temperature.

   B. **CORRECT:** Providing 100% oxygen will help prevent hypoxia due to muscle tremors and rigidity from increased lactic acid.

   C. **CORRECT:** Placing the client on a cooling blanket will help lower the rapidly rising temperature.

   D. Terminating surgery should occur as soon as the surgical team suspects malignant hyperthermia.

   E. **CORRECT:** Dantrolene IV is a muscle relaxant that treats malignant hyperthermia.

   Ⓝ *NCLEX® Connection: Physiological Adaptation, Medical Emergencies*

4. A. The nurse should monitor ABGs, CBC, and electrolytes for a client who has a systemic toxic reaction to a regional block.

   B. **CORRECT:** A systemic toxic reaction results in CNS depression. In this event, it is important to support the client's airway with maintaining patency and administering supplemental oxygen.

   C. Turning the client to the right side will not help with a systemic toxic reaction to a regional block.

   D. Manifestations of systemic toxic reaction include hypertension. Administration of a 500 mL IV bolus would exacerbate the problem.

   Ⓝ *NCLEX® Connection: Physiological Adaptation, Medical Emergencies*

5. A. The nurse should increase fluid intake to keep the client well-hydrated and to help replace cerebrospinal fluid.

   B. Applying pressure to the puncture site will not relieve the headache from cerebrospinal fluid leakage.

   C. **CORRECT:** Placing the head of the bed flat will decrease the intensity of the headache.

   D. Instructing the client to lie prone could worsen or not improve the client's headache pain.

   Ⓝ *NCLEX® Connection: Reduction of Risk Potential, Potential for Complications of Diagnostic Tests/Treatments/Procedures*

PRACTICE Active Learning Scenario

A nurse is preparing to administer moderate sedation to a client who will undergo a colonoscopy. What actions should the nurse plan for the client? Use the ATI Active Learning Template: Basic Concept to complete this item.

RELATED CONTENT: List three medications for and classifications of moderate sedation.

UNDERLYING PRINCIPLES: State the purpose of moderate sedation.

NURSING INTERVENTIONS: List two nursing actions for each: preprocedure, intraprocedure, and postprocedure.

PRACTICE Answer

Using the ATI Active Learning Template: Basic Concept

RELATED CONTENT
- Fentanyl (opioid)
- Propofol (anesthetic)
- Midazolam (benzodiazepine)

UNDERLYING PRINCIPLES: The purpose of moderate sedation is to relax the client to a point where he does not feel discomfort, yet he is able to respond to verbal stimuli, retains reflexes (gag reflex), and is easily arousable.

NURSING INTERVENTIONS

Preprocedure
- Instruct the client to be NPO for 6 hr before the procedure.
- Attach monitor equipment.
- Start IV access.
- Verify informed consent.

Intraprocedure
- Assess the level of consciousness.
- Monitor cardiac and respiratory status.
- Have an emergency cart and equipment available in the room.
- Have oxygen and suction equipment ready and available.

Postprocedure
- Continue to monitor vital signs and consciousness.
- Determine the ability to cough, breathe deeply, and swallow.
- Assess for nausea, vomiting, shortness of breath, and dizziness before discharge.

Ⓝ *NCLEX® Connection: Reduction of Risk Potential, Therapeutic Procedures*

UNIT 14 NURSING CARE OF PERIOPERATIVE CLIENTS

CHAPTER 95 *Preoperative Nursing Care*

Surgery can take on many forms, including curative, palliative, cosmetic, and functional.

There are three categories of inpatient surgical procedures based on acuity: emergent, urgent, or elective.

Outpatient or ambulatory surgery generally is an elective surgery that is not considered acute (cataract removal, hernia repair).

Preoperative care takes place from the time a client is scheduled for surgery until care is transferred to the operating suite. Assessment of risk factors is one of the major aspects of preoperative care. Preoperative care includes a thorough assessment of the client's physical, emotional, and psychosocial status prior to surgery.

RISK FACTORS

OF SURGERY
- Infection (risk of sepsis)
- Anemia (malnutrition, oxygenation, healing impact)
- Hypovolemia from dehydration or blood loss (circulatory compromise)
- Electrolyte imbalance through inadequate diet or disease process (dysrhythmias)

FOR SURGICAL COMPLICATIONS
- **Pregnancy:** Fetal risk with anesthesia
- **Respiratory disease:** COPD, pneumonia, asthma
- **Cardiovascular disease:** Heart failure, myocardial infarction, hypertension, dysrhythmias
- **Diabetes mellitus:** Decreased intestinal motility, altered blood glucose levels, delayed healing
- **Liver disease:** Altered medication metabolism and increased risk for bleeding
- **Kidney disease:** Altered elimination and medication excretion
- **Endocrine disorders:** Hypo/hyperthyroidism, Addison's disease, Cushing's syndrome
- **Immune system disorders:** Immunocompromise
- **Coagulation defect:** Increased risk of bleeding
- **Malnutrition:** Delayed healing
- **Obesity:** Pulmonary complications due to hypoventilation, effect on anesthesia, elimination, and wound healing
- **Some medications:** Antihypertensives, anticoagulants, NSAIDs, tricyclic antidepressants, herbal medications, over-the-counter medications
- **Substance use:** Tobacco, alcohol
- **Family history:** Malignant hyperthermia
- **Allergies:** Latex, anesthetic agents
- Inability to cope, lack of support system
- Disease processes involving multiple body systems
- **Older adult clients** Ⓖ
  - Age-related changes to hepatic and renal function alter clearance of anesthetic agents and opioids.
  - Co-morbidities (chronic disease processes, use of multiple medications)
  - Greater risk of adverse reactions to preoperative medications.
  - Less physiologic reserve than younger clients, which can cause decreased immune system response and decreased wound healing.
  - Reduction of muscle mass and the amount of body water places the older adult client at risk for dehydration.
  - Can have sensory limitations (poor eyesight, hearing loss), so the nurse must be alert to maintaining a safe environment.
  - Can have oral alterations (dentures, bridges, loose teeth) that pose problems during intubation.
  - Perspire less, which leads to dry, itchy skin that becomes fragile and easily abraded. Precautions need to be taken when moving and positioning these clients.
  - Have decreased subcutaneous fat, which makes them more susceptible to temperature changes.

PREOPERATIVE ASSESSMENT

Detailed history: Medical history, surgical history, tolerance of anesthesia, medication use, complementary or alternative practices (herbals), substance use, psychosocial history, and cultural considerations

Allergies: Medications, latex, contrast agents, and food products
- Allergies to banana or kiwi can indicate the client is at risk for a reaction to latex.
- Allergy to eggs or soybean oil is a contraindication to the use of propofol for anesthesia.
- Allergies to shellfish can result in a reaction to povidone-iodine.

Anxiety level: Regarding the procedure, support systems, and coping mechanisms

> Older adult clients can be more fearful due to financial concerns and lack of social support. Ⓖ

Baseline data: Head-to-toe assessment, vital signs, and oxygen saturations

Venous thromboembolism risk: Evaluation based on surgical procedure, client history, and anticipated time the client will be immobilized following surgery

DIAGNOSTIC PROCEDURES

Urinalysis: Renal function, rule out infection

Blood type and cross match: Transfusion readiness

CBC: Fluid status, anemia, infection/immune status

Pregnancy test: Fetal risk of anesthesia

Clotting studies: PT, INR, aPTT, platelet count

Electrolyte levels: Electrolyte imbalances

Serum creatinine and BUN: Renal status

ABGs: Oxygenation status

Chest x-ray: Heart and lung status

12-lead ECG: Baseline heart rhythm, dysrhythmias, history of cardiac disease; performed on all clients older than 40 years

PATIENT-CENTERED CARE

NURSING CARE

- Verify that the informed consent is accurately completed, signed, and witnessed.
- Administer enemas and/or laxatives the night before and/or the morning of the surgery for clients undergoing bowel surgery.
- Regularly check scheduled medication prescriptions. Some medications (antihypertensives, anticoagulants, antidepressants) can be held until after the procedure.

- Ensure that the client remains NPO for at least 6 hr for solid foods and 2 hr for clear liquids before surgery with general anesthesia (3 to 4 hr with local anesthesia) to avoid aspiration. Note on the chart the last time the client ate or drank. Ⓠᴱᴮᴾ
- Perform skin preparation, which can include cleansing with antimicrobial soap. If absolutely necessary, use electric clippers or chemical depilatories to remove hair in areas that will be involved in the surgery.
- Ensure that jewelry, dentures, prosthetics, makeup, nail polish, and glasses are removed. These items can be given to the family or stored safely.
- Cover the client with a lightweight cotton blanket heated in a warmer to prevent hypothermia. Hypothermia increases the chance for surgical wound infections, alters metabolism of medication, and causes coagulation problems and cardiac dysrhythmias.
- Establish IV access using a large-bore (18-gauge) catheter for easier infusing of IV fluids or blood products.
- Administer preoperative medications (prophylactic antimicrobials, antiemetics, sedatives) as prescribed.
  - Prophylactic antibiotics are administered within 1 hr of surgical incision.
  - If the client previously took a beta-blocker, administer a beta-blocker prior to surgery to prevent a cardiac event and mortality.
  - Have the client void prior to administration.
  - Monitor response to medications.
  - Raise side rails following administration to prevent injury.
- Ensure that the preoperative checklist is complete. **(95.1)**
- Confirm and verify the correct surgical site with the client and all health care team members before clearly marking the surgical site.

Informed consent

- Once surgery has been discussed as treatment with the client and significant other, family member, or friend, it is the responsibility of the provider to obtain consent after discussing the risks and benefits of the procedure. The nurse is not to obtain the consent for the provider in any circumstance.
- The nurse can clarify any information that remains unclear after the provider's explanation of the procedure. The nurse may not provide any new or additional information not previously given by the provider.
- The nurse's role is to witness the client's signing of the consent form after the client acknowledges understanding of the procedure.
- The nurse should determine if the client is
  - 18 years of age or emancipated.
  - Mentally capable of understanding the risks, reason, and options for surgery and anesthesia.
  - Under the influence of medication that affects decision-making or judgment (opioids, benzodiazepines, sedatives).

> ! Do not have the client sign the informed consent if medications have been administered.

- A legal guardian can sign the surgical consent form if the client is not capable of providing consent or if there is no family.
- Two witnesses may be required if the client is able to only sign with an "X," has vision or hearing impairments, or speaks English as a second language.
- Informed consent is required for surgical procedures, invasive procedures (biopsy, paracentesis, scopes), and any procedure requiring sedation or anesthesia, involving radiation, or that places the client at increased risk for complications.

PROVIDER RESPONSIBILITIES
- Obtain informed consent.
- To obtain informed consent, the provider must give the client the following.
  - Complete description of the treatment/procedure
  - Description of the professionals who will be performing and participating in the treatment
  - Information on the risks of anesthesia
  - Description of the anticipated benefits of the treatment/procedure
  - Description of the potential harm, pain, and/or discomfort that can occur
  - Options for other treatments
  - The right to refuse treatment

CLIENT RESPONSIBILITIES
- Give informed consent.
- To give informed consent, the client must do the following.
  - Give it voluntarily (no coercion involved).
  - Receive enough information to make a decision based on an understanding of what is expected.
  - Be competent and of legal age or be an emancipated minor. When the client is unable to provide consent, another authorized person must give consent.

NURSE RESPONSIBILITIES
- Witnesses informed consent.
- To witness informed consent, the nurse must do the following.
  - Ensure that the provider gave the client the necessary information.
  - Ensure that the client understood the information and is competent to give informed consent.
  - Notify the provider if the client has more questions or appears to not understand any of the information provided. (The provider is then responsible for giving clarification.)
  - Have the client sign the informed consent document.
  - Document questions the client has and notify the provider. Also document any additional reinforcement of teaching.
  - Provide a trained medical interpreter (not a family member or friend) and record the use of an interpreter in the medical record.

95.1 Preoperative checklist

ati Preoperative Checklist

	Yes	No	N/A	Initials
Allergies (list below)				
Operative permit correct/signed, dated, timed				
Authorization for treatment signed				
Anesthesia consent/signed, dated, timed				
Blood consent/signed, dated, timed				
ID bracelet correct and on client				
Blood bracelet correct and on client				
Height and weight recorded (height _____ /weight _____)				
Preoperative laboratory reports on chart				
ECG report on chart				
Chest x-ray report on chart				
Correct operative site marked with an X				
MAR/home medications				
History and physical report on chart				
Old records with chart				
Undergarments removed				
Hospital gown on client				
Operative area preparation				
Colored nailed polish removed				
Foley catheter placed				
Body piercing removed, if applicable				
Emboli stockings/elastic bandages applied				
Contact lens/glasses removed-deposition				
Dentures/partial plates removed-deposition				
Valuable jewelry removed-deposition				
Preoperative antibiotic given				
Preoperative teaching completed by _____				
Oxygen _____ liters per nasal cannula, _____% per face mask				

Allergies			
Preoperative medication given			
NPO since		Date	Time
Preoperative vital signs			
Comments			
Transported to OR per _____		Date	Time
Signed			

CLIENT EDUCATION

- Instruct the client about the purpose and effects of preoperative medications that will be administered.
- Teach the client postoperative pain control techniques (medications, immobilization, patient-controlled analgesia pumps, splinting)
- Demonstrate and teach the importance of splinting, coughing, and deep breathing.
- Demonstrate and teach the importance of range-of-motion exercises and early ambulation for prevention of thrombi and respiratory complications.
- Instruct the client about the purpose of antiembolism stockings and pneumatic compression devices to prevent deep-vein thrombosis.
- Teach the client bowel and skin preparations that will be completed (cleansing enema, preoperative shower with medicated soap).
- Instruct the client about invasive devices (drains, catheters, IV lines).
- Teach the client about the postoperative diet.
- Teach the client use of the incentive spirometer.
- Provide preoperative instructions (avoiding cigarette smoking, medications to hold, bowel preparation).
  - Clients who are taking acetylsalicylic acid should stop taking it for 1 week before an elective surgery to decrease the risk of bleeding.
  - Clients who take herbal medications (e.g., ginkgo biloba, ginseng, feverfew) should stop taking them 2 weeks before surgery to prevent hemorrhage or adverse effect to the anesthetic.
  - Medications for cardiovascular disease, pulmonary disease, seizures, and diabetes mellitus, some antihypertensive medications, and eye drops for glaucoma may be taken prior to surgery or a procedure.
  - Teach the client how to use a pain scale to rate pain level postoperative.
- Explain care and restrictions relative to the surgical procedure performed.

COMPLICATIONS

Complications during the postoperative period usually are related to the medications given preoperatively.

- For clients encountering severe anxiety and panic, reassurance will be necessary and sedation medications may be given. Nonpharmacological interventions, such as distraction, imagery, and music therapy, can be initiated.
- Ensure that measures are taken to prevent postoperative deep-vein thromboembolism by continuing anticoagulation therapy and/or antiembolism stockings, pneumatic compression devices, and range-of-motion exercises.
- Be alert for any allergic reactions the client has to medications.

Sedatives (benzodiazepines, barbiturates)
- Respiratory depression, drowsiness, dizziness
- NURSING CONSIDERATIONS
  - Monitor respiratory rate and oxygen saturation.
  - Administer oxygen.
  - Administer a reversal agent, flumazenil.

Opioids
- Respiratory depression, drowsiness, dizziness, constipation, urinary retention
- NURSING CONSIDERATIONS
  - Monitor respiratory rate and oxygen saturation.
  - Administer oxygen.
  - Administer a reversal agent, naloxone.
  - Perform prescribed intermittent catheterization.

IV infusions (0.9% NaCl, lactated Ringer's)
- Fluid overload, hypernatremia
- NURSING CONSIDERATIONS
  - Obtain preoperative cardiac and pulmonary history.
  - Monitor I&O closely.
  - Slow the IV fluid rate of infusion.
  - Administer prescribed diuretic.

Gastrointestinal medications (antiemetics, antacids, H_2 receptor blockers)
- Alkalosis, cardiac abnormalities (some H_2 receptor blockers), drowsiness
- NURSING CONSIDERATIONS
  - Obtain preoperative cardiac history.
  - Monitor for electrolyte abnormalities.

Application Exercises

1. A nurse is assessing a client's laboratory values before surgery. Which of the following results should the nurse report to the provider? (Select all that apply.)

   A. Potassium 3.9 mEq/L

   B. Sodium 145 mEq/L

   C. Creatinine 2.8 mg/dL

   D. Blood glucose 235 mg/dL

   E. WBC 17,850/mm³

2. A nurse providing preoperative teaching to a client who is to have abdominal surgery. Which of the following statements should the nurse make? (Select all that apply.)

   A. "Take your heart medication with a sip of water before surgery."

   B. "Splint the abdominal incision with a pillow when coughing and deep breathing."

   C. "Bed rest is recommended for the first 48 hr."

   D. "Antiembolism stockings are applied before surgery."

   E. "You may eat solid foods up to 4 hr before surgery."

3. A nurse is verifying informed consent for a client who is having a paracentesis. Which of the following actions should the nurse take? (Select all that apply.)

   A. Explain to the client the purpose of having the procedure.

   B. Inform the client of risks to having the procedure.

   C. Ensure the client understands information about the procedure.

   D. Witness the client signing the informed consent form.

   E. Determine if the client is capable of understanding the reason for the procedure.

4. A nurse is caring for a client who is scheduled for an exploratory laparotomy. The client's temperature is 39° C (102.2° F) orally. Which of the following actions should the nurse take?

   A. Inform the surgeon of the elevated temperature.

   B. Transfer the client to the preoperative unit.

   C. Apply ice packs to the groin.

   D. Encourage the client to increase intake of clear liquids.

5. A preoperative nurse is caring for a client who is having a colon resection. Which of the following actions should the nurse take?

   A. Encourage the client to void after preoperative medication administration.

   B. Administer antibiotics 2 hr prior to surgical incision.

   C. Remove hair using a manual razor.

   D. Remove nail polish on fingers and toes.

PRACTICE Active Learning Scenario

A preoperative nurse is planning preventative care for a client who is having a surgical procedure. What potential complications should the nurse include in the preventive plan of care? Use the ATI Active Learning Template: Basic Concept to complete this item.

RELATED CONTENT: List three preventions for potential complications. Explain the related cause and include one intervention for each complication.

Application Exercises Key

1. A. The potassium level is within the expected reference range.

   B. The sodium level is within the expected reference range.

   C. **CORRECT:** The nurse should report an elevated creatinine level, which can indicate impaired renal function.

   D. **CORRECT:** The nurse should report an elevated blood glucose, which needs treatment prior to surgery.

   E. **CORRECT:** The nurse should report an elevated WBC count, which indicates a need for antibiotic therapy before surgery.

   Ⓝ *NCLEX® Connection: Reduction of Risk Potential, Laboratory Values*

2. A. **CORRECT:** The nurse should teach the client to take certain cardiac and other medications as prescribed with a sip of water before surgery.

   B. **CORRECT:** The nurse should teach the client how to splint with a pillow to support the incision when coughing and deep breathing postoperatively.

   C. The nurse should teach the client the importance of early ambulation following abdominal surgery to prevent complications.

   D. **CORRECT:** The nurse should inform the client of the application of antiembolism stockings to prevent deep-vein thrombosis.

   E. The nurse should inform the client to stop eating solid food for 6 hr or more before surgery.

   Ⓝ *NCLEX® Connection: Reduction of Risk Potential, Therapeutic Procedures*

3. A. The provider should explain the purpose of the procedure.

   B. The provider should inform the client of risks to having the procedure.

   C. **CORRECT:** The nurse should ensure the client understands the information about the procedure.

   D. **CORRECT:** The nurse should witness the client sign the informed consent.

   E. **CORRECT:** The nurse should determine if the client is capable of understanding the reason for the procedure.

   Ⓝ *NCLEX® Connection: Reduction of Risk Potential, Therapeutic Procedures*

4. A. **CORRECT:** The nurse should immediately notify the surgeon of the elevated temperature to determine if canceling the surgery is necessary due to an underlying infection.

   B. Transferring the client to the preoperative unit is not an appropriate nursing action when there is a possible underlying infection.

   C. Applying ice packs to the client's groin is not an appropriate action for a temperature of 39° C (102.2° F).

   D. Increasing intake of clear liquids is not an appropriate action because the client should be NPO for at least 2 hr before surgery.

   Ⓝ *NCLEX® Connection: Reduction of Risk Potential, Therapeutic Procedures*

5. A. The client should void before administration of medication for relaxation or sedation to prevent the risk for falls.

   B. The nurse should administer antibiotics within 1 hr prior to the surgical incision as a prophylactic measure to prevent infection.

   C. The nurse should remove hair at the surgical site with electric clippers or use a chemical depilatory to prevent traumatizing the skin and increasing the risk for infection.

   D. **CORRECT:** The nurse should ensure the nail beds are visible for color and circulation by removing nail polish before surgery.

   Ⓝ *NCLEX® Connection: Reduction of Risk Potential, Therapeutic Procedures*

PRACTICE Answer

Using the ATI Active Learning Template: Basic Concept

RELATED CONTENT

Prevent respiratory depression.
- Caused by overmedication with benzodiazepines, barbiturates, or opioids.
- Administer a prescribed reversal agent, and monitor closely.

Prevent fluid overload.
- Caused by too much IV fluids and inability to readily excrete the fluids.
- Obtain a preoperative cardiac and pulmonary history, monitor I&O closely, slow the rate of IV fluids, and administer a prescribed diuretic.

Prevent deep-vein thrombosis.
- Caused by blood stasis in lower extremities due to absent muscle contractility.
- Apply antiembolism stockings and/or pneumatic compression devices, administer prescribed anticoagulants, and teach range-of-motion exercises.

Prevent infection.
- Caused by micro-organisms contaminating the surgical wound.
- Administer a prescribed prophylactic antibiotic within 1 hr before the surgical incision is made.

Ⓝ *NCLEX® Connection: Reduction of Risk Potential, Potential for Complications from Surgical Procedures and Health Alterations*

UNIT 14   NURSING CARE OF PERIOPERATIVE CLIENTS

CHAPTER 96 *Postoperative Nursing Care*

Transferring a client who is postoperative from the operating suite to the postanesthesia care unit (PACU) is the responsibility of the anesthesia provider, who is an anesthesiologist or certified registered nurse anesthetist. The circulating nurse will give the verbal hand-off report to the PACU nurse.

Postoperative care is usually provided initially in the PACU, where skilled nurses who are certified in advanced cardiac life support can monitor a client's recovery from anesthesia. In some instances, a client is transferred from the operating suite directly to the intensive care unit.

Initial postoperative care involves making assessments, administering medications, managing pain, preventing complications, and determining when a client is ready to be discharged from the PACU. During the immediate postoperative stage, maintaining airway patency and ventilation and monitoring circulatory status are the priorities for care. Postoperative clients who receive general anesthesia require frequent assessment of their respiratory status. Postoperative clients who receive epidural or spinal anesthesia require ongoing assessment of motor and sensory function.

A client who is stable and able to breathe spontaneously is discharged to a postsurgical unit or home if an outpatient surgical procedure was performed. A client discharged home must demonstrate ability to swallow and safely ambulate to the bathroom and wheelchair with assistance. A client who had an outpatient surgery should be accompanied by a significant other, family member, or other caregiver who can receive discharge instructions and transport the client home.

RISK FACTORS FOR COMPLICATIONS

Immobility: Respiratory compromise, thrombophlebitis, pressure ulcer

Anemia: Blood loss, inadequate/decreased oxygenation, impaired healing factors

Hypovolemia: Tissue perfusion

Hypothermia: Risk of surgical wound infection, altered absorption of medication, coagulopathy, and cardiac dysrhythmia

Cardiovascular diseases: Fluid overload, deep-vein thrombosis, arrhythmia

Respiratory disease: Respiratory compromise

Immune disorder: Risk for infection, delayed healing

Diabetes mellitus: Gastroparesis, delayed wound healing

Coagulation defect: Increased risk of bleeding

Malnutrition: Delayed healing

Obesity: Respiratory compromise, postoperative nausea and vomiting, wound healing, dehiscence, evisceration

Age-related: Respiratory, cardiovascular, and renal changes necessitate specific attention to the postoperative recovery of older adults. Ⓒ
- Older adult clients are more susceptible to cold temperatures, so additional warm blankets in the PACU can be required.
- Responses to medications and anesthetics can delay return of orientation postoperatively.
- Age-related physiologic changes (decreased liver and kidney function) can affect response to and elimination of postoperative medications. Monitor for appropriate response and possible adverse effects.
  ○ Older adults perspire less, which leads to dry, itchy skin that becomes fragile and easily abraded. The use of paper tape for wound dressings can be appropriate, as well as lifting precautions.
  ○ Older adults can be at risk for delayed wound healing because of possible compromised nutrition.

DIAGNOSTIC PROCEDURES

CBC: WBC (infection/immune status), Hgb and Hct (fluid status, anemia)

Metabolic profile: Serum electrolytes (electrolyte imbalances), BUN, and creatinine (renal function)

ABGs: Oxygenation status

Additional laboratory tests: Serum glucose, prothrombin time, INR based on procedure and associated health problems

PACU ASSESSMENT

Upon receiving a client from the operating suite, the nurse should immediately perform a full body assessment with priority given to airway, breathing, and circulation.

MONITORING AND MANAGEMENT

Airway

- An artificial airway (endotracheal tube, nasal trumpet, or oral airway) is left in place until a client can maintain an open airway without support.
- Assess blood oxygen saturation levels continuously (should be greater than 95% or at preoperative status).
- Assess respiratory pattern, rate, and depth to determine adequacy of oxygen exchange.
- Assess for symmetry of breath sounds and chest wall movement.
  - Absent breath sounds on the left can indicate the endotracheal tube has migrated down the right mainstem bronchus or that there is a pneumothorax.
  - Snoring or stridor (a high-pitched crowing type sound) can indicate poor oxygen exchange.
- Auscultate lung sounds.
- Administer humidified oxygen.
- Suction accumulated secretions if the client is unable to cough. Use a Yankauer suction for thick oral secretions or a large French suction catheter for nasopharyngeal or nasotracheal secretions.
  - Retained neuromuscular blocking agents can hinder the client's ability to cough and eliminate secretions.
  - Extubation of endotracheal tube is based on client's response to commands, ability to elevate head, and use of thoracic breathing.
  - As soon as the client follows commands, encourage coughing, deep breathing, and use of the incentive spirometer.

Circulation

- Observe for internal bleeding (abdominal distention, visible hematoma under/near the surgical site, tachycardia, hypotension, restlessness, increased pain) and external bleeding.
- Assess for hypervolemia and hypovolemia.
- Assess skin color, temperature, sensation, and capillary refill.
- Check mucous membranes, lips, and nail beds for cyanosis.
- Assess and compare peripheral pulses for impaired circulation and deep-vein thrombosis. Continue preventative deep vein thrombosis measures: sequential compression devices, antiembolism stockings, and prescribed anticoagulants or antiplatelet medications.
- Monitor ECG readings and apical and peripheral pulses to determine a pulse deficit, which can indicate a dysrhythmia. Qs
- Monitor fluid and electrolyte balance.

Vital signs

- Per agency protocol, obtain vital signs until stable (every 15 min) and assess for trends.
- Evaluate and treat the presence of hypotension and potential causes (anesthesia or other medications, cardiac depression, blood loss, pooling of blood in extremities, position changes).
- Report a blood pressure difference of 25% from baseline, a drop of 15 to 20 mm Hg in diastolic or systolic pressures, or a trending decrease in diastolic or systolic pressures by 5 mm Hg at each 15-min vital sign assessment.
- Evaluate and treat hypertension and potential causes (pain, hypoxia, bladder distention).
- Provide heated blankets when the client arrives after a temperature is obtained and reapply if the client is hypothermic. Causes of hypothermia include decreased body fat, age-related changes in the hypothalamus that regulates body temperature, and decreased environmental temperature in the surgical suite.

Positioning

- If the client responds to verbal stimuli, gradually elevate the head of the bed to semi-Fowler's position, if not contraindicated, to facilitate chest expansion.
- Maintain lateral position (right or left side) if the client is unresponsive or unconscious (risk of aspiration).
- Avoid placing a pillow under the knees or engaging the knee gatch of the bed, which can decrease venous return.
- Elevate legs and lower the head of the bed if hypotension or shock develops.

Response to anesthesia (sedation, nausea, vomiting)

- Monitor level of consciousness (weakness, restlessness, agitation, somnolence, irritability, change in orientation).
- Assess for movement of and sensation in extremities. Sensory function and voluntary movement of the extremities following a regional block should occur before transfer to another unit.
- Administer an antiemetic for nausea and vomiting after checking bowel sounds.

Input and output

- Monitor fluid and electrolyte balance following surgery.
  - Review postoperative laboratory findings (potassium, sodium, creatinine and BUN, hemoglobin and hematocrit).
  - Assess skin turgor and diaphoresis.
  - Review I&O during surgery and in PACU: emesis, drains, nasogastric (NG) tube, urine, estimated blood losses, IV fluids, blood products.
  - Administer isotonic IV fluids (0.9% sodium chloride, lactated Ringer's, dextrose 5% in lactated Ringer's) to maintain adequate cardiac output and fluid and electrolyte balance.
  - Administer prescribed blood products to treat hypovolemia (autologous blood, intraoperative blood salvage using a cell saver device, packed cells, fresh frozen plasma, albumin, platelets).
- Palpate bladder for distention.
- Monitor urinary catheters for patency.
- Observe color, consistency, odor, and amount of urine. Urine output less than 30 mL/hr can indicate hypovolemia.

Surgical wound, incision site, dressing

- Observe drainage tubes for patency and proper function.
- Check dressings for excessive drainage and reinforce as needed. Report excess drainage to the surgeon.
- Outline drainage spots with a pen, noting date and time. Report increasing drainage to the surgeon.

Pain

- Administer pain medication as appropriate, secondary to recovery status.
- Observe for respiratory depression and decreased oxygen saturation.

Mentition

- Monitor level of consciousness and mental status.
- Determine level of stimulation needed for arousal (pain, touch, verbal).
- Determine level of orientation compared to baseline.
- Older adult clients can experience acute confusion or delirium related to anesthesia or other medications, dehydration, hypoxia, blood loss, or electrolyte imbalance. Episodes of postoperative delirium can last 2 days or more in older adult clients. Ⓖ

ALDRETE SCORING

Monitor recovery from anesthesia by using the Aldrete scoring system. Each of five factors is given a score based upon observations of the client. The scores are totaled to determine the Aldrete score.

96.1 Modified Aldrete Scoring System

	ASSESSMENT/OBSERVATION	SCORE
Activity	Able to move four extremities	2
	Able to move two extremities	1
	Able to move no extremities	0
Consciousness	Fully awake	2
	Arousable	1
	Unarousable	0
Respiration	Breathe deeply and cough	2
	Dyspnea, hypoventilation	1
	Apneic	0
O₂ saturation	O_2 saturation maintained at 92% (minimum) on room air	2
	Inhaled oxygen is necessary to maintain O_2 saturation greater that 90%	1
	O_2 saturation level is less than 90% even though inhaled oxygen is being given	0
Circulation	Blood pressure is within 20% of preanesthesia level	2
	Blood pressure is 21% to 49% of preanesthesia level	1
	Blood pressure is within 50% of preanesthesia level	0

CRITERIA FOR DISCHARGE FROM PACU

The anesthesiologist must sign out the client before transfer to another unit or discharge to home.
- Aldrete score of 8 to 10
- Stable vital signs
- No evidence of bleeding
- Return of reflexes (gag, cough, swallow)
- Minimal to absent nausea and vomiting
- Wound drainage that is minimal to moderate
- Urine output at least 30 mL/hr

UNIT ASSESSMENT

Upon receiving the client from the PACU, the nurse should immediately perform a full body assessment with priority given to airway, breathing, and circulation. This assessment serves as a baseline to identify changes in postoperative status.

MONITORING AND MANAGEMENT

Airway

- Monitor oxygen saturation using a pulse oximeter.
- Assist with coughing and deep breathing at least every 1 hr while awake, and provide a pillow or folded blanket so the client can splint as necessary for abdominal incision.
- Contraindications to coughing include cosmetic, eye, or intracranial surgeries.
- Assist with the use of an incentive spirometer at least every 1 to 2 hr while awake to encourage expansion of the lungs and prevent atelectasis.
- Reposition every 2 hr, and ambulate early and regularly.

Positioning

- Do not put pillows under knees or elevate the knee gatch on the bed (decreases venous return).
- Encourage early ambulation with adequate rest periods to prevent cardiovascular disorders, deep-vein thrombosis, and pulmonary complications.

Fluid status and oral comfort

- A client who returns to the medical-surgical unit is given a prescription IV solution based on needs (hydration, electrolytes).
- Encourage ice chips and fluids as prescribed/tolerated.
- Provide frequent oral hygiene.

Pain

- If prescribed, provide continuous pain relief through the use of a patient-controlled analgesia pump. Epidural and intrathecal infusions are also used postoperatively.
- A preventative approach using around-the-clock scheduling is more effective than PRN medication delivery during the first 24 to 48 hr postoperatively.
- Assess pain level frequently, using a standardized pain scale.
- Encourage the client to ask for pain medication before pain gets severe.
- Assess for manifestations of pain, such as an increased pulse, respirations, or blood pressure; restlessness; and wincing or moaning during movement.
- Monitor for adverse effects of opioids, such as respiratory depression, nausea (encourage the client to change positions slowly), urinary retention, and constipation.
- Provide analgesia 30 min before ambulation or painful procedures.
- Assess for effectiveness of pain medication after administration.

Kidney function

- Output should equal intake.
- Monitor and report urinary output less than 30 mL/hr.
- Palpate bladder following voiding to assess for distention.
- Consider using a bladder scan to assess suspected retention of urine.

Bowel function

- Maintain the client NPO until return of gag reflex (risk of aspiration) and peristalsis (risk of paralytic ileus).
- Irrigate NG suction tubes with saline as needed to maintain patency. Do not move NG tubes in clients who are postoperative following gastric surgery as prescribed (risk to incision).
- Monitor bowel sounds in all four quadrants as well as ability to pass flatus.
- Advance diet as prescribed and tolerated (clear liquids to regular).

Thromboembolism

- Apply pneumatic compression devices and/or antiembolism stockings.
- Reposition every 2 hr, and ambulate early and regularly.
- Administer prescribed anticoagulants or antiplatelet medications.
- Monitor extremities for calf pain, warmth, erythema, and edema.

Incisions and drain sites

- Monitor drainage (should progress from sanguineous to serosanguineous to serous).
- Monitor the incision site. Expected findings include pink wound edges, slight swelling under sutures/staples, and slight crusting of drainage. Report any evidence of infection, including redness, excessive tenderness, and purulent drainage.
- Monitor wound drains with each vital sign assessment. Empty closed-suction drainage collection devices as needed to maintain compression. Report increases in drainage (possible hemorrhage).
- In most instances, the surgeon will perform the first dressing change. Subsequent dressing changes may be performed by the nurse using surgical aseptic technique.
- Use an abdominal binder as prescribed for clients who are obese or debilitated.
- Encourage splinting with position changes, coughing, and deep breathing.
- Administer prophylactic antibiotics as prescribed.
- Remove sutures or staples in 5 to 10 days as prescribed.

Wound healing

- Encourage the client to consume a diet high in calories, protein, and vitamin C.
- If the client has diabetes mellitus, maintain appropriate glycemic control.

Discharge teaching

- Teach the client the purpose, administration guidelines, and adverse effects of medications.
- Reinforce activity restrictions (driving, stairs, limits on weight lifting, sexual activity) with the client.
- Provide dietary guidelines, if applicable.
- Inform the client about treatment instructions (wound care, catheter care, use of assistive devices).
- Inform the client of emergency contact information and findings to report.

Hypoxia

Hypoxia is evidenced by a decrease in oxygen saturation.

NURSING CONSIDERATIONS
- Monitor oxygenation status, and administer oxygen as prescribed.
- Encourage coughing and deep breathing to prevent atelectasis.
- Position client with head of bed elevated, and turn every 2 hr to facilitate chest expansion.

COMPLICATIONS

Airway obstruction

Swelling or spasm of the larynx or trachea, mucus in the airway, or relaxation of the tongue into the nasopharynx can cause airway obstruction, often manifesting as stridor or snoring.

NURSING CONSIDERATIONS
- Monitor for choking; noisy, irregular respirations; decreased oxygen saturation values; and cyanosis. Intervene accordingly.
- Implement a head-tilt/chin-lift maneuver to pull the tongue forward and open the airway.
- Keep emergency equipment at the bedside in the PACU (resuscitation bag, suction equipment, airways).
- Notify the anesthesiologist, elevate head of bed if not contraindicated, provide humidified oxygen, and plan for reintubation with endotracheal tube.

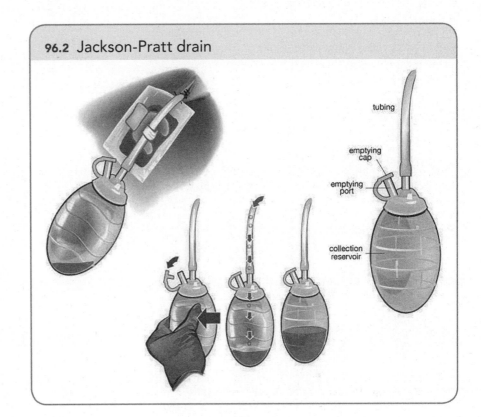

96.2 Jackson-Pratt drain

tubing

emptying cap

emptying port

collection reservoir

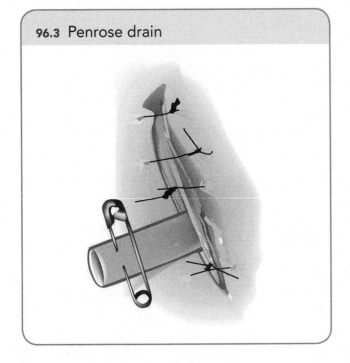

96.3 Penrose drain

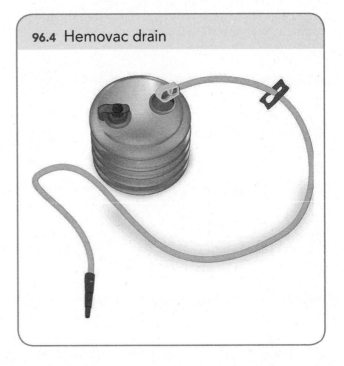

96.4 Hemovac drain

Hypovolemic shock

Postoperative shock can result from a massive loss of circulating blood volume.

NURSING CONSIDERATIONS
- Monitor for decreased blood pressure and urinary output, increased heart and respiratory rates, narrowing of pulse pressure, and slow capillary refill.
- Administer oxygen.
- Place the client in a supine position with legs elevated.
- Administer IV fluids and vasopressors as prescribed.

Paralytic ileus

Can occur due to the absence of GI peristaltic activity caused by abdominal surgery or other physical trauma

NURSING CONSIDERATIONS
- Monitor bowel sounds.
- Encourage ambulation.
- Advance the diet as tolerated when bowel sounds or flatus are present.
- The client can have an NG tube inserted to empty stomach contents.
- Administer prokinetic agents, such as metoclopramide, as prescribed.

Wound dehiscence or evisceration

- Caused by spontaneous opening of the incisional wound (dehiscence)
- Can progress to the protrusion of the internal organs through the incision (evisceration)

NURSING CONSIDERATIONS
- Monitor risk factors (obesity, coughing, moving without splinting, poor nutritional status, diabetes mellitus, infection, hematoma, steroid use).
- If wound dehiscence or evisceration occurs, call for help, stay with the client, cover the wound with a sterile towel or dressing that is moistened with sterile saline, do not attempt to reinsert organs, place in a low-Fowler's position with hips and knees bent, monitor for shock, and notify the provider immediately.

Deep-vein thrombosis

Caused by dehydration, stress response that leads to hypercoagulability of the blood, immobility, obesity, trauma, malignancy, history of thrombosis, hormones, and use of indwelling venous catheter

NURSING CONSIDERATIONS
- Prophylactic measures include administration of low-molecular-weight heparin, low-dose heparin, or low-dose warfarin; antiembolism stockings; pneumatic compression devices; range-of-motion exercises; and early ambulation.
- Avoid any form of pressure behind the knee with a pillow or blanket, which can cause constriction of blood vessels and decreased venous return.
- Avoid dangling the client's legs for long periods of time.
- Provide adequate hydration by administering IV fluids or encouraging increased oral fluid intake.

Application Exercises

1. A nurse is reviewing the health records of several clients in the postanesthesia care unit (PACU) to identify risk factors that can lead to postoperative complications. Which of the following clients are at risk for complications? (Select all that apply.)

   A. A client who has a WBC of 22,500/uL

   B. A client who uses an insulin pump

   C. A client who takes warfarin daily

   D. A client who has heart failure

   E. A client who has a BMI of 26

2. A nurse is caring for a female client who manifests indications of hypovolemia while in the PACU. Which of the following findings requires action by the nurse? (Select all that apply.)

   A. Urine output less than 25 mL/hr

   B. Hematocrit 48%

   C. BUN 24 mg/dL

   D. Tenting of skin over the sternum

   E. Apical pulse rate 62/min

3. A nurse is caring for a client who arrived in the PACU following a total hip arthroplasty. The client is not responding to verbal stimuli. Which of the following actions should the nurse perform first?

   A. Compare and contrast the peripheral pulses.

   B. Apply a warm blanket.

   C. Assess dressings.

   D. Place the client in a lateral position.

4. A nurse is planning care for a client to prevent postoperative atelectasis. Which of the following interventions should the nurse include in the plan of care? (Select all that apply.)

   A. Encourage use of the incentive spirometer every 2 hr.

   B. Instruct the client to splint the incision when coughing and deep breathing.

   C. Reposition the client every 2 hr.

   D. Administer antibiotic therapy.

   E. Assist with early ambulation.

5. A nurse is caring for a client who reports nausea and vomiting 2 days postoperative following hysterectomy. Which of the following actions should the nurse perform first?

   A. Assess bowel sounds.

   B. Administer antiemetic medication.

   C. Restart prescribed IV fluids.

   D. Insert a prescribed nasogastric tube.

PRACTICE Active Learning Scenario

A nurse is reviewing the health records of several clients to identify postoperative complications. What information should the nurse expect to find? Use the ATI Active Learning Template: Basic Concept to complete this item.

RELATED CONTENT: List three possible complications. Describe one cause and one intervention for each complication.

Application Exercises Key

1. A. **CORRECT:** An increased WBC indicates an underlying infection and places the client at risk for postoperative complications.

   B. **CORRECT:** An insulin pump indicates the client has type 1 diabetes mellitus and places the client at risk of postoperative complications, such as delayed wound healing.

   C. **CORRECT:** A client who takes warfarin daily is at risk for bleeding and postoperative complications, such as hemorrhage.

   D. **CORRECT:** A client who has a history of heart failure is at risk for complications, such as fluid overload or dysrhythmias.

   E. BMI 26 is within the expected reference range and does not place the client at risk for postoperative complications.

   Ⓝ *NCLEX® Connection: Reduction of Risk Potential, Potential for Complications of Diagnostic Tests/Treatments/Procedures*

2. A. **CORRECT:** Urine output less than 25 mL/hr is a manifestation of hypovolemia and requires intervention by IV fluid therapy.

   B. **CORRECT:** Hematocrit 48% indicates concentrated blood volume and is a manifestation of hypovolemia, requiring intervention by IV fluid therapy.

   C. **CORRECT:** BUN 24 mg/dL indicates decreased kidney function and can be a manifestation of hypovolemia, requiring intervention with IV fluid therapy.

   D. **CORRECT:** Tenting of skin indicates decreased or absent skin turgor due to dehydration, requiring intervention with IV fluid therapy.

   E. An apical pulse rate of 62/min is not a manifestation of hypovolemia.

   Ⓝ *NCLEX® Connection: Physiological Adaptation, Medical Emergencies*

3. A. Comparing and contrasting peripheral pulses is important to ensure adequate circulation, but it is not the first nursing action.

   B. Applying warm blankets to prevent hypothermia is important, but it is not the first nursing action.

   C. Assessing dressings for drainage is important to monitor the amount of drainage present, but it is not the first nursing action.

   D. **CORRECT:** The greatest risk to the client who is unresponsive or unconscious is injury from aspiration.

   Ⓝ *NCLEX® Connection: Reduction of Risk Potential, Potential for Complications of Diagnostic Tests/Treatments/Procedures*

4. A. **CORRECT:** Use of the incentive spirometer every 2 hr expands the lungs and prevents atelectasis.

   B. **CORRECT:** Incisional splinting with a pillow or blanket supports the incision during coughing and deep breathing, which prevents atelectasis.

   C. **CORRECT:** Repositioning the client every 2 hr will mobilize secretions and allow the client to deep breathe and expand the lungs to prevent atelectasis.

   D. Antibiotic therapy is used to prophylactically prevent or treat infection and does not prevent atelectasis.

   E. **CORRECT:** Early ambulation expands the lungs through deep breathing and prevents atelectasis.

   Ⓝ *NCLEX® Connection: Physiological Adaptation, Alterations in Body Systems*

5. A. **CORRECT:** Using the nursing process, the first step is to assess the client. Assessing bowel sounds is the priority action by the nurse.

   B. Administer an antiemetic medication can alleviate nausea and vomiting, but it is not the first nursing action.

   C. Restarting prescribed IV fluids will prevent dehydration, but it is not the first nursing action.

   D. Inserting a prescribed nasogastric tube can alleviate nausea and vomiting, but it is not the first nursing action.

   Ⓝ *NCLEX® Connection: Basic Care and Comfort, Nutrition and Oral Hydration*

PRACTICE Answer

Using the ATI Active Learning Template: Basic Concept

RELATED CONTENT

Paralytic ileus
- Caused by abdominal surgery or other physical trauma and absent gastrointestinal peristaltic activity
- Monitor bowel sounds, encourage ambulation, and insert nasogastric tube to empty stomach contents.

Wound evisceration
- Protrusion of the abdominal contents through the incisional wound of the abdominal cavity, caused by failure to splint when moving or coughing, delayed healing due to obesity or diabetes mellitus
- Call for help, cover the wound with sterile saline soaked dressings or towel, and position the client in semi-Fowler's position with hips and knees bent.

Airway obstruction
- Swelling or spasm of the larynx or trachea, mucus in the airway, or relaxation of the tongue into the nasopharynx can cause airway obstruction, often manifesting as stridor or snoring.
- Notify the anesthesiologist, provide humidified oxygen, elevate the head of the bed if not contraindicated, perform a head-tilt/chin-lift maneuver to open the airway, and plan for reintubation of the endotracheal tube.

Hypovolemic shock
- Caused by blood loss
- Monitor for decreased blood pressure and urinary output, increased heart and respiratory rates, narrowing of the pulse pressure, and slow capillary refill.
- Administer oxygen.
- Place the client in a supine position with the legs elevated.
- Administer IV fluids and vasopressors as indicated.

Ⓝ *NCLEX® Connection: Physiological Adaptation, Medical Emergencies*

References

Berman, A., Snyder, S., & Frandsen, G. (2016). *Kozier & Erb's fundamentals of nursing: Concepts, process, and practice* (10th ed.). Upper Saddle River, NJ: Prentice-Hall.

Burchum, J. R., & Rosenthal, L. D. (2016). *Lehne's pharmacology for nursing care* (9th ed.). St. Louis: Elsevier.

Dudek, S. G. (2014). *Nutrition essentials for nursing practice* (7th ed.). Philadelphia: Lippincott Williams & Wilkins.

Eliopoulos, C. (2014). *Gerontological nursing* (8th ed.). Philadelphia: Lippincott Williams & Wilkins.

Grodner, M., Escott-Stump, S., & Dorner, S. (2016). *Nutritional foundations and clinical applications of nutrition: A nursing approach* (6th ed.). St. Louis, MO: Mosby.

Halter, M. J. (2014). *Varcarolis' foundations of psychiatric mental health nursing: A clinical approach* (7th ed.). St. Louis, MO: Saunders.

Hinkle, J. L., & Cheever, K. H. (2014). *Brunner and Suddarth's textbook of medical-surgical nursing* (13th ed.). Philadelphia: Lippincott Williams & Wilkins.

Ignatavicius, D. D., & Workman, M. L. (2016). *Medical-surgical nursing* (8th ed.). St. Louis, MO: Elsevier.

Lilley, L. L., Rainforth-Collins, S., & Snyder, J. S. (2014). *Pharmacology and the nursing process* (7th Ed.). St. Louis, MO: Mosby.

Marquis, B. L., & Huston, C. J. (2015). *Leadership roles and management functions in nursing: Theory and application* (8th ed.). Philadelphia: Lippincott Williams & Wilkins.

Pagana, K. D. & Pagana, T. J. (2014). *Mosby's manual of diagnostic and laboratory tests* (5th ed.). St. Louis, MO: Elsevier.

Potter, P. A., Perry, A. G., Stockert, P., & Hall, A. (2013). *Fundamentals of nursing* (8th ed.). St. Louis, MO: Mosby.

Skidmore-Roth, L. (2016). *Mosby's 2016 nursing drug reference* (29th ed.). St. Louis, MO: Elsevier.

Touhy, T. A., & Jett, K. F. (2012) *Ebersole & Hess' toward healthy aging: Human needs and nursing response* (8th ed.). St. Lois, MO: Mosby.

Basic Concept

STUDENT NAME _____

CONCEPT_____   REVIEW MODULE CHAPTER_____

Related Content

(E.G., DELEGATION,
LEVELS OF PREVENTION,
ADVANCE DIRECTIVES)

Underlying Principles

Nursing Interventions

WHO? WHEN? WHY? HOW?

STUDENT NAME _____

PROCEDURE NAME _____ REVIEW MODULE CHAPTER_____

Description of Procedure

Indications

CONSIDERATIONS

Nursing Interventions (pre, intra, post)

Interpretation of Findings

Client Education

Potential Complications

Nursing Interventions

STUDENT NAME _____

DEVELOPMENTAL STAGE _____   REVIEW MODULE CHAPTER_____

EXPECTED GROWTH AND DEVELOPMENT

Physical Development	Cognitive Development	Psychosocial Development	Age-Appropriate Activities

Health Promotion

Immunizations	Health Screening	Nutrition	Injury Prevention

STUDENT NAME _____

MEDICATION _____ REVIEW MODULE CHAPTER_____

CATEGORY CLASS_____

PURPOSE OF MEDICATION

Expected Pharmacological Action

Therapeutic Use

Complications

Medication Administration

Contraindications/Precautions

Nursing Interventions

Interactions

Client Education

Evaluation of Medication Effectiveness

STUDENT NAME _____

SKILL NAME_____   REVIEW MODULE CHAPTER_____

Description of Skill

Indications

CONSIDERATIONS

Nursing Interventions (pre, intra, post)

Outcomes/Evaluation

Client Education

Potential Complications

Nursing Interventions

System Disorder

STUDENT NAME _____

DISORDER/DISEASE PROCESS _____ REVIEW MODULE CHAPTER_____

Alterations in Health (Diagnosis)	Pathophysiology Related to Client Problem	Health Promotion and Disease Prevention

ASSESSMENT

SAFETY CONSIDERATIONS

Risk Factors	Expected Findings

Laboratory Tests	Diagnostic Procedures

PATIENT-CENTERED CARE

Complications

Nursing Care	Medications	Client Education

Therapeutic Procedures		Interprofessional Care

Therapeutic Procedure

STUDENT NAME _____

PROCEDURE NAME _____ REVIEW MODULE CHAPTER_____

Description of Procedure

Indications

CONSIDERATIONS

Nursing Interventions (pre, intra, post)

Outcomes/Evaluation

Client Education

Potential Complications

Nursing Interventions